Oxford Medical Publications

Carleton's Histological Technique

Carleton's
HISTOLOGICAL
TECHNIQUE

FIFTH EDITION

by

R. A. B. DRURY
M.A., D.M.(Oxon.), F.R.C.Path.
Plymouth General Hospital, Plymouth

E. A. WALLINGTON
F.I.M.L.S.
Northwick Park Hospital, Harrow, Middlesex

Oxford New York Toronto
OXFORD UNIVERSITY PRESS
1980

Oxford University Press, Walton Street, Oxford OX2 6DP

OXFORD LONDON GLASGOW
NEW YORK TORONTO MELBOURNE WELLINGTON
KUALA LUMPUR SINGAPORE JAKARTA HONG KONG TOKYO
DELHI BOMBAY CALCUTTA MADRAS KARACHI
NAIROBI DAR ES SALAAM CAPE TOWN

© *Oxford University Press 1967, 1980*

First edition 1926
Second edition 1938
Third edition 1957
Fourth edition 1967
Fifth edition 1980

British Library Cataloguing in Publication Data

Carleton, Harry Montgomerie
   Carleton's histological technique. – 5th ed.
  1. Histology, Pathological – Technique
  I. Drury, Roger Anderson Brownsword
  II. Wallington, Eric Alfred
  III. Histological technique
  616.07'583   **RB43**   79–41733

ISBN 0–19–261310–3

*Printed in Great Britain by
Fletcher & Son Ltd, Norwich*

Preface to the fifth edition

On 7 January 1926 Harry Carleton wrote for the introduction to the first edition 'the aim of this book is to give the chief methods employed in the microscopical examination of human and other animal organs'. Today, over fifty years and four editions later, there is no reason to change this objective, but it has become more difficult to achieve. A golden age of histological methodology in the later part of the last century, during which many of the general and specialized dye staining techniques were developed, has been followed by an even more productive period in the middle decades of the twentieth century. Alternative methods of demonstrating the structure, and especially the function, of tissues have evolved which include amongst others, histochemistry and immunohistology, whilst fluorescence and electron microscopy have become complementary to the use of the conventional light microscope. A wide range of non-dye staining methods have emerged in the mid-twentieth century, and these are best used in conjunction with the established dye staining techniques of the nineteenth century.

The modern histologist needs to be aware of all new techniques and will use many of them, but much of the work of a histology laboratory still consists of dye staining of tissue sections. A technologist must be expert in the classical methods of the past and use the artistry and flair that are needed for successful dye staining, but scientific accuracy and training are essential for the more exact methods such as those of enzyme histochemistry. The authors of the present edition face the same problem of incorporating much new methodology whilst preserving all that is valuable from the past. We have continued to emphasize the importance of understanding the rationale of each method as difficulties can only be overcome by the well informed bench worker. Dogma and mystery now have no place in the histology laboratory.

New material in this edition owes much to experts in specialized fields. Immunohistology has emerged from a research tool into routine techniques that can use fixed tissues and great help has been given by Mr J. Burns in the preparation of this chapter. The growing respectability of histology as a science has taken the microscopist out of a world of subjective qualitative impressions into one of objective quantitative facts and this has been a stimulus to include a new chapter on quantitative methods for which we thank Dr C. S. Foster. Dr Alison Smithies has revised diagnostic cytology with emphasis upon the need for the satisfactory collection and preparation of specimens; without these, subsequent staining and examination cannot be completely successful. The whole text has been revised and additional sections and methods have been added, but only a few techniques have been deleted. The methods for special organs and tissues have been redistributed amongst other chapters and dye staining of ultrastructural organelles is now replaced by enzyme histochemistry or electron microscopy. Techniques for electron microscopy remain outside the scope of this volume, but Dr P. G. Toner has assisted with the introductory section on scanning electron microscopy. Many others have helped in the preparation of this edition and it is a pleasure to thank Professor H. A. Sissons, Mr W. Slidders, Miss Kathleen Page, Mr J. Chapman, and Mr R. A. Lambert for assistance with the text. Professor I. M. Roitt, Professor Deborah Doniach, Dr D. W. H. Barnes, Mr E. Lucas, Mr G. A. Harwood, and many commercial organizations provided illustrations, and our thanks are also due the editor of *Medical Laboratory Sciences*, Dr P. P. Anthony, and Messrs Churchill Livingstone for permission to publish some of the new figures. Others will recognize small details for which they were responsible; these are too numerous to list but are gratefully acknowledged. The completion of our work has been made possible by the active help and patient forbearance of our laboratory colleagues, by the secretarial assistance of Mrs Jacqueline West, and the guidance and support provided by the staff of the Oxford University Press.

Plymouth and London   R.A.B.D.
November 1979   E.A.W.

Contents

1 | The aims and methods of histology

The aims of histology

Histology is the study of tissues (from the Greek, *histos* = tissue; *logos* = word). Firstly, this involves the examination of the architecture and relationship of the different types of tissues, and secondly the detailed investigation of the structure of the individual cells—*cytology*. By combining this knowledge of microscopic anatomy and cellular composition much has been learnt about the physiological function of tissues and this has been amplified by more recent research into the histochemical reactions and ultrastructure of cells. Histology and cytology are closely interrelated, and in almost all histological preparations the components of individual cells will be studied. Ideally, microscopic examination of living tissues should be carried out, so that a true picture can be obtained, but only small primitive living animals can be examined in this way as most tissues are too thick or are not accessible for direct inspection. The majority of histological techniques are applied to killed tissues, preserved or 'fixed' in such a way as to retain the structure as closely as possible to that of the living tissues. It must be appreciated that the completed histological preparations of killed tissues show certain alterations of the cells and of the tissue as a whole; these changes, which we call '*artifacts*', may occur in any of the processes in the preparation of the specimen for microscopy, and the histologist must use methods which, for his particular purpose, cause the least tissue damage.

There are many different techniques for the preparation of tissues and many methods of examination. Most involve the preparation of *sections* that are examined by various types of microscopes, but no single method of examination, and certainly no single staining technique, will display all the cells of the tissue equally well, nor all the individual components within the cells. An advantage of histological techniques is that only small amounts of tissue are required and it may be possible to demonstrate morphology by dye staining, functional characteristics by histochemical or immunological methods, and ultrastructure by electron microscopy, all from the same specimen. Staining methods sometimes have no fully understood scientific basis, but an increasing number with a known chemical reaction are now being used; these histochemical techniques are not to be regarded as something distinct, only a more scientific and exact part of histology. Every histologist should know the reason why a technique is used in histology and how it works, in addition to remembering the details of the method. In a few cases we admit that we do not know, but in almost all histological techniques there are easily understood scientific reasons for what we do and how we do it. Recognition of the reasons behind the methods makes the whole subject more interesting and less of a mystery. Histological techniques remain something of an art, but are becoming more and more a science, and have not been superseded by the development of other biological scientific methods. They are capable of displaying beautifully the cellular details and some of the functional activities of the tissue, but it must be realized that histology has its weaknesses and not a few pitfalls.

The aim of the histologist is to obtain, within the time available, the greatest possible amount of information from the tissue. This will be achieved if workers appreciate that their techniques can cause alterations within the tissue; must be carried out with care, skill, and empathy; and need accurate and critical interpretation.

The methods of histology

METHODS OF PREPARATION

FRESH CELLS AND TISSUES

Cells that are suspended in a fluid, such as blood or lymph, may be seen by *direct examination* in a drop of the fluid. The fluid may require dilution with an isotonic solution such as normal saline. Cells that are grouped together in a loose tissue, as in subcutaneous connective tissue, may also be examined directly if the tissue is thin. If the tissue is thick, or in the case of a solid organ, cells can be separated from one another in a fluid medium like normal saline by *dissociation* or *teasing*. Fresh preparations show cells in their natural state, but suffer from difficulty in examination due to lack of contrast. This can be overcome by phase-contrast microscopy or vital staining.

Vital staining is a method of giving contrast and colour to the cytoplasm of cells. Ehrlich (1887, 1894) showed that certain parts of the living cell can be stained if the cells are dissociated in the staining solution (supra-vital staining) or by the injection of the dye into the living organism (intra-vital staining). These methods are ideal in that they demonstrate parts of living cells, but vital staining is limited by the fact that only certain cytoplasmic elements can be demonstrated. The nucleus is resistant to vital stains, and the permeability of the nuclear membrane towards dyes appears to be an indication of cell death. Vital staining has been widely used in experimental work, and can be a valuable control of cytological methods using fixed material but is now partly replaced by phase-contrast microscopy. Features of this method are described in greater detail in Chapter 6 [p. 108].

CYTOLOGICAL TECHNIQUES

Fluids containing cells, or tiny fragments of tissue such as aspirated bone marrow, are smeared upon a microscope slide, and the adherent cells are fixed in order to preserve their appearance. Organs or tissues can be smeared upon slides in the same way, and a number of the cells, depending upon the consistency and structure of the tissue, will adhere to the slide. The smears are stained to demonstrate cell structure, and finally mounted in a medium that gives a suitable optical refractility to the tissue. The examination of stained smears is the standard method in exfoliative cytology [p. 335]. The finding of atypical cells in body fluids and secretions may be suggestive or diagnostic of malignancy, and the recent great increase in diagnostic cytology is largely due to the development of the method by Papanicolaou (1943), although examination of body fluids for the detection of carcinoma cells dates back to the nineteenth century (Beale 1860).

For some organs, such as spleen or bone marrow, the *impression method* is used. This is done by touching the cut surface of the organ or piece of tissue with a slide; in this way, a little of the architectural arrangement of the tissue may be preserved in the imprint. Soft tumours may be rapidly studied by this method, which is still of value in the diagnosis of malignancy (Tribe 1973).

In smears or films the cells flatten and are effectively in two, rather than three, dimensions. They are larger than the same cells in tissue sections and cellular details are more easily seen. These are valuable features and smears can supplement sectional methods, thereby obtaining both cellular structural detail and architecture of the tissue. With tissue cultures and leucocyte cultures for chromosomes the use of films and smears is particularly appropriate.

SECTIONAL METHODS

These involve cutting the specimen into very thin translucent slices or sections, and have the advantage (in contrast to the methods mentioned above) that the architecture of the tissue—the relation of the cells to one another—is preserved. Three-dimensional tissues are deliberately converted into sections approximately one cell thick, and to see the cellular structure these are stained in various ways. The interpretation of thin sections requires experience, especially if the section is not a vertical cross-section. Oblique or tangential sections may give surprising appearances, and these are represented in FIGURE 1.1, which shows the shape of some of the sections that can be obtained by slices through a curved cylindrical object such as a banana in its skin. The accuracy of the various sectional methods is sufficiently great that most research and routine work in histology is carried out by one of them. An accurate reconstruction of a small piece of the tissue can be obtained by the examination of *serial sections*. The whole specimen is sectioned, and the sections retained in their correct order; the numbered, stained preparations are examined in sequence. With larger specimens serial sections may be an impossibility, but alternate sections, or sections retained at regular intervals (e.g. every tenth section) may give a good indication of the structure of the whole specimen; this is known as *step sectioning* [see p. 94].

Thick sections of fresh or fixed tissue may be cut freehand with a sharp knife or razor and by limiting staining to the surface, the histological structure can be seen. This technique (Terry 1928) has been of some value in rapid diagnostic work, and is still a quick and easy way of identifying tissues (Westwood and Hunt 1973), but is now superseded by sections cut on a microtome. Most sectional methods are based upon the conversion of the tissue into a uniform consistency suitable for sectioning. This alteration of tissue consistency may be done by *freezing*, though more commonly this is brought about by infiltrating and embedding the specimen with *paraffin wax, celloidin*, or *synthetic resins*. Frozen sections can be cut from fresh tissue in a cryostat refrigerated microtome, but tissue which is infiltrated and embedded in wax or other solid materials is 'fixed' to preserve the tissue, prevent diffusion from it and make it possible to prepare and stain suitable sections.

Most histological sections are 4–7 μm thick. The micrometre (μm) is a standard unit of measurement in histology and 1 μm equals one thousandth of a

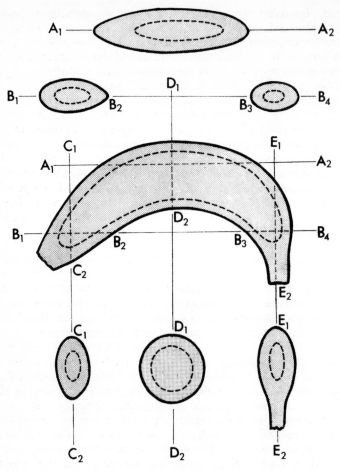

FIG. 1.1. Sections taken through a banana in its skin, showing variations in shape in different planes of section.

millimetre or one millionth of a metre. For techniques demonstrating large structures such as fat droplets, nerve fibres, and blood vessels, thicker sections in the range 10–25 μm are more successful. Sections 1 μm thick can be cut from tissues embedded in synthetic resins and these show more detail than thicker wax sections; they are intermediate between the conventional histological section and the 50–100 nm (0.05–0.1 μm) thick sections which are cut on the ultramicrotome for electron microscopy. In contrast, 300–400 μm thick sections of whole lungs or other organs designed for naked-eye examination can be cut on a large microtome after gelatin impregnation (Gough and Wentworth 1949), and are used for demonstration or teaching [p. 482]. Whilst most tissues are soft and require support before they can be sectioned, some are too hard, and bone usually needs decalcification [p. 200] before sections can be cut. Sections of undecalcified bone may be prepared from small specimens in order to determine if calcification of the matrix is normal. The use of dense embedding media and heavy microtomes has made this possible [p. 208].

The *staining of tissue sections* is required as tissues need contrast and colour for microscopical examination and the completed preparation must have a suitable refractive index. 'Staining' techniques will be considered in general in Chapter 7 [p. 125] and in detail in many of the other chapters. In brief, staining may be carried out by dyes, which may be coloured or induce fluorescence; by chemical reactions that produce coloured end-products; or by making tissue components opaque by metallic impregnation.

Non-staining techniques for tissue sections are used in addition to the traditional 'staining' methods. Modern histological techniques include fluorescent immunological methods, autoradiography, microincineration, and microradiography.

Fluorescent immunohistological methods are based on the use of fluorochrome-labelled antibodies [p. 323]. These have a high degree of specificity and can be used to demonstrate immune complexes and a wide range of cellular structures in tissues. The preparations are examined with the fluorescence microscope, which is capable of showing very small amounts of the fluorochrome.

Autoradiography demonstrates radioactive materials following the introduction of a labelled radioactive element into the tissue. This may be quickly incorporated into cells of the tissues and autoradiography will demonstrate the sites of radioactive isotopes by their ability to reduce the silver salts in a photographic emulsion. The technique was described by London in 1904, but the method in general use is that of Pelc (1947) and Doniach and Pelc (1950). In this, the photographic emulsion is stripped from special plates and applied to sections [p. 469]; after appropriate development, fixation, and mounting, the sites and approximate quantity of the radioactive isotope can be seen. All those who work with radioactive materials must remember that radioactivity is harmful, and special precautions are necessary when handling or disposing of radioactive substances. Radioactivity decays steadily, but may never completely disappear, so the duration of the radioactivity of an isotope is expressed as its 'half-life'; this is the time necessary for one half of the number of unstable atoms to disintegrate, after which the amount of radioactivity in the material is reduced by 50 per cent. The half-life of radioactive isotopes in biological use varies from a few hours to an enormous number of years.

Micro-incineration is believed to have been first carried out by Raspail in 1833. A section of tissue is mounted on a slide and heated in an electric furnace. The temperature is raised, slowly at first (Scott 1950), until all the organic matter has been burnt off, leaving a mineral skeleton of the tissue on the slide. This can be examined by reflected light or by dark ground illumination, and the sites of mineral deposition compared with a control section that has not been incinerated. Micro-incineration is reviewed by Glick (1949) and Horning (1951). Techniques such as histospectrography (Policard 1933) enable quantitative estimations of very small amounts of mineral materials to be made.

Microradiography is used to study the structure of histological sections by their absorption of X-rays, and it is also possible to obtain information on the actual chemical composition of the tissues concerned (Engström 1962).

Microradiography has particularly been applied to the study of calcified tissues (bone, cartilage, enamel, and dentine) when the presence of mineral material (hydroxyapatite) is responsible for virtually all the absorption of X-rays. If a thin section of bone is placed in close contact with a fine grain photographic emulsion and exposed to a beam of soft X-rays, the resultant picture shows the distribution of mineral material. A preparation of this type is known as a 'contact microradiograph', and is examined with an ordinary light microscope. Instruments for 'projection microradiography' have been developed, where the production of a magnified X-ray shadow allows direct enlargement of the negative. The measurement of the amount of mineral present in a given area of section is also possible. Bone specimens for microradiographic examination are usually prepared by sawing or by grinding and polishing after embedding in methyl methacrylate (Jowsey 1955). Relatively soft (20 kV) X-rays are used, and special photographic emulsions with a very fine grain are required.

Microradiographs of sections of soft tissues can give information on the protein content of tissues and the 'dry mass' of cells (Greulich 1960). For this work, very soft (5–10 kV) X-rays are needed. Microradiography is sometimes used to demonstrate the arrangement of blood vessels in a tissue, following their injection with radiopaque material.

METHODS OF EXAMINATION

MACROSCOPICAL METHODS

Histologists can learn much from the naked-eye examination of tissues. This is essential in the case of organs which are not uniform, because histological examination can only be made of parts of a large specimen and the appropriate selection of tissue blocks may be critical. The preparation of specimens for museum display (Kaiserling 1899; Wentworth 1947) and the demonstration of blood vessels or other anatomical structures by injection techniques (Tompsett 1970), are methods that supplement those of microscopic histology, whilst large paper-mounted sections of whole organs [p. 482] are intermediate links between gross and microscopic methods.

MICROSCOPICAL METHODS

The examination of intact tissue specimens with a low-power stereoscopic *dissecting microscope*, using reflected or transmitted light, will identify tissues and some of their components, such as the villi of the mucosa of the small intestine. The *phase-contrast microscope* converts differences of refractive index into patterns of light and shade and plays an important part in the examination of fresh and unstained cells and tissues. The *interference microscope* can be used to visualize cell details of living, unstained cells and by using it as an optical balance the weight of intracellular structures can be determined.

Smears and sections of tissues are translucent and are usually examined with a *conventional binocular microscope* using transmitted light. A wide range of magnification ($\times 20$ to $\times 1000$) is needed and it is an advantage if the microscope can also be used for some of the specialized types of light microscopy. High-intensity illumination is necessary for the indirect visualization of objects by *dark-ground microscopy* [p. 20] or for the examination of tissues that have a polarized or crystalline structure by the *polarized-light microscope* [p. 27]. A *fluorescence microscope* [p. 22] is used for sections that have been stained with fluorochrome dyes or have been treated with fluorescent-labelled antibodies in immunohistological techniques [p. 323]; these are methods which have a high degree of sensitivity.

Electron microscopes use a short wavelength beam of electrons that produce high resolution with high magnification. The *scanning electron microscope* [p. 32] demonstrates the surfaces of tissues and cells at low and high magnification and is a sophisticated extension of the examination of intact tissues by light microscopy using reflected illumination. *Transmission electron microscopes* [p. 29] examine ultra-thin sections with a highly magnified transmitted electron beam and have largely superseded light microscopy methods of stained sections for demonstrating the larger intracellular organelles such as mitochondria and the Golgi apparatus. A development of the transmission electron microscope is the *electron probe microanalyser* which gives a quantitative assessment of the chemical composition of tissues by passing a narrow electron beam through them, using a spectrometer to detect the X-rays that are given off (Carroll 1967).

METHODS OF RECORDING HISTOLOGICAL OBSERVATIONS

The final stage is reached when the histologist records the observations. Traditionally this has been in *qualitative* terms, using words to describe the structure of the tissues examined. With the development of colour photomacrography and photomicrography [p. 462] permanent *photographic records* can be kept or used for demonstration and teaching. *Quantitative* methods [p. 436], by which the numbers, sizes, and areas of histological structures can be expressed in absolute or comparative terms, are a more exact way of recording microscopical observations and can be applied to tissue sections. A feature of stained sections and tissue embedded in paraffin blocks is their permanence, and most histology laboratories will preserve blocks and sections for long periods of time.

REFERENCES

BEALE, L. S. (1860). *Arch. Med.* **2**, 44.
CARROLL, K. G. (1967). In In vivo *techniques in histology* (ed. G. H. Bourne). Williams and Wilkins, Baltimore.
DONIACH, I. and PELC, S. R. (1950). *Br. J. Radiol.* **23**, 184.
EHRLICH, P. (1887).*Biol. Zbl.* **6**, 214.
—— (1894). *Z. wiss. Mikr.* **11**, 25.
ENGSTRÖM, A. (1962). *X-ray microanalysis in biology and medicine.* Amsterdam.
GLICK, D. (1949). *Techniques of histo- and cytochemistry.* Interscience, New York.
GOUGH, J. and WENTWORTH, J. E. (1949). *J. roy. micr. Soc.* **69**, 231.
GREULICH, R. C. (1960). In *X-ray microscopy and X-ray microanalysis.* Proceedings of the 2nd International Symposium (eds. A. Engström, V. Cosslett, and H. Pattee). Amsterdam.
HORNING, E. S. (1951). In *Cytology and cell physiology* (ed. G. H. Bourne), 2nd edn. Oxford.
JOWSEY, J. (1955). *J. sci. Instrum.* **32**, 159.
KAISERLING, C. (1899). *Verh. dtsch. Ges. Path.* **2**, 203.
LONDON, E. S. (1904). *Arch. Élect. méd.* **12**, 363.
PAPANICOLAOU, G. N. and TRAUT, H. F. (1943). *The diagnosis of uterine cancer by the vaginal smear.* Commonwealth Fund, New York.
PELC, S. R. (1947). *Nature (Lond.)* **160**, 749.
POLICARD, A. (1933). *Protoplasma (Wien)* **19**, 602.

Raspail, F. V. (1833). Quoted by Lison, L. (1936). *Histochimie animales*. Gautier-Villars, Paris.

Scott, G. H. (1950). In *Microscopical technique* (ed. by R. McClung-Jones), 3rd edn. Cassell, London.

Terry, B. T. (1928). *J. Lab. clin. Med.* **13**, 550.

Tompsett, D. H. (1970). *Anatomical techniques*, 2nd edn. Livingstone, Edinburgh.

Tribe, C. R. (1973). *J. clin. Path.* **26**, 273.

Wentworth, J. E. (1947). *J. techn. Meth.* **27**, 201.

Westwood, P. J. and Hunt, A. C. (1973). *J. clin. Path.* **26**, 723.

2 | Microscopy

The light microscope, now 400 years old, is the standard instrument for the examination of histological preparations. Within the last 50 years the development of the electron microscope has enormously expanded our knowledge of cellular structure but has not superseded the light microscope. Using natural daylight, or artificial visible light, the resolution of the light microscope is limited by the wavelength of its light source [p. 17]. With visible light of wavelength 400–800 nm it is not possible to resolve two separate points that are closer together than half the wavelength. Thus an object smaller than 0.2 µm is unlikely to be seen clearly, even if the optics of the microscope are perfect. Shorter wavelength light rays, such as ultraviolet light, allow a higher resolution to be obtained but as these rays are invisible the magnified image must be projected on to a fluorescent screen or photographed. In the fluorescence microscope the invisible ultraviolet rays are converted by the specimen into visible light rays and this is a light microscope technique. A stream of electrons has such a short wavelength that the magnification of the electron microscope is not limited by the wavelength factor. Thus there are two main types of microscopy *light microscopy* and *electron microscopy*. In histological laboratories at least three microscopes are usually found, the conventional light microscope, the fluorescence microscope, and the electron microscope. Every histologist should know the basic theory and structure of these microscopes, and should understand the defects and limitations of lenses and some of the special techniques of microscopy. These will be briefly described; fuller accounts are given by Casartelli (1965), Barer (1968), and Culling (1974). Specialized techniques are considered by Chayen and Denby (1968).

In all types of microscopy there must be a system of visualization of the object so that it can be observed directly by the human eye, or on a cathode-ray tube, or seen as a photograph. Visible light, with a wavelength of 400–800 nm, represents only part of the wavelengths that can be used in microscopy. These are compared with the sizes of the objects examined by microscopes in Table 2.1, and the resolution of some of the microscopes used by histologists is also shown. For the measurement of size the metric system is universal and this is included in the larger group of measurements known as the International System of Units which is abbreviated SI from the French *Système International d'Unités*. The development of the SI system has been described by Baron (1973), Baron *et al.* (1974), and *Journal of Clinical Pathology* (1970). For the measurement of length in histology we use the millimetre (mm), which is one thousandth part of a metre; the micrometre (µm), one thousandth part of a millimetre; and the nanometre (nm), one thousandth part of a micrometre (Table 2.2). The micrometre (µm) is the same length as the micron (µ), and the nanometre (nm) is the same as the millimicron (mµ). The Ångstrom unit (Å) is one tenth of a nanometre. Microns, millimicrons, and Ångstrom units have now been superseded and their use is being discontinued as the SI system becomes widely accepted.

Table 2.1 Wavelengths, sizes of biological structures, and resolution of microscopes

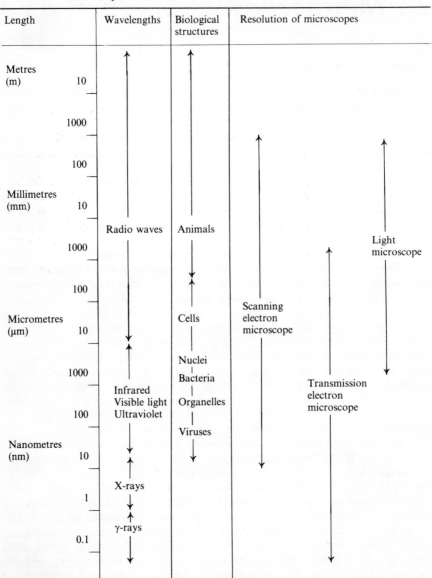

Length	Wavelengths	Biological structures	Resolution of microscopes
Metres (m) 10			
1000			
100			
Millimetres (mm) 10			
1000	Radio waves	Animals	Light microscope
100			
Micrometres (µm) 10		Cells	Scanning electron microscope
1000		Nuclei	
	Infrared	Bacteria	Transmission electron microscope
100	Visible light	Organelles	
	Ultraviolet		
Nanometres (nm) 10		Viruses	
1	X-rays		
0.1	γ-rays		

The light microscope

GENERAL PRINCIPLES OF LIGHT MICROSCOPY

THE FORMATION OF THE IMAGE

The simple microscope may be considered to have two convex lenses, one as the objective and the other as the eyepiece. The path of light through these is shown in FIGURE 2.1. The objective (O) magnifies the illuminated specimen SP

Table 2.2. Units of length (SI units)

SI Unit	Length in metres	Equivalent
Metre (m)	1	
Millimetre (mm)	$0.001\ (1 \times 10^{-3})$	
Micrometre (μm)	$0.000001\ (1 \times 10^{-6})$	Micron (μ)
Nanometre (nm)	$0.000000001\ (1 \times 10^{-9})$	Millimicron (mμ)
	$0.0000000001\ (1 \times 10^{-10})$	Ångstrom (Å)

to produce a real inverted image S_1P_1; to do this, the specimen must be farther away from the objective than the focal length of the objective lens. The eyepiece (E) is close to the image S_1P_1, within the focal length of the eyepiece lens; a magnified upright virtual image of S_1P_1 is produced by the eyepiece and will be seen by the observer's eye at S_2P_2. Thus the specimen has been magnified twice but inverted only once for visual examination.

These basic principles apply to all light microscopes, and the condenser and light source are only used for the satisfactory illumination of the specimen.

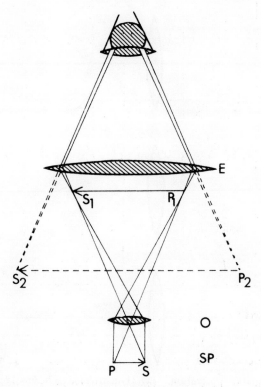

FIG. 2.1. The path of light through a simple microscope. E = eyepiece; O = objective; SP = specimen.

Translucent thin sections are usually used for histological techniques, and these are examined by *transmitted* light; the light source is below the specimen and is passed (transmitted) through the specimen into the microscope. Opaque objects must be examined by *reflected* light; thick uncleared specimens, metals, etc. are illuminated from above and light is reflected upwards by the specimen into the microscope.

MICROSCOPE LENSES AND THEIR DEFECTS

The objective and the eyepiece have been considered to be simple convex lenses, but in practice these, and the condenser, are compound structures made up of several convex and concave lenses. These are designed to overcome the optical defects or aberrations of colour or form that are inherent in simple lenses.

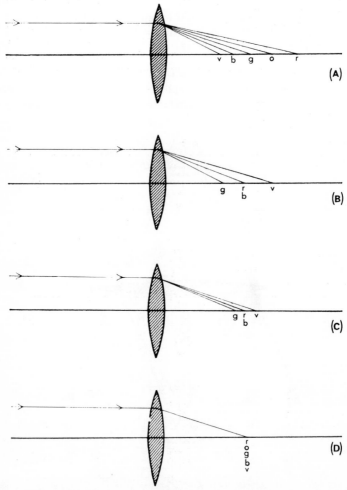

FIG. 2.2. Chromatic aberration. (A) Uncorrected chromatic aberration. (B) Achromatic objective. (C) Fluorite objective. (D) Apochromatic objective. (b) = blue, g = green, o = orange, r = red, v = violet.)

Axial aberrations

Chromatic aberration is the production of a coloured spectrum of light by a lens. When light passes through glass or other substances the blue end of the spectrum is refracted more than the red; this breaks the white light into a secondary spectrum of colours [FIG. 2.2A]. An *achromatic* objective is corrected for two colours, usually red and blue, which are focused to the same point. Green light is brought to a shorter focus and violet light to a longer focus [FIG. 2.2B]. By the use of *fluorite* in the objective the spread of the secondary spectrum is much reduced, though the type of correction is the same as that of an achromatic objective. A fluorite objective has a short secondary spectrum of the achromatic type [FIG. 2.2C] and the use of the term 'semi-apochromatic' is best avoided. An *apochromatic* objective is fully corrected for three colours and by the design of the lens and by the use of fluorite the formation of a secondary spectrum is almost completely eliminated and all colours are brought to the same focus [FIG. 2.2D].

Spherical aberration is another defect of a single lens, due to its curved surface. Light rays passing through the periphery of a lens will be refracted to a greater extent than those passing through the central part and images are brought into focus at different points along the axis [FIG. 2.3A]. These different

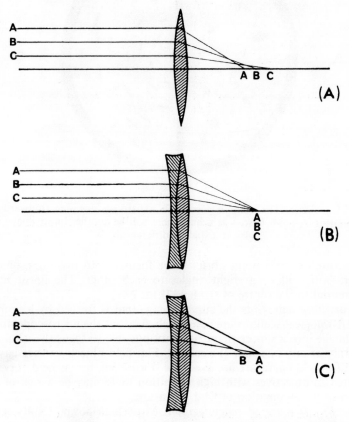

FIG. 2.3.   Spherical aberration. (A) Uncorrected spherical aberration.
(B) Corrected spherical aberration. (C) Zonal aberration.

image planes can be brought to one point by the use of a compound lens [FIG. 2.3B], though in practice it may be found that lenses that have been corrected for spherical aberration still contain zones with a different focus from the rest. This residual defect is called zonal aberration [FIG. 2.3C]. Uncorrected spherical aberration can be reduced by cutting off the outer light rays with an opaque diaphragm, thus using the central part of the lens only; this is commonly done in cheap photographic lenses, but is not usually applicable to microscopy.

Off-axial aberrations

Coma is an aberration which causes a point object to be seen with a flare, like the tail of a comet. The flare is radial to the centre of the field, and may point inwards or outwards [FIG. 2.4A].

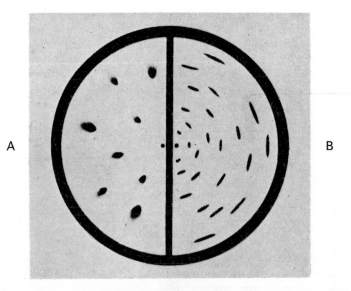

A   B

FIG. 2.4. (A) Coma. The point is seen with a flare on one side (outward coma). (B) Astigmatism. A point is seen as a line; there will be another linear image at right angles at a slightly different focus.

Astigmatism causes a point object to be focused into two lines, one above the other; both will be at right angles to each other. The linear image is circumferential to the centre of the field [FIG. 2.4B].

Field curvature represents the curved image that is formed by a simple lens system. Histological sections are completely flat, but the microscope may convert the image into a saucer-shape; it is not possible to focus the whole of the field sharply at any one time [FIG. 2.5A]. Flat-field objectives that have been corrected for field curvature are available [FIG. 2.5B], but as field curvature is accentuated in objectives with high definition there may be a risk of loss of resolution in the elimination of field curvature.

Chromatic difference of magnification. Most high-power (× 40 or more) objectives have slightly different magnifications for different colours of the spectrum. They tend to magnify blue and violet most, and red the least. A dark object will tend to show a red fringe on its outer side and a blue fringe on the inner side. Chromatic difference of magnification is corrected by the use of a compensating eyepiece.

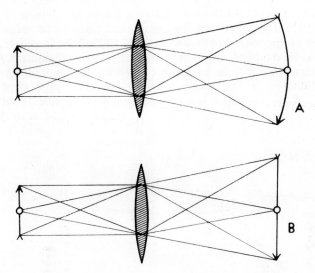

FIG. 2.5. Field curvature. (A) Uncorrected. (B) Corrected (flat-field).

EYEPIECES

Huygenian eyepieces are the simplest form of eyepieces in common use; they are cheap, but do not correct for chromatic difference of magnification. This type of eyepiece can be identified if it is not marked, by removing it from the microscope and holding it up to the light; a blue fringe is seen inside the diaphragm.

Compensating eyepieces are compound lenses with a chromatic difference of magnification which is equal and opposite to that of high-power objectives. They are essential for use with apochromatic objectives, but they also improve the performance of most high-power achromatic objectives. Low-power objectives have no significant chromatic difference of magnification, but in order to avoid the necessity of changing eyepieces each time the objective is changed a chromatic difference may be introduced into them; the same compensating eyepiece can then be used with all the objectives of the microscope. When held up to the light a red fringe will be seen in a compensating eyepiece.

Eyepieces for binocular microscopes must be accurately paired, with equal centration, magnification, and field in order to reduce eye-strain. Interocular distance should be accurately adjusted, and the microscopist should sit at the correct height for the eyepieces to come to the exact height of the observer's eyes.

OBJECTIVES

The three main types of objective, achromatic, fluorite, and apochromatic, have already been described. Every objective has a fixed working distance, focal length, magnification, and numerical aperture. The working distance is

the distance between an object in focus and the front of the lens. Long working distances are necessary for dissecting microscopes. The focal length of a
simple lens is the distance from the centre of the lens to the point at which
parallel rays of light are brought to a sharp focus; in the compound lenses of
most objectives this is the distance between an object in focus and a point
approximately halfway between the component lenses. The magnification is
dependent upon the focal length, and is equal to the tube length of the microscope divided by the focal length of the objective. The magnification of a low-
power objective with a focal length of 16 mm and a standard tube length of
160 mm is $160/16 = 10$. The *numerical aperture (NA)* is a product of the size of
the aperture of the front lens. $NA = n$ multiplied by the sine of half the angle
of aperture, where n is the refractive index of the medium between the lens and
the object. In FIGURE 2.6 the NA is equal to $n \times$ sine of angle at O; the sine of
angle at O is $\dfrac{r}{H}$ and the $NA = n \times \dfrac{r}{H}$.

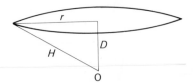

FIG. 2.6. The calculation of the numerical aperture of a lens. (r = radius of the lens.
O = object in focus. D = working distance. H = hypotenuse.)

As the distance H is always greater than the radius r, the numerical aperture
is invariably less than the refractive index of the intervening medium. The
refractive index of air is 1.0, and the NA of dry objectives must be less than
1.0. Immersion oil has a refractive index of 1.51, and the NA of oil immersion
objectives are about 1.3. A high numerical aperture increases resolution, but
diminishes the thickness of section that is in focus at one time (depth of focus)
and increases field curvature. Tables 2.3 and 2.4 show the characteristics of
objectives in use in histology, together with the magnification of microscope
optical systems.

Table 2.3 Characteristics of microscope objectives

Focal length (mm)	NA	Magnification	Working distance (mm)	Diameter of field (mm)	Depth of field (μm)
25	0.15	× 5	23	3.2	20
16	0.28	× 10	7	1.6	10
4	0.74	× 40	1	0.4	2
2	1.3	× 100	0.25	0.15	1

These figures apply to a standard tube length of 160 mm. With binocular
microscopes there is usually an additional magnification of × 1.25 in the binocular head.

Table 2.4 Magnification of microscope optical systems

Objective Focal length (mm)	Primary magnification	Final magnification			
		Eyepieces			
		×6	×8	×10	×15
25	×5	30	40	50	75
16	×10	60	80	100	150
4	×40	240	320	400	600
2	×100	600	800	1000	1500

The *resolution* of a lens is its capacity to demonstrate closely set points as clearly distinct images; the greater the detail that can be defined, the higher the resolving power. It is dependent upon the wavelength of the light (λ) and the numerical aperture of the objective (NA). The minimum resolvable distance between two points (i.e. the maximum resolution of the lens) is given by the formula

$$r = \frac{0.6\,\lambda}{\text{NA}}$$

and is about 0.2 μm with the light microscope under ideal conditions (Table 2.5).

Table 2.5 The approximate limits of useful magnification and resolution

Objective		NA	Useful magnification limit	Resolution (μm)
Focal length (mm)	Magnification			
25	×5	0.15	×150	2
16	×10	0.28	×280	1
4	×40	0.74	×740	0.4
2	×100	1.3	×1300	0.2

It has already been seen that the numerical aperture cannot exceed 1.0 in air and 1.5 in oil; thus the only way to increase resolution is to use energy of shorter wavelength, as in the electron microscope. Using visible light, the maximum useful magnification is approximately 1000 times the numerical aperture (Table 2.5). Beyond this there is only empty magnification that does not show any more detail, as two points are not separated sufficiently for the human eye to be able to appreciate them as different images. With a micro-projector there may be a very high final magnification, but no more detail can be produced on the screen (in practice this is less) than can be seen by looking through the microscope.

CONDENSERS

The substage condenser should have the same numerical aperture as the objective in use, and should form a true image of the light source. The Abbe condenser is simple and cheap, but it is not suitable for critical microscopy. An achromatic condenser corrected for spherical and chromatic aberration is needed for objectives with high resolution. For histology it is particularly useful to have a condenser with a top lens that can be swung out of the path of light, thus filling the whole field with light when very low-power objectives are used. The use of the 'flip-top' accessory lens converts a long focal length low NA condenser into a short focal length high NA condenser that is suitable for higher magnifications. The dark-ground condenser is described later [p. 21].

ILLUMINATION

The use of daylight, once preferred by histologists, has been superseded by artificial light, which is more constant and available at all times. Microscopes with built-in, variable, high-intensity light sources are convenient for histology and for photomicrography.

Critical illumination

The illumination is said to be critical when an image of the light source is focused upon the object plane and the illuminating rays are symmetrically disposed about the long axis of the microscope. The diameter of this area should cover the whole field under examination and the illumination must be of even intensity.

Köhler illumination

High intensity microscope lamps may have a small light source that is not sufficient to fill the whole of the field with light. They are usually supplied with an auxiliary lens and iris diaphragm which increases the apparent size of the light source. With Köhler illumination the auxiliary lens of the lamp focuses the enlarged image of the lamp on to the iris diaphragm of the sub-stage condenser. The adjustable iris diaphragm of the lamp is then closed and focused on to the object plane by means of the substage condenser. The resolving powers of critical and Köhler illumination are similar, but Köhler illumination has the advantage of providing a variable and evenly illuminated field of view, and is displacing critical illumination for most purposes. The light source and the condenser should be set up in the following way.

1. Switch on the microscope illumination and ensure that the light intensity is safe for visual work.
2. Half close the iris diaphragm (field diaphragm) in front of the light source.
3. Place a slide on the microscope stage and rack the substage condenser up until it nearly touches the slide.
4. Open the substage condenser diaphragm to its full extent.
5. Focus the preparation using × 10 objective.
6. Close the substage diaphragm.
7. Adjust the lamp condenser until a sharp image of the light source is obtained on the substage diaphragm.
8. Open the substage diaphragm to its full extent.
9. Check that the object is still in focus.
10. Move the substage condenser until the circle of light, limited by the field diaphragm, is in focus.

11. By manipulating the centring screws on the substage condenser, centre the illuminated circle.
12. Adjust the field diaphragm so that the circle of light is just larger than the field to be examined.
13. Remove the eyepiece and view the back lens of the objective. Close the substage diaphragm until its diameter coincides with the diameter of the back lens of the objective.
14. Replace the eyepiece.

NOTE

If the microscope has integral illumination, steps 6–9 may be omitted.

MICROMETRY

The size of a cell or part of a histological preparation can be accurately measured with stage and eyepiece micrometers. The stage micrometer is a 1 or 2 mm scale marked into 1/10 mm and 1/100 mm divisions; the distance between the small divisions is 10 µm. The eyepiece micrometer rests upon the field stop in the eyepiece, and its scale is calibrated by examining the stage micrometer with an appropriate objective. By simple calculation the size of an object between a certain number of eyepiece scale divisions is determined; if, with a particular microscope optical system, 10 eyepiece divisions correspond with 1 stage division, 1 eyepiece division equals 1 µm, and an object 6 eyepiece divisions in length measures 6 µm.

Micrometry may also be performed by projecting the image of a stage micrometer through the microscope on to a screen or on to squared paper. Magnification can also be determined; if the 1 mm scale extends over a length of 8 cm on the screen the magnification is × 80. Accurate measurements can be obtained with a haemocytometer; the small squares are 1/400 mm², and their sides are 50 µm long. A histological section can be superimposed upon an England Finder (used for identifying a microscope field, page 463); approximate measurements can be read off directly, as the small squares have sides 1000 µm long, divided into quarters.

MICROSCOPES FOR HISTOLOGY

At least two different microscopes are needed for histology. A *staining microscope* should always be available in the laboratory for the assessment and control of staining techniques whilst these are in progress. This should be a simple monocular instrument that can be used standing up; a mechanical stage is undesirable, and low-power eyepiece and objectives are usually sufficient. The staining microscope must be completely portable, and daylight is often used; daylight is still preferable to artificial light for the control of certain techniques such as metachromatic staining. If blue or other filters are used they must always be in place to ensure uniformly constant results. The *working microscope* for the examination of the mounted sections has to be more complex. Prolonged microscopy calls for a binocular head and a high intensity artificial light source, preferably built-in. A histologist needs a very low-power objective (× 3 or × 5) for scanning the whole section, and the condenser should be fitted with a swing-out top lens. A mechanical stage is desirable, and is essential for cytology; it must have a wide traverse in both directions for the examination of large sections. Long working distance eyepieces are valuable to those who wear spectacles. Versatility and ease of operation are special virtues in a microscope for histology, as this will be used for very low-power and for high-power work; the continual changing of eyepieces and condenser setting should not be required, except for very critical work.

The stereoscopic dissecting microscope

The low-power dissecting microscope plays a useful part in laboratories that examine tissues and may provide a link between naked-eye examinations and high-power microscopy. It consists of two separate low magnification microscopes which are mounted at an angle of about 15 degrees. Controls are simple, and usually consist of only a single coarse adjustment. Illumination can be either by transmitted or incident light or both, and although it might be anticipated that two matched microscopes would be expensive, the dissecting microscope is cheap to buy and simple and robust in use.

The dissecting microscope, being two angled microscopes, has strong stereoscopic qualities, and the depth of an object appears to be increased. The image is reversed so that it appears upright, and moving the object and dissection becomes natural and easy. Because the object planes are at an angle to each other only the centres of both the fields will be in focus at the same time but this disadvantage is largely overcome by the large depth of focus. Magnification is normally not more than × 100, and this represents the approximate limit of magnification as the NA of the objectives is not usually more than 0.1; a choice of magnifications is provided by two or three paired objectives or zoom-lens attachments giving infinite variation. The working distance is long, usually between 5 and 10 cm. Photography is a problem as it is difficult to produce and to project or view stereoscopic micrographs. Photography through one of the eyepieces can be easily achieved but the stereoscopic quality is lost.

A stereoscopic dissecting microscope can be useful to the histologist for the identification of tissue and for orientation before it is trimmed and processed prior to paraffin embedding. In the past histologists have not been as interested in surface topography as in cellular structure of sections, but the increasing use of the dissecting microscope and (at the other end of the scale of sophistication) of the scanning electron microscope [p. 32] has brought about a revival in the examination of cellular surfaces.

THE DARK-GROUND MICROSCOPE

In the dark-ground method of illumination no direct rays of light from the condenser enter the microscope. Objects are visible not because they are traversed by direct light rays entering the microscope, but because they cause diffraction and reflection of indirect light rays into the microscope.

Diffraction is a peculiar phenomenon which may be expressed, in Bayliss' words, as 'the property of light waves to bend round corners'. Dust seen in a beam of sunlight is an example of diffraction. This is due to the fact that light waves bend around each particle of dust, forming a diffraction halo around it. In order to see the particles it is necessary that the line of vision is at right angles—or at any rate obliquely directed—to the beam of sunlight. If you face the beam of light you will see nothing except dazzle. It is important to avoid getting direct light rays into your eyes, as these will mask the diffracted rays formed around the dust particles.

The principle of the dark-ground condenser can be illustrated by the simple paraboloid condenser of Siedentopf. As shown in FIGURE 2.7 this condenser is a single lens with plane upper and lower surfaces and slightly convex sides; a black disc masks the centre of the lower surface, and only a ring of light can enter around the edge. The dark-ground condenser is closely applied to the undersurface of the slide, in place of the normal substage condenser; a layer of cedarwood oil—not air—must be present between them. The path of light passes outside the aperture of the microscope objective, and a clean slide will appear black and empty. Solid particles will cause diffraction, refraction, and reflection of light rays, and some of these will enter the objective of the microscope causing the particles to be brilliantly illuminated against a black background.

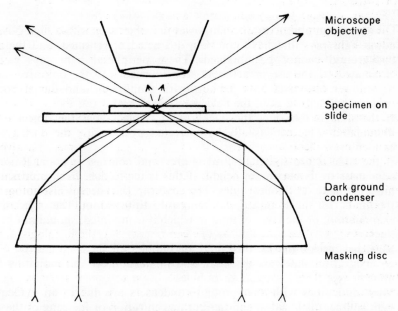

Microscope objective

Specimen on slide

Dark ground condenser

Masking disc

FIG. 2.7. Dark-ground condenser. The broken lines represent rays diffracted by an object into the microscope.

A dark-ground condenser is constructed so that the alteration of the light rays takes place at a definite distance above it. This means that the thickness of the slide and the coverslip are important if clear details are to be obtained. The appropriate slide thickness is usually stated with each dark-ground condenser (frequently this is 1.2 mm) and slides within 0.1 mm of this should be used. The dark-ground condenser is used for the detection of spirochaetes, trypanosomes, and other micro-organisms in body fluids. It is more valuable for the examination of fresh specimens than for sections, but may be used with sections in fluorescence microscopy.

Adjustment of the dark-ground condenser

1. A powerful lamp is needed. Modern halogen lamps are excellent.
2. Use the plane side of the microscope mirror, and adjust the condenser of

the light source so that it throws an image of the lamp on to the centre of the mirror.

3. The dark-ground condenser must be accurately centred. The upper surface is usually engraved with one or more concentric circles; focus these with the 16 mm objective and centre the condenser with the two centring screws. Adjust the plane mirror until the top of the condenser shows a dark disc surrounded by a ring of light that is uniform and of equal width all round.

4. Add several drops of cedar wood oil to the upper surface of the condenser. The specimen, mounted on a slide of the correct thickness, is placed on the stage and the condenser racked upwards until the slide and condenser are completely joined by a thin layer of oil. It is important to avoid air bubbles in this oil seal.

NOTES

1. Oil-immersion objectives or high-power dry objectives with a high NA will admit light rays that have not been diffracted or reflected, and the dark background cannot be obtained. These peripheral light rays can be eliminated by the use of a funnel stop inserted into the objective. Some high-power objectives have a built-in iris diaphragm, and this should be progressively closed until the field is just darkened.

2. If the slide is too thin, the background is black, but the object is not illuminated. This can usually be corrected by lowering the dark-ground condenser.

3. If the slide is too thick the field is grey and contrast is poor. Raise the condenser to its maximum height; if this is ineffective, fresh preparations must be made on thinner slides. The coverslip thickness is also important, the limits (for most condensers) being 0.15 to 0.18 mm. The object under examination, or the layer of fluid in which it is mounted, should not be too thick.

4. Scratches, grease marks, dust, and air bubbles all show up clearly. Clean coverslips and slides are essential, and immersion oil and mounting fluid must be free from dust and air bubbles.

5. Most difficulties with dark-ground condensers are due to an inadequate light source, thick slides, and inaccurate centration or focusing of the condenser.

THE FLUORESCENCE MICROSCOPE

Fluorescence is the property of some substances which, when illuminated with light of a certain wavelength, causes them to emit rays of a different and longer one. In fluorescence microscopy a fluorescent specimen is illuminated with invisible ultraviolet light; light rays of longer wavelength within the spectrum of visible light are given off and these are seen as various colours against a black background. If the new light waves persist after the stimulating light is cut off this is known as phosphorescence. Fluorescence was first applied to microscopy by Köhler in 1904, using ultraviolet light of very low wavelength and complicated quartz optical equipment. Hamperl (1934) described naturally-occurring fluorescent substances in histological specimens, and Haitinger (1938) used fluorochrome dyes to induce fluorescence in animal and plant tissues. Fluorescence techniques have become widely used in research and fluorochrome dye methods are routinely employed for the demonstration of tissue components, bacteria, fungi, and heavy metals in sections and for the identification of malignant cells in exfoliative cytology. Fluorescence microscopy is the basis of immunofluorescent techniques for the demonstration of antigens and antibodies in tissues and sera. This important application of fluorescence microscopy is described in Chapter 17, page 323.

Fluorescence is not strong in comparison with visible light or the strength of the ultraviolet light source, but it appears to be bright owing to its sharply localized wavelength and the contrast with a dark background. FIGURE 2.8 shows that strong ultraviolet light may only induce weak peaks of visible fluorescence but these are sufficient for microscopical examination. The wavelengths of ultraviolet rays, visible light, and infrared rays are also shown in FIGURE 2.8. Wavelengths are stated in nanometres; a nanometre (nm) is one thousandth of a micrometre (μm).

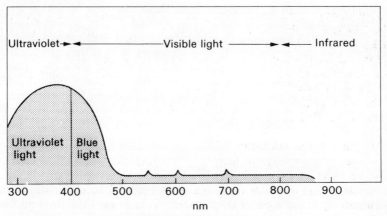

FIG. 2.8. Diagrammatic representation of intense ultraviolet and blue light and three peaks of visible light given off by the fluorescent dye acridine orange.

Ultraviolet light (below 400 nm) is commonly used (the exciting source) for fluorescence microscopy, but fluorescence may be produced by visible light rays of much longer wavelength than ultraviolet light. The fluorescence of eosin solutions in daylight is an example of this, and fluorescent paints are used for road signs and stage scenery to increase the visual impact. Hicks and Matthaei (1955) have drawn attention to the fact that it is possible to induce strong fluorescence with certain fluorochrome dyes with blue light (400–500 nm) in the visible spectrum.

There are two types of fluorescence. *Primary* natural fluorescence (autofluorescence) is the capacity of some substances to fluoresce intrinsically. Examples are vitamin A, riboflavine, porphyrins, and chloroplasts in plants. Tissues may have a general blue fluorescence, and this is more strongly seen in some components such as elastic fibres. Primary fluorescence may cause confusion in the interpretation of the results of staining methods; control sections that have not been stained but have otherwise been treated as the test section must be compared with the test section in fluorescence microscopy. Certain substances such as mercury, iron, and iodine destroy (quench) natural fluorescence, and quenching of some fluorochrome dyes occurs when they are combined with tissue components, making them unsuitable for histological techniques. It is possible to quench unwanted fluorescence in certain histological methods, but it should be remembered that fixatives containing heavy metals such as mercury are unsuitable.

Secondary (or induced) fluorescence is produced after the interaction of substances that are not naturally fluorescent with a fluorochrome dye (acridine orange, auramine, thioflavine-T, etc.). Secondary fluorescence will demonstrate certain tissue components in sections, and the brilliant induced fluorescence of acid-fast bacilli when combined with auramine, or malignant cells with acridine orange, enables them to be seen quickly with low-power magnification and is used as a screening method for their detection. There are several advantages of the secondary fluorescence that is induced in fluorescence microscopy techniques. One is the fact that very small amounts of fluorescent material produce visible fluorescence, and it is possible to demonstrate tissue components that are present in very low concentration with small amounts of a fluorescent dye; these can even be added to living cells without causing toxic damage. The method is very sensitive and gives good contrast; small variations in visible transmitted light are not discernible, but fluorescence can accentuate these differences so that they are easily seen. Resolution and localization may not be as exact as that given by visible light techniques, as the fluorescence is given off in all directions and appears diffused. Like natural fluorescence, induced fluorescence is quenched by impurities such as heavy metals; it is also sensitive to minor changes in pH and buffered fluorochrome dye solutions are necessary for successful results in some techniques.

Apparatus for fluorescence microscopy

A completely dark room is desirable. It is essential to eliminate or reduce background light, and a photographic dark room is suitable. Brilliant fluorescence depends upon maximum contrast and this is greatly reduced if there is much background light in the room, and blinds in a working laboratory are often inadequate. The equipment consists of a light source emitting ultraviolet or blue light, a microscope, and a filter system.

LIGHT SOURCE

For critical work a high-pressure mercury lamp and starter unit are required and these are the most expensive items that it will be necessary to buy for fluorescence microscopy unless a complete fluorescence microscope designed for the purpose is purchased. Ultraviolet lamps need to be warmed up before use and have a limited life. The mercury arc is small and may not be large enough to fill the whole field of view with even light; Köhler illumination [p. 18] can be used to overcome this. Carbon arcs give off a large amount of ultraviolet light and projector lamps and high-intensity microscope lamps may give off enough blue light (400–500 nm) for routine fluorescence microscopy. Halogen lamps are now fitted in several modern microscopes with built-in high-intensity illumination systems, and these give off sufficient blue light for routine histological methods using fluorochrome dyes such as thioflavine-T (for amyloid [p. 225]), acridine orange (for malignant cells [p. 348], mucins [p. 253], and fungi [p. 253]) and auramine-rhodamine (for acid-fast bacilli [p. 396]). A halogen lamp is satisfactory for routine stained sections, for dark-ground·microscopy, polariscopy, and simple fluorescence microscopy. Such a versatile light source saves duplication of equipment and is particularly convenient for diagnostic work as there is no delay caused by warming up the lamp. These lamps have a long life if they are not run at maximum intensity, and it should be remembered that the brightness of the light is greatly increased in a binocular microscope if a monocular tube is used. Fluorescence microscopy with a tungsten–halogen lamp is described by Heimer and Taylor (1972) and practical details for the use of a tungsten–halogen microscope as a fluorescence microscope for routine laboratory use are given by Taylor, Heimer, and Tomlinson (1973).

Incident light fluorescence is now replacing transmitted light in fluorescence microscopes. This depends upon the use of an interference beam splitter (or dichroic mirror) which reflects light of a wavelength less than 500 nm and transmits light of a higher wavelength. Brumberg (1959) put forward the concept of fluorescence microscopy of objects using light from above, and the

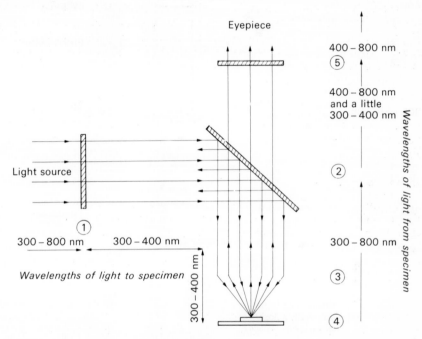

FIG. 2.9. Path of light through an incident light fluorescence microscope. 1. Exciter filter. 2. Interference beam splitter. 3. Objective. 4. Specimen. 5. Barrier filter.

beam splitting mirror is a multilayer interference filter which reflects 90 per cent of the exciting illumination and transmits about 90 per cent of the light from the specimen. The wavelengths of the reflected and transmitted light can be varied by the use of interchangeable dichroic mirrors (Ploem 1967). In theory the need for exciter and barrier filters (see below) are not necessary if the beam splitter reflects only the short-wave excitation component of the light and transmits only the longer-wave fluorescence light from the specimen, but in practice such precision is not realized and filters are needed. An incident light microscope with a suitable light source can be modified for incident light fluorescence (Lea and Ward 1974). The path of light in an incident light fluorescence microscope is shown in FIGURE 2.9.

FILTER SYSTEM

Two filters are needed for fluorescence microscopy. An *exciter filter*, placed between the light source and the specimen, is ultraviolet transmitting but cuts out visible light. Commercial mercury vapour lamps emit much of their ultraviolet light at about 365 nm, and this wavelength is widely used in fluorescence microscopy. For pure ultraviolet illumination the exciter filter should cut out all light above 400 nm, but if blue light is also used the filter can allow light up to 500 nm to pass through. The specimen is now illuminated with ultraviolet light [see Fig. 2.10] and will fluoresce, giving off some visible light.

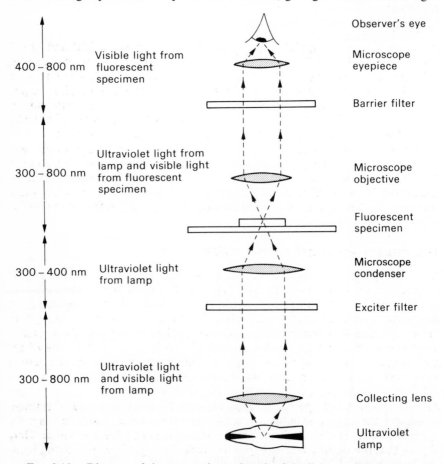

		Observer's eye
400 – 800 nm	Visible light from fluorescent specimen	Microscope eyepiece
		Barrier filter
300 – 800 nm	Ultraviolet light from lamp and visible light from fluorescent specimen	Microscope objective
		Fluorescent specimen
300 – 400 nm	Ultraviolet light from lamp	Microscope condenser
		Exciter filter
300 – 800 nm	Ultraviolet light and visible light from lamp	Collecting lens
		Ultraviolet lamp

Fig. 2.10. Diagram of the type and wavelength of the light passing through a transmission fluorescence microscope using ultraviolet light

In order to protect the eyes from the damaging effects of ultraviolet light, and to reduce non-specific fluorescence so that the fluorescent object is seen as a bright object against a dark background, an eyepiece filter is essential. This is the *barrier filter*, which is ultraviolet absorbing and will only allow visible light rays to pass through the eyepiece; all light below 400 nm (for ultraviolet fluorescence) and 500 nm (for blue light fluorescence) must be absorbed by the barrier filter. Thus the exciter filter and the barrier filter are complementary, and together they should absorb all ultraviolet and visible light; only the fluorescent light rays given off by the specimen between the two filters are seen by the eye. In the presence of a fluorescent specimen no fluorescence should be seen if the two filters are reversed. FIGURE 2.10 shows the filter system with the wavelengths of the light passing through a fluorescence microscope.

A wide range of filters is now available commercially and these are described by Holborow (1970), Pearse (1972), and Nairn (1976). The filters should be complementary and must be appropriate for the wavelength of the light source and the excitation wavelength of the fluorescent compound that is employed.

MICROSCOPE

It was originally thought that glass absorbed all ultraviolet light and quartz optics were used by Köhler (1904). However, it is now recognized that glass only cuts off light rays below 300 nm, and microscopes with standard glass optical systems are satisfactory for fluorescence in the 365 nm region. A polished metallic reflector mirror has been recommended, and is useful for detailed microscopy, but the silvered glass mirror is often adequate. A binocular head absorbs a lot of light and an upright monocular microscope may be employed. High numerical aperture objectives increase light transmission, and the same applies to the condenser, which is left fully open. Some workers use a dark-ground condenser, and, although it will have been appreciated from the consideration of the filter system that a black background is obtained with a standard condenser, a dark-ground condenser is preferable for oil-immersion objectives.

THE POLARIZED LIGHT MICROSCOPE

A ray of light consists of electromagnetic waves vibrating in all directions at right angles to the path of the ray of light itself. In polarized light the waves are caused to vibrate in one plane only. The classical way of doing this is by interposing prisms of calcite (Nicol prisms) in the path of the beam of light. In the microscope two Nicol prisms are used (polarizer and analyser). One is fitted below the substage condenser; the other is installed in the tube of the microscope or in the eyepiece. The analyser must be capable of rotation through 90 degrees. Each prism is a rhombohedron diagonally cut and cemented with Canada balsam. When the diagonals of the sectioned prisms are parallel polarized light passed through both. If the analyser is rotated through 90 degrees the rays transmitted by the lower prism will not pass through the upper; the field is now dark and this position is called *crossed Nicols*. Only objects that are doubly refractile (i.e. intrinsically capable of polarizing light) are illuminated.

Objects fall into two groups in regard to their polarity:

1. Isotropic or singly refractile. These do not change the direction of the beam and are not illuminated when examined with crossed Nicols.
2. Anisotropic (birefringent or doubly refractile). These alter the direction of the vibration of the beam of light when examined with crossed Nicols, and some of this light passes through the analyser, causing the object to be seen brightly against a dark background.

Isotropic substances are common; they include glass, certain crystals, and most animal cells and tissues. Anisotropic objects comprise crystals such as talc, and vegetable fibres like cotton and linen. Cotton fibres from cotton wool or from a laboratory white coat can be used as control material when setting up the microscope for polariscopy. Tissue substances which are doubly refractile include collagen fibres and bone matrix, striated muscle, cholesterol, red blood corpuscles after Zenker fixation (especially if partly lysed or poorly preserved), and certain pigments such as formalin pigment. Plant tissues provide more examples of birefringency than those of animals. The polarizing microscope can be a useful means of identification of tissue components and of exogeneous and endogenous crystals, especially when combined with special staining techniques and with histochemistry.

The discovery and commercial manufacture of polarizing compounds has simplified polariscopy and made it cheaper. Polaroid is a substance composed of very fine, elongated crystals, all orientated in the same direction, enclosed in a cellulose film, and mounted between two glass discs. A pair of these constitute polarizer and analyser. A special microscope is not required, and almost any monocular and most binocular microscopes can be adapted so that the substage and the eyepiece discs can be rotated.

NOTES

1. Source of light. This must be more powerful than for ordinary microscopy, as the light reaching the specimen is reduced by half and the light reaching the eye is further reduced, almost to zero. A high-intensity light source is essential. Coloured filters and diffusing filters should be removed. A completely black background can usually be obtained, but may not be necessary for routine work, and a dark room is seldom required.
2. Glass is normally isotropic, but stressed glass may be birefringent. This applies to slides and coverslips, and also to the lenses of the microscope. If one of the latter is under strain the field cannot be completely darkened. Most polariscopy on histological material is done with the × 10 (16 mm) and × 40 (4 mm) objectives, and each should be tested for extinction. Occasionally slides and coverslips may show birefringency, especially if they have been put under strain by being flamed.
3. The apparatus can be easily tested with a few cotton or linen fibres in an aqueous mount. These should be brilliantly birefringent against a black (or dark) background.

THE PHASE-CONTRAST AND INTERFERENCE MICROSCOPES

If two unstained structures of almost the same refractive index (RI) are examined by ordinary illumination it will be found that they are indistinguishable from each other. Small colourless granules in the cytoplasm of living cells are an example of this. The basis of phase-contrast microscopy is the exaggeration of minute differences in RI by advancing or retarding light waves, thus converting them into differences of amplitude which are seen as variations in brightness. Two rays of light striking the same point of a screen will reinforce or interfere with each other according to the relative positions of their wavelengths; light waves of similar phase reinforce each other to produce a combined light of double the amplitude (or brightness), whilst if one ray of light is retarded by exactly half a wavelength it will interfere or subtract from the other ray to produce no light. Smaller phase differences will produce smaller alterations of amplitude and a picture will be built up of a pattern of different brightnesses.

A method that can reveal cellular structure of living cells due to differences in the refractive indices of the components of the cell is obviously of great value in cytology, and can be applied to haematology and microbiology. Phase-contrast microscopy is of limited value for the examination of fixed and stained material as these processes alter the refractive index of the cellular constituents.

Interference microscopy differs from phase contrast in that it does not depend upon the object producing the interference in the light rays but generates its own interfering rays. These are emitted by a plate of birefringent material which is placed above the condenser, and eventually recombine to form the image. The interference microscope can be used as a phase-contrast microscope for the examination of parts of living cells, but can also be used as an optical balance. An increase in refractive index can be accurately measured, and from this dry mass can be estimated. The principles of interferometry and the use of the interference microscope in histology have been described by Chayen (1967).

The electron microscope

It has already been stated that the wavelength of visible light (400–800 nm) limits the resolving power of the light microscope to 0.2 μm under optimal conditions. In an attempt to find alternative sources of illumination, X-rays with a short wavelength (0.5 nm) were investigated but these could not be focused and were unsuitable for microscopy. In 1923 it was shown that a beam of electrons could be focused by a magnetic or an electric field and the electron microscope became a possibility. When electrons are accelerated through an electrical potential difference their wavelength is inversely proportional to the square root of the voltage. The wavelength of a 50 kV electron beam is $1.23 \text{ nm}/\sqrt{50\,000}$ which equals 0.0055 nm; this is one hundredth of the wavelength of X-rays and one hundred thousandth that of visible light. Magnetic lenses have a small numerical aperture, and using the formula [p. 17] for resolution

$$R = \frac{0.6 \text{ wavelength}}{\text{numerical aperture}} \quad \text{or} \quad \frac{0.6 \times 0.0055 \text{ nm}}{0.01} = 0.33 \text{ nm.}$$

A resolution of 0.5 nm (5 Å) is guaranteed for many electron microscopes and two objects separated by 0.1 nm (1 Å) can be resolved. The depth of field of a microscope lens is inversely proportional to its numerical aperture and the low NA of the electromagnetic lens gives the electron microscope a large depth of field. This can be at least 100 times greater than a light microscope with a high NA objective, giving excellent sharpness of detail in electron micrographs of rough surfaces. Two types of electron microscope are used in histology, the *transmission* electron microscope and the *scanning* electron microscope. The general principles of these instruments and their applications and developments will be described.

THE TRANSMISSION ELECTRON MICROSCOPE (TEM)

The transmission electron microscope (FIG. 2.11) has similarities to the light microscope. Both have condenser lenses to concentrate the incident beam

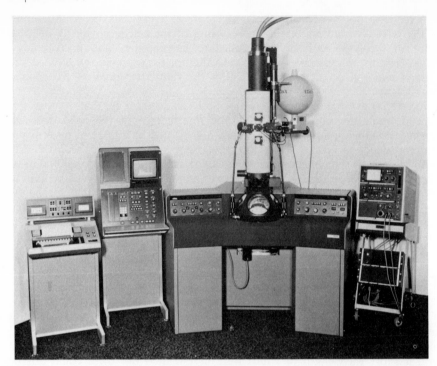

FIG. 2.11.   The transmission electron microscope (Philips type EM 400 with scanning and X-ray analysis attachments).

upon the specimen and in the electron microscope this passes through the specimen to be focused by electromagnetic lenses to form an enlarged image on a fluorescent screen. The transmission electron microscope may have a magnification range of 1500–200 000 and a resolution of better than 0.5 nm, compared with the light microscope's magnification of 30–1500 and resolution of 200 nm, but it is more complex, expensive, and difficult to maintain. For the electrons to reach their acceleration speed without deflection by air molecules, a high vacuum is needed and as the specimen is in this vacuum living objects cannot be examined. A very stable power supply is required and the microscope has its own power unit for the accelerating voltage and for the lenses. By changing the amount of current to a lens the magnification is altered, making it a continuously variable focal-length lens similar to a zoom lens system. Finally a water cooling system is needed. A diagrammatic cross-section of a transmission electron microscope is shown in FIGURE 2.12.

The final image is seen on the fluorescent screen through an observation window, and very fine focus can be obtained with a low power binocular. The photographic chamber is below the fluorescent screen which can be tilted out of the electron beam so that the image falls on the photographic plate or film. In contrast to the light microscope, the high resolution of the electron microscope enables further detail to be seen by enlargement of electron photomicrographs.

An introduction to electron microscopy techniques has been given by Nunn (1970). More detailed information on the principles and use of the electron

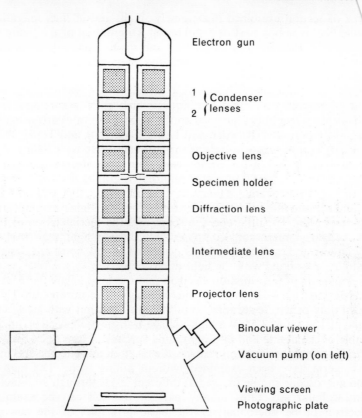

Electron gun

1 ⎰ Condenser
2 ⎱ lenses

Objective lens

Specimen holder

Diffraction lens

Intermediate lens

Projector lens

Binocular viewer

Vacuum pump (on left)

Viewing screen
Photographic plate

FIG. 2.12. Diagram of the main components of a transmission electron microscope.

microscope has been described by Agar, Alderson, and Chescoe (1974), on fixation and tissue processing by Glauert (1974), on ultramicrotomy by Reid (1974) and on staining methods by Lewis and Knight (1977).

It will be readily appreciated that many of the difficulties that are encountered in light microscopy are greatly increased in electron microscopy. In addition to the usual histological artifacts the vacuum dehydrates all tissues and these are examined with all fluids removed. The usual fixatives for electron microscopy are glutaraldehyde or osmium tetroxide and after dehydration the tiny tissue specimens are embedded in methacrylate or in an epoxy resin such as Epon 812. Very thin sections, often about 60 nm thick, are cut on the ultramicrotome [p. 82] which is fitted with an advance mechanism of between 5 and 200 nm in order to cut sections within that range of thickness. Thicker sections (500–2000 nm) may also be cut at the same time for histological staining for light microscopy [p. 105], in order to compare with the electron micrographs. Colours have no real place in electron microscopy, but contrast in increased by staining with heavy-metal salts such as lead citrate, lead hydroxide, and/or uranyl acetate. More specialized techniques such as histochemistry and autoradiography can also be used. The very thin sections are picked up on wire grids or meshes covered by a very thin film of plastic.

The area of section examined is extremely small, and at high magnifications the whole field is only a part of a single cell. Orientation of the tissue and the identification of the cells may be difficult and require many separate examinations of different tissue blocks. Satisfactory preparations require immediate examination and photography.

Normal and pathological histological structure has been studied with the electron microscope and rapid techniques which allow a specimen to be examined within a few hours have led to the greater use of electron microscopy for diagnostic purposes (Rowden and Lewis 1974; Carr and Toner 1977). For histological purposes low-power electron photomicrographs (× 2000 to × 10 000) are often more valuable for comparison with light microscopy than high-power (× 50 000 to × 100 000) electron photomicrographs, and an electron microscope with an effective range of magnification between × 1000 and × 25 000 may be as valuable as a more expensive instrument with a higher magnification and greater resolution. The differences in scope and the specialization of the techniques of electron microscopy compared with those of light microscopy will be readily understood, and the methods described in this book are designed for the histologist working with the light microscope.

Developments in transmission electron microscopy include the *high-voltage microscopes* and the *electron probe microanalyser*. The normal 100 kV instrument can only penetrate sections 50 to 100 nm thick but with an accelerating potential of 500 kV to 3 MeV a high-voltage transmission electron microscope is capable of examining and photographing specimens 1μm thick. In addition, the great speed of the electrons reduces the beam damage to the specimen and living bacteria have been examined without killing them. The high-voltage electron microscope can be focused at different levels through an intact cell, so that intracellular structures in any part of the cell can be examined. In the electron probe microanalyser the basic principles of the conventional transmission electron microscope are used to analyse very small amounts of elements in the specimen (Chandler 1977). Electrons are focused into a narrow beam about 100 nm in diameter, and when this hits the specimen X-rays are given off. Elements produce characteristic wavelengths whereby they can be identified, and an X-ray spectrometer [FIG. 2.11] can not only pick these up, but can also count them and give a quantitative analysis of the elements that are present in exact situations within tissues.

THE SCANNING ELECTRON MICROSCOPE (SEM)

Electron microscopy can be employed in the same way as light microscopy to examine specimens by transmitted or by incident light. An incident electron beam is used in the reflection scanning electron microscope and the reflected electrons produce a topographical view of the *surface contours* of the specimen [FIG. 2.13]. Like the conventional transmission electron microscope, the scanning electron microscope image is not limited by the wavelength of light and its depth of field is 200 times greater than the corresponding light microscope. The transmission light microscope will produce a two-dimensional image of a thin section that has a higher resolution and a far greater magnification than the light microscope, and the scanning electron microscope also has a higher resolution and a greater depth of field than the dissecting light microscope. High magnifications are always available with the scanning electron microscope though these may not always be used in biological specimens. Details of

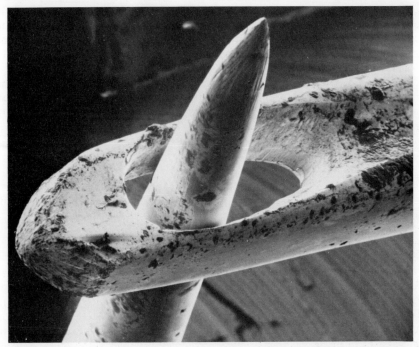

FIG. 2.13. Scanning electron micrograph of the point of a needle through the eye of a needle. (×150.) Reproduced by permission of Eastman Kodak Company.

the principles and techniques of scanning electron microscopy have been described by Hayat (1973).

The three dimensional image of the scanning electron microscope is instantly appreciated because it mimics our own natural visual perception, giving us a subjective experience as well as an image for scientific analysis. A grasp of surface topography does not come so readily from the conventional two dimensions of the histological section and the scanning electron micrograph is an invaluable aid for teaching and a regular feature of popular television documentaries. The scanning and transmission electron microscopes have several features in common. In both there is a column maintained at high vacuum and a source of electrons in the form of an electron gun. The electron beam is brought to a focus by the condenser lens system, forming a bright illuminating spot on the specimen. In the scanning electron microscope the focused spot is not static, as in the transmission electron microscope, but moves to and fro across the specimen surface in a rectangular grid pattern, or *raster*, controlled by the action of a set of scanning coils, activated by an electron scan generator [FIG. 2.14]. As the focus spot passes across the specimen surface line by line, secondary electrons are generated by the impact of beam with the specimen surface and the intensity of this signal of secondary emission fluctuates according to the topographical detail of the specimen surface. This reflected signal is picked up by an electron collector close to the specimen and is amplified and displayed on a cathode-ray tube. Thus the electron beam in the microscope probes the details of the specimen surface by screening it line by line and the secondary emission produced by this probe is

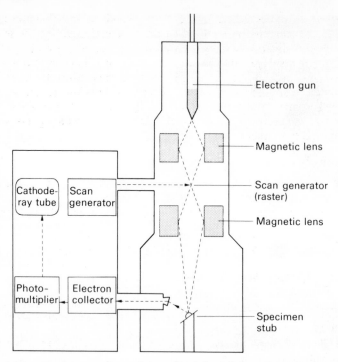

FIG. 2.14. Component parts of the reflecting scanning electron microscope.

simultaneously displayed line by line on a television screen, building up a faithful replica of the surface detail of the specimen. A permanent micrograph can be obtained by photographing the image on the screen with a conventional camera. The image produced by the scanning electron microscope is thus built up, not through an image-forming electron lens, but through a system of television electronics. The magnification is not controlled by altering the strength of an image-forming lens but by varying the ratio between the width of the displayed screen, which is constant, and the width of the raster, or grid pattern on the specimen surface, which is controlled by the microscope scanning coils. Thus if the width of the area scanned is 0.1 mm and the width of the displayed screen is 10 cm, the magnification is 1000. Resolution is not controlled by the quality of the image-forming lens but by the spot size which may be about 10 nm (100 Å) or less, and spot sizes down to 0.5 nm (5 Å) are now possible, although ultra-high vacuum conditions are essential.

Tissues for scanning electron microscopy require fixation and dehydration and are finally coated with a thin layer of metal such as gold, carbon, or palladium, in a vacuum evaporator. Smears of cells can also be examined. Tissues that have been prepared for examination with the scanning electron microscope can be reprocessed by resin embedding and studied as sections by the conventional transmission electron microscope. In this way a full range of comparisons can be made in almost any specimen by the techniques of light microscopy, surface scanning, and transmission electron microscopy.

Scanning electron microscopy has been mainly used for the examination of the surface of cells or tissues but it is important to realize that a scanning microscope can also be used to examine tissue sections. The section is placed in the same position, but the electron collector is relocated below the specimen so that it now collects the transmitted electron signal instead of the secondary reflected emission signal. The specimen is scanned as before on a grid system and the image is displayed on the screen line by line, building up a scanning transmission picture of the section which corresponds to the familiar transmission electron microscope image. It is likely that the advanced research electron microscope of the future will be a *scanning transmission electron microscope* rather than an upgraded version of the existing conventional transmission electron microscope.

REFERENCES

AGAR, A. W., ALDERSON, R. H., and CHESCOE, D. (1974). *Principles and practice of electron microscope operation*. North-Holland, Amsterdam.

BARER, R. (1968). *Lecture notes on the use of the microscope*, 3rd edn. Blackwell, Oxford.

BARON, D. N. (1973). *J. clin. Path.* **26**, 729.

——, BROUGHTON, P. M. G., COHEN, M., LANSLEY, T. S., LEWIS, S. M., and SHINTON, N. K. (1974). *J. clin. Path.* **27**, 590.

BRUMBERG, E. M. (1959). *Biophysics* **4**, 97.

CARR, I. and TONER, P. G. (1977). *J. clin. Path.* **30**, 13.

CASARTELLI, J. D. (1965). *Microscopy for students*. McGraw-Hill, London.

CHANDLER, J. A. (1977). *X-ray microanalysis in the electron microscope*. North-Holland, Amsterdam.

CHAYEN, J. (1967). In *In vivo techniques in histology* (ed. G. H. Bourne). Williams and Wilkins, Baltimore.

—— and DENBY, E. F. (1968). *Biophysical technique*. Methuen, London.

CULLING, C. F. A. (1974). *Modern microscopy*. Butterworths, London.

GLAUERT, A. M. (1974). *Fixation, dehydration and embedding of biological specimens*. North-Holland, Amsterdam.

HAITINGER, M. (1938. *Fluoreszenzmikroscopie*. Leipzig.

HAMPERL, H. (1934). *Virchows Arch. path. Anat.* **292**, 1.

HAYAT, M. A. (1973). *Principles and techniques of scanning electron microscopy: biological applications*. Van Nostrand-Reinhold, New York.

HEIMER, G. V. and TAYLOR, C. E. D. (1972). *J. clin. Path.* **25**, 88.

HICKS, J. D. and MATTHAEI, E. (1955). *J. Path. Bact.* **70**, 1.

HOLBOROW, E. J. (1970). *Standardization in immunofluorescence*. Blackwell, Oxford.

JOURNAL OF CLINICAL PATHOLOGY (1970). *Editorial* **23**, 818.

KÖHLER, A. (1904). *Z. wiss. Mikr.* **21**, 219.

LEA, D. J. and WARD, D. J. (1974). *J. clin. Path.* **27**, 253.

LEWIS, P. R. and KNIGHT, D. P. (1977). *Staining methods for sectioned material*. North-Holland, Amsterdam.

NAIRN, R. C. (1976). *Fluorescent protein tracing*, 4th edn. Churchill–Livingstone, Edinburgh.

NUNN, R. E. (1970). *Electron microscopy: microtomy, staining and specialised techniques*. Butterworths, London.

PEARSE, A. G. E. (1972). *Histochemistry, theoretical and applied*, 3rd edn., Vol. 2. Churchill Livingstone, Edinburgh.

PLOEM, J. (1967). *Z. wiss. Mikr.* **68**, 129.

REID, N. (1974). *Ultramicrotomy*. North-Holland, Amsterdam.

ROWDEN, G. and LEWIS, M. G. (1974). *J. clin. Path.* **27**, 505.

TAYLOR, C. E. D., HEIMER, G. V., and TOMLINSON, A. H. (1973). *A guide to the choice of optical equipment and reagents for immunofluorescence techniques*, Broadsheet 76. Association of Clinical Pathologists, London.

3 | Preparation and fixation of tissues

Preparation

The reception, recording, handling, and dissection of specimens are important preliminaries to the application of histological techniques and are best carried out in rooms designed for these purposes. The equipment of these rooms should include sinks of suitable dimensions and some form of under-sink waste-disposal unit. Extractor fans are essential and these should be appropriately sited to carry formalin and other fumes away from workers in this area.

A dissecting table made of teak or similar hard wood with a working surface of 45 × 35 cm is very useful and may be stood in a sink beneath a mixertap for hot and cold water. Wood or cork are commonly used as actual cutting surfaces but these are not ideal and fragments from either may become adherent to tissues and appear in the final section. Rubber pads of various dimensions are used in the food industry and are very suitable for the dissection of histological specimens [p. 503]. The surface of these pads is smooth and does not chip; it is hard but not unduly damaging to knife edges and the material is very durable. A pad of suitable size laid on a table such as that described above makes a very satisfactory dissection bench.

Instruments for the dissection of specimens should include thin-bladed knives 20–30 cm in length, scissors (including bowel and coronary types), probes, scalpels and razor blades, a stainless-steel rule, forceps in various sizes, and sponges (the synthetic fibre variety are adequate). Scales for the weighing of specimens should be adjacent to the dissection area as should an X-ray viewing box, small bandsaw and a stereoscopic dissecting microscope. A first-aid box and an eye-wash bottle should also be at hand in the dissection area together with disinfectant for the preliminary treatment of infected material and instruments.

Scrupulous cleanliness is necessary during the dissection of tissues to avoid the transfer of fragments from one specimen to another. It should be the rule for the cutting board and instruments to be thoroughly cleaned before proceeding from one specimen to the next and for small biopsies and solid specimens such as lymph nodes to be dealt with before bulky or fatty tissues such as large ovarian cysts and mastectomy specimens. Attention to these points should reduce the incidence of translocation of tissue and contamination artifacts. Another form of contamination that can occur at dissection is the deposition of starch granules (glove powder) in tissues. These are seen in haematoxylin and eosin stained sections as pale pink-staining rounded bodies 10–15 μm in diameter, often having a central speck of black material. They are strongly periodic acid–Schiff positive and display Maltese cross birefringence in polarized light [FIG. 3.1]. The powdering and donning of gloves away from the dissection area and the washing of gloved hands before dissection will reduce the incidence of this artifact.

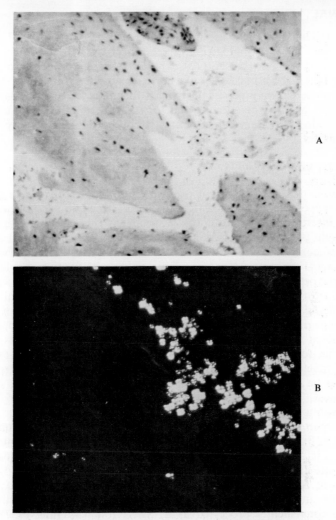

Fig. 3.1. (A) Starch glove powder in cleft of synovial tissue. Haematoxylin and eosin (HE). × 100. (B) As A, polarized light.

Most histopathology departments provide containers of fixative to operating theatres, clinics, and wards, and specimens received in the laboratory may be quite adequately fixed, partially fixed, or almost completely unfixed according to the size of the specimen and time elapsed since removal.

It is very difficult to cut satisfactory blocks from unfixed tissue without their becoming distorted and requiring further trimming after fixation. With bulky, unfixed material such as some hysterectomy or mastectomy specimens it is better to make appropriate incisions to allow penetration of the fixative and then to immerse the specimen in a large volume of fixative for some hours before dissection and selection of blocks.

Special preparatory procedures for certain organs and tissues are given below.

ADRENAL

Autolytic changes take place in the adrenal soon after death. The old term 'suprarenal capsule' originated from the fact that at autopsy the gland was often found to be a thin cortical capsule containing semi-liquid debris. For cellular detail the adrenals should be fixed within an hour or two of death, though some enzymes persist unchanged for much longer periods. Blood vessels ramify around the adrenal, and for some histopathological changes (e.g. arteritis; also secondary carcinoma) it is not advisable to remove all the surrounding fat.

ALIMENTARY CANAL

Fixation is the most important problem. Autolytic changes take place in the gastric mucosa almost immediately the blood circulation ceases, and are rapid in the intestine. In human autopsy specimens the gastro-intestinal mucosal epithelium is almost always desquamated, leaving only the ghost architecture of the mucosal structure or the bases of the glands. For the preservation of the oesophageal or gastric mucosa a large volume of fixative should be passed down the oesophagus into the stomach immediately after death; formal-saline is satisfactory. It is more difficult to fix the whole of the intestinal canal without opening the body and perfusing the intestine, but fixative can be injected into the peritoneal cavity. This usually gives patchy fixation, dependent upon the amount of fixative injected and the number of loops of intestine that are accessible to the fixing fluid. Human surgical specimens and experimental animal material should be distended or perfused with the fixative. The stomach can be opened and pinned out upon a cork board with the mucosa uppermost. The intestine can also be pinned out in this way or opened and sewn with a continuous thread on to a frame on which it is fixed and stored vertically in the fixative. Packing viscera with cotton wool or surgical gauze soaked in fixative is not advisable as these flatten the mucosal folds and may leave an imprint of the mesh of the gauze on the specimen. Blocks for histology are taken after fixation, and if the specimen is required for photography or for museum preservation longitudinal blocks should be selected from the cut edge. Long (up to 15 cm) strips of gastric or intestinal mucosa can be conveniently processed as a 'Swiss roll' (Magnus 1937); these are wound into coils taking care to roll all specimens in the same direction so that the proximal end is identifiable (especially important in the stomach). Use fine pins to hold them together and process, embed and cut as a roll. The villi of the small intestine are particularly delicate and must be handled gently to avoid damage.

AMPUTATED LIMBS

Skin is practically waterproof and an effective barrier to most fixatives, and amputated limbs should be promptly dissected and parts required for examination placed in fixative. If early dissection is not possible, the limb may be immersed in a tank of 10 per cent formal-saline or wrapped in a waterproof covering and kept in a refrigerator at 4 °C. The usually well-intentioned practice of temporarily storing such specimens in a 'deep freeze' at −20 to −40 °C will inevitably result in the production of gross artifacts in the tissues through the formation of large ice crystals [FIG. 3.2].

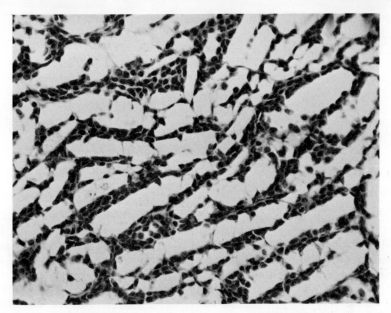

FIG. 3.2. Disruption of tissue by ice crystals. HE. × 250.

EYE

The eye is a composite organ made up of layers of different consistencies that tend to separate during fixation and sectioning. Fixation in 10 per cent formal-saline should be carried out immediately after removal to prevent drying of the cornea and to reduce autolytic changes in the retina. After 48 hours fixation the eye is opened in the horizontal plane with a razor blade. The eye should not be opened or frozen before fixation and fixative should not be injected into the chamber (Ashton 1967).

Cellulose nitrate [p. 69] is the recommended embedding medium for eyes. Paraffin-wax sections can be of reasonable quality though showing more re-tinal separation and distortion than in celloidin or low viscosity nitrocellulose (LVN) sections. Celloidin–paraffin-wax double embedding [p. 71] is a useful compromise procedure for eyes.

LUNG

Special measures are necessary to preserve the size and shape of lungs and the epithelium of the bronchial tree. This is commonly done by the intratracheal injection of fixative before opening the thorax by passing a tube or cannula through the mouth or exposed trachea.

Gravity, or a syringe with a pressure of less than 100 mm of mercury is used to inject 10 per cent neutral formal-saline until resistance is encountered.

Alternatively, if the trachea and lungs are carefully removed from the body, satisfactory results can be obtained if fixative is injected into the trachea until the lungs are life-size. Heppleston (1953) found that there was no danger of rupturing alveolar walls if the removed lungs were distended with neutral formal-saline until they were of ante-mortem size.

In both techniques, the trachea is tied off after injection and the lungs immersed in fixative for 48 hours. If the pleura is damaged during removal, and this may be impossible to avoid if there are extensive pleural adhesions, these techniques will be partly or completely unsuccessful.

Another method of fixing whole lungs after their removal from the body is by inflation with formalin vapour and many devices have been described for this purpose. One of these, where the lung is caused to 'breathe' the vapour above heated formalin has been described by Wright *et al.* (1974), and excellent preservation of pulmonary architecture may be obtained by the use of this apparatus [see p. 437].

For a review of fixation methods used in the study of pulmonary emphysema see Silverton (1964, 1965).

LYMPHATIC TISSUE

Lymph nodes and spleen are difficult to fix satisfactorily and if the capsule is intact may be affected by autolysis in the deeper parts no matter how promptly fixed. Spleen commonly shows a narrow rim of subcapsular fixation beyond which the fixative has not penetrated. Small lymph nodes (less than 5 mm thick) may be fixed intact, but larger lymph nodes, lymphatic tumours, and spleen should be sliced to allow penetration of the fixative. This should be done with a very sharp, long flat knife, not a scalpel, with the slices being carefully laid in a suitable container of fixative, avoiding bending of the slices. In the case of soft tumours and spleen it may be necessary to commence fixation with the tissue intact and to bisect it later the same day after a few hours fixation, by which time the tissue has begun to harden and will retain its shape.

PITUITARY

Median sagittal sections of the pituitary give good pictures of the anterior lobe, stalk, and posterior lobe. For studies of the anterior lobe horizontal sections are more informative as cytology is not uniform throughout the lobe; it is advisable to include in the section the lateral wings since these contain most of the acidophil cells.

For the preparation of bone marrow see page 205, and muscle, page 191.

Selection of blocks

The thickness of tissue blocks selected for sectioning is related to the processing procedure employed and for routine paraffin blocks using automatic tissue processors and 16–24 hour schedules this should not exceed 3–4 mm. The surface area of the block is generally governed by the size of the cassettes used in the processing machine, the size of the microtome chuck, and the standard 76×26 mm glass slide. Several blocks of small surface area may be processed and embedded together as one composite block, but only if they are of similar consistency. It is unwise, for example, to embed together a piece of dense bone and a piece of soft cellular tissue, no matter how small the former.

It is common practice to indicate the opposite side to the intended cutting surface of a block by marking with carbon ink. The ink may not remain confined to this one surface though, but flow through vessels and spaces to the cutting surface and appear in sections as a dark pigment. When marking blocks in this way it is advisable to mop the surface with a paper towel before application of the ink and to use the minimum quantity of ink possible. Indication of the cutting surface of solid tissues may also be given by making a shallow V-shaped cut with a razor blade on the opposite side.

Fixation

The increasing use of histochemical and immunohistological techniques which require sections of unfixed tissue means that a proportion of specimens entering the laboratory will not be in fixative and will require immediate attention. Ideally the laboratory should be given warning when these investigations are envisaged and co-operation between clinician, operating theatre, and laboratory is essential.

It is convenient if the fresh specimen is large enough to be divided into portions as required for enzyme histochemistry, immunohistology, or electron microscopy as well as into blocks for paraffin-wax embedding for routine purposes. When the specimen is too small to be divided a decision as to the best fixative or treatment has to be taken in the light of available information and clinical diagnosis and this problem has been discussed by Dawson (1973). In practice, the great majority of specimens sent to histopathology laboratories are still prepared as paraffin-wax sections following standard fixation procedures. Special preliminary treatments and fixation methods will be given in the appropriate chapters.

AIM OF FIXATION

The aim of fixation is the preservation of cells and tissue constituents in a condition identical to that existing during life and to do this in a way that will allow the preparation of thin, stained sections. Clearly, since material for histological examination is removed from the body, this aim can never be completely fulfilled; methods now available for the preparation of tissue sections are essentially a compromise between the limitations of the technique and the desire to preserve and demonstrate every tissue component in a completely life-like manner.

In practice, the purpose of fixation is: (1) to prevent or arrest autolysis and bacterial decomposition and putrefaction; (2) to so coagulate the tissue as to prevent loss of easily diffusible substances; (3) to fortify the tissue against the deleterious effects of the various stages in the preparation of sections, e.g. dehydration, clearing, and wax impregnation (tissue processing); and (4) to leave the tissues in a condition which facilitates differential staining with dyes and other reagents.

AUTOLYSIS

Autolysis means 'self-destruction' and is caused, after the death of cells, by the action of intracellular enzymes whose normal behaviour is altered, causing the breakdown of protein and eventual liquefaction of cells. Autolytic changes are independent of any bacterial action, are retarded by cold, greatly accelerated by keeping at 37 °C and almost inhibited by heating the tissue to 57 °C (Cruickshank 1911).

Autolysis affects the highly specialized cells of complex organs such as brain and kidney more rapidly and seriously than, for example, elastic fibres and collagen. On microscopical examination, the cell nuclei of autolysed tissue may show condensation (pyknosis), fragmentation (karyorrhexis), or lysis and eventual disappearance (karyolysis). The cytoplasm may become swollen and granular and the whole tissue subsequently converted to a granular, homogeneous mass with loss or great alteration of the usual staining reaction. Autolysis causes desquamation of epithelium, the cells splitting away from their basement membranes [FIG. 3.3]. In addition, substances of diagnostic significance, e.g. glycogen, may diminish in quantity or diffuse out of the tissue in the absence of prompt and suitable fixation.

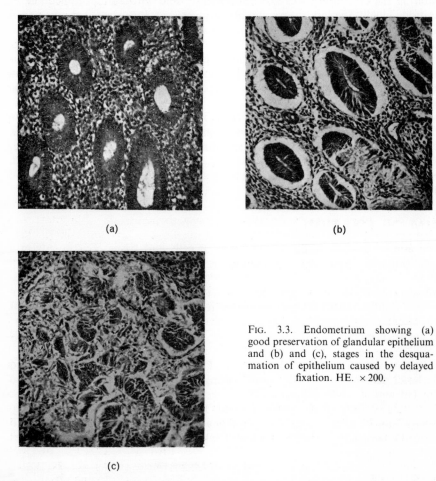

(a)

(b)

FIG. 3.3. Endometrium showing (a) good preservation of glandular epithelium and (b) and (c), stages in the desquamation of epithelium caused by delayed fixation. HE. × 200.

(c)

BACTERIAL DECOMPOSITION

Bacterial decomposition causes changes in the tissues that are very similar to those of autolysis and is brought about by the presence of multiplying bacteria in the diseased tissues at time of death (as in septicaemia) or by bacteria normally present in the body in life such as the non-pathogenic organisms inhabiting the intestines.

EFFECTS OF FIXATION

One of the most important effects of fixation is the coagulation of tissue proteins and constituents, thus minimizing their loss or diffusion during tissue-processing. But in addition, the fixative should safeguard the tissue against the damaging effects of tissue-processing and the combined effects of coagulation and hardening of tissues by the fixative helps to withstand the disrupting qualities of hypertonic and hypotonic solutions. If fresh, unfixed tissue were to be washed in running water, severe and irreparable damage and lysis of cells would result, but if the tissue were to be first fixed in Zenker's fluid, then subsequent immersion in water is both necessary and harmless. It is worth-while to keep in mind that the coagulation of tissue structures, although necessary, in itself constitutes a major artifact, since the living cell is fluid or semi-fluid in nature.

Fixation aids optical differentiation of cells and tissue constituents by altering their refractive indices in varying degrees. This is of value, since the refractive index of some elements of the cell is so close to that of surrounding structures as to render them invisible in the living state when examined with an ordinary microscope.

Fixation has a marked effect on the subsequent staining of tissues, generally facilitating the action of dyes. Some fixing agents have a specially beneficial effect on the application of certain dyes, while others are inhibitory to their action. For example, carmalum [p. 428], a nuclear stain, stains less strongly after formalin than after mercuric chloride fixation. Sometimes, a fixing agent may act as a direct link between a particular tissue component and the stain, and when this is the case, the fixative is said to act as a mordant [p. 117]. An example of this is the treatment of tissue with potassium dichromate as a preliminary stage in the demonstration of myelin with haematoxylin [p. 363].

COMMON FIXING AGENTS

In considering the following list of substances, from which a large variety of fixatives may be prepared, it is necessary to bear in mind that no single substance or known combination of substances has the ability to preserve and allow the demonstration of every tissue component. Because of this, some fixatives have only special and limited application and most are mixtures of two or more reagents designed to make use of the special features of each. Sometimes such mixtures are chemically incompatible (oxidizing and reducing agents) though none the less effective.

Much attention has been given to the osmotic pressure of tissue cells in relation to fixative solutions but in general, and irrespective of osmotic pressures, precipitant fixatives such as mercuric chloride shrink cells while non-precipitant fixatives such as formalin do not. However, in practice, salts such as sodium chloride or sodium sulphate are often recommended for inclusion in fixatives, particularly with those of relatively low powers of penetration.

FORMALDEHYDE (H.CHO)

Formaldehyde is a gas which is soluble in water to a maximum extent of 40 per cent by weight and is sold as such under the name of formaldehye (40 per cent), or *formalin*. It contains 10–14 per cent added methanol as a stabilizer. The concentrated solution is nearly always acid and certainly becomes acid on storage through the production of formic acid. Neutralization of the solution is desirable and is often effected by allowing the (diluted) solution to stand over magnesium or calcium carbonate, or, more satisfactorily, by the addition of buffer salts [p. 49].

Concentrated acid formalin should not be treated with magnesium or calcium carbonate as the consequent release of carbon dioxide has been shown to be responsible for a serious explosion in the laboratory (*Gazette of the Institute of Medical Laboratory Technology* 1965).

The concentrated solution of formalin sometimes becomes turbid on keeping through the production of para-formaldehyde; this decreases the strength of the solution, but does not prevent its use if removed by filtration. Formalin should be colourless. Yellow solutions are likely to be contaminated with ferric iron derived from metal containers used for bulk storage and transit. Sections of tissue fixed in iron-containing formalin will give a positive Prussian blue reaction and samples of formalin suspected of being contaminated may be tested by the same method [p. 264].

Formalin is unsuitable for use as a concentrated solution and is diluted with tap water, physiological saline or buffer-salt solutions, commonly in the proportions of 10 parts formalin to 90 parts diluent. These solutions contain 4 per cent formaldehyde, but in order to avoid the confusion of the past and in keeping with the now established practice, all references in this book to concentrations of formalin solutions will mean dilution of the concentrated solution in the proportion indicated. For example, 10 per cent formal-saline will mean 10 parts formalin to 90 parts physiological saline (4 per cent formaldehyde in physiological saline).

Formalin gives off an unpleasant vapour that causes irritation to the eyes and respiratory epithelium, particularly distressing to some individuals. For this reason, some system of forced ventilation should be a feature of any room used for the dissection of formalin-fixed tissues and all containers should be provided with well-fitting, corrosion-resisting lids. In addition, rubber gloves or an efficent barrier cream should be worn when handling formalin-fixed material, for while some workers appear to be immune from its effects, others will suffer an unpleasant 'formalin dermatitis' after immersion of hands in this solution.

Formalin has a beneficial hardening effect on tissues but causes little, if any, shrinkage. Shrinkage is produced when tissues are subjected to paraffin embedding [p. 58].

Formalin fixes proteins by forming additive compounds without precipitation. It is virtually without effect on carbohydrates although preserving glycogen when this is held by fixed protein. Lipids are generally well preserved (though not fixed) by formalin but Baker (1958) points out that some types of lipid may be lost if treatment with formalin is prolonged. Formalin favours the staining of acidic structures (nuclei) with basic dyes and diminishes the effect of acid dyes on basic structures (cytoplasm).

GLUTARALDEHYDE ($(CH_2)_3CHO.CHO$)

Since its introduction as a fixative for use in ultrastructural studies and cytochemistry by Sabatini, Bensch, and Barrnett (1963) glutaraldehyde has become a standard fixative for electron microscopy. It is generally employed as a primary fixative followed by secondary fixation in osmium tetroxide [p. 47].

Chambers, Bowling, and Grimley (1968) suggested that glutaraldehyde might be used as a fixative in routine histopathology but it does not appear to have any significant advantages over formalin for this purpose and like formalin, has the disadvantage of somewhat poor penetration into larger pieces of tissue. In addition, sections fixed in glutaraldehyde tend to give a generalized positive reaction with the periodic acid–Schiff method and the reagent is much more costly than formalin.

MERCURIC CHLORIDE (CORROSIVE SUBLIMATE: HgCl₂)

Mercuric chloride is a white crystalline substance, soluble in water at room temperature to about 7 per cent and in alcohol to 33 per cent. It is extremely poisonous and is corrosive to metals. Containers for mercuric chloride should never have metal lids and metal instruments for handling tissues should be protected by dipping in hot paraffin wax. As a precaution, containers should bear a printed 'Corrosive-Poison' label and Lendrum (1943) suggested that mercuric chloride and mercuric chloride–formalin mixtures be coloured with very dilute acid fuchsin to draw attention to the nature of the substance and to prevent confusion with colourless, plain formalin solutions.

Mercuric chloride is a powerful protein precipitant and penetrates and hardens tissue fairly quickly. It shrinks but does not distort tissue and fixes both nucleus and cytoplasm well, favouring the staining of both components, especially the latter, with acid dyes. It is used in conjunction with other fixing agents, particularly formalin, potassium dichromate, and acetic acid but almost invariably produces a brown to black granular deposit, distributed uniformly throughout the tissue. This so-called 'mercury pigment' is soluble in alcoholic iodine and does not affect subsequent staining after removal. It is removed either during dehydration of tissue blocks by the addition of 0.25–0.5 per cent iodine to 70–80 per cent alcohol or by the treatment of sections before staining as follows:

1. Remove wax from paraffin sections by treatment with xylene.
2. Wash in absolute alcohol.
3. Treat with 0.5 per cent iodine in 70 per cent alcohol, 3–5 minutes.
4. Rinse briefly in tap water.
5. Treat with 2.5 per cent sodium thiosulphate ('hypo') until bleached, 30 seconds–two minutes.
6. Wash in running tap water, five minutes.
7. Proceed with staining.

It is often recommended that both the above methods should be used, on the grounds that the first treatment may not be completely effective and that this artifact pigment in the tissue may cause difficulty in section-cutting as well as damage to the microtome knife. In practice, however, with paraffin wax and cellulose nitrate embedded material, there is little or no evidence to support this theory and the treatment of sections only with iodine is sufficient. The pigment is removed by being converted by iodine into mercuric iodide which is soluble in alcohol. The brown coloration of the section is removed by the bleaching action of sodium thiosulphate, or by treatment with alcohol. Lugol's iodine and 5 per cent sodium thiosulphate are often used for the removal of 'mercury pigment' but while effective for this purpose, it has been shown (Baker 1958) that some mercuric chloride–protein complexes are soluble in potassium iodide (an ingredient of Lugol's iodine) and solutions containing this should not be used on mercuric chloride fixed tissues. The 5 per cent sodium thiosulphate, while not generally harmful, is at least wasteful, for a solution of half that concentration is just as effective in bleaching the iodine colour from the section.

In spite of its excellent properties as a fixative, mercuric chloride is rapidly falling into disuse because of the dangers of pollution of the environment by the disposal of waste fixative solutions. Porter (1972) discusses this problem and suggests either the discontinuance of the use of this reagent or its conversion to the safer mercuric sulphide before disposal. It would appear that there is no non-toxic substance with the same fixation properties as mercuric chloride.

POTASSIUM DICHROMATE ($K_2Cr_2O_7$)

Potassium dichromate is an orange crystalline substance used as a 2.5–5 per cent solution in water. A saturated aqueous solution contains about 12 per cent at room temperature.

The pH of potassium dichromate solutions profoundly affects the type of fixation (Baker 1958) and on the less acid side of the critical pH range (3.4–3.8) the cytoplasm is homogeneously fixed and mitochondria, but not nucleoprotein are preserved. On the more acid side, potassium dichromate acts like chromic acid, both nucleus and cytoplasm being precipitated with destruction of mitochondria.

Potassium dichromate is used in conjunction with other substances to make several important fixatives and is also commonly used alone, on formalin fixed tissues and sections, for its mordanting effects in subsequent staining procedures.

Tissues fixed in potassium dichromate should be washed in running water before proceeding to alcohol to prevent the formation of an insoluble precipitate. Prolonged (days to weeks) exposure of tissue to this reagent causes most tissue to become brittle with consequent difficulty in sectioning, particularly if embedded in paraffin wax.

CHROMIC ACID (H_2CrO_4)

Chromic acid is prepared by dissolving the dark red crystals of the anhydride (CrO_3) in distilled water. A 2 per cent solution is convenient for the preparation of fixatives. It precipitates proteins and fixes carbohydrates, and, being a powerful oxidizing agent, should not generally be mixed with alcohol or formalin.

After fixation in chromic acid, tissues should be washed in running water before treatment with alcohol. Failure to do so may result in the formation of an insoluble precipitate in the tissues.

PICRIC ACID ($C_6H_2(NO_2)_3OH$)

Picric acid is a bright yellow crystalline substance usually supplied damped with water because of its explosive properties if heated or detonated. It is sparingly soluble in water (about 1 per cent at room temperature) but more so in alcohol (nearly 5 per cent) and benzene (10 per cent).

Picric acid precipitates nucleoproteins and causes much shrinkage but little hardening. It enhances results with cytoplasmic stains and is a useful constituent of fixatives for glycogen. After fixation in picric acid, tissues are transferred directly to alcohol. No valid evidence exists to support the claim that picric acid–protein complexes are soluble in water, but since the excess picric acid is more soluble in alcohol there is little point in using water for the purpose (Baker 1958).

OSMIUM TETROXIDE (OsO₄)

Osmium tetroxide, commonly referred to as 'osmic acid', is supplied as pale yellow crystals in sealed tubes of 0.5 or 1 gramme and is used as a 0.5 to 1 per cent solution in water. It is a costly chemical and the vapour from both crystals and solution is irritant and dangerous. Exposure of the eyes to the vapour should be avoided by the use of close-fitting goggles, and containers of the solution should be kept tightly stoppered. Preparation of the solution should be carried out as follows:

Remove the label and all traces of gum from the tube with water, but not hot water. Dry the tube with a clean cloth, score with a glass file and break in the middle, dropping the two halves with contents into a dark-glass bottle containing the appropriate amount of pure distilled water. The crystals may take some time to dissolve but heat should not be used to hasten solution. The bottle should have a glass stopper and be stored in a cool place.

Osmium tetroxide is easily reduced to the grey or black lower oxide by light, warmth or organic matter and once-used solutions should not be returned to the stock bottle. An effective way of preventing reduction is by the addition of one drop of saturated aqueous mercuric chloride to each 10 cm³ of solution.

Like formalin, osmium tetroxide forms additive compounds with protein. Most lipids including myelin are blackened by the reduction of the osmium tetroxide to the lower oxide. Its penetration is poor and fixation is liable to be uneven. Minute objects, smears of cells, and thin sections may be fixed by the vapour, without immersion in the fluid. While little used for general histological and histopathological work, mainly because of its cost and restrictions in use, osmium tetroxide has recently enjoyed a revival as a fixative (particularly in buffered solutions) for material to be examined with the electron microscope.

ACETIC ACID (CH₃COOH)

Pure acetic acid is called 'glacial' because it solidifies at about 17 °C if water free. It is a colourless liquid of pungent odour and is used in many fixing mixtures, often to complement the action of other ingredients. It swells collagen fibres, precipitates nucleoprotein and may have a solvent action on some cytoplasmic granules [p. 172].

ETHYL ALCOHOL (ETHANOL: C₂H₅OH)

Ethyl alcohol is a colourless, inflammable liquid, boiling at 78 °C and when anhydrous, mixes with xylene without cloudiness. It is a powerful dehydrating agent and causes shrinkage and hardening. It coagulates protein but not nucleoprotein, precipitates glycogen and dissolves many, but by no means all, lipids.

STOCK SOLUTIONS

It will be found convenient to keep stock solutions of the above common fixing agents for the preparation of mixtures. Suggested concentrations are given below.

Formalin: 40 per cent formaldehyde.
Glutaraldehyde: 25 per cent solution.
Mercuric chloride: saturated aqueous solution.
Potassium dichromate: 5 per cent aqueous solution.
Chromic acid: 2 per cent aqueous solution.
Picric acid: saturated aqueous solution.
Osmium tetroxide: 2 per cent aqueous solution.
Acetic acid: glacial acetic acid.
Ethyl alcohol: absolute ethyl alcohol [but see p. 58].

The foregoing reagents are those most commonly used, alone or as mixtures, for the fixation of tissues. Many other substances have been and a few still are used for special purposes. Acetone is used sometimes in histochemical investigations [p. 300], trichloracetic acid is an ingredient of the 'Susa' fixative [p. 51] as well as being a decalcifying agent [p. 203], zinc chloride has been suggested as a cheaper substitute for mercuric chloride in Zenker's fluid (Russell 1941), 7 per cent sulphosalicylic acid has been recommended by Gurjar (1955) and 2–10 per cent glyoxal has been proposed as an odourless substitute for formalin (Wicks and Suntzeff 1943).

COMMON FIXATIVES AND THEIR USES

Fixatives may be divided into two main groups according to their uses.

1. *Micro-anatomical fixatives*, which aim at accurately preserving the relations of tissue layers and large aggregates of cells to one another. Most of the routine work of normal and pathological histology is done with such fixatives.
2. *Cytological fixatives*, which are intended to preserve constituent elements of the cells themselves. Penetrative power, the ability to work with large masses of tissue, lack of hindrance to cutting or staining—essentials from the micro-anatomical point of view—are sacrificed towards this end. Thus with Flemming's fluid [p. 53] the outermost and inner portions of the block may be badly fixed while an intermediate zone shows admirable fixation.

As in any system of arbitrary classification, there is a certain amount of overlap in grouping fixatives in this way but this is unimportant if it is realized that certain micro-anatomical fixatives may be used cytologically and vice versa.

When considering the practical application of fixatives it is necessary to be clear as to the actual purpose of the investigation, the size, type and freshness of the tissue, the sectioning process and the staining technique it is desired to employ. No fixative is ideal for all tissues and all techniques and in histopathology particularly, where fresh tissue is not always available, fixation is often a matter of compromise between expediency and the best method. Furthermore, a fixative may give different results with tissues from different species, and in diagnostic work the need for a certain fixative may not be apparent until later.

In some cases it is possible to modify the effect of a given fixative by subsequent treatment of tissue blocks or sections with other fixing agents [see p. 54].

The volume of the fixative used should be at least 10 times that of the tissue, and the suggested duration of fixation quoted below applies to blocks 3–4 mm in thickness, not to whole specimens. An obvious prerequisite is that containers for specimens should be of sufficient size. They should also be straight-sided, without shoulders or neck. This will allow the subsequent removal of specimens placed in too small a jar with minimal further damage.

10 PER CENT FORMAL-SALINE

Formalin   100 cm^3
Sodium chloride   8.5 g
Tap water   900 cm^3

A layer of 'marble chips' (calcium carbonate) in the container assists in the neutralization of the formic acid produced by the formalin. A more certain means of avoiding the acidity of formalin is by the use of buffer salts.

BUFFERED 10 PER CENT FORMALIN (pH 7.0)

Formalin   100 cm^3
Tap water   900 cm^3
Acid sodium phosphate, monohydrate ($NaH_2PO_4.H_2O$)   4 g
Anhydrous disodium phosphate (Na_2HPO_4)   6.5 g

The use of 2 per cent calcium acetate to neutralize formalin solutions has been recommended by many authors but Luna and Gross (1965) found that this could cause an artifact simulating areas of calcification in soft tissues. Experiments carried out by one of us confirmed Luna and Gross's results [FIG. 3.4].

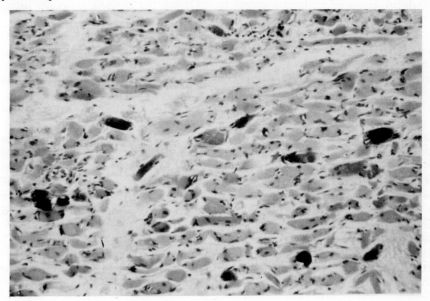

FIG. 3.4.   Basiphilic staining of muscle, simulating calcification. HE. × 100.

Ten per cent formal-saline is the most widely used histological fixative. It imparts a firm consistency to tissue without excessive hardening and is tolerant in terms of duration of fixation. It is usually possible to restore, or partially restore, the natural colour of tissues after formalin fixation; this is of special value in the preparation of museum specimens. It is undoubtedly the best fixative for the preservation of red blood cells, particularly when used as a neutral buffered solution.

Prolonged immersion in formalin (months to years) while not affecting the sectioning qualities of the tissue, may result in some loss of ability to stain with basic stains although results with certain silver impregnation techniques may be improved. Thin blocks of tissue are adequately fixed in 10 per cent formal-saline in 24–48 hours, but it is necessary to be aware that the *optimum duration* of fixation is *7–10 days*. A comparison of sections from blocks fixed for 1 day and 7 days respectively will readily confirm this fact. It should also be noted that better tissue preservation will be seen in frozen and celloidin sections than in paraffin sections of formalin fixed tissues. This is because a fundamental weakness of formalin fixation is its inability to produce a coagulum of tissue structures sufficiently robust to withstand the rigours of paraffin embedding without damage (Mallory 1938; Lillie 1965).

After formalin fixation, tissues containing altered blood may show an artifact pigment (formalin pigment). This is a brown, granular material, extracellular and birefringent. It is more commonly found in, but not confined to, tissues obtained post mortem and is progressive in its deposition, often being absent after a few hours' immersion in formalin but widely and heavily deposited in the tissues after several days. The pigment is caused by the action of acid formalin on blood and is avoided by the use of neutral buffered solutions. It may be removed from sections by treatment (in a jar) with a saturated alcoholic solution of picric acid for 20 minutes or longer (Barrett 1944). The general appearance and properties of the pigment are similar to those of malaria pigment [p. 261] but the latter is generally intracellular.

Ten per cent formal-saline is a micro-anatomical fixative. It allows a wide variety of staining methods to be applied and gives good results with haematoxylin. Occasionally, and for no clear reason, a peculiar artifact is seen in sections fixed in formal-saline and stained with haematoxylin and eosin. This takes the form of complete or partial failure of nuclei to stain with haematoxylin which instead, take up eosin, with consequent loss of distinction of nuclear margins. The artifact, which is most noticeable in lymphoid and epithelial tissue, is extremely patchy in its distribution and curiously, occurs most in tissues which were promptly and apparently properly fixed. It is rarely, if ever, seen in post-mortem tissues, although autolysed. Bayley (1949) has described this artifact as 'pink disease' and advocates the use of 2 per cent acetic acid in 10 per cent formalin as means of avoiding its occurrence or, when present, the treatment of de-waxed sections with 1 per cent hydrochloric acid in absolute alcohol for 1 hour immediately before staining with haematoxylin, but see page 132.

No special after-treatment is required after formalin fixation and tissues may be transferred firectly to 70 per cent alcohol before embedding or may be sectioned by the freezing method.

MERCURIC CHLORIDE–FORMALIN (FORMAL-SUBLIMATE)

Saturated aqueous mercuric chloride   900 cm³
Formalin   100 cm³

An excellent micro-anatomical fixative. It shrinks tissue, but without the distortion (in paraffin sections) of formal-saline. A superior preservation of the cytoplasm is obtained as well as brilliant staining with acid dyes and enhanced metachromasia. It is generally less suitable than formal-saline with silver impregnation techniques for nerves fibres and cells, though perfectly satisfactory reticulin fibre impregnation may be obtained.

Blocks are fixed for 12–24 hours, but contrary to the widely held view, much longer treatment does not result in a consistency of tissue that makes sectioning difficult, and staining may be improved (Lendrum *et al.* 1962).

Formal-sublimate is especially useful as a secondary fixative after primary treatment with formal-saline [p. 54] and its major disadvantages are its severe corrosive action on metals and its increasing cost.

Tissues should be transferred to 70–90 per cent alcohol after fixation and the 'mercury pigment' removed from sections as described on page 45.

SUSA FIXATIVE (HEIDENHAIN 1916)

Mercuric chloride   45 g
Sodium chloride   5 g
Trichloracetic acid   20 g
Acetic acid   40 cm³
Formalin   200 cm³
Distilled water   800 cm³

Much praised as a general fixative, especially for biopsy material, Susa (a contraction of the German words 'sublimat' and 'saure') is a good micro-anatomical fixative but gives an indifferent to poor preservation of red blood cells, particularly with post-mortem material. For reasons not clear, elastic fibres stain poorly with Weigert's (1898) elastic fibre stain after Susa. The number of ingredients is a disadvantage and the mixture has little advantage over the simpler formal-sublimate described above.

Blocks are fixed for 3–24 hours and are transferred directly to 95 per cent alcohol. Immersion in more aqueous solutions would result in swelling of collagen fibres. Quite often, 'mercury pigment' is not apparent after fixation in Susa but it is nevertheless a wise precaution to treat sections with iodine and 'hypo' as described above.

ZENKER'S FLUID (ZENKER 1894)

Mercuric chloride   5 g
Potassium dichromate   2.5 g
Sodium sulphate   1 g
Distilled water   100 cm³
Acetic acid   5 cm³ *added immediately before use*

The stock solution, without acetic acid, keeps well.

Zenker is an efficient micro-anatomical fixative and is used as much for its beneficial effect on staining, particularly with cytoplasmic and fibre stains, as for the quality of tissue preservation. It is more useful with fresh material than with post-mortem tissues and red blood cells are not well preserved.

Blocks are fixed for 3–18 hours and are then washed in running water to remove excess dichromate. 'Mercury pigment' is removed from sections as described on page 45.

HELLY'S FLUID OR ZENKER-FORMAL (HELLY 1903)

The acetic acid is omitted from Zenker's fluid and in its place, 5 cm³ of formalin is added immediately before use.

Helly's fluid is an excellent fixative in spite of the theoretical objection to the mixing of an oxidizing agent (potassium dichromate) and a reducing agent (formalin). Helly is particularly suitable for use with bone marrow, spleen, lymph glands, pituitary, and pancreas where an accurate preservation of cytoplasm as well as nuclei is desired.

Blocks should be fixed for 6–24 hours, washed in running water, and 'mercury pigment' removed as with Zenker's fluid. Helly may be used as a micro-anatomical or cytological (cytoplasmic) fixative and like formal-sublimate, may be usefully applied as a secondary fixative after 10 per cent formal-saline [p. 54].

BOUIN'S FLUID (BOUIN 1897)

Saturated aqueous picric acid	75 cm³
Formalin	25 cm³
Acetic acid	5 cm³

The mixture keeps well.

Bouin causes partial or complete lysis of red blood cells and collagen fibres may be swollen. It does not cause excessive hardening and gives brilliant staining with cytoplasmic stains. Glycogen is well preserved, particularly with an alcoholic variant of the above mixture but the kidney is badly preserved and some cytoplasmic granules may be dissolved. Bouin's fluid is a micro-anatomical fixative or a cytological (nuclear) fixative when used for the demonstration of chromosomes.

Blocks are fixed for 6–24 hours and transferred to 70 per cent alcohol. The yellow staining of tissues is sometimes an advantage with very small specimens but should be removed from sections by treatment with alcohol followed by 2.5 per cent sodium thiosulphate before using basic aniline dyes, otherwise a precipitate will be formed.

CARNOY'S FLUID (CARNOY 1887)

Absolute alcohol	60 cm³
Chloroform	30 cm³
Acetic acid	10 cm³

Carnoy is a rapidly penetrating and acting fixative. Its main use is for the quick fixation (and partial dehydration) of tissues for urgent diagnosis. It has been used for the study of chromosomes which are well preserved, but it causes lysis of red blood cells and much shrinkage. Glycogen is preserved but some cytoplasmic granules may be dissolved. Blocks not thicker than 3 mm should be fixed for 30–90 minutes and then transferred to 95 per cent or absolute alcohol. A micro-anatomical or cytological (nuclear) fixative.

SANFELICE'S FLUID (SANFELICE 1918)

Solution A
Formalin   128 cm³
Acetic acid   16 cm³
Solution B
1 per cent chromic acid   100 cm³

Mix 9 cm³ of solution A with 16 cm³ of solution B immediately before use.

This is an excellent fixative for mitotic figures and chromosomes generally. Small pieces, not thicker than 3 mm, should be fixed for 12–24 hours followed by washing in running water. A cytological (nuclear) fixative.

FLEMMING'S FLUID (FLEMMING 1884)

1 per cent chromic acid   15 cm³
2 per cent osmium tetroxide   4 cm³
Acetic acid   1 cm³ or less

Appropriate amounts of the ingredients should be mixed before use. Penetration may be uneven and cause excessive blackening of superficial layers with incomplete fixation and subsequently poor staining of the innermost cells. Page (1970) successfully used Flemming's fluid as a secondary fixative for the demonstration of myelin following primary formalin fixation. She found that used in this way, fixation was more even and overfixation rare.

Small pieces, 2–3 mm thick, should be fixed for 12–48 hours followed by washing in running water. With full acetic acid content this is a nuclear fixative; lipids are blackened by the osmium tetroxide. Alum haematoxylin nuclear stains do not take readily after this fixative and safranin is often used instead.

LEWITSKY–BAKER MODIFICATION OF FLEMMING'S FLUID (BAKER 1956)

Prepare Flemming's fluid but without acetic acid and with 0.75 per cent sodium chloride in water as solvent in place of distilled water. The same restrictions as to size of specimen apply but this mixture gives superior preservation of cytoplasmic constituents to the traditional 'Flemming minus acetic acid'. After 12–24 hours' fixation, transfer tissue to running water. A cytological (cytoplasmic) fixative, this and other chrome–osmium mixtures, give the best results with tissues of invertebrates and lower vertebrates. Helly's fluid is recommended for mammalian tissues.

ORTH'S FLUID (ORTH 1896)

Formalin   10 cm³
Muller's fluid (potassium dichro-
mate, 2.5 g, sodium sulphate, 1 g,
distilled water, 100 cm³)   100 cm³

Orth's fluid does not keep and should be freshly prepared. The mixing of formalin and Muller's fluid results in a mixture especially useful for its mordanting effect on cytoplasmic constitutents such as mitochondria, and in the chromaffin reaction [p. 280].

Blocks should be fixed for 24–48 hours before washing in running water or further chromation in 2.5 per cent potassium dichromate in distilled water. Prolonged treatment with potassium dichromate, though sometimes desirable, almost inevitably results in a tendency to brittleness and difficulty in sectioning paraffin wax embedded material, particularly with soft, solid tissues such as spleen and brain.

TREATMENT OF TISSUES AFTER FIXATION

10 per cent formal-saline	
Buffered 10 per cent formalin	70 per cent alcohol
Bouin	

Formal-sublimate	80–90 per cent alcohol
Susa	95 per cent alcohol
Carnoy	95 per cent or absolute alcohol

Zenker	
Helly	
Sanfelice	
Flemming	Wash in running water 12–24 hours
Lewitsky–Baker	
Orth	

SECONDARY FIXATION

It has been shown (Wallington 1955) that tissues fixed initially in 10 per cent formal-saline are still susceptible to the effects of other and more vigorous precipitant fixatives and such treatment has been called 'secondary fixation'. Mercuric chloride-formalin and Helly's fluid are particularly useful as secondary fixatives and tissues so treated will show general improvement in preservation and staining. The method originally described recommended the incorporation of a secondary fixative as the first stage in automatic processing schedules [p. 67], thus permitting the initial fixation of specimens to be conveniently effected with 10 per cent formal-saline but with treatment of selected blocks with a more desirable fixative, the remainder of the specimen being stored in formalin.

POST-CHROMING AND POST-MORDANTING

Post-chroming and post-mordanting are methods designed to facilitate the preservation and subsequent staining of a particular tissue component and entail the treatment of tissue blocks (after fixation) or sections, with a chrome salt. The method is often made use of as an aid to demonstration of mitochondria and myelin [pp. 180 and 363].

POST-FIXATION

Leach (1945) showed that some tissue proteins are protected or 'masked' by fatty substances which prevent the complete penetration of most fixatives and that this protein is subsequently lost, with impairment of tissue preservation, after the removal of the protecting fatty substance during clearing with fat solvents.

Leach recommended that tissues should be fixed, dehydrated, and cleared in a fat solvent and then 'post-fixed' in absolute alcohol before re-clearing and wax impregnation.

PRESERVATION AND STORAGE OF TISSUES

Tissues fixed in formalin that are not immediately required for sectioning are often allowed to remain in the unchanged fixative, sometimes for several years. This results in a progressive impairment of the staining qualities although the use of buffered neutral solutions will retard this effect. Another common practice is to use 70 per cent alcohol as a preserving fluid after fixation and washing out of the fixative. Lendrum (1941) recommends a 30 per cent solution of glycerol after fixation in formal-sublimate and washing in water, while Lillie (1965) has used 10–20 per cent diethylene glycol for preserving tissues. Owen and Steedman (1956) recommend the use of 1 per cent Phenoxetol (a derivative of ethyleneglycol monophenolether) [p. 501] which is bactericidal and fungicidal. This substance has amply fulfilled its early promise as an excellent preservative for fixed tissue (Steedman 1963) but Owen and Steedman stress that thorough fixation is a prerequisite for the use of these (and all) preserving fluids which are intended to maintain the effects of fixation without alteration.

Better than any preserving fluid is (where possible) implementation of a decision to prepare a properly mounted museum specimen or an embedded tissue block.

REFERENCES

ASHTON, N. (1967). Association of Clinical Pathologists Broadsheet No. 59.
BAKER, J. R. (1956). *Quart. J. micr. Sci.* **97**, 621.
—— (1958). *Principles of biological microtechnique.* Methuen, London.
BARRETT, A. M. (1944). *J. Path. Bact.* **56**, 135.
BAYLEY, J. H. (1949). *J. Path. Bact.* **61**, 448.
BOUIN, P. (1897). *Arch. Anat. micr. Morph. exp.* **1**, 225.
CARNOY, J. B. (1887). *Cellule* **3, 276.**
CHAMBERS, R. W., BOWLING, M. C., and GRIMLEY, P. M. (1968). *Arch. Path.* **85**, 18.
CRUICKSHANK, J. (1911). *J. Path. Bact.* **16**, 167.
DAWSON, I. M. P. (1973). Fixation: what should the pathologist do? In *Fixation in histochemistry* (ed. P. J. Stoward) p. 193. Chapman-Hall, London.
FLEMMING, W. (1884). *Z. wiss. Mikr.* **1**, 349.
GAZETTE OF THE INSTITUTE OF MEDICAL LABORATORY TECHNOLOGY (1965). *Annotation* **9**, 171.
GURJAR, N. V. (1955). *Br. med. J.* **i**, 230.
HEIDENHAIN, M. (1916). *Z. wiss. Mikr.* **33**, 232.
HELLY, K. (1903). *Z. wiss. Mikr.* **20**, 413.
HEPPLESTON, A. G. (1953). *J. Path. Bact.* **66**, 235.
LEACH, E. H. (1945). *J. Path. Bact.* **57**, 149.
LENDRUM, A. C. (1941). *J. Path. Bact.* **52**, 132.
—— (1943). *Br. med. J.* **ii**, 644.
—— FRASER, D. S., SLIDDERS, W., and HENDERSON, R. (1962) *J. clin. Path.* **15**, 401.
LILLIE, R. D. (1965). *Histopathologic technic and practical histochemistry*, 3rd edn. McGraw-Hill, New York.
LUNA, L. G. and GROSS, M. A. (1965). *Am. J. med. Technol.* **31**, 412.
MAGNUS, H. A. (1937). *J. Path. Bact.* **44**, 389.
MALLORY, F. B. (1938). *Pathological technique.* W. B. Saunders, Philadelphia.
ORTH, J. (1896). *Berl. klin. Wschr.* **33**, 273.

OWEN, G. and STEEDMAN, H. F. (1956). *Quart. J. micr. Sci.* **97**, 319.

PAGE, K. M. (1970). *J. med. Lab. Technol.* **27**, 1.

PORTER, D. D. (1972). *Arch. Path.* **94**, 279.

RUSSELL, W. O. (1941). *J. tech. Meth.* **21**, 47.

SABATINI, D. D., BENSCH, K., and BARRNETT, R. J. (1963). *J. cell. Biol.* **17**, 19.

SANFELICE, F. (1918). *Ann. Inst. Pasteur* **32**, 363.

SILVERTON, R. E. (1964). *J. med. Lab. Technol.* **21**, 187.

—— (1965). *Thorax* **20**, 289.

STEEDMAN, H. F. (1963). Personal communication.

WALLINGTON, E. A. (1955). *J. med. Lab. Technol.* **13**, 53.

WEIGERT, C. (1898). *Zbl. allg. Path. path. Anat.* **9**, 289.

WICKS, L. F. and SUNTZEFF, V. (1943) *Science* **98**, 204.

WRIGHT, B. M., SLAVIN, G., KREEL, L., CALLAN, K., and SANDIN, B. (1974). *Thorax* **29**, 189.

ZENKER, K. (1894). *Münch. med. Wschr.* **41**, 532.

4 | Tissue processing

The examination of tissues with the microscope usually requires a slice of the tissue thin enough to transmit light and the preparation of such thin slices is called section-cutting, or microtomy. In most cases, the tissue must undergo preparatory treatment before being sectioned, entailing impregnation of the specimen with an embedding medium to provide support and a suitable consistency for microtomy. This preparatory treatment is known as tissue-processing.

Just as there is no perfect fixative for tissues, so is there no perfect embedding medium and a variety of methods and materials are available for this purpose, each having special advantages and limitations. They may be grouped as follows:

1. *The paraffin wax method* involves the dehydration of tissues and their impregnation with molten paraffin wax which is subsequently allowed to solidify by cooling. This is the most commonly used embedding medium in both normal and pathological histology. Cutting qualities are good, the blocks are durable and their storage presents no special problem.
2. *Ester wax* (Steedman 1960) has a lower melting point than the paraffin wax usually used for embedding but is harder when solid. It is therefore especially suitable for cutting thin (2–3 µm) sections with minimal shrinkage of tissues.
3. *Water soluble waxes* (polyethylene glycol waxes) may be used as embedding media, tissues being transferred directly from aqueous fixatives to the wax for infiltration, thus avoiding the need for dehydration and clearing. Shrinkage of tissue is reduced in this way but the cutting and manipulation of sections is more difficult than with paraffin wax and blocks must be kept in a dry atmosphere.
4. *Cellulose nitrate (celloidin and low viscosity nitrocellulose (LVN))* embedding methods entail the dehydration and impregnation of tissues with solutions of cellulose nitrate in a suitable solvent, commonly a mixture of alcohol and ether. The solvent is subsequently allowed to evaporate to produce a block of the required consistency. No heat is used and the method is particularly suitable for large pieces of bone and brain and where the resilience of the medium helps to avoid the separation of layers of tissue of differing consistency, as with the eye.
5. *Double-embedding* is a combination of the paraffin and cellulose nitrate methods designed to use the virtues of each.
6. *Synthetic resins* are used particularly for the preparation of sections for the electron microscope, for 0.5–2 µm sections for examination with the light microscope and for embedding specimens of undecalcified bone for microtomy, sawing, or grinding.
7. *Freeze drying*, and 8, *freeze substitution* methods of preparation of tissues are used mainly in histochemical investigations.

9. *Gelatine* and other aqueous media are used mainly to support tissue to be cut on the freezing microtome and in the Gough and Wentworth method [p. 482].

GENERAL PROCEDURE

1. Precise identification of the specimen should be ensured at all stages by the use of suitable labelling. This may be effected by a typewritten, pencilled, or carbon-inked slip of paper or thin card which is carried through with each specimen within the container.
2. Small fragments of tissue, e.g. endometrial curettings, or friable material should be wrapped in a square of bandage or thin paper or placed in specially made metal containers to avoid loss of fragments or 'contamination' of other specimens.
3. Glass-stoppered, wide-mouth jars are preferable to narrow-neck corked tubes for manual tissue processing and the volume of reagent used should be at least 20–50 times that of the specimen.
4. The size of specimens to be processed will vary considerably from one millimetre or less in diameter to several centimetres and it is essential that consideration be given to the thickness of the block when determining the duration of the various stages of processing. In practice, with automatic tissue processing machines, a schedule is adopted where the duration of the various stages is adequate for the largest pieces of tissue but without damaging effects on the smallest specimens.

PARAFFIN WAX EMBEDDING

DEHYDRATION

Paraffin wax will not penetrate tissues in the presence of water so dehydration is an essential preliminary in the process. This is effected by immersion of the tissue in ethyl alcohol and it is usual to begin with a dilution of the alcohol in water, e.g. 70 per cent alcohol, to prevent the distortion that would accompany the direct transference of tissue from an aqueous medium such as 10 per cent formalin, to absolute alcohol. On the other hand, dehydration, clearing and wax impregnation will inevitably cause shrinkage and hardening of tissues no matter what technique is used or what fixative has preceded processing. Shrinkage may be kept to a minimum by careful choice of processing schedules but there is little doubt that more paraffin embedded tissues cause difficulty in cutting through insufficient time in alcohol, clearing agent and wax than is the case where tissues are allowed to remain for a longer time in these reagents. It is unfortunate that it is the already hard material, such as dense fibrous tissue and bone, that is often given too short a period in these processes in the mistaken belief that cutting will be easier. Imperfect impregnation is the inevitable result of such treatment and while, given a sharp knife, hardness does not in itself prevent successful section cutting, inadequately impregnated tissue certainly does.

In practice, dehydration is carried out either in stoppered glass jars or in tissue processing machines. Industrial Absolute Alcohol 74 OP (99.24 per cent, SG 0.7974) is commonly used in preference to the more costly Dehydrated Alcohol, BP, the use of which is also subject to the surveillance of Customs and Excise authorities. Unless otherwise indicated, future references to absolute alcohol will be to the industrial product.

A commonly used range of dehydrating solutions is 70 per cent, 90 per cent, and two or three changes of absolute alcohol. Sometimes, with particularly soft and delicate tissues such as embryos, a first stage of 50 per cent alcohol is recommended but the point of entry to the dehydration schedule is closely related to the fixative used. For example, after Carnoy's fluid and other alcoholic fixatives the usual and correct progression is directly to 90–95 per cent or even absolute alcohol. Susa fixed material is transferred to 90 per cent alcohol because lower grades of alcohol would cause swelling of fibrous tissue. Where tissues have been washed in water after fixation, as with potassium dichromate fixatives, it is usual to transfer to 70 per cent alcohol.

Various reagents have been recommended for use as dehydrating agents instead of, or in conjunction with, ethyl alcohol (ethanol). Some of these are acetone, pyridine, dioxane (diethylene dioxide), butyl alcohol (butan-1-ol), isopropyl alcohol (propan-2-ol), and Cellosolve (2-ethoxyethanol).

The time required for dehydration will vary from a few minutes to many hours and a selection of processing schedules for different tissues and conditions is given on page 66.

The frequency with which alcohol is renewed will of course largely depend on the use given to it, and sometimes a 10 mm layer of anhydrous copper sulphate is placed in the last jar of absolute alcohol as an indicator of water. If using the cheap industrial alcohol, however, the regular and frequent replacement of the last jar of absolute alcohol in the sequence should ensure thorough dehydration at all times. (If, for example, four jars of absolute alcohol are in use, then number one should be discarded, number two should become number one, number three becomes number two, number four becomes number three and number four will contain the fresh alcohol.)

When transferring tissues from one container to another they should be handled with care, brought to rest on blotting paper and the operation carried out over a flat clean surface and not over sink or floor.

CLEARING

Alcohol is scarcely miscible with paraffin wax and so after dehydration it is necessary to treat tissue blocks with a reagent that mixes with both substances and which may in turn be eliminated in the process of wax impregnation. This step has come to be known as clearing because most but not all the reagents used for this purpose raise the refractive index of tissue rendering it more or less transparent. This is incidental to the main purpose of replacement of the alcohol by a wax solvent.

As with fixatives and embedding media, there are a number of clearing agents available, each with their advocates, each with advantages and disadvantages. The following are commonly used and will meet all but the most special requirements.

NB—Clearing agents are volatile and mostly toxic and inflammable. They should be kept in containers with well-fitting lids and exposure to their vapour avoided.

Xylene (SG 0.863, b.p. about 140 °C) is widely used in histological technique for removing wax from sections prior to staining as well as a clearing agent for tissues and sections. It is rapid in its action, renders tissue transparent and is readily eliminated in the paraffin oven. Blocks up to 3 mm thick may be cleared in as little as 15–30 minutes but any prolonged exposure may make solid, soft tissues such as brain and spleen rather brittle. Xylene is highly inflammable.

Toluene (SG 0.866, b.p. 110 °C) is very similar in its properties to xylene. It may be recommended as a general purpose clearing agent.

Benzene (SG 0.879, b.p. 80 °C) was formerly popular as a clearing agent but because of its toxic vapour is now rarely used.

Chloroform (SG 1.489, b.p. 61 °C) is more expensive than the foregoing (approximately four times more costly than benzene). Its high specific gravity makes it heavy and inconvenient to handle in bulk but it is non-inflammable. Chloroform is considerably slower in its action than xylene or toluene, both in replacement of alcohol and in being eliminated from blocks in the wax oven, but it has little hardening effect and because of this is widely used in histopathology especially with brain and bone. Tissues float at the surface of chloroform and are not made so translucent as with toluene and xylene.

Cedar wood oil (SG 0.927, b.p. 168–237 °C). This is the thin fluid and not the thicker variety used for oil immersion objectives in microscopy. It is expensive but has certain advantages as a clearing agent, for while slow, it has a very gentle action and little if any hardening of tissue is caused even after prolonged immersion. In addition, complete dehydration is not a prerequisite with this clearing agent as is the case with the above and it is probably the only example where the tissue block may smell of, and contain, residual clearing agent after embedding in wax, without detriment to the cutting qualities. Cedar wood oil makes tissue transparent and takes a long time to be eliminated in the wax oven. Because of this, it is common practice to soak tissues in xylene or toluene for about 30 minutes after clearing in cedar wood oil in order to displace the latter and speed up the process of wax impregnation.

Cedar wood oil sometimes partially solidifies, through the formation of needle-like crystals. This is thought to be due to contamination with acetic acid and other impurities, and Popham (1950) recommended the addition of 0.5 cm^3 xylene to each 40 cm^3 cedar wood oil to redissolve, or prevent the formation of the mass.

WAX IMPREGNATION

The function of wax impregnation is to remove clearing agent (wax solvent) from the tissues and for them to be completely permeated by the paraffin wax which is subsequently allowed to harden to produce a block from which sections may be cut.

Ideally, the consistency of any solidified embedding medium should be exactly the same as the particular specimen which it encloses. Unfortunately, this state of affairs is rarely achieved because of the infinitely wide variation in consistency of tissues and the impracticability of using a large variety of embedding media.

The hardness of paraffin wax when set is indicated by its melting point. Thus, wax with a melting point of 45–50 °C is soft, while waxes which melt at 55–60 °C are of correspondingly harder consistency. Choice of wax will depend on the average temperature in the working area, the nature of the material to be embedded, and the thickness of section required. It would be very difficult, for example, to cut thin (3–5 μm) sections from 45 °C melting point wax in a hot climate. In Great Britain, for a wide variety of tissues, wax with a melting point of 56–8 °C is most commonly used for general-purpose paraffin embedding.

Paraffin wax is obtained in the process of oil refining and is sold by laboratory suppliers in a range of melting-points and in tablets, pellets, or granules. Best quality histological wax is filtered in the course of preparation but it is nevertheless advisable to re-filter before use.

Several substances have been recommended as additives to paraffin wax to improve the consistency and cutting characteristics of the block. For a comprehensive account of the properties of paraffin wax and additives see Steedman (1960) and Lamb (1973). Mixtures that are available commercially include paraffin wax–microcrystalline (cosmetic) wax mixtures as well as several examples of 'plastic waxes' which are mixtures of paraffin wax and synthetic rubber. These latter are more expensive than plain paraffin wax but make section cutting somewhat easier, sections ribboning well with rather less tendency to wrinkle than plain wax.

Specimens may be impregnated with molten wax in glass jars, in the special saucepan-like containers that are a feature of some wax ovens, or in the wax baths of tissue processing machines. To avoid an accumulation of tissue debris and the possibility of a fragment of tissue from one batch of embedding becoming part of a subsequent batch, these containers should be regularly emptied and cleaned and the wax filtered if to be used again.

Stock wax for embedding may be kept in jugs in an oven maintained at 2–3 °C above the melting point of the wax or in one of the specially made wax dispensers. These are electrically heated containers holding several litres of molten paraffin wax and incorporating a filter and a tap to deliver wax into the embedding mould. They are especially convenient when using the Peelaway or Tissue-Tek systems [p. 63].

The duration and number of changes of wax necessary for impregnation will vary with the size and consistency of the specimen but as the temperature of the wax oven will cause shrinkage and hardening of tissue, the time in the oven should be kept to a minimum *consistent with thorough impregnation*. It has already been pointed out [p. 58] that generally more difficulty is met in section cutting through inadequate processing than through tissues having been longer than is strictly necessary in dehydration, clearing, and wax infiltration stages. Moreover, residual clearing agents in an embedded tissue block will render the production of good sections impossible, but keeping tissues for a longer time in wax is not necessarily harmful. Lendrum (1951) described a processing schedule designed to give especially good sections which uses long dehydration and clearing stages with combinations of ethyl and butyl alcohol, aniline oil, acetone, and benzene, and recommended that wax impregnation should occupy *1–20 days, or more*. The teaching of experience will determine a suitable duration for this and other stages of tissue processing. The schedules to be given subsequently are guides.

Tissues are generally transferred directly from clearing agent to pure paraffin wax but sometimes, with fragile specimens it is recommended that graded mixtures of clearing agent and wax be used as an intermediate step. However, with specimens where it is considered desirable to use this manoeuvre an embedding medium other than paraffin wax would probably be preferable.

VACUUM IMPREGNATION

Evaporation of clearing agent, impregnation with paraffin wax and removal of trapped air in specimens occur more quickly and completely if carried out at reduced pressure. The time required for complete impregnation may be reduced by half and the air contained in blocks of lung is difficult to remove by any other means.

Reduced pressure is obtained by use of the so-called vacuum embedding oven, a common pattern of which consists of a circular brass well closed at the top by a thick plate-glass lid with a rubber washer to make an air-tight seal. (The life of the rubber ring will be prolonged if it is removed when the oven is not in use.) The chamber is set in a water-filled container which is electrically heated and maintained at a temperature 2–3 °C above the melting point of the wax. At the top of the chamber is a connection to the vacuum line and an air-admittance valve.

The reduction of pressure is obtained by an electric vacuum pump, a water pump, or a simple hand pump. A reduced pressure of 40–65 kPa is adequate for most purposes and some form of dial gauge or column manometer should be incorporated in the apparatus. If a water pump be used, a large, thick-walled vessel should be interposed between pump and chamber to lessen the risk of water being sucked into the containers should the pump be inadvertently turned off while still in direct connection with the chamber.

Technique

To evacuate.
1. Place tissues (from clearing agent) in fresh molten wax in an open jar.
2. Secure lid and make sure that the washer is flat in its seating.
3. Close air-admittance valve.
4. Start pump and check reduction of pressure on the gauge. When at the appropriate level (40–65 kPa), isolate pump by means of a stopcock or tap. Turn off pump.

To re-admit air.
1. *Slowly* open air-admittance valve to bring pressure in the chamber into equilibrium with that of the atmosphere—the glass lid may be removed when this is done.

Neither reduction or increase of pressure should be carried out abruptly because of the danger of rupture of delicate membranes such as alveoli of lung or thin-walled cysts.

EMBEDDING

Having been completely impregnated with wax, it is necessary to obtain a solid block containing the tissue. This is done by filling a mould of suitable size with molten paraffin wax, orientating the specimen in the mould to ensure its being cut in the right plane, and finally cooling the mass to promote solidification.

This stage in the processing of paraffin wax blocks and their preparation for the microtome can be a time-consuming operation and this was recognized by Orchin (1967) who analysed embedding procedures in respect of the number of steps involved, time, and the cost of materials.

Nowadays, most large histopathology laboratories use one or another of the metal or plastic embedding moulds such as Tissue-Tek II [p. 503] or Peel-away [p. 503]. Both can be recommended. The former has the advantage that specimens are processed in the plastic cassettes which form the surround to the embedded block with the cassettes being numbered with pencil prior to processing. A disadvantage is that special adaptors are required for microtome chucks to receive these blocks. Peelaway embedding moulds are made in five sizes from 8 × 8 mm cutting area to 22 × 40 mm. After solidification of the block (with included label), the plastic mould is peeled away and discarded. The block is clamped directly into the chuck of the microtome.

Both these systems are greatly superior to the older method of using two L-shaped pieces of metal to enclose multiple blocks and labels and entailing the subsequent separation, trimming, mounting on wood or metal holders, and the de-mounting of blocks after cutting.

With both Tissue-Tek II and Peelaway systems, the recurrent expenditure on plastic cassettes and embedding moulds should be more than compensated by the saving in man-hours and greater productivity.

The embedding of tissues has been further facilitated by the introduction of equipment combining a wax dispenser, heated platform for orientation and embedding, and cooled platforms for solidification of wax blocks, all in one unit. An example of such equipment is the Tissue-Tek II embedding centre [FIG. 4.1].

A further refinement in embedding is the use of temperature-controlled, electrically-heated forceps. These are very convenient and materially reduce the fire-hazard associated with gas burners in the vicinity of inflammable substances.

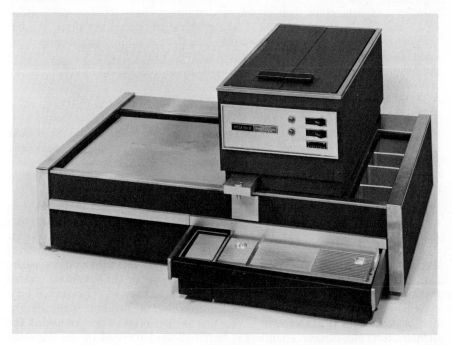

FIG. 4.1.   Tissue-Tek II embedding centre (Ames Company).

Technique

1. Metal moulds should be lightly smeared with glycerol to prevent adhesion of the wax on solidification.
2. Almost fill the mould with fresh filtered wax.
3. With warmed, but not too hot, smooth-tipped forceps, firmly but gently and without squeezing, orientate the specimen so that the intended cutting surface is pressed against the base of the mould.
4. Place the identifying label adjacent to the specimen, causing it to adhere to the inside edge of the mould.
5. After a skin of wax has formed completely over the surface of the block its solidification should be hastened by careful immersion in cold water, or by refrigeration. This step is not, as is sometimes stated, designed to prevent crystallization, since solid paraffin wax is essentially a crystalline substance. Rather, the induced solidification is to prevent the formation of large and irregular crystals and to ensure that the structure of the wax block is as finely crystalline and homogeneous as possible.

   The block should be allowed to cool in water for at least 15 minutes and large blocks may require an hour or more for complete solidification, for paraffin wax is a very poor conductor of heat.
6. When the block is completely solid it may be removed from the mould. This may happen spontaneously where glycerol has been used but if the block should stick in a metal mould, a sharp tap of the base plate against the bench usually causes separation.

STORAGE OF PARAFFIN BLOCKS

If properly fixed, dehydrated, cleared, and impregnated, tissues embedded in paraffin wax will retain their cutting and staining characteristics indefinitely. Of course, blocks should be stored in a cool rather than a hot place and cut surfaces protected from dust and vermin, but there is no doubt that if tissue is intended for microscopical examination at some future date it keeps better in the form of a paraffin block than in any fixative or preserving fluid.

AUTOMATIC TISSUE PROCESSING

The time required for the reagents used in processing to penetrate tissues may be considerably reduced if the tissue be: (1) suspended in the fluid; (2) continuously agitated; and (3) moved from one reagent to another when desirable and not merely when the restrictions of normal working hours make this possible. These requirements are met in the automatic tissue processing machines now widely used in histological laboratories throughout the world.

Several types of machine are available but the three features of suspension, agitation and automatic changeover of tissues at pre-set intervals are common to each [FIG. 4.2].

Tissue blocks not more than 5 mm thick together with an identifying label are placed in the metal or plastic containers provided with the machine, taking care that the label does not block the perforations in the container. Small fragments of tissue are first wrapped as described in page 58. The desired time cycle is selected and with the tissue basket attached, the machine is started, the first beaker being either fixative or the first in the series of reagents used for dehydration. No further attention is required until the end of the sequence when the tissues are in wax before embedding.

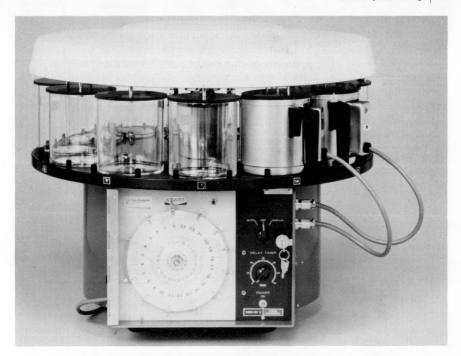

FIG. 4.2.   Tissue-Tek II tissue processor (Ames Company).

In addition to the fully automatic machines, there are available devices for tissue processing providing the features of suspension and agitation of tissues. While lacking automatic changeover and thus the potential speed of processing of the larger equipment, these units are very useful for the effective and convenient processing of multiple blocks, particularly where a longer duration in reagents is required.

ULTRASONIC VIBRATIONS

A means of speeding up tissue processing has been described in preliminary reports by Gagnon and Katyk (1959, 1960) who used ultrasonic vibrations (37 000 Hz) to aid the penetration of reagents used in fixation, decalcification and paraffin wax embedding. Processing was very rapid by this method but there was apparently a tendency for artifacts to be caused, particularly at the edges of the specimen.

SCOPE OF PARAFFIN EMBEDDING

Paraffin wax is the most widely used embedding medium and offers the advantages of reasonable speed of processing, a good consistency for serial sectioning, a wide range of section thickness and a durable block. Tissues are of course considerably hardened and shrunken by the method and an alternative procedure is preferable for some specimens. Dense cortical bone, for example, is difficult to cut in paraffin wax and large pieces of brain, where thick sections are required, is better suited to cellulose nitrate embedding or frozen sectioning. With some animal tissues, notably the liver and spleen of rodents, there is a marked tendency for cracks to appear in sections, sometimes after cutting. Several processing schedules have been devised to overcome this tendency and this material will benefit from special treatment [see p. 71].

The usual range of dimensions of blocks for paraffin wax embedding is 3–5 mm thick × 10–20 mm × 10–40 mm but very much larger blocks (5–10 cm × 10–15 cm) may be prepared from some tissues given a suitable microtome and very much extended processing schedules. For methods designed for the preparation of 'giant' sections of paraffin embedded material see Moore (1951a) and Oakley and Miller (1954).

Table 4.1. Outline of processes in paraffin wax embedding

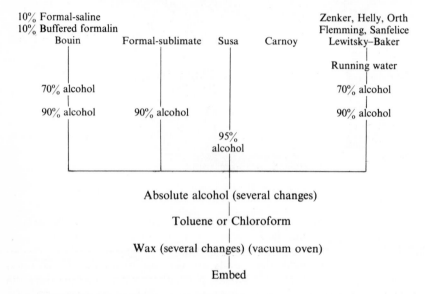

10% Formal-saline				Zenker, Helly, Orth
10% Buffered formalin				Flemming, Sanfelice
Bouin	Formal-sublimate	Susa	Carnoy	Lewitsky–Baker

70% alcohol — Running water — 70% alcohol

90% alcohol — 90% alcohol — 90% alcohol

95% alcohol

Absolute alcohol (several changes)

Toluene or Chloroform

Wax (several changes) (vacuum oven)

Embed

SPECIMEN PROCESSING SCHEDULES

It must be emphasized that the specimen schedules given below are merely guides and are subject to modification to suit circumstances and the type of work being carried out. For example, the first standard manual process would be unnecessarily long with a block only 1 or 2 mm in size while it might be very much too short for a specimen 5 × 10 × 1 cm. As has been shown above, the fixative used will govern the point of entry to the processing schedule and room temperature will affect the rate of penetration of the various reagents, heat generally accelerating and cold retarding the process.

Routine manual process (blocks 3–5 mm thick)

1. Fixation
2. Wash in water if necessary.
3. 70 per cent alcohol alcohol—during day, 3–8 hours.
4. 90 per cent alcohol—overnight, 16 hours.
5. Absolute alcohol I, two hours.
6. Absolute alcohol II, three hours.
7. Absolute alcohol III, three hours.
8. Toluene or chloroform—overnight, 16 hours.

9. Three changes of paraffin wax, 3 × 1 hours.
10. Embed in fresh wax.

Rapid manual process (blocks not thicker than 3 mm)

1. Fix in Carnoy's fluid, 30–60 minutes.
2. Absolute alcohol I, 30 minutes.
3. Absolute alcohol II, 30 minutes.
4. Absolute alcohol III, 30 minutes.
5. Xylene or toluene, 15–30 minutes (until clear).
6. Three changes of paraffin wax, 3 × 20 minutes, in vacuum oven.
7. Embed.

NOTE

Dehydration and clearing may be carried out in the wax oven using well stoppered containers.

Routine automatic process (blocks 3–5 mm thick)

1. 70 per cent alcohol	three hours
2. 90 per cent alcohol	three hours
3. Absolute alcohol I	one hour
4. Absolute alcohol II	one hour
5. Absolute alcohol III	two hours
6. Absolute alcohol IV	two hours
7. Toluene I	$1\frac{1}{2}$ hours
8. Toluene II	$2\frac{1}{2}$ hours
9. Wax bath I	three hours
10. Wax bath II	three hours
	22 hours

It is a common and useful procedure to transfer blocks from the second wax bath on the machine to a third change of wax in the vacuum oven before embedding.

48-hour automatic process (blocks 3–5 mm thick)

1. 10 per cent formal-saline I	four hours
2. 10 per cent formal-saline II	four hours
3. 70 per cent alcohol	four hours
4. 90 per cent alcohol	four hours
5. Absolute alcohol I	four hours
6. Absolute alcohol II	four hours
7. Absolute alcohol III	four hours
8. Absolute alcohol IV	four hours
9. Chloroform I	four hours
10. Chloroform II	four hours
11. Wax bath I	four hours
12. Wax bath II	four hours
	48 hours

Transfer blocks from the second wax bath on the machine to the vacuum embedding oven for at least one further change of wax before embedding.

Some automatic tissue processing machines incorporate a delayed-start mechanism whereby the routine week-day cycle may be used at week-ends, the tissue blocks remaining in the first beaker of the sequence until automatically transferred to the next to begin the cycle on completion of the selected delay period of up to 24 hours.

ESTER WAX EMBEDDING

Ester wax (Steedman 1960) is a mixture of diethylene glycol distearate, glyceryl monostearate and 300 polyethylene glycol [p. 503]. Although having a low melting point (45–7 °C) the block is hard when set, has a small crystal size and enables sections to be cut as thin as 1 μm at a room temperature of 18–20 °C. The wax is soluble in alcohol and xylene and ribbons of sections are permeable to aqueous solutions of basic dyes.

Ester wax offers particular advantages for the preparation of thin (1–3 μm) sections of tissue without the shrinkage that would be caused by the much higher impregnation temperature required by paraffin wax of suitable hardness for the purpose. In addition, ester wax gives superior support, and wax to tissue adhesion with hard, smooth material such as insects and cortical bone. No special conditions are necessary for the storage of ester wax blocks but it is approximately eight times more expensive than paraffin wax.

Technique (modified from Steedman 1960)

Fixed tissues, not exceeding 5 mm in thickness are processed as follows:

1. 70 per cent Cellosolve (2-ethoxyethanol), eight hours.
2. 90 per cent Cellosolve, overnight.
3. Pure Cellosolve I, 2½ hours.
4. Pure Cellosolve II, 2½ hours.
5. Pure Cellosolve III, three hours.
6. Cellosolve–ester wax 50 : 50, overnight at 37 °C.
7. Impregnate with ester wax using at least three changes of one hour each. Occasional stirring or shaking is helpful.
8. Embed, using freshly melted wax in metal L-pieces. Keep the surface of the block molten until the deeper part has solidified. This is to prevent rapid contraction of the surface and the admission of air. Do not immerse the block in water.

NOTES

1. It may be necessary to regulate the temperature of the oven at 48–50 °C to keep the wax completely molten.
2. A brief period (10–15 minutes) in the vacuum oven, immediately before embedding will help remove any trapped air in the specimen.

WATER-SOLUBLE WAX EMBEDDING

Solid polyethylene glycols (water waxes) of suitable molecular weight may be used as embedding media. They are readily soluble in water and tissues may thus be impregnated immediately following fixation in aqueous solutions. This allows the possibility of the demonstration of lipids in sections prepared without freezing and also results in much reduced shrinkage since the use of dehydrating and clearing agents is generally avoided. Unfortunately, water-soluble waxes do not readily penetrate tissues rich in fatty material and these require treatment with a fat solvent prior to impregnation. Miles and Linder (1953), however, convincingly demonstrated the reduction in shrinkage obtained by the use of this medium with teeth and associated tissues, when the demonstration of lipid was not the prime object.

Polythylene glycol waxes are difficult to prepare in pure form and samples of varying hardness and melting point are available and are designated by the approximate molecular weight of the substance, 1500 being generally used for embedding.

After impregnation, blocks of tissue are embedded and allowed to solidify at room temperature or in a refrigerator, but not by immersion in water. A warm and humid atmosphere may cause difficulty in section cutting and the manipulation and flattening of sections is hampered by the solubility of the wax in the solutions normally used for this purpose. Blocks must be stored away from moisture but may be protected by coating with paraffin wax.

The several disadvantages noted above have precluded the general use of water-soluble wax as an embedding medium but the greatly improved methods now available for the preparation of frozen sections are mainly responsible for the virtual obsolescence of the method.

CELLULOSE NITRATE (CELLOIDIN AND LVN) EMBEDDING

Celloidin and low viscosity nitrocellulose (LVN) are both forms of cellulose nitrate. LVN, being less viscous, penetrates tissue more readily and may be used in higher concentrations than celloidin, giving a harder block and the possibility of thinner sections.

Fixed and dehydrated tissues are impregnated with ascending concentrations of celloidin or LVN dissolved in a mixture of absolute alcohol and ether. Clearing agents are not required and no heat is used in the process. After impregnation, tissues are embedded in a thick solution of the cellulose nitrate, the final consistency of the block being regulated by controlled evaporation of the solvent. Blocks are stored in alcohol.

The *advantages* of celloidin and LVN embedding are: (1) considerable reduction in shrinkage of tissue due largely to the absence of heat in the process; (2) improved cutting qualities of large blocks of dense tissue such as bone, due to reduced hardening, and the plasticity of the medium; (3) the facility of preparation of sections of brain where thick sections are often required and where the shrinkage and distortion occasioned by paraffin embedding are to be avoided; and (4) the superior cohesion of tissue layers of different consistency as in the eye, where, in paraffin sections, the retina, choroid, and sclera often become separated and distorted.

The *disadvantages* of celloidin and LVN embedding are: (1) the slowness of the method, it generally requiring several weeks for complete impregnation and hardening of the block; (2) restrictions in thickness of sections, it being difficult to cut thinner than 10 μm; (3) being a non-ribboning medium the preparation of serial sections is a laborious process; (4) it is inconvenient and space-consuming to have to store blocks in jars of alcohol; and (5) the high flammability of the embedding medium.

GENERAL PROCEDURE

Cellulose nitrate, formerly in the shape of hard, transparent shreds in water, is nowadays supplied as soft white fragments damped with alcohol, often *n*-butyl alcohol. (It is usual to discount the weight of the damping alcohol when preparing solutions.) Both celloidin and LVN may explode if detonated when dry.

Solutions of the required strength are commonly made in a mixture of absolute alcohol and anhydrous ether although other solvents such as amyl acetate have been used and Yates and Slater (1964) use LVN in concentrations of 10, 20, 30, 40, and 50 per cent in Cellosolve (2-ethoxyethanol) for the embedding of brain and spinal cord. Wide-mouth jars with well-fitting lids should be used and Ferreira and Combs (1951) recommend that solutions should be stored in the dark, having found that light-affected LVN caused fading of blocks of mordanted central nervous system material.

As with the other processing schedules already given, the following are only intended as a guide. Generally, larger rather than smaller pieces of tissue are selected for cellulose nitrate embedding and since the solutions do not penetrate readily, the duration of each stage is long compared with paraffin wax embedding. Certainly, no harm will befall tissue left in the various mixtures for periods considerably in excess of those quoted and is more likely to be beneficial. Steedman (1960) rightly stresses that 'rapid celloidin methods, especially those involving heat, should be avoided, since they tend to defeat the purpose of using celloidin by nullifying at least some of its advantages'.

Celloidin method

Thoroughly fixed (perhaps decalcified) and dehydrated tissues of 5–8 mm thickness are treated as follows. Thicker blocks may require longer.

1. Absolute alcohol and ether, equal parts, 24 hours.
2. 2 per cent celloidin in absolute alcohol–ether, 5–7 days.
3. 4 per cent celloidin in absolute alcohol–ether, 5–7 days.
4. 8 per cent celloidin in absolute alcohol–ether, 3–4 days.
5. Embed in 8 per cent celloidin either in individual paper boxes or, with multiple blocks, *en masse* in a tray of suitable size. In both cases, the blocks are covered to a depth of 30–40 mm, leaving a margin of at least 10 mm at each side of the tissue. The paper box should be placed in an air-tight container while the tray containing multiple blocks should by covered by a sheet of plate-glass. Before covering either container, a small dish of ether may be placed alongside the blocks to promote the dispersion of the numerous air bubbles that will have been introduced into the celloidin during pouring. In an hour or two, when the bubbles have dispersed, the ether is replaced with chloroform, the vapour from which facilitates the hardening of the block but without the formation of a hard outer skin and a soft centre. Re-seal the container and allow hardening to continue (replacing the chloroform as necessary) until the block has the consistency of hard rubber; this may take several days. At this stage, individual blocks may be cut out from the celloidin mass and are either given further treatment with chloroform or placed in 70 per cent alcohol for storage prior to cutting.

LVN method

The generally higher concentrations of cellulose nitrate used in LVN embedding may result in cracking of sections and it is advisable to incorporate a plasticizer in the embedding medium. Chesterman and Leach (1949) have used tricresylphosphate for this purpose while Moore (1951b) used oleum ricini (castor oil) with LVN embedded, chrome mordanted central nervous system material, a stringent test.

Thoroughly fixed and dehydrated blocks of 5–8 mm thickness are treated as follows. Thicker blocks may require longer.

1. Absolute alcohol and ether, equal parts, 24 hours.
2. 5 per cent LVN in absolute alcohol–ether, plus *either* 1 per cent tricresylphosphate *or* 0.5 per cent oleum ricini, 3–5 days.
3. 10 per cent LVN plus plasticizer, 3–5 days.
4. 20 per cent LVN plus plasticizer, 2–3 days.
5. Embed in 20 per cent LVN plus plasticizer in a paper box, leaving a margin of at least 10 mm at each side of the tissue. Place in a container, seal tightly and allow air bubbles to disperse. Harden block by exposure to chloroform vapour followed by immersion in 70 per cent alcohol in which the block is stored prior to cutting as in celloidin embedding.

NOTE

Chrome or osmium treated tissues embedded in cellulose nitrate have a strong tendency to stick to the bottom of the container in which they are embedded (Anderson 1929). To prevent this and possible damage to the specimen on removal of the hardened block, a sheet of aluminium or tin foil should be placed on the bottom of the container before pouring in the cellulose nitrate and embedding the blocks.

CELLOIDIN–PARAFFIN DOUBLE EMBEDDING

The combination of cellulose nitrate (celloidin or LVN) and paraffin wax is a useful compromise embedding method. This is designed to produce the improved cohesion of tissue layers and plasticity given by celloidin with the facility of cutting ribbons of sections from a dry, durable block that is characteristic of paraffin wax. The method is particularly useful with bone, brain, muscle, and tissues from laboratory animals.

Peterfi's (1921) method

1. Transfer thoroughly dehydrated tissue from absolute alcohol to 1 per cent celloidin in methylbenzoate for three changes of 24 hours each. The tissue will be 'cleared'.
2. Give three changes of toluene, up to eight hours each change.
3. Impregnate with several changes of paraffin wax.
4. Embed.

NOTES

1. Dry celloidin does not dissolve readily in methylbenzoate and may require several days for complete solution. It should be kept in tightly-stoppered containers.
2. Double embedding is not a rapid method although small pieces of porous

tissue may well be completely infiltrated with celloidin–methylbenzoate in less than the 72 hours of the standard method. The duration of treatment with toluene is always in relation to the duration in celloidin–methylbenzoate.

3. Russell (1956) described a modification of Peterfi's method adapted to an automatic tissue processing machine schedule (47 hours) which is especially beneficial for those tissues that are prone to cracking, such as the liver and spleen of small experimental animals; Ball (1957) used 3 per cent and 20 per cent LVN in methylbenzoate before wax impregnation of small blocks of undecalcifed iliac crest material for sectioning by the Sellotape method [p. 209].

4. Another, simpler method of double embedding, it to treat tissues after dehydration in absolute alcohol with alcohol–ether (equal parts) followed by 1 or 2 per cent cellulose nitrate in alcohol–ether. The cellulose nitrate is hardened with chloroform before impregnation with paraffin wax.

AQUEOUS MEDIA AND GELATINE EMBEDDING

Frozen sections are generally prepared without the tissue being impregnated with an embedding medium. In some cases, however, it is necessary to use a means of embedding, particularly with multiple fragments such as curettings, and to prevent the disintegration of sections after cutting and before mounting on a slide as with cystic structures and lung. Gelatine is most commonly used for this purpose.

Gelatine embedding

1. Fixed tissue is washed for up to 24 hours in running water.
2. Impregnate with 12.5 per cent gelatine at 37 °C for 24 hours.
3. Transfer to 25 per cent gelatine at 37 °C for a further 24 hours.
4. Embed in 25 per cent gelatine using a paper or metal-foil box, or metal or plastic embedding moulds.
5. Allow to cool and solidify, preferably in the refrigerator at 4 °C.
6. Trim the block with a thin, sharp blade and further harden by placing in 10 per cent formalin in which blocks may be stored.

NOTES

1. It is essential to thoroughly wash out the fixative before impregnation to prevent premature hardening or 'fixation' of the gelatine.
2. To prepare the medium: dissolve 25 g good quality gelatine in 75 cm^3 of 1 per cent phenol in distilled water at 37 °C. (The phenol is to prevent the growth of micro-organisms.) Filter through gauze at 37 °C. The 12.5 per cent solution is prepared by dilution of the above with 1 per cent phenol.
3. Since gelatine is slow to freeze, the size of tissue and block should be kept to a minimum.
4. Oakley (1937) in describing the use of gelatine embedding for the preparation of frozen sections of the eye, warned that if 25 per cent gelatine be used more than twice, it either fails to solidify or sets and stains unevenly.
5. For details of the Gough and Wentworth method for preparing paper-mounted sections of gelatine embedded whole organs see page 482.

AGAR EMBEDDING

Agar has been used for the embedding of unfixed and fixed tissue and Cook and Hotchkiss (1977) have described a method using a solution of agar in neutral buffered formalin to aggregate fragments of tissue prior to routine processing and embedding in paraffin wax. This method also prevents the possibility of loss of very small fragments of tissue during processing.

Agar does not generally stain with haematoxylin and eosin, unlike gelatine, which is very prone to stain particularly with basic dyes.

GUM

In the absence of gelatine or agar embedding, the consistency for frozen sectioning of many tissues may be improved by soaking for some hours in a thick solution of gum arabic in water. The formation of 'ice-crystal' artifacts [p. 38] may be reduced by the use of gum, but sections should be well washed after cutting as residual gum may interfere with some staining reactions.

SYNTHETIC RESIN EMBEDDING

It is axiomatic that the thinner the sections required, the harder will be the embedding medium necessary for the purpose. For example, the minimum thickness generally obtainable with cellulose nitrate embedded material is 10 μm, while with paraffin wax, melting at 56 °C (which is harder than cellulose nitrate) sections of 3–4 μm may be obtained. However, when considering the thickness of sections necessary for examination with the electron microscope (0.005–0.1 μm) it will be appreciated that the embedding media described so far are not suitable for the preparation of such thin sections. To meet this need, use is made of synthetic resins (acrylic, polyester, and epoxy resins).

In addition to their uses in ultra-microtomy, these substances, separately or in mixtures, and sometimes with plasticizers or other additives to improve cutting characteristics, have proved their value in more general ways. Using these media, the preparation of sections at 1μm for examination with the light microscope is becoming a routine procedure in histopathology and the sectioning of exceptionally hard material such as undecalcified bone is best carried out after synthetic resin embedding [p. 210].

It is noteworthy that in addition to the facility of preparation of thin sections, superior preservation of tissue structures and lack of distortion are seen in tissues embedded in these materials.

Among the first to describe a method of embedding using synthetic resins were Newman, Borysko, and Swerdlow (1949) who used butyl methacrylate and since that time a large variety of synthetic resins and mixtures of resins have been used.

A reliable resin embedding method for the preparation of 1–2 μm sections for light microscopy is given below.

Sims's (1974) glycol methacrylate embedding method

Fixed tissues, not exceeding 2 mm in thickness are processed as follows.

1. Dehydrate in 70 per cent and 90 per cent alcohol for 30 to 60 minutes in each followed by four changes of absolute alcohol for 30 to 60 minutes in each change.

2. Impregnate in freshly prepared Solution A (hydroxyethyl methacrylate 80 cm³, butoxyethanol 8 cm³, and benzoyl peroxide 0.5 g) for 16 to 48 hours, replacing the solution two or three times during the period. Tissues should be translucent when impregnated.

3. Polymerize in a mixture of 42 parts solution A and 1 part solution B (polyethylene glycol-400 8 cm³ and N,N-dimethylaniline 0.5 cm³). Tissues should be in filled, air-tight plastic moulds as the presence of oxygen inhibits polymerization which should take 30 to 45 minutes at room temperature. Embedding moulds should be partially immersed in cold water during polymerization to disperse the heat produced and prevent the formation of bubbles.

NOTES

1. Preparation of solutions A and B, infiltration and polymerization should be carried out in a fume cupboard as toxic vapours are evolved. Skin contact should be avoided.
2. Hardness of the block may be varied by altering the concentrations of polyethylene glycol and butoxyethanol. Murgatroyd (1976) produced a softer block by doubling the quantity of solution B (accelerator and plasticizer).
3. For the microtomy of this material see page 105.

FREEZE DRYING AND FREEZE SUBSTITUTION

Freeze drying of tissues prior to embedding and the freeze substitution method of processing are special procedures used mainly in histochemical investigations. Tissues may be finally embedded in paraffin wax, polyethylene glycol wax, ester wax, or a synthetic resin.

FREEZE DRYING

Since fixation of tissues with chemicals and the subsequent use of dehydrating and clearing agents may cause alteration, loss or displacement of enzymes and other substances, their use is not generally acceptable to the histochemist. Freeze drying is a means of avoiding these deleterious effects for, theoretically, only water is removed from the tissue, there being no alteration in arrangement or quantity of any other tissue component. The method consists of the following basic steps:

1. Immediate freezing of very small pieces of fresh tissue by immersion in isopentane cooled by liquid nitrogen to about −150 °C. This is called 'quenching'.
2. Transfer of the specimen to the drying chamber where, at a temperature of −30 to −60 °C and under vacuum (0.01 mm Hg), the ice (tissue water) is removed by sublimation, the water vapour being absorbed by phosphorus pentoxide or other drying agent.
3. Impregnation with the embedding medium under reduced pressure.

The quenching must be carried out immediately on perfectly fresh tissue before autolytic changes can occur, otherwise the purpose of the whole procedure will be unfulfilled. The size of the specimen must be small (about 1 mm) to ensure that freezing will be virtually instantaneous. Larger pieces may be rendered useless by slower freezing and the formation of the ice-crystal artifact described on page 38.

The drying of the specimen under vacuum may be done in apparatus constructed in the laboratory workshop or in commercially produced tissue driers, a modern example of which employs thermo-electric cooling [p. 101] and integral embedding facilities, drying tissues in 4–12 hours according to the size of the specimen.

The embedding medium should be degassed before use and it should be noted that even though embedded, freeze dried tissues are not fixed, and exposure of the cut surface of the tissue to the atmosphere will result in absorption of moisture and deterioration of the specimen. Blocks should be stored in a desiccator in a cool place.

FREEZE SUBSTITUTION

This is a compromise method which aims at the preservation of labile substances achieved with the freeze drying method, but without the need for much special equipment, and in a way more suited to routine use. It consists of the following steps:

1. Initial quenching of small pieces of tissue as in freeze drying.
2. Simultaneous fixation and removal of ice from tissue by immersion in an ice solvent such as absolute alcohol or acetone, at low temperature (-60 to $-70\,°C$) for several days. (Feder and Sidman (1958) added 1 per cent mercuric chloride to the alcohol and 1 per cent osmium tetroxide to the acetone to augment the fixing action of these solvents.)
3. Gradual raising of temperature and completion of the embedding process at the appropriate temperature.

REFERENCES

ANDERSON, J. (1929). *How to stain the nervous system.* Livingstone, Edinburgh.
BALL, J. (1957). *J. clin Path.* **10**, 281.
CHESTERMAN, W. and LEACH, E. H. (1949). *Quart. J. micr. Sci.* **90**, 431.
COOK, R. W. and HOTCHKISS, G. R. (1977). *Med. Lab. Sci.* **34**, 93.
FEDER, N. and SIDMAN, R. (1958). *J. biophys. biochem. Cytol.* **4**, 593.
FERREIRA, A. V. and COMBS, C. M. (1951). *Stain Technol.* **26**, 81.
GAGNON, J. and KATYK, N. (1959). *Rev. canad. Biol.* **18**, 346.
—— —— (1960). *Arch. Anat. path.* **8**, 203.
LAMB, R. A. (1973). Waxes for histology. In *Histopathology, selected topics* (ed. H. C. Cook) p. 123. Bailliére Tindall, London.
LENDRUM, A.C. (1951). In *Recent advances in clinical pathology* (ed. S. C. Dyke) 2nd edn. Churchill, London.
MILES, A. E. W. and LINDER, J. E. (1953). *J. roy micr. Soc.* **72**, 199.
MOORE, G. W. (1951a). *J. med. Lab. Technol.* **9**, 86.
—— (1951b). *J. med. Lab. Technol.* **9**, 105.
MURGATROYD, L. B. (1976). *Med. Lab. Sci.* **33**, 67.
NEWMAN, S. B., BORYSKO, E., and SWERDLOW, M. (1949). *Science* **110**, 66.
OAKLEY, A. H. and MILLER, J. W. (1954). *Am. J. clin. Path.* **24**, 996.
OAKLEY, C. L. (1937). *J. Path. Bact.* **44**, 365.
ORCHIN, J. C. (1967). Modern techniques in histology. In *Progress in medical laboratory technique 4* (ed. F. J. Baker). Butterworths, London.
PETERFI, T. (1921). *Z. wiss. Mikr.* **38**, 342.
POPHAM, R. E. (1950). *Stain Technol.* **25**, 113.
RUSSELL, N. L. (1956). *J. med. Lab. Technol.* **13**, 484.
SIMS, B. (1974). *J. Micros.* **101**, 223.
STEEDMAN, H. F. (1960). *Section cutting in microscopy.* Blackwell, Oxford.
YATES, P. O. and SLATER, R. (1964). Personal communication.

5 | Microtomy

Details have been given in the preceding chapter for the preparation of tissues for microtomy and most of the stages involved in this preparation depend only on the adherence to suitable time schedules with appropriate reagents and may be carried out automatically. The production of good quality sections from embedded material, however, is by no means an automatic process and it is unfortunate that the time spent on careful preparation of tissue is sometimes wasted by subsequent poor technique and unsatisfactory equipment at the stage of section cutting. The damage and disfigurements that may be caused to previously well preserved tissue during attempts to cut good sections are many and varied and the appearance under the microscope of such sections may give rise to serious difficulty or error in interpretation.

To become competent with the different types of equipment available, to be able to prepare properly-sharpened knives and to produce blemish-free sections from a wide variety of tissues prepared in various ways, takes a long time, a lot of patience, and an awareness of the many factors that can influence the cutting of sections.

Sections are prepared on an instrument known as a microtome of which various types are available. Common features of all types are separate and firm supports for knife and tissue-block and a feed mechanism designed to advance the specimen a predetermined number of micrometres on each cutting stroke. The thickness of sections produced during microtomy may range between a fraction of one micrometre (ultra-microtomy) and several hundred micrometres. The most common range is 3–8 μm, but while both maximum and minimum thicknesses are limited by the consistency of the tissue and embedding medium, the relation of the thickness of the section to the nature of the tissue should also be taken into account. Generally, the looser the texture of the tissue or organ, e.g. de-fatted adipose tissue or normal lung, the thicker can sections be made. Furthermore, thick (15–50 μm) sections of such material are not only easier to cut but they are often more informative than thin ones. On the other hand, a dense richly cellular tissue such as spleen requires a thin (3–5 μm) section for microscopical examination.

Microtomes

A careful consideration of the type of specimen to be sectioned will help in the choice of an appropriate microtome. All have their limitations with no single model being suitable for all types of embedding media and specimens.

Rotary, rocking, and sledge microtomes are widely used for paraffin wax embedded material while the Jung KM [p. 80] and the sliding microtome [p. 78] are used principally for sectioning undecalcified bone and cellulose nitrate embedded tissue respectively.

The position and function of the various controls should be well understood and the manufacturer's instructions carried out before putting any microtome into use. Regular cleaning and lubrication of bearings and moving parts is essential and the microtome should always be covered when not in use.

CAMBRIDGE ROCKING MICROTOME

Introduced more than 90 years ago, modern versions of this microtome are small, lightweight instruments which are very suitable for class-work and the teaching of microtomy. The knife is fixed, with the edge uppermost, while the object moves against the knife in the arc of a circle, producing a slightly curved surface to the block. This cutting stroke is spring-operated and somewhat less controllable than with other types of microtome. The Cambridge rocking microtome is simple to operate, has a minimum of moving parts, is

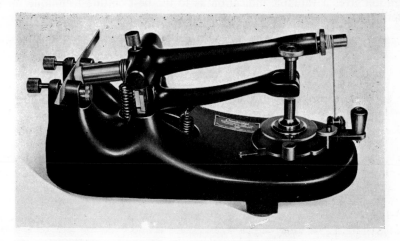

FIG. 5.1.   Cambridge rocking microtome (Cambridge Medical Instruments Ltd.).

consequently easy to maintain and some models have been in use for many years. Although it is not suitable for large blocks of hard materials, admirable sections may be produced from smaller blocks of paraffin embedded tissue and the design lends itself to the production and manipulation of ribbons of sections.

Because of the lightness of the machine and rather jerky, pulling action required to operate the feed mechanism, the microtome may tend to move about on the bench during operation. This may be prevented by placing the microtome on a mat of non-slip material such as sponge-rubber. A larger and heavier version of the rocking microtome, incorporating a rotary drive (see below) and retraction of the specimen arm on the return stroke, is now widely used in cryostats [p. 102] as well as for paraffin wax embedded material.

ROTARY MICROTOMES

Rotary microtomes are so-called because the feed mechanism is actuated by turning a wheel at one side of the machine. In all models, the knife is fixed, edge uppermost and the object moves against the knife according to the thickness selected, rising and falling vertically. One rotation of the operating wheel produces a complete cycle of downwards cutting-stroke, an upwards return stroke and activation of the advance mechanism. The downwards travel of the block holder is not spring assisted and is under greater control of the operator than with the rocking microtome. Several examples of this type are available (sometimes called Minot microtomes from the name of the originator), the main differences being in size and weight. The mechanism is usually encased to prevent access of dust and dirt.

The feed activation of rotary microtomes lends itself to power-drive attachments and apparatus has been described where the fly-wheel was connected to a treadle or electric motor (thus allowing both hands to be used for manipulation of sections). These aids may be advantageous for certain types of work, particularly the preparation of multiple sections from a single block, but often, with a wide variety of tissues, the 'feel' of the block obtained by manual operation gives a valuable indication as to the best cutting technique for the material.

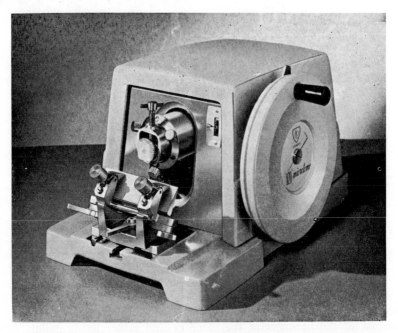

FIG. 5.2.   Rotary microtome (British American Optical Co Ltd.).

Rotary microtomes are good general purpose instruments. They are used mainly for paraffin wax embedded material and are well suited to the production of serial sections. A special knife-holder, allowing the knife to be set at an oblique angle to the specimen, may be used on some models for cutting cellulose nitrate embedded tissues.

SLIDING AND BASE SLEDGE MICROTOMES

The sliding microtome is used mainly for the cutting of cellulose nitrate embedded tissue with the obliquely-set knife being drawn across the surface of the object.

The base sledge microtome is a large, heavy instrument with a fixed knife beneath which travels the object mounted in a heavy sliding base containing the feed mechanism. This base (or sledge) is moved to and fro on runners against the knife to produce sections, the feed mechanism being either automatic or activated manually on each cutting stroke. It is an instrument with a wide range of uses, being suitable for cellulose nitrate embedded tissues (the knife may be set obliquely), while a freezing chamber may be substituted for the several types of large and small holders for paraffin wax blocks that are available.

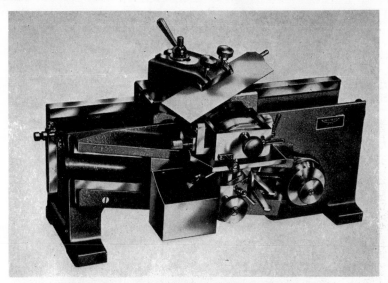

FIG. 5.3.   Sliding microtome (Reichert–Jung).

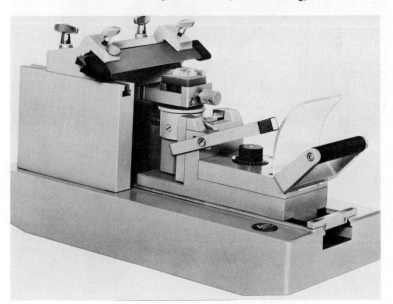

FIG. 5.4.   Base sledge microtome (E. Leitz Ltd.).

Base sledge microtomes are much used in pathology laboratories where specimens for microtomy are often large and hard. They are particularly suitable for cutting bone and teeth, and Moore (1951) described the use of these microtomes for the preparation of thin sections of large paraffin wax embedded embryos.

While less convenient than the rotary or rocking type microtomes for serial

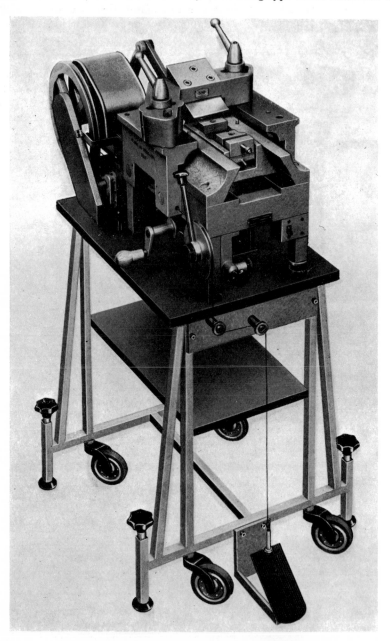

Fig. 5.5. Jung KM microtome (Reichert–Jung).

section work, good ribbons of sections may be obtained from wax embedded material with the sledge microtome when the knife is set at right-angles to the direction of travel of the object.

Although designed for special purposes, the *Jung KM* is essentially a base sledge microtome. It may be hand-operated or power-driven and its massive construction and near-perfect rigidity of both knife and object holder combine to allow the production of thin, flat sections from the hardest of biological materials.

FREEZING MICROTOMES

These are designed for the preparation of 'frozen' sections of fixed or unfixed tissues, usually without preliminary embedding. The object stage is connected to a cylinder of compressed carbon dioxide for rapid cooling of the specimen and provision is also made for cooling the knife. The movement of the knife

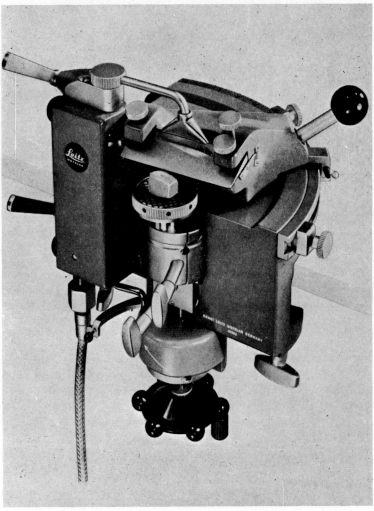

FIG. 5.6.   Freezing microtome (E. Leitz Ltd.).

horizontally across the surface of the specimen also activates the feed mechanism which is commonly in steps of 5 μm. It is not possible to prepare ribbons of sections with the freezing microtome and the production of serial sections is difficult. For the use of thermo-electric cooling devices and refrigerated microtomes (cryostat) see pages 101 and 102.

ULTRA-MICROTOMES

Ultra-microtomes are instruments especially designed for preparation of the very thin sections necessary for examination with the electron microscope. They differ from the conventional microtomes described above in: (1) the fineness and precision of the feed mechanism which is activated either by mechanical means or by electrically controlled thermal expansion to give a thickness range of 5–100 nm (0.005–0.1 μm); and (2) the specially prepared knives (usually of plate-glass) used to cut the very small 'blocks' of tissue which are embedded in a hard synthetic resin such as Araldite.

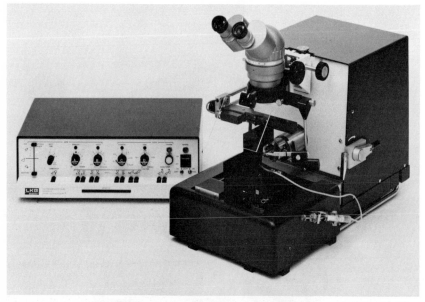

Fig. 5.7.   Ultra-microtome (LKB Ltd.).

The several models of ultra-microtomes currently available vary in performance characteristics but usually incorporate a low-power binocular microscope mounted above the object to aid orientation, automatic and manual cutting action and provision for cutting 'thick' (1–2 μm) sections for examination with a light microscope.

Microtome knives

Regardless of the type of microtome or embedding medium, and notwithstanding the skill of the microtomist, the production of good quality sections depends ultimately on a properly sharpened knife; attempts at section cutting with an unsatisfactory knife edge are wasteful of time and valuable or irreplaceable material.

Microtome knives are made from steel although prepared glass is used for cutting in ultra-microtomy. They are available in various types and sizes according to the microtome and embedding medium used. They are identified by their profile [FIG. 5.8] as follows:

Profile A is biconcave (hollow ground on both sides) and is generally used for wax embedded sections.

Profile B is planoconcave (hollow ground on one side) and is mainly used for cellulose nitrate embedded material. Planoconcave knives are available in greater or lesser degrees of concavity.

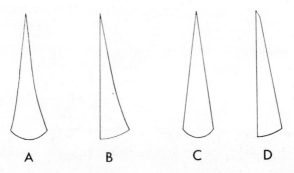

FIG. 5.8. Microtome knives seen in profile. A = biconcave; B = planoconcave; C = wedge shape; D = tool edge.

Profile C is wedge shaped (plane surface on both sides) and has wide application in microtomy. It is used for wax embedded tissue with any microtome, for hard, cellulose nitrate embedded tissue, for cutting frozen sections and for synthetic resin embedded specimens.

Profile D is described as a tool edge. It is intended for exceptionally hard materials such as wood, plastics, and undecalcified bone.

Razor blades and somewhat thicker disposable blades mounted in suitable holders have been used for section cutting but these have generally limited application.

While the various types of knife are mainly used for the purposes indicated, it should be appreciated that variation in conditions (or lack of the appropriate knife) may determine otherwise. The overriding consideration is effectiveness in operation and while a profile D knife would not be best for brain embedded in celloidin, a slightly biconcave knife (Heiffor type) may be effectively used in some types of cryostat for cutting frozen sections.

Most microtome knives are provided with a detachable handle which screws in to one end of the blade. An exception is the Heiffor type which is used with the Cambridge rocking microtome. In this case, the handle is fashioned from the same piece of metal as the blade and is an integral part of the knife.

Since the actual cutting edge of a microtome knife is not the point at which the two sides meet but a point formed by a greater angle than this [FIG. 5.9], some means of maintaining this cutting facet or bevel is required. This is achieved during manual sharpening by the fitting of a device known as a honing bevel or knife-back. It consists of a semicircular sheath which fits over the base of the knife and extends the full length of the blade. Honing bevels were previously made from slotted metal tubing but are now usually made from plastic material which is at least as hard-wearing as the metal, is cheaper and much lighter in weight, which last is an important consideration, especially in the handling of the larger (240 mm) knives during sharpening.

In practice, planoconcave and wedge-shaped knives require a knife-back for sharpening and profile D knives require a back of special shape. Biconcave knives do not require a honing back as will be apparent from study of their profile.

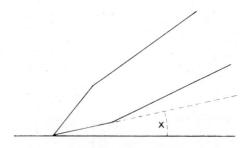

FIG. 5.9.   Cutting face (bevel) of microtome knife. X = clearance angle.

Since the purpose of the knife-back is to maintain the actual cutting facet during sharpening (wearing away of metal), it will be appreciated that not only should each knife have its own knife-back but this should always be fitted to the knife in the same way, for, unfortunately, microtome knives are not always completely straight and true and if they were, this condition is not always maintained during sharpening. It is most important, therefore, that both edge and knife-back should wear at an equal rate and in the same way.

It is advisable to choose a knife with as broad a base as the knife clamps of the microtome will allow, to obtain rigidity, and a length of blade that will give alternative cutting positions without projecting dangerously at either end. (Knife guards are available, or may be made from rubber tubing to cover the exposed corners of the knife.)

When not in use or being sharpened, the knife should be kept in its box, while the handle should be attached and used for all handling of the knife. The knife should be carefully cleaned after use (disposable paper tissues are convenient) and if to be stored, should be smeared with anti-corrosion oil or grease.

KNIFE SHARPENING

A blunt or damaged knife edge will cause many and varied faults in sections or will fail to cut any sections at all. Bluntness is caused through the edge becoming rounded and damage takes the form of large (macroscopic) or small (microscopic) nicks, teeth, or serrations caused by breaking or rearrangment of the metal edge. In practice, there is a wide range of conditions between the perfect edge and the badly damaged and blunted knife and no small part of the microtomist's skill lies in the quick appreciation of the state of the edge from observation of sections during cutting, coupled with the knowledge and ability to apply the required treatment. Sometimes, however, the extent of the damage caused by an imperfect knife is not apparent even in haematoxylin and eosin stained sections and is only revealed after the use of special stains [FIG. 5.10].

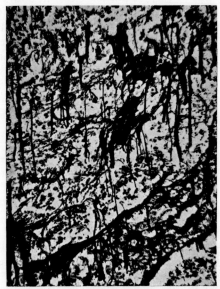

FIG. 5.10. A blunt knife has caused connective tissue fibres to become re-orientated in the direction of travel of the knife. Silver impregnation. × 100.

A knife edge viewed by reflected light and magnified about 60 times should not show any indentations or projections of the edge, but be straight. On the other hand, a perfectly straight knife edge is not in itself indicative of sharpness for if the cutting bevel has become too broad, bluntness is inevitable. The extent to which blemishes in the knife edge will be transferred to the section depends to a certain extent on the tissue, the embedding medium, and thickness of cutting, for while a damaged knife edge may not cause obvious tears or scores in a 15 μm frozen section of uterus, they will almost certainly be present in a 5 μm paraffin wax section of densely cellular tissue such as spleen.

Various tests are suggested for establishing the condition of a microtome knife but are of limited reliability. Certainly the knife should feel sharp, should show no macroscopic or microscopic nicks or teeth and, according to some microtomists, should easily cut a detached human hair. These tests are useful but the experienced microtomist will gain most information from the naked-eye appearance of the first sections produced with a knife of doubtful sharpness.

Knife sharpening consists of two operations; one is honing, where the knife edge is moved over a hard surface which is either itself abrasive, or has abrasive material applied to the surface, the other is stropping or polishing on a softer surface such as leather or cork, with and without the addition of fine abrasive.

HONING

An excessively broad cutting facet and the presence of nicks are indications for honing and the preparation of a new edge. When carried out manually, the hone takes the form of a rectangular block, either of abrasive material (carborundum, Belgian yellow stone, Arkansas stone) or of plate-glass on which is applied aluminium oxide of various particle sizes. In both cases, water or light oil is used as a lubricant and the knife (with honing bevel fitted) is moved edge first up and down the hone, with light pressure only. In most cases the blade will be longer than the width of the hone and therefore, side as well as forward travel of the knife is necessary to bring the entire length of the edge into contact with the abrasive surface. Manufactured hones of suitable size for the manual honing of long (240 mm) knives are not readily available but glass plates may be cut to individual requirements and, if of correct size, will help to avoid the curved edge that is inevitable with knives sharpened on too narrow a honing surface.

The coarseness of the abrasive used initially will depend on the condition of the knife edge and the larger the size of the irregularities in the edge, the greater the need for a coarse rather than a fine abrasive to reduce the time and effort necessary to remove the requisite amount of metal. Progression is made from coarse to fine abrasive as the number and size of irregularities of the edge diminish.

Manufactured hones and hones prepared from quarried stone vary in their abrasive quilities, carborundum being very much coarser than, for example, a Belgian stone.

Aluminium oxide in a range of particle sizes is used as an abrasive when honing with glass plates, the finest grades being less than 0.5 µm average particle size. Water or oil is used as a vehicle for these powders.

Both knife and plate should be thoroughly cleaned before proceeding from one abrasive to another and hones should be kept scrupulously clean and protected from dust. If chipped, cracked, or curved, they should be re-ground or discarded.

AUTOMATIC KNIFE SHARPENERS

The past decade has seen the increasing use of machines designed for sharpening microtome knives and current models of these machines use copper or glass plates, have automatic turn-over of the blade, pressure control, and provision for selection and reproduction of the correct setting of the edge in relation to the honing surface, thus disposing of the need for honing bevels.

Though expensive, these machine are efficient, save valuable man-hours for the actual cutting of sections and are undoubtedly a wise investment for any histological laboratory.

STROPPING

In some cases, particularly after machine sharpening, where the final abrasive used is extremely fine, no further treatment is required before using the knife for section cutting. It is common practice however, in spite of theoretical objections, for stropping to be carried out after honing to give further refinement to the knife edge. The objectors to stropping claim that the fine edge produced by honing will be impaired by the softer materials used for stropping, but in fact, many accomplished microtomists will maintain a very sharp edge for a long time and will prepare many sections by frequent stropping of the knife.

Stropping consists of moving the knife with edge trailing (opposite direction from honing) lightly over the surface of leather which may be impregnated with fine abrasive such as jeweller's rouge. Strops may either be mounted on a solid base or be of the flexible or hanging type, the latter being pulled as taut as possible in use, to prevent rounding of the edge. Cork of suitable texture, mounted on a board will also provide an effective stropping surface. As with hones, strops should be protected from dust and dirt when not in use and a sheath made from polythene film makes a suitable covering.

CONTAMINATION

It is important that knives should be thoroughly cleaned after honing or stropping for it has been shown (Taggart 1970) that traces of metal dust remaining on the knife edge may be transferred to the section during cutting and subsequently give a false-positive Prussian blue reaction for ferric iron.

SAFETY PRECAUTIONS

All knife sharpening, both honing and stropping, should be done in the most secluded part of the laboratory. Strops should never be sited near to a door and serious accidents may be avoided if restraint is exercised in approaching a person who is intently engaged in knife sharpening.

Section cutting

The preparation of blemish-free sections from animal tissues depends on: (1) properly prepared tissue; (2) a suitable microtome in good condition; (3) a sharp knife; and (4) the skill of the microtomist. The first three criteria may be provided, the fourth may only be gained by practice and the following should be considered as a general guide and supplement to practical section cutting.

The general specification of microtomes has been given, but, regardless of the type of machine chosen, some thought should be given to the position of the microtome on the bench and the posture of the microtomist. Rocking and rotary microtomes lend themselves to low (75–85 cm) benches and a sitting position. The chair should be firm and swivelling chairs are less satisfactory. The larger, base sledge microtomes are less convenient to operate than the foregoing and some microtomists find it more satisfactory to stand at a higher (92 cm) bench with these machines. A trial of various positions should be made but the cutting area should be well lit, away from doors and open windows, and, preferably, remote from the constant passage of other workers.

RELATION OF KNIFE TO OBJECT

The basic principle of advancement of the specimen against the knife edge at a predetermined thickness is common to all microtomes with any embedding media. Provision is made on most microtomes for variation of the position of the knife in relation to the object. Most important are the angles of tilt and slant.

SLANT AND TILT OF KNIVES

SLANT OF THE KNIFE

The slant of a microtome knife may be defined as the angle its edge makes with the line of section or direction of travel of the object.

In FIGURE 5.11A the object presents a square face to the knife edge. For the preparation of ribbons of sections, two edges of the block must be parallel to

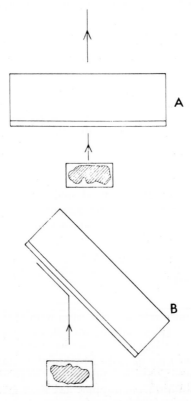

FIG. 5.11. Slant of microtome knives. A = nil slant, knife edge parallel to object; B = 45 degree slant.

each other as well as to the knife edge. This position is commonly used with wax embedded material especially with rocking and rotary microtomes which do not usually have provision for alteration of the slant of the knife.

In FIGURE 5.11B the knife has been positioned obliquely to the block. This position is used extensively with cellulose nitrate embedded material and with wax embedded, narrow strips of hard material on sliding and base sledge microtomes.

TILT (OR INCLINATION) OF THE KNIFE

Knife-tilt is defined as the angle between the surface of the block and a line bisecting the edge of the knife [FIG. 5.12].

Where knife-tilt is adjustable, an engraved scale will be found on the knife holder of the microtome although this may register quite arbitrary values and

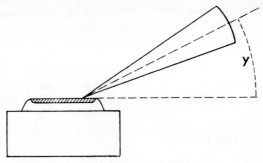

FIG. 5.12   Tilt of microtome knives. y = angle of tilt, here 30 degrees.

not actual degrees of tilt. In practice however, less tilt is used with soft objects than with hard and there must always be sufficient clearance to avoid compression of the object against the back of the knife after passing the edge. Tilt angle may vary between 10 and 40 degrees according to the shape of the knife and, particularly, depending on the angle of the cutting facet [FIG. 5.9]. In practice, the critical value is the angle between the object and lower cutting facet. This is commonly called the clearance angle, is usually between 3 and 10 degrees and in turn, governs the angle of tilt according to the profile of the knife.

RATE OF CUTTING AND TEMPERATURE

Both the slant and the tilt of the knife are important factors in microtomy; no less important are the rate of cutting and the ambient temperature, the latter especially with wax embedded tissues.

RATE OF CUTTING

Each embedding medium has an optimum cutting rate for a given thickness of section and, being aware of this, may be quickly determined. Soft tissue embedded in a soft medium (brain in celloidin) requires a slow, smooth action and too fast and forceful a rate will cause badly compressed sections. On the other hand, the cutting of ribbons of sections from a paraffin wax embedded specimen requires a more brisk and rhythmic rate of cutting. The combined variation in the consistency of tissues and embedding media and required thickness of section is almost infinite, but the most suitable combination of knife slant, tilt, and cutting rate should, with practice, be readily found.

TEMPERATURE

The air temperature of the laboratory has some effect on section cutting, particularly with wax embedded tissue and in warm weather it may be necessary to cool the block to prevent softening of the wax and to allow thin sections to be prepared. A convenient way to cool tissue blocks is by the application of an ice-bag. These may be easily prepared by sealing a small amount of water in a sachet made from polythene film. This is frozen in the refrigerator and used repeatedly as required. It avoids the swelling effects of direct contact of tissue with water and reduces the possibility of rusting of the microtome.

Less frequently, the surrounding temperature is too low, resulting in failure of sections to ribbon or an inability to cut sections of the requisite *thickness* because of the hardness of the embedding medium. This may be remedied by warming the atmosphere locally with a Bunsen burner, electric lamp, or fire, or by breathing on the block before each section is cut (a combination of warmth and moisture). It should be noted however, that applied heat and moisture, or removal of a source of cooling, will result in expansion of the object and a section thickness greater than the setting of the feed mechanism.

ORIENTATION OF THE BLOCK

Most microtomes have provision for orientation of the specimen to allow the presentation of a particular area of the tissue to the knife edge but in practice, blocks of embedded tissue are usually trimmed with parallel upper (cutting) and lower (base) surfaces and are affixed so that the cutting surface lies parallel to the surface of the object holder.

PARAFFIN WAX, CELLOIDIN-PARAFFIN, AND ESTER WAX EMBEDDED TISSUE

PREPARATION OF THE BLOCK

The increasing use of plastic embedding moulds and systems such as Peelaway and Tissue-Tek [p. 63] where blocks are clamped directly into the microtome chuck avoids the necessity for block-shaping and mounting on to a suitable holder. For paraffin blocks embedded in other ways proceed as follows.

With the cutting surface of the tissue uppermost, pare away surplus wax from the sides of the block using a straight-edged scalpel, old table knife, or Heiffor-type microtome knife. The two edges to be presented to the knife should be parallel and trimmed so as to leave a 2–3 mm margin of wax: the other two sides may be trimmed closer to the tissue. Upper and lower surfaces of the block should be parallel and flat.

One or more corners may be cut off the block to aid orientation and easier separation of individual sections from a ribbon. The depth of the block will depend on the thickness of the tissue and will generally amount to the thickness of the tissue plus 2–4 mm of underlying embedding medium. A shallow block will be more stable than a deeper block when in the microtome with less likelihood of vibration on striking the knife.

Wooden blocks of suitable size to fit the microtome chuck may be used as object holders and should be made from hard-wood with plane surfaces, one of which may be scored to promote adhesion of the specimen. To fix a paraffin wax block to a wooden block, place some wax shavings on the surface of a wooden block, heat a metal spatula or other broad flat blade in the flame of a Bunsen burner and with the wax block in one hand and the hot spatula in the other, melt the wax shavings and lower the base of the block on to the spatula for a second before withdrawing the blade. Press down firmly on the block and complete the adhesion by applying the hot blade to the four sides of the wax block at the junction with the wooden block.

Object holders for some rocking and rotary microtomes consist of a metal platform or cylinder. These may be heated in a flame and then pressed directly to the base of the wax block to effect union.

PREPARATION OF MICROTOME AND TRIMMING OF SPECIMEN

Screw back the feed mechanism of rocking and rotary microtomes, lower the object clamp of base sledge microtomes. Fix the object in the clamp, tighten securely, and check that the paraffin block will be correctly orientated in relation to the knife edge. Secure the knife in the knife clamps, selecting an appropriate angle of tilt.

Operate the coarse adjustment of the feed mechanism or raise the object to just short of the knife and begin trimming the block (removal of surplus wax above the tissue and exposure of the complete surface area of the specimen). This trimming or 'roughing down' of the block is performed at a thickness setting of 12–15 µm with an old knife kept for the purpose. Even such old 'rough' knives should be sharpened occasionally as the too vigorous removal of thick slices with an exceedingly blunt knife may cause small pits in the surface of soft tissue [FIG. 5.13].

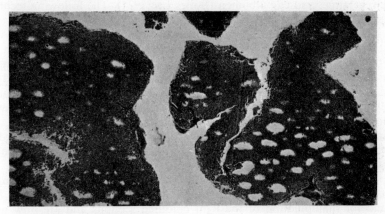

FIG. 5.13. Holes in a paraffin section of soft, cellular tissue caused by trimming the block with a blunt knife at too great a thickness. HE. × 15.

Very small specimens should be trimmed with great care and it is at this stage of section preparation that unsuspected foci of calcification will be revealed. These should on no account be excavated from the specimen but treated as described on page 208.

CUTTING OF SECTIONS

Replace the old knife with one reserved for actual section cutting noting that the latter may have a broader blade than the rough knife, necessitating the screwing back or lowering of the object. Select the required thickness setting (commonly 5 µm, but see page 76) and begin cutting.

With a sharp knife, a correctly adjusted microtome and properly processed material, sections will be cut and, with a brisk cutting rate, will adhere to one another in the form of a ribbon. The first section of the ribbon should be gently held with fine forceps and guided away from the knife as succeeding sections lengthen the ribbon.

MANIPULATION AND MOUNTING OF SECTIONS

When sufficient sections have been cut or when the ribbon is 10–15 cm in length it is detached from the knife by inserting a scalpel blade or needle between it and the knife edge taking care to avoid scraping the latter. It is then laid on a piece of black paper (the wrapping of X-ray or photographic film) prior to mounting on a glass slide.

Glass slides are available in various sizes, the most commonly used being 76 × 26 mm with a thickness of 1–1.2 mm. As received from the suppliers they are rarely clean enough for use and should be immersed in 1 per cent hydrochloric acid in 70 per cent alcohol and subsequently polished with a clean, fluff-free cloth.

During cutting, paraffin sections are always compressed and usually wrinkled and need to be flattened and mounted on slides before staining. Adhesives are not usually necessary. Nevertheless, many adhesive mixtures and ways of using them have been described and substances that have been recommended as adhesives range from quince jelly to garlic water and include sugar, gum, starch, gelatine, and egg albumen (Bolles Lee 1921). The following technique of flattening and mounting sections is widely used.

A strip of sections, or individual sections cut from a ribbon are gently lowered on to the surface of water 5–10 °C below the melting point of the wax. The sections will float, expand slightly, and become flatter. Wrinkles that remain may be removed by gentle stretching with fine (but not sharply pointed) forceps. Dip a clean slide in the water obliquely, the upper part above the surface slightly forward, the lower submerged portion tilted backwards. Draw the section towards the slide with forceps or needle and as the selected edge of the section touches the glass, remove the slide and section with an upward and forward motion. Confirm or alter the arrangement of the section on the slide (allowing space for a label) and stand up the slide to drain.

Specially designed, electrically heated, temperature controlled floating-out baths are made. These have black painted interiors to give a convenient background for manipulation of the light coloured sections and are now widely used.

When the use of an adhesive is advisable, e.g. with tissues given long mordanting in chrome salts or with brain or bone, the simplest method is to add the adhesive to the water in the floating-out bath. Separate stock solutions of 1 per cent gelatin and 1 per cent potassium dichromate should be prepared and added in a concentration of 0.002 per cent of each to the volume of water in the floating-out bath. Fresh water and adhesive should be used daily, and during the use of the bath the surface of the water should be frequently cleaned by skimming with a sheet of thin paper. When used as described, this adhesive does not take up stains.

The most commonly used adhesive is a mixture of egg albumen and glycerol. Traditionally made with the white of hen's eggs mixed with an equal volume of glycerol (Mayer 1883), it is now often prepared with dried egg albumen, flake, or powder. Concentrations vary from 2.5 per cent in equal parts of 0.5 per cent sodium chloride and glycerol (Faulkner and Lillie 1945) to 20 per cent in distilled water (Allan 1949). The mixture is smeared very thinly on a slide before mounting the section, either from a bowl of warm water as above or by floating the section on a little water added to the adhesive on the slide, the section being flattened by gentle heat from a flame or hot plate.

After the section has been mounted on a slide and most of the water drained away, thorough drying is essential. This may be done at room temperature but more quickly with greater heat. Methods used are: (1) drying for 16–24 hours in an incubator at 37 °C; (2) in an oven or on a hot plate at 45–50 °C for two hours or more; or (3) in an oven or on a hot plate at a temperature high enough to melt the wax (55–65 °C) for 30–60 minutes. There is some conflict of opinion, however, about the effect of melting the wax in the drying process and some authors stress that this should never be allowed to occur. Smith (1962) has described the shrinkage and distortion caused by the use of high temperatures (56–65 °C) and emphasizes the need for standardization in the laboratory (whatever the temperature used) to attain consistent results. On the other hand, Humason (1962) after warning of the damage caused by excessive heat, recommends that sections of lymphoid tissue and brain should be dried at 60–65 °C to avoid cracking. There is no doubt, however, that poorly fixed tissue is most likely to be damaged by heating and, in fact, the drying of sections of well prepared material at a temperature which just melts the wax is effective, should not produce gross artifacts and is widely practised.

SERIAL SECTIONS

Serial sectioning consists of the preparation of consecutive sections at a uniform thickness throughout the entire mass of the specimen. They are used in the teaching of histology, in embryological research and for the reconstruction of anatomical models.

The sectioning technique is little different from that in routine work but certain precautions should be observed and preparations made, for a 5 mm thick block of tissue should yield 1000 (5 μm) sections when cut serially. If the block is small enough, however, one or more strips of several sections may be mounted on one slide and the possibility of using a slide larger than 76 × 26 mm should be considered. Obviously, a ribboning medium is desirable for the purpose and paraffin wax is mainly used for serial work.

Before commencing, choose as draught-free a position for cutting as possible, for ribbons of sections are easily disturbed or damaged and as well as being kept in strict sequence, sections should all be the same way up. An inverted section is recognizable by the lower surface of a paraffin section always being shinier than the upper surface. Have available boxes, with lids, to receive the ribbons which should be laid on sheets of paper or cardboard, labelled to indicate the order in the sequence—the accidental loss of a section being indicated by a space of one (or more) sections between preceding and succeeding sections. The observance of this rule is especially important in embryological research work. Nothing is more misleading than 'serial' sections not in series although, to the practised eye, the gap is often evident.

The trimming or 'roughing down' of the block, practised routinely, will not apply in serial sectioning where the first portion of tissue to be exposed (however small) will be mounted. Accurate orientation of the block before cutting is therefore essential.

A uniform cutting rate should be used but if a halt in cutting is necessary, the feed mechanism should be retarded to avoid the cutting of an exceptionally thick section on resumption. This is because the block is compressed somewhat on meeting the knife and then expands afterwards. This expansion and contraction is of little account with a steady cutting rate. If time is allowed for the block to expand further however, a thicker section is inevitable and the series will comprise sections of unequal thickness which is undesirable.

Sections may be mounted as described earlier, arranging the sections on the slide with special care (see also Sack 1963). Strips of sections should be of equal length and one corner of the slide selected as a reference point to indicate the order, being marked with a diamond pencil as soon as it has received its full complement of sections. Decide in advance on the size of cover glass to be used, bearing in mind that sections expand on flattening and should not extend fully to any edge of the slide. This allows more convenient handling and avoids the edge of the slide or cover glass being included if the section is photographed.

The preparation of serial sections requires meticulous care, is time consuming and entails the subsequent examination of several hundred slides. These facts should be recognized before embarking on such work.

A compromise between strict serial sectioning and routine cutting (where a few sections only are cut from the block) and which is used particularly in pathology, is to prepare step sections at intervals through the block. This is done by cutting a few (2–4) sections, then trimming away, say, 50–100 μm of tissue, then cutting a further 2–4 sections and so on. Sections should be labelled to indicated the interval between each cutting.

CLASS SECTIONS

Less exacting than serial section work is the preparation of sections for general teaching purposes. This involves the cutting of 50–200 sections which are mounted singly and these do not require to be cut strictly serially although, in fact, not to do so only results in the waste of possibly rare material.

To conserve space, sections may be mounted on coverslips which are loaded into specially made racks, dried in an oven, stained *en masse*, and subsequently mounted on slides. Alternatively, the mica-slip method may be used. As many serial sections as possible are mounted on 76 × 50 mm albumenized mica-slips. When dry, these may be kept unstained until required. Staining is done as for slides and the mica-slip is then cut up into individual sections with fine scissors. To mount, place the mica-slip, section upwards, on a drop of mounting medium on a slide, add another drop of mountant, and apply a coverslip.

DIFFICULTIES IN SECTION CUTTING

Most difficulty in section cutting is caused through a blunt or damaged knife, poorly processed material, a maladjusted or worn microtome, or inappropriate choice of embedding medium and the remedy for each of these is self evident. Sometimes however, a less than perfectly prepared block is received for sectioning when time does not permit the complete re-processing of the material. In such cases the following procedures may prove useful in the preparation and flattening of sections.

The application of ice to the block is generally helpful but not invariably so and solid blood clot may be made more difficult to cut by this treatment. Instead, soaking the exposed surface of the tissue in cold running water is helpful and the addition of 0.2 per cent 'Teepol' (or other wetting-agent) to the water imparts a better consistency for cutting. Badly processed fibrous tissue and muscle will benefit from this treatment or by soaking in a mixture of 9 parts 60 per cent alcohol to 1 part glycerol (Baker 1942), but note that this, and other softening fluids, will cause superficial swelling of the tissue and should be used with discretion.

Some tissue cuts well but wrinkles excessively and the preliminary flattening of the section on the slide with 0.2 per cent 'Teepol' before transferring to warm water (Whiting 1958) removes wrinkles and is less damaging to the section than the use of alcohol for the same purpose.

When non-calcified tissues fragment during cutting and the above treatments fail, a complete section may sometimes be obtained by painting the surface of the block with 0.5 per cent celloidin in alcohol–ether, allowing this to dry and then cutting the section which may require a higher temperature than usual for flattening. Another way is to apply Sellotape [p. 209] to give support to the section or, gummed paper which is stuck to the surface of the block and removed during flattening of the section in water (Hart 1962). These 'tape' methods are intended primarily for the preparation of sections of undecalcified bone which is a special problem. Difficulties in the preparation of sections of soft tissues are generally easier to prevent than to remedy but see TABLE 5.1.

STORAGE OF SECTIONS

Unstained paraffin sections mounted on slides and properly dried may be stored indefinitely if protected from dust and scratches [but see p. 222]. Specially designed slide storage cabinets may be used and those that hold slides in an upright position, one against another, are less space consuming than others where slides are laid flat in shallow drawers. Whatever method is used, it is advisable to ensure that floor or shelves are strong enough to support the considerable weight of an accumulation of many slides. Cardboard boxes or trays are commonly used for the temporary storage of slides and for their movement within the laboratory.

ESTER WAX BLOCKS

These are prepared for cutting in the same way as paraffin wax with leading and trailing edges of the block parallel to each other and the knife edge.

An appropriate cutting rate is essential with Ester wax and Steedman (1960) recommends a rate of 30–50 sections per minute.

Sections are flattened on water at 40–45 °C, mounted on albumenized slides and dried at 40–45 °C.

CELLULOSE NITRATE EMBEDDED TISSUE

PREPARATION OF THE BLOCK

The hardened block is trimmed to leave a margin of 10 mm around the tissue, thus facilitating handling during cutting and subsequent staining. The depth of the block should be 10–20 mm, according to the thickness of the tissue. Upper and lower surfaces of the block should be parallel and flat.

The trimmed block is attached by means of an adhesive to a hard-wood or

Table 5.1 Faults in section cutting and their remedy

Fault	Cause	Remedy
Ribbon is curved instead of straight	Either the edges of the block are not parallel to one another and to the knife, or, if one border of the section is crumpled, the knife edge is dull at that point	1. Pare away wax until edges of the block are parallel 2. Move knife along until the edge presented is uniformly sharp
Ribbon curls upward as sections are cut	The tilt of the knife is too great	Reduce tilt
Sections cut well individually but do not adhere together to form a ribbon	The wax is too hard for the temperature at which sections are being cut, or the rate of cutting is too slow	1. Coat the leading edge of the block with soft (45–50 °C) wax 2. Warm the room, or place a lighted Bunsen burner or lamp close by 3. Cut sections more rapidly
Sections crumple	The paraffin wax is too soft or the knife is blunt	1. Cool block by application of ice 2. Sharpen the knife
Sections are longitudinally scratched	Knife edge is serrated or is coated with debris from previous sections. Tissue contains small foci of calcification	1. Hone the knife 2. Clean the knife edge 3. Apply surface decalcification
Sections cut sometimes thick, sometimes thin	Faulty feed mechanism which may lack oil. Knife is improperly clamped or the block holder is loose. The block is not securely attached to the object holder and 'springs' under pressure of the knife	Obvious

Table 5.1 Faults in section cutting and their remedy—*continued*

Fault	Cause	Remedy
There are thick and thin zones in each section (chatters)	The knife vibrates owing to hardness of the object, or excessive tilt, or movement caused by play on slides of the microtome (especially sledge type)	Soften the block if possible, or use a heavier knife and a less worn microtome
Resistance is felt when the block is near the downward limit of its travel (with rotary and rocking microtomes)	Tilt of the knife is insufficient, the paraffin block being pressed against the base of the knife towards the end of the stroke	Increase the tilt
Sections of uneven thickness are produced and a harsh metallic note is emitted on contact of knife and object	Tilt of the knife is too great and a second section may be cut with the feed mechanism disengaged, the block having expanded to its original size	Reduce the tilt
Width of sections much less than that of block	Knife edge, though perhaps smooth, has too broad a cutting facet	Hone or re-grind to reduce angle of cutting facet
Sections crumble into fragments	Bad processing or unsuitable medium	Apply a thin film of dilute celloidin to surface of the block each time a section is cut, or re-process
Sections have tight irremovable wrinkles across their surface (most common with tissues such as lymph node and brain)	Knife or object holder being moved with too much force and too quickly	Cut more slowly, using less force

plastic object holder, the surface of which is scored to promote adhesion and the area of which should be at least as great as the underside of the specimen block. The traditional adhesive for the purpose is the thickest solution of celloidin or LVN but a commercial adhesive such as Durofix [p. 503] may be used with success. In either case, the object holder is thoroughly cleaned before application of the adhesive while the underside of the specimen block may be softened by brief immersion in alcohol–ether. Specimen and support are pressed firmly together. The object holder with attached block is now inverted in a shallow dish of 70 per cent alcohol and a weight applied to maintain contact of the two surfaces. Satisfactory adhesion will take from one to two hours.

Almost immediate attachment of block to object holder may be obtained by using one of the 'instant-setting glues' (Eastwood 1977).

SECTION CUTTING

A sliding or base sledge microtome is most suitable for sectioning cellulose nitrate embedded material.

The object holder with attached specimen is clamped securely in the chuck of the microtome and oriented so that the knife (wedge or planoconcave profile) is parallel to and above the surface of the specimen. The knife is positioned obliquely to produce a shearing effect, the slant being about 45 degrees. The optimum tilt of the blade will vary with the angle of its cutting facet and the consistency of the tissue. The consistency of embedding medium and tissue will also determine the type of knife used and generally, with a softer block, a planoconcave knife is necessary while with a harder block (high concentration LVN) a wedge profile knife will be satisfactory.

The complete surface area of the tissue is exposed by a series of cutting strokes with the thickness regulator set at 20 μm. The action should be slow and smooth, the knife and specimen being constantly wetted with 70 per cent alcohol either by the use of a pipette or dropping bottle, or from a special reservoir with drip-outlet which may be attached to the microtome. (Some microtomes incorporate a tray to receive excess alcohol or one may be made by the user from metal or plastic to surround the object stage and prevent the washing away of oil or grease from moving parts.)

The thickness selected for sectioning will vary with the material and the purpose of the investigation but will commonly be in the 15–25 μm range. It is rarely possible to cut at less than 10 μm. Sections are unrolled or flattened while on the knife and are transferred to a dish of 70 per cent alcohol with brush or forceps to await staining.

It is necessary to preserve and identify the sequence of cut sections, this may be done by placing each section on a sheet of thin paper (toilet paper) cut slightly larger than the size of the section, each or some of which may be numbered with Indian ink. A pack of such sections may be kept together in alcohol by enclosing in a folder or envelope of polythene film. For the manipulation and staining of cellulose nitrate sections, singly and in series, see page 135.

After cutting, the blocks, which should never be allowed to dry, are returned to 70 per cent alcohol for storage. Alcohol should be mopped up from the microtome and the machine oiled; knives should also be carefully dried.

PREPARATION OF FROZEN SECTIONS

Frozen sections have important advantages over sections prepared in other ways. They are desirable or obligatory for the following purposes:

1. In surgical pathology where a section may be required and a diagnosis made in a few minutes, during the course of an operation.
2. For the demonstration of lipids, most, but not all of which are dissolved by the reagents used in the paraffin wax and cellulose nitrate methods.
3. In histochemistry, especially with unfixed tissue, where the use of processing reagents would result in loss or alteration of the substances to be demonstrated, particularly enzymes.
4. For demonstration of the components of the central nervous system, to avoid shrinkage and to allow better penetration of stains.
5. In fluorescent antibody techniques [p. 323].
6. For the preparation of sections of material such as tendon that would be difficult to cut or flatten after paraffin embedding.

While the freezing method is very much quicker than other forms of microtomy and the sections lack the artifacts produced by tissue processing, it is not an ideal method. One important disadvantage is that after cutting, blocks of tissue must either be stored in a low temperature cabinet, or in a jar of fixative or preservative at room temperature, or processed to make a paraffin block which latter, though providing more convenient storage, introduces artifacts that were avoided by freezing in the first instance.

It is impossible to prepare ribbons of frozen sections and serial sectioning is more difficult than with wax embedded material. In addition, the preparation of very thin sections (1–3 μm) is not as readily accomplished as when the tissue is embedded in wax or a synthetic resin.

PREPARATION OF MATERIAL

Specimens for cutting on the freezing microtome should not exceed 3 mm in thickness, for as the size of the specimen increases, so does the time required for freezing and the probability of the formation of ice-crystal artifacts.

Ten per cent formal-saline gives a particularly satisfactory consistency to tissues for frozen sectioning. No after-treatment is required and blocks may be placed on the microtome directly from the fixative.

Mercuric chloride-containing fixatives will damage the microtome knife, being corrosive to metal. Tissues so fixed should be treated with iodine–alcohol to remove mercury pigment and well washed in running water.

Chrome salts should be washed out in water and tissues fixed in alcohol (although rarely required for freezing, since it is likely that the alcohol was used expressly to avoid water) should also be well washed because alcohol inhibits freezing.

The consistency imparted to tissues by being frozen is usually satisfactory for sectioning without a supporting medium but, for convenience in handling, small multiple fragments such as uterine curettings require embedding in gelatine or agar [p. 72] and lung, skeletal muscle, and papillomata, though cutting without difficulty, need the support of an embedding medium to prevent disintegration of sections.

MICROTOMY

Frozen sections are prepared either with a special freezing microtome or by the adaptation of one or another of the microtomes already described.

The low temperature necessary is obtained by: (1) compressed carbon dioxide; (2) with thermo-electric cooling devices (thermo modules); by a refrigerated microtome (cryostat); or (4) dichlorofluoromethane aerosol sprays which have replaced ethyl chloride sprays.

CO_2 Freezing microtomes

A narrow bore, stoutly covered flexible hose connects the valve of the cylinder to the object holder of the microtome which is hollow and provided with holes or slots at the edge to allow the escape of the expanding, vaporizing carbon dioxide which cools the specimen. Most freezing microtomes have provision for a knife-cooling device (from a separate source of CO_2).

With cylinders not fitted with an internal tube, the valve should always be above the level of the object stage of the microtome to ensure the *liquid* CO_2 enters the stage. Cylinders fitted with an internal tube (syphon) should be stood upright, below the microtome. Freshly charged cylinders of CO_2 (without an internal tube) may contain some water. This should be 'blown off' by opening the valve briefly, with the cylinder inverted, *before connecting to the microtome*. Liquid CO_2 is at a pressure of about 7000 kPa and the possible consequences of the connecting tube becoming blocked are obvious. This tube should, therefore, be as short as possible, ideally 20–30 cm, although a greater length than this will be necessary to allow movement with a base sledge microtome. Securely tighten the tube connections, making sure that the fibre washers give a gas-tight fit.

TECHNIQUE

1. Lower the object holder to give clearance between the top of the tissue block and the knife edge. Place the specimen on the stage on a drop of water or gum, or on a small piece of wet blotting paper or gauze. This is to secure adhesion between tissue and the stage.
2. Insert the knife in the clamps and tighten securely, a wedge profile knife being most suitable.
3. Bring the surface of the tissue to just below the knife edge, using the coarse feed adjustment.
4. Adjust the feed mechanism to the desired setting (usually 10–15 µm).
5. Open the valve on the cylinder and then operate the lever controlling the admittance of CO_2 to the object stage. Do this in short bursts of one or two seconds' duration with a similar interval between bursts. Operate the knife-cooler (if fitted) in a similar fashion. Observe the tissue, which will whiten as freezing proceeds, from below upwards. Immediately before the block is completely white, cease freezing.
6. Operate the microtome and cut sections.

NOTES

1. Given a sharp knife, the most important factor in the preparation of frozen sections is the correct assessment of the optimum temperature and consistency of tissue for cutting, the best temperature unfortunately being of short duration when using intermittent CO_2 cooling.
2. If the tissue is too cold, the sections split into fragments and the knife

makes a characteristically harsh sound as it passes through the hard block. The remedy is to wait a while for slight thawing or to warm the tissue by application of the finger to the surface of the block.
3. If the tissue is too warm, the sections will accumulate on the knife edge in a pulp and will be difficult or impossible to deal with, while the block may be swept off the stage by the impact of the knife. The tissue should be re-frozen.

MOUNTING OF SECTIONS

With CO_2 microtomes, sections are removed from the knife with the finger or a moistened brush and transferred to a bowl of distilled water. They are then stained either by lifting the sections from one solution to another by means of a bent glass rod or after being first mounted on slides. This may be done in a variety of ways, two of which are as follows.

1. An albumenized slide is lowered into the bowl and the section manipulated so that one edge rests against the surface of the slide. Allow the free end of the section to unfold and then carefully withdraw the slide. Stand the slide upright to drain and allow the section to dry completely. This may take 15–20 minutes and is indicated by the section becoming uniformly opaque white.
   Poulding (1959) recommends the addition of 0.1 per cent liquid detergent to the water to help the flattening of frozen sections.
2. Leach's method. Place clean slides in 2.5 per cent gelatine in 1 per cent phenol at 37 °C for a few minutes. Wipe one side of the slide clean and allow the other side to dry at room temperature away from dust. Float the section on to the slide, drain off surplus fluid and allow to become nearly dry at room temperature. Place the slides for five minutes in a closed jar containing a little 40 per cent formaldehyde, the vapour from which acts on the gelatine and causes adhesion of the sections.
   Unmounted frozen sections may be stored in 5 per cent formal-saline.

Thermo-electric cooling devices

A more recent development in the preparation of frozen sections of both fixed and unfixed tissues is the use of thermo-electric cooling devices. These consist of layers of dissimilar semi-conducting materials through which is passed low voltage, direct current. This results in either heat loss or heat gain, depending on the direction of the current (Peltier effect). The series-connected thermo-elements are surmounted by a metal plate which forms the stage for the specimen while beneath the elements is a water-cooled 'heat sink' to dissipate the heat produced.

Variation of the electric current fed to the stage alters the temperature of stage and specimen and allows the optimum cutting temperature to be readily determined for any tissue. Initial cooling of the *stage* is quick (−30 °C in about 30 seconds) and with current and water coolant continuously applied, the selected temperature may be maintained indefinitely. Some tissues, however, particularly those rich in lipid such as brain, may require several minutes after switching on the current to reach a temperature low enough to permit sectioning; they should be pre-cooled before affixing to the stage.

Additional units may be used for cooling the knife and are essential with unfixed tissue (Hardy and Rutherford 1962) and an anti-roll plate may be used to keep sections flat as with the cryostat.

The initial cost of thermo-elements and power-pack should be set against the cost of purchase or hiring of gas cylinders and the recurrent expenditure for CO_2, but the equipment can be used with virtually any microtome which need not be restricted to frozen section work only, as is the case with the cryostat.

The cryostat

The growth of histochemistry and the need for a more satisfactory method for the preparation of thin sections of unfixed tissues has resulted in the development and extensive use of cold microtomes or cryostats (Pearse 1960; Hollands 1962) [FIG. 5. 14].

As has been noted above, a major disadvantage of the CO_2-freezing microtome is the constantly changing temperature of the tissue caused by repeated freezing, following application of CO_2, alternating with thawing—caused by the higher ambient temperature. This freezing and thawing results in: (1) inactivation of some enzymes; and (2) an inability to prepare multiple sections of uniform thickness.

Originally described by Linderstrom-Lang and Mogensen (1938), the cold microtome or cryostat consists of a microtome contained within a refrigerated

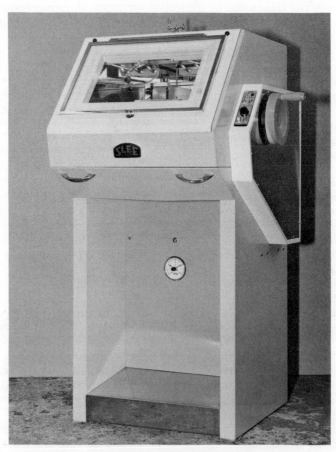

FIG. 5.14.   Cryostat (Slee Medical Equipment Ltd.).

cabinet designed to operate at -5 to $-30\,°C$. In the earlier models, openings in the cabinet were provided for the (gloved) hands of the microtomist to make the necessary manipulations. Contemporary models have completely external controls, a small opening being used for the removal of sections.

The kind of microtome used in a cryostat is relatively unimportant. Most rotary types are modified for this purpose by the use of stainless steel components. This avoids corrosion of parts and also substantially increases the cost of the instruments. The Cambridge rocking microtome is widely used in Great Britain and its simple construction and few moving parts allow trouble-free operation at low temperature.

All cryostats incorporate an anti-roll plate either of plastic material (with a low coefficient of friction) or in the form of a glass plate coated by spraying with a similar material. Its purpose is to keep the sections flat on the knife blade for subsequent direct mounting on to a slide or coverslip, or delivery down a metal chute into a container of reagent. The correct positioning of the anti-roll plate in relation to the knife is essential and requires careful adjustment.

A clearance of 70 μm to accommodate the section can be obtained by the following method (Sandison 1965). A length of Sellotape is placed sticky-side upwards on the bench and the guide is placed upon this with its working-side upward. The Sellotape is trimmed on either side to give 3 mm margins, and these are brought forward over the edges on the working face. When the face of the guide plate is in position the Sellotape acts as stops giving 70 μm clearance through which the section slides.

As with any other form of frozen sectioning, the exact temperature best suited to the preparation of sections in a cryostat will vary according to the type of tissue and the thickness of section required. In general, a cabinet temperature of -15 to $-20\,°C$ provides suitable conditions for a wide range of tissues. Where lower temperatures are required, e.g. with fatty material, additional cooling may be effected by the application of solid CO_2 to either knife or object holder, for although cryostats are provided with a means of regulating the thermostat, this is not effective quick enough for the microtomist confronted with tissue requiring a lower temperature than the setting in use.

Fixed tissue may not yield such good sections as immediately frozen fresh tissue, this being due to: (1) the tissue being affected by artifacts of fixation; and (2) an inferior consistency at the low temperature of the cryostat due to the added water (ice) from the fixative.

Fresh frozen sections (cryostat technique)

Blocks of fresh tissue up to 3 mm thick, not larger than the block holder platform, are selected. Fatty tissue should be trimmed away as much as possible as fat thaws more quickly than other tissues. Small fragments can be handled more easily if they are included in a block of solid tissue such as rat liver. It must be remembered that unfixed diseased tissues may carry a risk of infection and require strict bacteriological technique.

The block is mounted in a small quantity of 1 per cent glucose or water on the platform of the chuck standing vertically on the bench, and must be immediately frozen (quenched). This can be carried out in various ways, but liquid carbon dioxide from a cylinder or solid carbon dioxide (dry ice) are satisfactory. By holding two large pieces of dry ice in thickly gloved hands on opposite sides of the block holder the tissue will be rapidly frozen without artifacts; loud vibration may take place at first. The chuck with the frozen tissue is transferred to the microtome maintained at -15 to $-20\,°C$ in the refrigerated chamber. The window is closed and the block is trimmed to its full face, using one end of the knife. The coarse feed control must be advanced slowly or the block may be detached or the knife edge damaged. The knife is kept clean by making upward sweeps with a brush introduced through the porthole. The knife is now moved to give a fresh cutting edge and sections are cut (usually at 4–5 μm) with the anti-roll guide plate in position.

A section is cut and the anti-roll plate is removed. The section is picked up from the surface of the knife on to a slide or coverslip carried through the porthole on a suction holder. The section should adhere to the slide or cover-slip which is briefly dried against the back of the hand. For enzyme techniques, incubating medium is delivered straight on to the unfixed section on the slide. Alternatively, unmounted sections are allowed to fall direct from the cryostat microtome knife into a dish of the incubating medium. For conventional histo-logical staining techniques (HE, etc.) and for some enzyme methods, dry mounted sections are fixed in 5 per cent acetic acid in absolute ethyl alcohol (Wolman's fixative). The tissue block may be stored in the refrigerated cham-ber for a limited time, and it is advisable to do this until satisfactory mounted preparations of the histochemical reaction have been obtained. Alternatively, the tissue block can be thawed, placed in fixative and processed as a routine paraffin block.

Complete de-frosting of the apparatus will be required from time to time, depending partly on the frequency of opening the cabinet and local humidity. All parts of the microtome and fittings should be cleaned, dried and lubricated with suitable low-temperature oil or grease where necessary.

Aerosol sprays

Aerosol sprays of dichlorofluoromethane (under various trade names) may be used for freezing small pieces of tissue but are slower in action than carbon dioxide. They may occasionally be useful with 'difficult' paraffin wax-embedded tissues in high ambient temperatures.

Rapid frozen section technique

The precise method used for the preparation of sections for diagnosis within a few minutes from receipt of the specimen will depend on the pathologist, the time and equipment available and, to a certain extent, on the tissue to be examined. Whatever method is adopted, frequent practice with a variety of tissues is a condition of success and while speed is the keynote of the opera-tion, a good section prepared in say, eight minutes will be of more help to all concerned than an unrecognizable offering produced in four minutes.

PREPARATION OF SECTIONS

With the carbon dioxide microtome, it is usual for the tissue to be fixed in hot (80–90 °C) or boiling 10 per cent formal-saline for 1–2 minutes before placing on the microtome and cutting. In practice, boiling water is just as effective and lacks the obnoxious fumes of formalin.

Sections are received into a bowl of distilled water containing 0.1 per cent wetting agent and are mounted on to an albumenized slide, drained, blotted with a hard filter paper, and dried by holding high over a Bunsen flame.

Cryostat sections are cut unfixed, mounted on slides as described above, and fixed before staining.

STAINING

Three main methods are used. One is a rapid haematoxylin and eosin stain using a vigorous nuclear haematoxylin such as Mayer's, Harris', or Cole's [p. 139] for one or two minutes with or without differentiation, followed by 'blue-ing' in tap water substitute [p. 142], counterstaining in eosin in alcohol (which also dehydrates), completion of dehydration, clearing in xylene, and mounting in resinous media.

The second method aims at a haematoxylin and eosin effect (blue nuclei and pink cytoplasm) by the use of a rapidly acting single solution such as the Solochrome cyanine RS mixture of Hyman and Poulding (1961).

The third and most rapid method of staining frozen sections is by the use of a simple aqueous solution of thionin, methylene blue, or toluidine blue followed directly by application of coverslip and examination. Such preparations are not permanent and lack the clarity of sections which are dehydrated and cleared prior to mounting in a resinous medium.

NOTE

In all three of the above methods a preliminary de-fatting of the tissue, by treatment of the section with absolute alcohol and xylene followed by rehydration, will improve the clarity of staining and give an appearance more akin to that of an HE stained paraffin section of similar material.

SYNTHETIC RESIN EMBEDDED TISSUE

The techniques of ultra-microtomy are outside the scope of this book. For details of the preparation, microtomy, and staining of material for examination with the electron microscope see Glauert (1974), Reid (1974), and Lewis and Knight (1977). Thin (1 μm) sections of resin embedded tissue for examination with the light microscope may be cut on an ultra-microtome with glass knives or on a conventional sledge or rotary microtome using wedge or D-profile steel knives [p. 83]. A slow, steady cutting stroke is essential. Sections are mounted on a drop of water on a slide, dried on a hotplate, and stained with routine histological stains without removal of the embedding medium (Lee 1977). For details of the microtomy of resin embedded, undecalcified bone see page 210.

FREEZE-DRIED TISSUE

The section cutting technique used with freeze-dried material will be that appropriate to the particular embedding medium used which may be paraffin wax, water soluble wax or, possibly, a synthetic resin. The fact that the tissue is dehydrated but not fixed however, means that special procedures have to be adopted for 'floating-out' and mounting of cut sections and for the storage of blocks after cutting.

MANIPULATION OF SECTIONS

No special microtome is required and sections are cut at 5–7 μm. Sections are mounted directly on a warmed albumenized slide and gently flattened by pressure of finger or thumb. (If not precluded by the nature of the investigation, sections may be floated on the surface of an appropriate fixative.)

STORAGE OF BLOCKS

After cutting, the exposed surface of the tissue is protected by coating with molten paraffin wax and the block stored (preferably at 4 °C) in a desiccator over calcium chloride or other drying agent.

REFERENCES

ALLAN, R. D. (1949). *Bull. Inst. med. Lab. Technol.* **14**, 185.

BAKER, J. R. (1942). *J. roy. micr. Soc.* **61**, 75.

BOLLES LEE, A. (1921). *The microtomist's* vade mecum, 8th edn. Churchill, London.

EASTWOOD, H. (1977). *Med. Lab. Sci.* **34**, 271.

FAULKNER, R. R. and LILLIE, R. D. (1945). *Stain Technol.* **20**, 99.

GLAUERT, A. M. (1974). *Practical methods in electron microscopy*, Vol. 3. Part I. North Holland, Amsterdam.

HARDY, W. S. and RUTHERFORD, T. (1962). *Nature (Lond.)* **196**, 785.

HART, P. (1962). *J. med. Lab. Technol.* **19**, 115.

HOLLANDS, B. C. S. (1962). In *Progress in medical laboratory technique* (ed. F. J. Baker), Vol. 1. Butterworths, London.

HUMASON, G. L. (1962). *Animal tissue techniques*, p. 60. W. H. Freeman, San Francisco.

HYMAN, J. M. and POULDING, R. H. (1961). *J. med. Lab. Technol.* **18**, 107.

LEE, R. L. (1977). *Med. Lab. Sci.* **34**, 231.

LEWIS, P. R. and KNIGHT, D. P. (1977). *Practical methods in electron microscopy* (ed. A. M. Glauert), Vol. 5, Part II. North Holland, Amsterdam.

LINDERSTROM-LANG, K. and MOGENSEN, K. R. (1938). *C.R. Lab. Carlsberg, Sér. chim.* **23**, 27.

MAYER, P. (1883). *Mitth. Zool. Stat. Neapel* **4**, 521.

MOORE, G. W. (1951). *J. med. Lab. Technol.* **9**, 86.

PEARSE, A. G. E. (1960). *Histochemistry, theoretical and applied*, 2nd edn. Churchill, London.

POULDING, R. H. (1959). *J. med. Lab. Technol.* **16**, 58.

REID, N. (1974). *Practical methods in electron microscopy*, Vol. 3, Part II. North Holland, Amsterdam.

SACK, O. W. (1963). *Stain Technol.* **38**, 315.

SANDISON, A. T. (1965). Association of Clinical Pathologists Broadsheet No. 49.

SMITH, A. (1962). *Stain Technol.* **37**, 339.

STEEDMAN, H. F. (1960). *Section cutting in microscopy*. Blackwell, Oxford.

TAGGART, M. E. (1970). *J. med. Lab. Technol.* **27**, 36.

WHITING, G. (1958). *J. med. Lab. Technol.* **15**, 204.

6 | The theory and practice of staining

HISTORICAL

The foundations of histology were laid before the advent of staining methods. Early attempts to stain tissues, such as those of Leeuwenhoek (1719) using saffron, were neither wholly successful nor followed up by others (Conn 1948), and specimens were examined unstained. Crudely dissociated tissues or rough free-hand sections were examined in water, and by the middle of the nineteenth century accurate descriptions of the microscopical structure of tissues had been published (Kölliker 1852). From this time the development of the dye industry took place, and the application of commercial dyes to histology enabled details of cellular structure, previously invisible, to be seen and studied. Staining techniques originate from the second half of the last century, and many methods have changed little since that time.

Carmine staining was first introduced by the botanists Göppert and Cohn (1849), but they only achieved a diffuse coloration of the tissues. The first use of a selective nuclear stain may be attributed to Gerlach (1858) who was attempting to stain nerve cells. After initial failure '. . . a section of cerebellum, hardened in potassium bichromate, was left by oversight in an exceedingly dilute solution of ammoniacal carmine, and when found 24 hours later was beautifully stained, the nerve fibres and the nerve cells being differentiated' (Gustav Mann 1902).

Gerlach also discovered regressive staining [p. 116] by differentiation in weak acetic acid. Haematoxylin was first used as an unsatisfactory watery extract, but two years later Böhmer (1865) combined haematoxylin with alum as a mordant [p. 117] and obtained more specific staining. The aniline dyes were later developed for industrial use, and these dyes, together with haematoxylin, still comprise the commonest stains used in histology. Most of the old historical stains still persist, and though carmine is now less used for histology, it is still retained by zoologists for the staining of whole preparations (entire organisms) such as cestodes, medusae, etc. Present-day staining methods are commonly modifications of classical methods; techniques of recent origin are mainly histochemical methods giving coloured reactions for the identification of specific chemical structures and enzymes.

OBJECTIVES OF HISTOLOGICAL STAINING METHODS

As tissues and their constituent cells are usually transparent and colourless, different structures cannot be easily distinguished from each other when examined with the conventional light microscope. Successful histological techniques used for the distinction of tissue components commonly cause two changes in the tissue, either an alteration of *contrast* or an alteration in *colour*.

Changes in tissue contrast can be brought about by microscopical methods, such as phase contrast or the use of polarized light. These make parts of the tissue grey or black and the same result can be achieved by impregnation methods, whereby opaque silver or other metallic compounds are deposited upon the surfaces of cells, commonly fibres. More often, histological staining methods depend on the production of colours in the tissues by dye-staining; this modifies the wavelength of the light that has been passed through the stained tissue, thereby imparting colour into the tissue and its cells. The coloration of tissues by the dyes used in staining solutions is due to the absorption of light by the dye. A yellow dye will absorb red and blue and transmit yellow, so the stain solution or the tissue components stained by the dye appear yellow. A blue–red stain will absorb yellow and appear blue–red. If a tissue component is stained by the yellow dye and the blue–red dye, it will absorb all colours and appear to be black.

Successful staining methods are both *specific* and *sensitive*. Specificity or selectivity is the ability to discriminate between individual tissue components and to colour one or a few of these, leaving the others unstained. It is obviously important if one wishes to demonstrate a particular component that the stain should select that component and no others; diffuse staining is imprecise and is unsuitable for histological techniques. Sensitivity is the capacity of the stain to demonstrate a tissue substance in low concentration. All staining methods have a threshold below which it is not possible to demonstrate the component and if the threshold of a staining technique is high, this indicates that the sensitivity is low and that small amounts of the tissue component will not be demonstrated by the technique although they are present. A satisfactory staining method is one which combines high sensitivity with high selectivity.

'STAINING' PROCESSES EMPLOYED BY HISTOLOGISTS

Several different types of 'staining' process are used to give tissues contrast or colour, usually both, before they are examined with the microscope. The main types of 'staining' technique employed by a histologist are shown in Table 6.1, and although it is not usual to include metallic impregnation techniques or histochemical methods as staining techniques, these will all be considered together as they achieve, in different ways, the same objectives of alterations of light intensity and wavelength as do the classical dye-staining methods. This table may give some insight into the way 'staining' substances combine with tissues; some of these reactions are completely understood, though others remain obscure.

VITAL STAINING

Living cells can be stained by dissociation in the staining fluid (supra-vital staining) or by injection of the dye into the living organism (intra-vital staining). These methods are not applicable to fixed sectioned tissues, but may be used as a valuable control for comparison with stained sections. The staining of living cells received its main stimulus from Paul Ehrlich, who first used methylene blue and later introduced neutral red (Ehrlich 1887, 1894). Vital staining demonstrates cytoplasmic structures by the phagocytosis of particles of dye into the cytoplasm, or by the staining of pre-existing cellular components. The nuclear membrane of the living cell is impermeable to dyes, and it is not possible to stain the living nucleus. The demonstration of cells of the

Table 6.1 The main types of staining processes used in histology

Staining process	Demonstration of	In	By
1 Vital staining			
(a) Phagocytosis of particulate substances	RE cells	living tissues	trypan blue
(b) Specific staining of living structures	mitochondria	living cells	Janus green
2 Elective solubility	fat droplets	frozen sections	Lysochromes, such as Sudan stains
3 Production of coloured chemical substances			
(a) Stable compounds	ferric iron	all sections	Perls' method
(b) Unstable compounds	enzymes	specially prepared sections	Histochemical methods
4 Metallic impregnation			
(a) Intracellular structures	melanin	all sections	Fontana's silver
(b) Fibrils	reticulin	all sections	silver methods
5 Staining with dyes			
(a) General chemical and physical actions	tissue structures	all sections	haematoxylin and eosin
(b) Metachromasia	cartilage; amyloid	all sections	thionin; crystal violet
(c) Local formation of a dye	DNA	paraffin sections	Feulgen reaction

reticulo-endothelial (RE) system by vital staining with trypan blue is an example of cytoplasmic phagocytosis; this stain is colloidal, and fine suspensions, such as Indian ink, are taken up by RE cells and other cells with phagocytic capacities. True vital staining of cellular components is shown by the staining of mitochondria by Janus green. Nile blue will stain lipid inclusions, but does so by simply dissolving in the fat—an example of elective solubility that will be discussed in the next paragraph.

STAINING BY ELECTIVE SOLUBILITY

One of the easiest understood ways by which stains combine with tissues is by simple solution in tissue fluids. Aqueous stains are unsuitable because water is widely distributed throughout cells and the staining would be too diffuse. Substances that dissolve in tissues are known as lysochromes. Almost all the lysochromes are lipid-soluble and are used in histology for the demonstration of lipids in tissue sections. Fat droplets can be electively coloured by stains in alcoholic (often 70 per cent) solutions if the stain is more soluble in the fat than in the alcohol; the amount of stain that is taken up by the fat is determined by the partition coefficient that applies to the stain in the presence of the two solvents. If the coefficient favours the fat the uptake will be strong.

Successful histological staining by solution is mainly confined to fat stains, and the lysochromes must be brightly coloured, highly soluble in lipids and have no affinity for any other cellular structures except by elective preferential solubility.

STAINING BY THE CHEMICAL PRODUCTION OF COLOURED SUBSTANCES IN TISSUES

Some staining techniques use pale or colourless solutions which react with tissue components to produce coloured substances. The resulting coloured end-products of these reactions are either: (1) true dyes; or (2) coloured chemical products that are not dyes. Many of these methods, especially those of the second group, are *histochemical techniques* involving clearly understood chemical reactions with a high specificity. These contrast with the staining methods using natural or synthetic dyes [p. 111] which have a less precise physicochemical basis and far less chemical specificity.

An example of the first group is Schiff's reagent, used in the PAS reaction [p. 237] and the Feulgen reaction [p. 160]. The straw-coloured or colourless solution is converted into a purple dye by the presence of aldehydes in the tissues.

The second group of histochemical reactions have a final reaction product that is coloured but is not a dye. The simplest way that this is produced is by the chemical combination of a tissue constituent with a chemical substance in a pale or colourless solution. Perls' reaction for iron [p. 264] is an example of such a reaction. Potassium ferrocyanide combines with ferric ions to form potassium ferric ferrocyanide (Prussian blue); this is a simple chemical reaction and the product, Prussian blue, is not a dye and is not used as such, but only as an insoluble, deeply coloured, visible deposit. If more tissue components gave such clear-out, specific coloured chemical reactions histological staining would be more easily understood and might be more precise. Another variant of this kind of coloration of tissues is seen in enzyme histochemistry. Enzymes do not combine with chemical substrates to produce coloured end-products; they react upon them, either: (1) changing the substrate into a coloured substance at the site of enzyme activity; or (2) producing a colourless compound that can be substituted by a coloured compound in a second-stage reaction.

The end-result of all these methods is similar, involving the production of a coloured final reaction compound which in some ways resembles the coloured solution obtained in a colorimetric chemical analysis, and the intensity of the reaction is proportional to the quantity of the active reagent in the tissues. The success of these chemical reactions in histological sections is dependent upon the preservation of the active cellular constituents in their original situations within the cell and at their original concentration; special precautions have to be taken to avoid the loss of labile (unstable) substances like glycogen or enzymes. It must also be appreciated that the end-products should be opaque or deeply coloured as pale colours like yellows or pinks may not have sufficient colour contrast for accurate microscopy.

METALLIC IMPREGNATION

Some metallic compounds can be reduced by tissues to the metallic state, producing an opaque, usually black, deposit. Solutions of ammoniacal silver

$[Ag(NH_3)_2]OH$ are suitable for histology as they are readily reduced and the deposited silver is stable. Tyrosine derivatives such as melanin, and phenolic compounds such as those found in the granules of the Kultschitzky cells of the intestinal glands have the capacity of reducing ammoniacal silver to form a visible deposit. Such cells are called argentaffin cells, whilst those that cannot reduce ammoniacal silver directly, but do so with the addition of an extraneous reducer, are known as argyrophil cells.

Metallic impregnation is also a standard method for the demonstration of fibrils. In this we believe that there may be some direct reduction of the ammoniacal silver, but that this is too small to be visible. However, nerve and other fibres such as reticulin combine with ammoniacal silver and this transparent unreduced silver can be deposited upon the fibre as opaque metallic silver by a photographic developer or some other reducing agent in a second stage of the technique. Thus, staining by metallic impregnation may be a one-stage technique if the reducing agents in the tissues are powerful enough, but the impregnation of fibrils will usually require a second-stage reduction analogous to argyrophil cells. By the use of sensitizing agents and by variations of the silver methods, many cellular structures, pigments, spirochaetes, and fungi can be demonstrated by metallic impregnation.

STAINING WITH NATURAL AND SYNTHETIC DYES

The largest number of staining techniques fall into this group. The mechanism of dye staining is less clearly understood than most of the methods described in the previous groups of staining methods, but the structure and mode of action of dyes have been extensively studied in the textile industry. The application of the knowledge of the structure and action of commercial dyes to histology has enabled us to understand many of the factors involved in the combination of dyes with tissues.

The structure of dyes used in histology

There are two main types of dyes used in histology, natural and synthetic.

Natural dyes, which include carmine and haematoxylin. Carmine is obtained from cochineal, the dried bodies of the female insect, *Dactylopius cacti*, that lives on Central American succulent plants. Carminic acid is obtained by boiling cochineal in water and extracting with benzene after chemical purification; a crude form, carmin, is prepared by precipitation of cochineal with potassium aluminium sulphate. Haematoxylin is extracted from the wood of a small tree, *Haematoxylon campechianum* (logwood), which originated in Mexico and has been cultivated in Jamaica. Haematoxylin is one of the most widely used dyes in histology and will be described later but in its natural form it has little or no staining capacity and requires oxidation to haematein, either naturally by contact with air or chemically with an oxidizing agent such as sodium iodate or mercuric oxide.

Synthetic dyes are a large group of organic compounds that were originally produced from coal in the coal-gas industry; more recently petroleum oils have become an important alternative source. The primary products include hydrocarbons, such as benzene, toluene, and naphthalene, or phenols, such as phenol and cresols. A large group of synthetic dyes are derived from benzene [FIG. 6.1] which is a resonating molecule with three possible alternative struc-

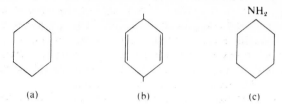

(a)   (b)   (c)

FIG. 6.1. Benzene ring structure of dye compounds. (a) Benzene. (b) Quinone. (c) Aniline.

tural formulae. Resonance is associated with absorption of light and with the production of colour and, although benzene is a colourless substance, it has an absorption band in the ultraviolet band and would appear coloured if our eyes were sensitive to ultraviolet light. In order to make a coloured compound from benzene it is necessary to make certain chemical changes and colour-bearing chemical configurations are known as *chromophores*. There are three main groups of chromophores—the quinonoid ring, usually para-, sometimes ortho- [FIG. 6.2(a) and (b)], the azo-coupling [FIG. 6.2(c)], and the nitro-group, NO$_2$ [FIG. 6.2(d)]. Quinone [FIG. 6.1(b)] is an important chromophore-

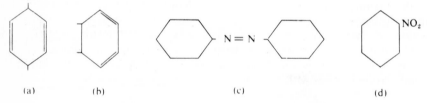

(a)   (b)   (c)   (d)

FIG. 6.2. Chromophores. (a) Paraquinonoid ring. (b) Orthoquinonoid ring. (c) Azo-coupling. (d) Nitro-grouping (nitrobenzene).

bearing compound and is coloured yellow but the presence of a quinonoid ring in more complex organic compounds produces brilliant darker colours. Compounds which contain chromophores are known as *chromogens* and can colour tissues and textiles; however, the resulting colours are not 'fast' and can be easily removed by washing in simple solutions. This can be understood by the fact that chromogens dissolve to form solutions of molecules whereas satisfactory dyes dissolve as ions; to convert a chromogen into a true dye it is necessary to introduce an ionizing group and these ionizing groups are called *auxochromes*, which increase the intensity of the colour. Auxochromes are either basic or acidic and are the parts of the dye that determine the staining action of the whole molecule. The most important basic auxochrome is the amino- group ($-NH_2$) and dyes containing the aniline ring [FIG. 6.1(c)], which formed the original basis of the dye industry, are still used for many staining techniques in histology. Acidic auxochromes include the sulphonic group $-SO_3$, the carboxyl group $-COOH$, and hydroxyl group $-OH$. The greater the number of basic or acidic auxochromes that a dye compound contains determines the strength of its basic (cationic) or acidic (anionic) dye characteristics. Dyes that have a basic and an acidic group are basic as the basic group predominates, but is weakened by the presence of the acidic group. Dyes contain additional chemical groups called *modifiers* which have the effect of altering the colour of the dye. These may be methyl ($-CH_3$) or ethyl ($-C_2H_5$) and have the effect of making the colour of the dye deeper. Thus, rosaniline differs from pararosaniline by having a single methyl group which modifies the colour into a slightly bluer shade. If the hydrogens of the basic amino-auxochromes are replaced by methyl or aryl (a benzene ring with one or more substitutions) groups, the dye becomes bluer. Crystal violet is an example of a dye with multiple modifying groupings.

Thus a dye is made up of an organic compound that is coloured by a chromophore and is ionized by an auxochrome, the final colour being altered or strengthened by a modifier. The structures of the main groups of dyes that are used in histology are described by Lillie (1977) and Baker (1958, 1966). It is sufficient to state here that the quinonoid dyes include basic and acid fuchsin, crystal violet, aniline blue, eosin, thionin, methylene blue, neutral red, and the natural dyes haematein (the active oxidized constituent of haematoxylin [FIG. 6.3(a)] and carminic acid. The azo-dyes are a smaller group of which orange G [FIG. 6.3(b)], Congo red, and trypan blue are of special importance in histology. The nitro-dyes are the smallest group and include picric acid (trinitrophenol [FIG. 6.3(c)]) and aurantia.

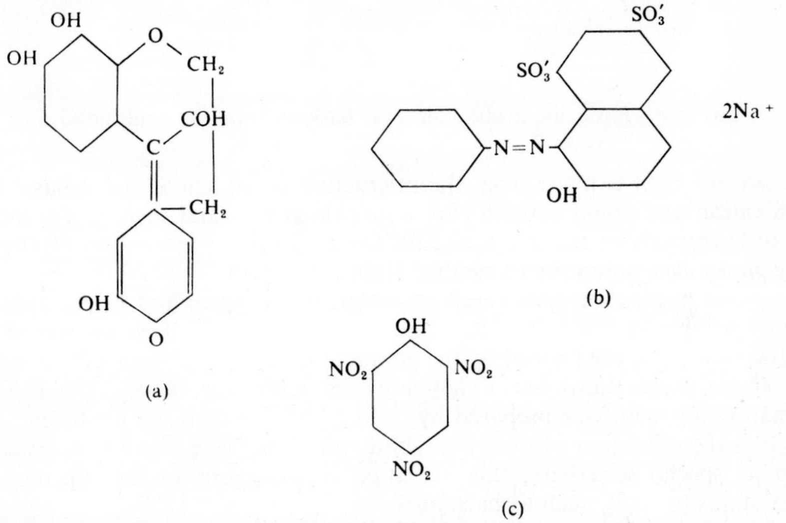

FIG. 6.3   The structures of dyes. (a) Quinonoid dye (haematein). (b) Azo-dye (orange G). (c) Nitro-dye (picric acid).

BASIC, ACIDIC, AND NEUTRAL DYES

When basic or acidic dyes go into solution, they ionize, and a typical basic dye gives cationic or positively charged dye ions and negatively charged colourless chloride ions, whilst an acidic dye gives anionic or negatively charged coloured dye ions and positively charged colourless sodium ions. These terms 'basic' and 'acidic' applied to dyes have no relevance to pH and it would be better if the term 'cationic dye' was used for a basic dye and 'anionic dye' for an acidic dye. In practice it is usually found that cationic basic dyes are slightly acid in reaction due to chloride radicles, whereas anionic acid dyes are sodium salts and may be slightly alkaline.

A *basic stain* is a dye, such as basic fuchsin which is composed of a coloured rosaniline base and the colourless acidic Cl radicle [FIG. 6.4(a)].

An *acidic stain* is one in which the acidic component of the dye molecule is coloured, the base being colourless, usually sodium. Acid fuchsin is the sodium salt of an acidic sulphonated derivative of rosaniline [FIG. 6.4(b)].

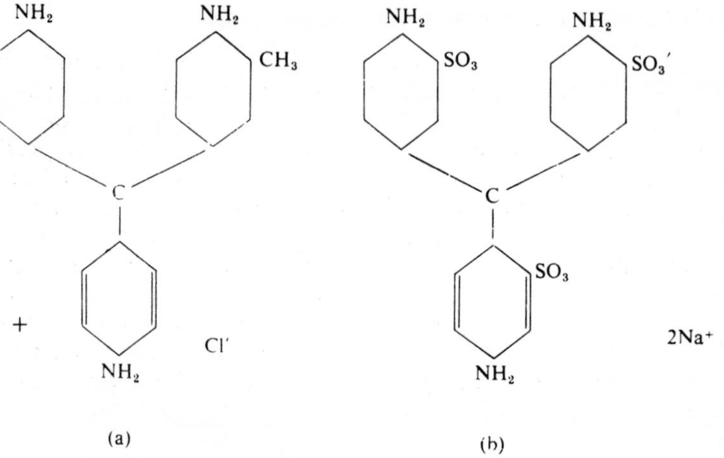

FIG. 6.4. Basic and acidic stains. (a) Basic fuchsin. (b) Acid fuchsin.

A *neutral stain* is made from the interaction of an acidic and a basic dye. Both cation and anion contain chromophoric groups and there is a coloured dye in both parts of the dye molecule. Owing to the combination of already large molecules, solutions of neutral stains are often colloidal. Neutral dyes are soluble in alcohol, only rarely in water, whilst basic and acidic dyes are usually soluble in both. The Romanowsky dyes are the best known of the neutral stains and are formed by the interaction of polychrome methylene blue and eosin; these stains are widely used as stains for blood. The original Romanowsky stain was prepared by chance with an oxidized methylene blue and it is the oxidation of methylene blue into methylene azure that gives the stain its special selectivity; this oxidation is analogous to the 'ripening' of other stains [p. 118], such as haematoxylin.

An *amphoteric stain* is made from a dye which is cationic below a certain pH (the iso-electric point) and anionic above it. Carminic acid is amphoteric with an iso-electric point of pH 4.5.

Basic stains colour acidic tissue components such as nuclei. Acidic stains will combine with basic structures such as cytoplasm. Neutral dyes have, as expected, an affinity for acidophilic and basiphilic elements in the cell, and certain tissue components also react with the compound neutral stain, thus giving a triple staining effect.

COLOURLESS LEUCOBASES

Some dyes can easily be reduced and if the chromophore is destroyed in this process the dye loses its colour. Quinonoid ring double bonds are broken and take up hydrogen. Such leuco-dyes (e.g. leuco-methylene blue) can become recolourized by oxidation in a vital staining technique. Conversely cell structures that have been vitally stained by methylene blue can become colourless (converted into leucobase) if the oxygen tension falls, and may be recoloured by exposure to oxygen. Schiff's reagent (a leuco-fuchsin) is not a true leucobase as it is not used as a test for oxidizing agents, though it resembles leucobases in becoming coloured by the reconstitution of its chromophore.

METACHROMATIC STAINING

Certain tissue components combine with dyes to produce a colour different from the colour of the original dye and different from the colour produced in the rest of the tissue. This was first described by Jürgens and others in 1875 and is known as metachromasia; dyes that act in this way are said to be metachromatic. A substance that can alter the colour of a metachromatic dye is a chromotrope. The term orthochromatic may be used to denote a tissue that does not cause metachromasia or a dye that is not metachromatic.

Metachromatic dyes have more than one absorption spectrum, and these must be sufficiently different to give a marked colour contrast between the orthochromatic and the metachromatic tissue-dye compounds. The most important metachromatic tissue components are cartilage, connective tissue and epithelial mucins, mast cell granules and amyloid. The dyes that are metachromatic are mainly thiazines [FIG. 6.5] such as toluidine blue and thionin,

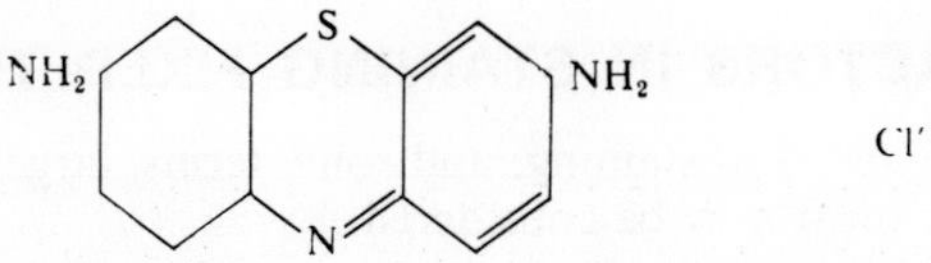

FIG. 6.5.   Thiazine dye structure (thionin).

though a triphenylmethane dye, methyl violet, is widely used. The colour contrast using these dyes is blue–red. The absorption spectrum of toluidine blue with an orthochromatic tissue is maximum at about 630 nm and the staining result is blue; with a metachromatic substance the absorption maximum is 480–540 nm and the colour is red. In addition to the red staining, known as γ-metachromasia, toluidine blue may stain tissues violet or purple, and this is called β-metachromasia. The results of metachromatic staining may be expressed as alpha (α), which is blue, negative; beta (β), which is violet or purple, slightly positive; and gamma (γ), which is red, strongly positive.

The thiazine dyes act by the production of differently coloured polymers and Michaelis and Grannick (1945) have shown that the monomers are blue and the polymers are red. Intermediate dimers and trimers are violet, corresponding with the colours of β-metachromasia. To enable metachromasia to take place there must be free electronegative groups (usually sulphate or carboxyl) on the surface of the tissue; these are present in highly sulphated acidic polysaccharides, and Lison (1936) believed that metachromasia was a specific test for acid mucopolysaccharides. A decrease in the number of acidic groupings, or their loss by protein binding, is associated with a fall in metachromasia.

A curious feature of metachromasia is the fact that alcohol converts the polymerized (metachromatic) form of a dye into the monomeric (ortho-chromatic) form. Metachromasia is usually lost if the section is dehydrated in alcohol after staining, though Hughesdon's (1949) technique [p. 250] is an exception and permanent preparations can be obtained. Water is necessary for most metachromatic staining and Sheppard and Geddes (1944) have suggested that water is incorporated into the dimeric form of a metachromatic dye, though Ramalingam and Ravindranath (1971) studied the effects of alcohol dehydration on protein polysaccharide metachromasia and concluded that alcohol does not abolish the metachromatic reaction of toluidine blue.

FLUORESCENT STAINING

Dyeing in industry, and most histological stains use coloured solutions that cause colour reactions which are visible in daylight or ordinary artifical light. Fluorochromes are quinonoid dyes with the usual chromophores and auxo-chromes, which behave as acidic or basic dyes, but have the capacity of altering ultraviolet light into visible light when combined with tissues. Thus fluorescent staining is similar to ordinary colour dyeing, but we recognize the tissues that have combined with the fluorochrome by the use of ultraviolet light, and not by the colour that is produced in daylight. Fluorochromes are not more specific than non-fluorescent dyes but a valuable feature is that they are highly sensitive; bright high-contrast fluorescent staining is produced by very small quantities of a fluorochrome bound to a tissue. Fluorescence is discussed in Chapter 2 [p. 22].

GENERAL FACTORS IN STAINING FIXED TISSUES

Certain factors involved in staining, and some terms, largely derived from the dyeing of textiles, must now be considered.

THE EFFECTS OF FIXATION UPON STAINING

Fixation assists the interaction of tissues and dyes. Chromatin is probably split into DNA and protein by fixation, allowing the DNA to be stained by a basic dye. Mercuric chloride, formaldehyde, and ethyl alcohol appear to act in this way. Proteins are also more easily stained after fixation; formaldehyde and mercuric chloride favour basic dyes, whilst trichloroacetic acid, picric acid, and chromium compounds facilitate the action of acidic dyes. After fixation with ethyl alcohol or acetic acid, both basic and acidic dyes are taken up by the tissues easily. Blockage of carboxyl groups, with preservation of amino groups is the probable explanation of a fixative that assists an acidic dye, whilst the reverse action favours a basic dye. The action of fixatives is considered in further detail in Chapter 3 [p. 43].

PROGRESSIVE AND REGRESSIVE STAINING

A *progressive* staining technique is one in which the different elements in the tissues are coloured in sequence, and at the end of the correct time in the staining solution a satisfactory differential coloration of the tissues is achieved. A *regressive* technique is one in which the tissue is first over-stained (obliterating cellular details) and then de-stained or differentiated by removing excess stains from unwanted parts of the tissue. Regressive staining is now far more commonly employed than the older progressive method. This is because it is difficult to obtain sufficiently intense progressive staining of one part of a cell without some staining of the other cell structures; the latter gives a diffuse result which obscures details. By differentiation it is possible to remove stain from the more lightly stained sites, still leaving a strong enough staining of other structures to give selective and clearly detailed results.

DIRECT AND INDIRECT STAINING

Many of the aniline dyes (e.g. methylene blue, eosin) stain tissues perfectly if these are placed in a simple aqueous or alcoholic solution of the dye. This is known as *direct* staining [FIG. 6.6(a)]. Many stains, including haematoxylin, require an additional intermediate substance known as a *mordant* before satisfactory combination with tissues takes place; these are *indirect* stains [FIG. 6.6(b)]. The dye and the mordant unite to form a coloured *lake*, and

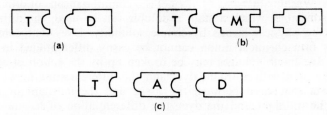

FIG. 6.6. Direct and indirect staining. (a) Direct staining. (b) Indirect staining with mordant. (c) Indirect staining with accentuator. (T = tissue; D = dye; M = mordant; A = accentuator.)

the mordanted dye combines with the tissue to form a tissue–mordant–dye complex; this is insoluble in ordinary aqueous or alcoholic solvents, allowing subsequent counterstaining and dehydration to be easily carried out. In histological staining methods the dye and the mordant are either used together (e.g. haematoxylin with potassium alum in Ehrlich's haematoxylin) or the mordant may be used first before the tissue is passed into the staining solution (e.g. the preliminary iron alum bath before Heidenhain's haematoxylin). Iron, aluminium, and chromium compounds are mordants which combine with dyes to form basic stains; the metallic mordant attaches itself, both to the dye and to the tissue, by chemical bonds.

Accentuators [FIG. 6.6(c)] differ from mordants, though they increase the staining power of the dyes with which they are used. They do not form lakes with dyes, and they are not essential for the chemical union of the dye with the tissue. Potassium hydroxide in Loeffler's methylene blue and phenol in carbol thionin and carbol fuchsin act as accentuators, increasing the intensity and selectivity of staining. Accentuators are often acids or alkalis which are added to anionic (acidic) dyes and cationic (basic) dyes respectively, for example potassium hydroxide in Loeffler's methylene blue. By adding acid to an anionic dye the staining is intensified by increasing the ionization of basic groups of tissues. If alkali is added to a cationic dye, the ionization of acidic groups is increased. Phenol is used as an accentuator in carbol thionin and carbol fuchsin, but the mode of action is not clearly understood.

Accelerators used in the metallic impregnation techniques for the nervous system (e.g. chloral hydrate and veronal in Cajal's methods) also appear to act in the same way as accentuators.

Trapping agents hold dyes in combination with tissues or bacteria; tannic acid and iodine are examples. Laveran (1899) showed that a blood smear stained with methylene blue/eosin selectively retained the methylene blue in the chromatin after treatment with tannic acid. The finding of Gram (1884) that certain bacteria stained with gentian violet and iodine resisted alcoholic decolorization is also due to the trapping action of iodine on the bacteria–dye complex. It is believed that the iodine does not alter the capacity of the dye to react with bacteria but tends to hold the dye and thus prevents it escaping from the tissue during differentiation.

DIFFERENTIATION

De-staining or differentiation of an over-stained tissue in a regressive technique can be brought about by washing in simple solutions, or by the use of acids and oxidizing agents. Mordants and some dyes can also act as differentiating agents. Washing in water or alcohol is a common means of differentiation, and any solvent in which a stain is soluble can be used; the differentiating fluid acts by physical means by simple solubility. Dyes that combine with tissues by firm chemical union cannot be easily differentiated in this way, but their dye–tissue linkages may be broken up by the action of acids; these are usually used with mordant dyes and the differentiating agent may then either break the union between the tissue and the mordant or the bonds between the mordant and the dye. The differentiation of haematoxylin dye lakes with acids breaks the mordant–dye link by reconstituting the hydroxyl group of the dye which was lost when it combined with the mordant; the acid also depresses the ionization of acidic groups in the tissues, thereby breaking the tissue–mordant linkage. Oxidizing agents act differently, oxidizing the dye into a colourless compound. Mordants used for differentiation break up the insoluble dye–mordant–tissue complex by the partial redistribution of the dye into a soluble dye–mordant lake that disperses in the differentiating fluid, leaving only part of the dye in the tissue as a stain. Dyes can act as differentiators if they have a stronger affinity for the tissue constituents than the dyes with which these have already been stained; thus a stronger dye, such as orange G, can displace another less avid stain and produces the same effect as simple de-staining.

RIPENING OF STAINING SOLUTIONS

A number of staining solutions are only effective after exposure to air, light, and (often) warmth for a period of weeks or months. Haematoxylin is a well-known example; it is useless as a nuclear stain when freshly prepared, but it becomes active after some weeks of storage. This is due to the oxidation of haematoxylin into haematein, and can be quickly accomplished by the addition of an oxidizing agent (sodium iodate, mercuric oxide, potassium permanganate). It is advisable to artificially ripen only part of the haematoxylin in the staining solution, allowing the excess haematoxylin to ripen naturally. This allows the stain to be used at once, but the continued oxidation maintains the activity of the stain for several months; otherwise the completely ripened solution quickly becomes ineffective by further oxidation into inactive compounds. The gradual ripening of a staining solution with increased staining activity, followed by steady deterioration, can mean that the time required for the staining of tissues will vary considerably over a period of time; it is wise to label each staining solution with its date of preparation.

THE CLASSIFICATION AND STANDARDIZATION OF DYES

It has already been seen that the majority of dyes used in histology have one of the three main chromophoric groups—the quinonoid ring, the azo-group, or the nitro-group. The quinonoid dyes are such a large and important group that they are subdivided into classes with particular types of quinonoid structure. Table 6.2 shows the chemical classification of dyes used in histology.

Table 6.2. Chemical classification of dyes used in histology

Chromophore	Structure	Cationic dye (basic dye)	Anionic dye (acidic dye)
Quinonoid ring	Triarylmethane	Rosaniline dyes Crystal violet	Acid fuchsin Aniline blue
	Haematein		Haematein
	Xanthene	Pyronin	Eosin Phloxine
	Thiazine	Thionin Methylene blue	
	Oxazine	Cresyl violet Celestine blue	
	Azur	Neutral red Safranin	Azocarmine
Azo-group	Monazo-		Orange G Tartrazine
	Diazo-	Bismark brown	Congo red Biebrich scarlet
Nitro-group	Nitro-		Picric acid Martius yellow

The greatest use of dyes is in the textile industry where the dyer classifies them according to their mode of application, such as direct or mordant dye, or according to their general chemical character—acid or basic dye. Dyes may also be classified according to their use in specific commercial applications, such as the dyeing of wool. In this there are two main groups of dyes, small molecule anionic dyes that diffuse readily into the wool fibre, producing a very level or uniform dyeing effect (levelling dyes) or large molecule anionic dyes that diffuse slowly to the fibre and are resistant to extraction during subsequent felting processes (milling dyes).

Not only is the classification of dyes a complex problem but their names also create difficulties. Some dyes have names that are descriptive of a colour, such as light green, whilst others, such as aniline blue, convey some chemical information as well. Many dyes have names which are followed by numbers and letters and the letter 'R' after the name of a dye indicates that it is redder than a related dye and '2R' is even more red. 'B' usually indicates a bluish colour and 'G' (gelb) and 'Y' both indicate a yellowish colour. A uniform nomenclature for dyes is particularly important in view of the existence of several synonyms for one dye. For example, Sudan IV, a stain for lipid, also may be called scarlet red, scharlach R, oil red IV, fat ponceau R or LB, or cerotine ponceau 3B. There are many synonyms for orange G but conversely other dyes with similar names like phloxine G and phloxine B are not similar to each other. This confusion can be avoided by the use of the Colour Index which is a system of dyeing indexing introduced by the Society of Dyers and Colourists of Bradford, England in 1924. This is now prepared in conjunction with the American Association of Textile Chemists and Colorists (1971, 1975). The Colour Index is in six volumes. Volumes 1–3 list dyes, pigments, and textile developers according to their methods of application to textiles. Volume 4 states chemical compositions and sets out a numerical list of Colour Index numbers, together with patent information. Volume 5 is an alphabetical, commercial, and generic-name index. The sixth volume is a supplement published in 1975. Dyes can be accurately identified by their Colour Index numbers and the Colour Index number of all dyes mentioned in this book is given on page 501. Valuable progress towards the standardization of the dyes used in histology has also been made by the American Biological Stain Commission (Lillie 1977). Certified dyes can be used with confidence and newly certified dyes are listed in the Commission's journal, *Stain Technology*.

Very large numbers of biological stains are available from manufacturers throughout the world, though the routine work of histology is done with a moderately small number of these. With the progressive knowledge of chemical composition of dyes, and the more rational identification of them, quality is now generally good and in most cases samples are tested by manufacturers, not only for chemical identity but also in the histological technique for which the dye is generally used. Despite this, variation in staining characteristics from batch to batch and manufacturer to manufacturer does occur and the testing of new batches in the user's laboratory, with known control material, is strongly recommended. Most histology laboratories will not have facilities for the analysis or identification of dyes as these are usually carried out by spectrophotometric, chromatographic, and electrophoretic methods. In spectrophotometry an absorption spectrum of the wavelength of light that is absorbed by the dye is produced. The wavelength of the absorption spectrum is measured in nanometres (nm) or in Ångstrom units (1 Å = 0.1 nm), and is characteristic of the dye, providing an accurate means of identification. It will also determine whether dyes are homogeneous or consist of a mixture of dyes. The individual components of mixtures of dyes can be separated by chromatography in which different substances diffuse at different rates, becoming separated into bands. This is particularly valuable if spectrophotometric analysis has only shown one component as this may mask the presence of a second component. Finally, electrophoresis produces results which in some ways are similar to those of chromatography but these also give an indication of the nature and strength of the electrophoretic charge on the component dyes. Various aspects of the purification and standardization of dyes were discussed at a conference sponsored by the Biological Stain Commission in 1974 and the report (Mowry and Kasten 1975) describes the subjects discussed, the conclusions, and the recommendations.

THE MODE OF ACTION OF DYE STAINING

Chemical and physical reactions hold dyes in tissues, and both processes commonly take place at the same time.

CHEMICAL DYE STAINING REACTIONS

A dye must ionize in solution to produce coloured cations or anions which are capable of uniting with proteins and other tissue constituents to form coloured compounds. A typical basic dye is positively charged (cationic) at pH ranges that are used in histology, and an acidic dye is negatively charged (anionic); an amphoteric dye has an uncharged point (isoelectric point) within the pH range and is basic below and acidic above this pH (Table 6.3).

Table 6.3. Ionization of basic, acidic, and amphoteric dyes

	pH								
	3	4	5	6	7	8	9	10	
Crystal violet	+	+	+	+	+	+	+	+	Basic dye (cationic)
Orange G	−	−	−	−	−	−	−	−	Acidic dye (anionic)
Haematein	+	+	+	+	−	−	−	−	Amphoteric dye

In the same way, electrically charged groups are present in the proteins and other components of tissues. At ordinary pH range tissue constituents, like dyes, are basic, acidic, or amphoteric (Table 6.4). DNA, RNA, and phospholipid are acidic due to their phosphoryl groups, and mast cells, cartilage, and some mucous secretions of glands contain acidic sulphuryl and carboxyl groups. Collagen, red blood corpuscles, and the granules of eosinophil leucocytes are basic due to the predominance of basic amino groups, whilst the amphoteric proteins of cell cytoplasm and muscle contain a balance between acidic carboxyl and hydroxyl groups and basic amino groups. Small changes in pH will make amphoteric substances in tissues basic or acidic, whilst larger changes alter the electrical charges of basic or acidic tissue components.

Table 6.4. Ionization of tissue components

Basic (+)	Acidic (−)	Amphoteric
Collagen	DNA, chromatin	Cytoplasm
Red blood corpuscles	RNA	Muscle
Granules of eosinophil leucocytes	Myelin	
	Cartilage	
	Mucous secretions	
	Mast cell granules	

As dyes and tissues are both ionized, they will react together, and do so in direct staining techniques; electropositive stains unite with electronegative tissues and vice versa. Mordanted dyes act as basic stains in indirect staining methods. The differentiation of acidic and basic staining by acids and alkalis is due to ionic changes brought about by the changes in pH; both the stain [p. 118] and the tissue will be affected. For instance, the addition of alkali diminishes the ionic dissociation of basic amino groups and increases the dissociation of carboxyl groups, thus making the proteins of cell cytoplasm and muscle negatively charged; acids will have the reverse effect and proteins will become positively charged. The intensity and 'fastness' or grip of a stain depends upon the avidity of its ionized radicles for tissue components and from the number and strength of these chemical bonds. Carboxyl groups are only weakly acidic whilst phosphoryl groups are stronger and the sulphuryl groups are stronger still; thus sulphonated dyes (acid fuchsin, orange G) have strong affinity for the basic groups of proteins, which are in plentiful supply, and will unite with them to form powerful bonds that require strong differentiation. These sulphonated dyes will successively compete for ions in tissues, and will even displace less avid dyes that have already combined with tissues, thereby staining or differentiating the first dye. Mordanted dyes combine with tissue in the same way as direct basic stains, but the metallic mordant forms a firm tissue–metal–dye linkage.

Successful dye staining by chemical interaction can be briefly described as a presentation of fixed tissues with ionized chemical groups to staining solutions with different and opposite charged radicles that have an affinity for each other.

PHYSICAL DYE STAINING

Dyes can combine with tissues by *adsorption*, which is the property of solid objects, especially when in a state of fine division, to attract and hold other substances on their free surfaces (Bayliss 1906); such stains can usually be differentiated in water or alcohol. Physical factors that are important include the *density* and *permeability* of the tissues. Dense tissue substances that have a large amount of protein chain per unit volume hold a large amount of dye and will remain coloured after less dense tissues have been decolourized by differentiation. Similarly, highly permeable tissues will be quickly stained and quickly differentiated, whilst less permeable substances require longer to take up a stain and more resistant to differentiation. Closely woven or 'close knit' tissues (Gurr 1962) have a tight meshwork of molecular protein chains that first resist penetration, then resist differentiation of dye. Moreover, tissue substances may change their permeability with age; Lendrum *et al.* (1962) described staining methods for fibrin of different ages which are based upon the fine structure of fibrin becoming more open as the fibrin ages and thus more capable of holding dyes with larger molecules. This principle has also been applied to the staining of amyloid (Lendrum, Slidders, and Fraser 1972). It has already been seen that dye staining is sometimes due to solubility [p. 109]; the Sudan fat stains are the best examples of these and they will not be discussed further here. Finally, it must be re-emphasized that dye staining is usually brought about by a mixture of physical and chemical affinities between the dye and the tissue constituents.

THE SCIENTIFIC CONTROL OF STAINING METHODS

It has been shown that histological staining can be accomplished by precise chemical reactions, but is still carried out by less exact chemical and physical processes. This means that staining methods will vary considerably according to a large number of different factors and explains the numerous modifications of staining techniques that have been developed. The techniques described in the following chapters have all been tested, but every histologist has had the discouraging experience of a method that gives poor or even negative results. This may be due to unreactive tissues; unsuitable fixation; to differences in the composition and solubility of the dyes; to the inadequate ripening or the deterioration of a staining solution; to variations in the temperature or pH of tap water or stains; and to many other factors.

This lack of scientific precision in dye staining means that a histologist must be prepared to control his own methods in order to obtain the best results. A method which works well in one country may not be satisfactory in another country, or even in a different part of the same country, if climatic conditions vary or the composition or pH of tap water alters. The directions given in a staining technique should be carefully followed, but usually represent a compromise and should not be regarded as inviolable. The laboratory should hold a stock of mounted unstained paraffin sections of tissues known to contain special tissue elements, pathological changes, bacteria, metals, etc.; these are used as *control sections* and are stained at the same time and in exactly the same way as the sections under investigation. This is best achieved by placing the slide with the test section back to back with the slide of the control section; the two slides are treated identically, being stained, differentiated, etc., for the same lengths of time. These controls avoid the frustration of staining for special structures, such as glycogen or acid-fast bacilli, and then being unable to tell whether the tissue contained no glycogen or acid-fast bacilli, or whether the technique was a failure; a glance at the control section will decide this. Every laboratory worker should be able to make controlled variations of a technique. Multiple haphazard alterations of a staining method may by chance give excellent results, but it is then usually impossible to reproduce the technique. Changes in a staining method must be made one at a time, in an orderly and carefully recorded fashion. A large number of sections should be cut from the same tissue block, and a series of variations of each step of the method should be made, one by one, with only one change in each section. By keeping the rest of the technique constant these sections will show which part of the method was defective and how it can be corrected. Occasionally it is required to stain a foreign substance or a rare pathological change which is not present to any appreciable amount in normal tissues or in the laboratory control sections. In these cases an artificial 'tissue block' can be made of gelatine containing the substance under examination (Cameron 1930), or the material may be injected into a laboratory animal, and the tissues used for control sections.

In the laboratory it is essential to appreciate the strengths and the limitations of the methods in use. By an understanding of the modes of action of staining and their applications to histology, it is possible to obtain the best results and to recognize the cause and the cure of failures when they occur.

REFERENCES

BAKER, J. R. (1958). *Principles of biological microtechnique*. Methuen, London.
—— (1966). *Cytological technique*, 5th edn. Methuen, London.
BAYLISS, W. M. (1906). *Biochem. J.* 1, 175.
BÖHMER, F. (1865). *Ärztl. Intelligenzbl. (Munich)* 12, 539.
CAMERON, G. R. (1930). *J. Path. Bact.* 33, 929.
CONN, H. J. (1948). *The history of staining*, 2nd edn. Biotech Publications, Geneva, New York.
EHRLICH, P. (1887). *Biol. Zbl.* 6, 214.
—— (1894). *Z. wiss. Mikr.* 11, 250.

GERLACH, J. VON (1858). *Wiss. Mitth. Phys.*; med. Soc. Erlangen.

GÖPPERT, H. R. and COHN, F. (1849). *Bot. Z.* **7**, 681.

GRAM, C. (1884). *Fortschr. Med.* **2**, 185.

GURR, E. (1962). *Staining animal tissues, practical and theoretical.* Leonard Hill, London.

HUGHESDON, P. E. (1949). *J. roy micr. Soc.* **69**, 1.

JÜRGENS, R. (1875). *Virchows Arch. path. Anat.* **65**, 189.

KÖLLIKER, A. (1852). *Manual of human microscopic anatomy.* London.

LAVERAN, M. A. (1899). *C. R. Soc. Biol. (Paris)* 2nd series, **1**, 249.

LEEUWENHOEK, A. VAN (1719). *Epistolae physiologicae.* Delphis. Cited by Lewis, F. T. (1942). *Anat. Rec.* **83**, 229.

LENDRUM, A. C., SLIDDERS, W., and FRASER, D. S. (1972). *J. clin. Path.* **25**, 373.

—— FRASER, D. S., SLIDDERS, W., and HENDERSON, R. (1962). *J. clin. Path.* **15**, 401.

LILLIE, R. D. (1977). *H. J. Conn's biological stains*, 9th edn. Williams and Wilkins, Baltimore.

LISON, L. (1936). *Histochimie et cytochimie animales.* Gautier-Villars, Paris.

MANN, GUSTAV (1902). *Physiological histology.* Clarendon Press, Oxford.

MICHAELIS, L. and GRANNICK, S. (1945). *J. Am. chem. Soc.* **67**, 1212.

MOWRY, R. W. and KASTEN, F. H. (1975). *Stain Technol.* **50**, 65.

RAMALINGAM, K. and RAVINDRANATH, M. H. (1971). *Stain Technol.* **46**, 221.

SHEPPARD, S. E. and GEDDES, A. L. (1949). *J. Am. chem. Soc.* **66**, 2003.

SOCIETY OF DYERS AND COLOURISTS (1924). *Colour index* (ed. F. M. Rowe) 1st edn. The Society of Dyers and Colourists, Bradford, England.

—— (1971–5). *Colour index*, 3rd edn. The Society of Dyers and Colourists and the American Association of Textile Chemists and Colorists. Lund Hymphries, London.

7 | General staining procedures

Equipment and materials
GENERAL STAINING EQUIPMENT

Ideally, a special bench with a suitable sink should be reserved for staining. The dimensions of the sink should be ample in area but shallow in depth, preferably not more than 15 cm deep. An efficient overflow should be incorporated in the sink which should be served with cold water and provided with two taps. A slide-washing tray may be placed in the sink and if made of metal, must be rustless. A white background is desirable during the staining of sections and Crawford (1952) described a slide-washing tray made from white Perspex and allowing an efficient flow of water. The solubility of this substance in chloroform is a minor disadvantage. Whatever the type of slide-washing tray used, scrupulous cleanliness is essential to avoid contamination of slides from a build-up of the many and varied living things that abound in dirty laboratory sinks.

A staining rack made from two pieces of stout glass rod, about 4 cm apart, and fastened at the ends by rubber tubing, or specially designed and adjustable clips, may rest on the bench over the sink. This is used for staining sections individually by application of stains and reagents from dropping bottles or pipettes. It is not convenient for these racks to be a fixture on the staining bench.

A Bunsen burner should be available in the staining area and a hot plate, 37 °C incubator and 60 °C oven should be near at hand.

Attention should be given to the lighting of the staining area. Bright daylight is good but is not consistently available while the yellow light given by low wattage tungsten-filament lamps may give a false (naked-eye) impression of the depth of eosin staining. With fluorescent lighting, 'colour matching' tubes are recommended.

It is common practice for sections to be stained by one person, for examination by another and it is important that any colour filters (or lack of them) should be the same in the microscopes of both. (The commonly used 'yellowish' eosin appears a quite different shade if viewed through a blue filter.)

Suitable objectives for the staining microscope are × 3, × 10, and × 40 and it is useful to have Polaroid discs available for substage and eyepiece, for the examination of birefringent material [p. 27].

The type of container used for stains and reagents will depend: (1) on the number of sections to be stained daily (and the number of people to stain them); and (2) on the variety and complexity of the staining methods used. In general practice, sections will be stained either in two's or three's, or in batches of 10–30, or more. In the first case, a dropping bottle rack holding one dozen 60 cm^3 capacity bottles will be found convenient. Such a rack might contain the following:

1. Xylene.
2. Xylene–absolute alcohol.
3. Absolute alcohol.
4. 90 per cent alcohol.
5. 70 per cent alcohol.
6. Acetone.
7. 1 per cent hydrochloric acid in 70 per cent alcohol.
8. Haematoxylin.
9. 1 per cent aqueous eosin.
10. 0.5 per cent iodine in 70 per cent alcohol.
11. 2.5 per cent sodium thiosulphate ('hypo').
12. 1 per cent aqueous neutral red.

Glass-lidded jars are used for stains and are made to accommodate one or two slides, or grooved to hold six slides (Coplin jars) or ten slides. It should be noted that the lids of these jars do not generally provide completely air-tight closure.

Polythene wash bottles ('squeeze bottles') are useful for distilled water and reagents applied frequently to individual sections as with 1 per cent acetic acid in trichrome staining [p. 184].

For staining multiple mounted sections, stainless steel or plastic slide racks are available. These may hold 10 to 20 slides or may be made larger to individual requirements. Square or rectangular dishes are used to contain stains and reagents for use with these racks which may be made of glass or suitable plastic material.

Racks may also be made to hold coverslip preparaions which affords a convenient way of staining many (50–100) class sections in one operation. The coverslips are mounted on slides on completion of the staining process.

Very small Coplin jars (Columbia jars) are available for staining a small number of coverslip preparations and 10 cm³ beakers may be used for the same purpose, as well as with the costly reagents often used in histochemical methods. Chaffey and Spain (1962) designed a plastic tray to hold coverslip preparations for the latter purpose.

The transfer of slides or coverslips from one staining reagent to another by mechanical means is now widely practised and several varieties of staining machine are available. These follow the general pattern of tissue processing machines but carry slide-racks instead of tissue containers and they may be programmed for brief immersion periods in the various solutions. Good results may be obtained with haematoxylin and eosin staining of sections [p. 141] and with Papanicolaou's method on smears [p. 345] and staining machines have become standard equipment in many histopathology and cytology laboratories.

Most cellulose nitrate sections and some frozen sections are stained before attachment to a slide, being transferred from one dish to another before placing on a slide and mounting with a coverslip. Standard procedures for these sections are given on page 135.

Coverslips of various sizes will be necessary, the range depending on the scope of the work in hand and the average size of tissue block selected for sectioning. The most commonly used sizes in histopathological technique are 22 × 22 mm, 26 × 22 mm, 32 × 22 mm, and 40 × 22 mm, while with smears of cells, rather longer coverslips such as 50 × 22 mm may be used. Circular coverslips of 22 mm diameter are available and are especially suitable for use with the small racks described above, and for preparations requiring 'ringing', with the aid of a turntable.

The standard thickness of coverslips in Great Britain is 0.13–0.16 mm which is designated as No. 1 thickness. These are suitable for the microscope objectives commonly used in histology and are reasonably robust.

Coverslips may be stored in 1 per cent hydrochloric acid in 70 per cent alcohol before drying and polishing with a fluff-free cloth such as nylon or silk. Any with visible blemishes should be discarded.

PREPARATION OF STAINS

Dyes may be purchased in quantities ranging from one or two grammes to several hundred grammes, depending on the concentration in the stain and frequency of use. They should be marked with the date of receipt and stored in a cool place away from strong light in air-tight containers. Dyes in solid form generally keep well but it is unwise to assume that an aged sample will perform as well as was the case many years previously, and preliminary testing is advisable. It is wise to assume that all dyes are toxic substances.

Distilled water is used for aqueous stains unless otherwise stated and solvents generally should be pure, although Industrial Absolute Alcohol (74 OP) may be used for most alcoholic stains. Exceptions will be noted.

Instructions regarding heating and filtering should be meticulously followed in preparing stains. They should be kept in hard glass bottles, of dark glass where indicated. Stoppers should be tightly fitting and made of glass or plastic rather than rubber or cork. All bottles should be fully labelled with 'spill-proof' labels and should bear the date of preparation. All stains should be kept in a cool rather than a warm place and some require filtering before use, even if filtered immediately after preparaion.

MOUNTING AND RINGING MEDIA

MOUNTING MEDIA

Mounting media are syrupy fluids used between section and coverslip. Most of them set quite firmly, preventing movement of the coverslip. Their refractive index should be as near as possible to that of glass (1.518). Two main types are available: these are (1) resinous media, for preparations dehydrated and cleared in xylene; and (2) aqueous media, for mounting sections directly from water, where treatment with alcohol or xylene would be detrimental to the stain.

Mountants are usually applied to sections in drops from the end of a glass rod which is dipped into a jar of the medium. Glass rods remain in these jars which have loose-fitting glass lids. These are not ideal, the mountant being subject to: (1) contamination with dust and dirt; and (2) alteration in consistency and thickening of the medium through evaporation of the solvent, especially if only used occasionally. A way of avoiding these faults is to dispense the medium from stock bottles into screw-cap, open-ended collapsible tin tubes (rather like toothpaste tubes). With the screw cap in position, mountant is poured into the tube to within about 1 cm of the opening which is then carefully flattened, folded, and pinched with a pair of pliers, to secure a leak-proof seal. In this way, the mountant is kept free from evaporation of the solvent and will be found easy to apply from the nozzle of the tube. The tubes are discarded when empty but are cheap and well worth the cost in terms of greater efficiency. Small plastic 'oil cans' are also used for applying mounting media to sections and are superior to glass rods and bottles.

Of the many different types of mounting media available, a small selection of general utility is given below; all of these have been in use for some years and it is noteworthy that no mounting medium can be deemed satisfactory until after some years have elapsed without alteration of the medium, or adverse effect on staining or section. This explains the marked reluctance of histologists to commit their valuable preparations to a new mounting medium that has not passed a long and stringent probationary period. For a review of histological mounting media, see Lille *et al.* (1950, 1953), and Greco (1950).

In the past, mounting media were generally prepared in the laboratory, but nowadays it is common practice to purchase the prepared media, thus avoiding the rather tedious and sticky procedure of mixing the ingredients and the slow and sometimes inefficient filtering to remove dirt.

Resinous Media

Xylene-balsam (RI 1.524)

About 60 per cent by weight of the dried natural resin, Canada balsam, is dissolved in xylene in the incubator or paraffin oven. When dissolved, the solution is filtered through a soft filter paper and the desired consistency obtained by the controlled evaporation of the solvent.

Xylene-balsam should be kept in a dark glass bottle. A few lumps of 'native' calcium carbonate (marble chips) in the stock bottle will help maintain a neutral reaction. Xylene-balsam darkens with age and exposure to light and does not preserve stains as well as the following media. Sections are mounted from xylene.

Colophonium-Turpentine (RI 1.52)

The prepared medium has a syrupy consistency and contains about 50 per cent colophonium resin by weight in Turpentine, BP (or xylene). With either solvent, sections are mounted from xylene and placed on a hot-plate at about 60 °C for 2–3 minutes. The slide is removed and while still warm, air bubbles are removed by gentle pressure on the coverslip with a mounting pin. The slide is then dipped in xylene to wash away surplus media and is dried and polished.

Euparal (RI 1.483)

A proprietary mixture of eucalyptol, sandarac, camsal, and paraldehyde which is available in two versions. One of these is termed colourless (actually, pale yellow) while the other is green (Euparal vert) and contains a copper salt designed to enhance haematoxylin staining. The lower refractive index of this medium is of value for the examination of unstained preparations while the ability to mount sections from 95 per cent alcohol is very convenient where treatment with absolute alcohol and xylene is damaging to stains or embedding media (see mounting of cellulose nitrate embedded sections, page 136).

Euparal is a recommended mounting medium, setting fairly quickly and causing little if any, fading of stains.

DPX and BPS synthetic resin mountants (Kirkpatrick and Lendrum 1929, 1941)

A mixture of distrene (a polystyrene), a plasticizer (tricresyl phosphate), and xylene, called DPX, was introduced in 1939 and later modified by the substitution of a more satisfactory plasticizer, dibutylphthalate (butyl, phthalate, styrene = BPS).

These colourless, synthetic resin mounting media are now available commercially and have generally replaced xylene–balsam. They preserve stains well and dry quickly, when surplus mountant may be peeled off the preparation after cutting round the coverslip with a razor blade or scalpel. They are not recommended for use with thick (e.g. cellulose nitrate) sections where there is a danger of retraction of the mountant on drying. Sections are mounted from xylene.

Aqueous Media

Kaiser's (1880) glycerol-jelly (RI approximately 1.47)

PREPARATION

Gelatine	10 g
Distilled water	60 cm^3
Pure glycerol	70 cm^3
Phenol (crystals)	0.25 g

Dissolve the gelatine in the water in a beaker placed in a water-bath before adding the glycerol and phenol. When completely mixed, and while still fluid, decant into small screw-cap jars. For use, melt by placing in the paraffin oven or in warm water.

Originally intended as an embedding medium, glycerol-jelly has for long been the standard mountant where dehydration and clearing in xylene is precluded, as with lipid stains. The need to melt the mountant before use, the tendency for stains to fade and the lack of hardness of the set mountant have combined to make this less popular in recent years. Preparations mounted in glycerol-jelly should be ringed.

Apathy's (1892) mountant (RI 1.52)

PREPARATION

Pure gum arabic (crystals, not powder)	50 g
Pure cane sugar	50 g
Distilled water	50 cm^3
Thymol	0.05 g

Dissolve with the aid of gentle heat and store in tightly stoppered jars, or screw-cap collapsible tubes.

Von Apathy described this mountant for use with methylene blue stained preparations of nerves. It sets quite hard, scarcely requiring ringing and has a higher refractive index than most aqueous mounting media.

Lillie and Ashburn (1943) modified the above mixture by doubling the quantity of distilled water and this mountant, plus 50 g potassium acetate *or* 10 g sodium chloride (Highman 1946), is effective in preventing the 'bleeding' of metachromatic stains for amyloid [p. 222]. It is also recommended as a general purpose aqueous mountant.

Temporary Mountants

A mixture of equal parts pure glycerol and distilled water (RI 1.397) may be used as a temporary mountant with fresh or watery preparations while thickened cedar wood oil (RI 1.52) is suitable with dehydrated specimens.

Mountants for Fluorescence Microscopy

Some mountants fluoresce when subjected to short wavelength light, this property interfering with the examination of sections and smears specially prepared for fluorescence microscopy. Mountants lacking this defect are available commercially but not all are entirely satisfactory. Recommended mounting media for fluorescence microscopy will be given with the appropriate staining technique.

RINGING MEDIA

Fluid and semi-fluid mounts, including those media which fail to set completely hard should be sealed at the margins of the coverslip to prevent seepage or evaporation of the mountant, to immobilize the coverslip, and to prevent sticking of slides on storage.

Ringing media may be solid, being melted for use and applied with a bent wire, or fluid, being applied with a fine brush, the medium hardening by evaporation of the solvent.

For a solid medium, paraffin wax may be used or, preferably, Kronig's (1886) cement which is composed of two parts paraffin wax to 7–9 parts powdered colophonium resin. The two ingredients are mixed together by heating and are filtered, while hot, into a metal container. The cement is re-melted for use.

Several fluid ringing media are available commercially and cellulose adhesives such as Durofix [p. 503] may be used for the purpose as may nail varnish, the bottles of which usually incorporate a suitable brush, the contents being in a range of interesting colours.

As the name implies, ringing is most easily accomplished when using circular coverslips and a specially designed turntable.

For a description of the technique applicable to small larvae, insects, and helminths see Furse (1955).

LABELLING OF SLIDES

When sections are attached to slides, the latter should bear the laboratory or case number of the section. This is most effectively applied with a diamond writing pencil and not only provides ready identification of the section but also helps to avoid the damage or partial loss of sections caused by wiping the 'wrong' side of the slide.

Unstained sections kept in reserve are sometimes numbered with a coloured grease-pencil thus avoiding an indelible marking of slides which might be cleaned and re-used. In actual practice however, labour costs are currently so high that it is probably more economical to discard unwanted unstained slides and to use new slides, purchased at quantity rates.

In pathology, it is a general rule for a paper label, bearing the patient's name, section number, and staining method used, to be attached to the slide, covering the diamond pencil number. Self-adhesive labels are available and may be printed with the name of the department or institution. Modern adhesives are very effective and these labels (in reels of 1000) are infinitely superior to individual, water-soluble gummed labels which often become detached on drying and which are less convenient and possibly dangerous in application.

FADING OF STAINED SECTIONS

With the mounting media described above, nearly all stained sections should retain their colour for many years if protected from strong light. However, the exposure of sections to strong sunlight by leaving on the bench will rapidly bleach sections, whatever the mounting medium. Prolonged exposure to an intense light-source such as the carbon arc of some microprojectors will also cause focal bleaching of sections while microradiographs, which require a strong light for examination under the microscope, should be protected by using a heat-absorbing filter.

Transferring stained sections from a broken slide to a new one

The following method quoted by Clayden (1948) from an anonymous source is very useful when slides bearing rare or irreplaceable sections are broken.

TECHNIQUE

1. Remove the coverslip from the section by soaking in warm xylene.
2. Treat further with xylene to dissolve all residual mountant.
3. Cover the whole slide with a mixture of butyl acetate, six parts and Durofix [p. 503] one part.
4. Harden the film in a 37 °C incubator for 15–30 minutes.
5. Cut the film from around the section with a sharp scalpel blade.
6. Immerse the whole slide in cold water until the film and section float off.
7. Mount on a clean, grease-free slide, and wipe off excess water.
8. Place in a 37 °C incubator until completely dry.
9. Remove remaining film by washing carefully with butyl acetate.
10. Wash thoroughly in xylene.
11. Mount in a synthetic resin mountant.

Standard staining methods

GENERAL METHOD

The mode of action of dyes and ways of applying stains to histological sections have been considered in the previous chapter. Further consideration should be given to the following practical details.

1. The *temperature* of the working area and the stain solutions will influence the duration and intensity of staining. A simple example of this is the staining of the tubercle bacillus with carbol-fuchsin [p. 398] where the time required for satisfactory staining decreases as the temperature of the stain is raised.
2. The presence or absence of *embedding medium* will not only influence the manipulation of the section during staining, but may result in coloration of the embedding medium and obscuring of detail in the section (see below).

3. The *thickness* of the section will profoundly influence staining and the duration of staining with, for example, haematoxylin and eosin, will be different with a 5 μm paraffin section compared with a 25 μm cellulose nitrate section of the same material. Furthermore, it is difficult to apply differential trichrome stains to thick sections successfully.

4. *Washing in water* is a procedure occurring in many staining methods but results may be affected by the pH of the laboratory water supply. This varies widely from country to country and indeed, within quite short distances in the same country. In the methods to be given below, a clear distinction will be made between washing in tap water, or tap water substitute (where an alkaline solution is required or is not harmful) and washing in distilled water, where the latter is desirable or essential.

OUTLINE OF PROCEDURE FOR STAINING PARAFFIN SECTIONS

Paraffin sections are nearly always stained on the slide after attachment thereto by the methods described on page 92.

Before staining, certain preparatory treatment of sections is necessary and involves the following steps. The reagents are either poured from drop bottles over the sections (in which case the slide should be flooded at least once, tilted, and flooded again), or the slides are placed in jars or dishes of the solutions.

For the preparation of large numbers of sections (e.g. for class work) the mica-slip or coverslip methods are recommended [p. 94].

Study of FIGURE 7.1 will indicate the steps necessary in the preparation of paraffin sections for staining and in their return to xylene, prior to mounting and examination. The function of each step is as follows.

Removal of paraffin wax

Because paraffin wax is poorly permeable to stains its removal with a solvent is necessary and xylene is used for this purpose. One or two minutes immersion in each of two changes of xylene is usually sufficient for sections up to 10 μm in thickness and removal of the wax will be promoted by warming the slide before immersion.

Sometimes, this treatment does not completely remove the wax from sections and Nedzel (1951), Hamperl (1961), and Vlachos (1968) referred to residual paraffin wax being the cause of birefringence of cell nuclei, particularly of lymphocytes and tumour tissue. In addition, failure to completely remove the wax from sections will result in impairment of staining and it is possible that the 'Pink Disease' artifact [p. 50] may be caused by incomplete removal of wax from sections. Vlachos stated that in some cases, treatment of sections with xylene for one hour at 60 °C might be necessary to remove all wax and improve staining.

Removal of xylene with absolute alcohol

Xylene is not miscible with aqueous solutions and low-grade alcohols and it is therefore necessary to remove this with absolute alcohol. One half to one minute in each of two changes of absolute alcohol is adequate for the purpose.

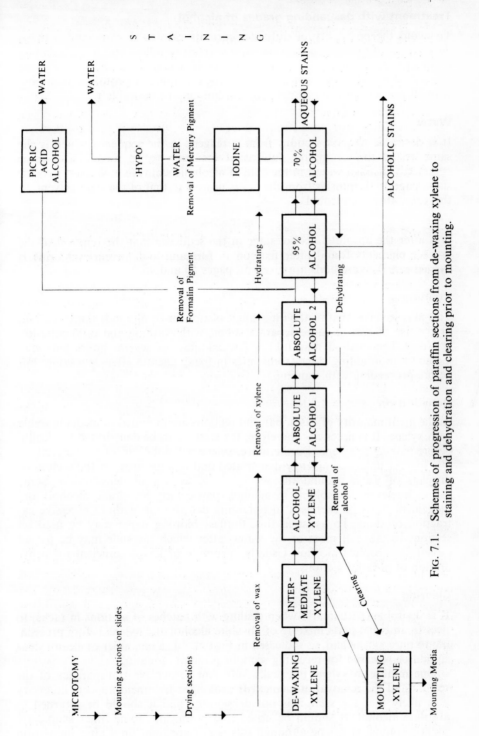

FIG. 7.1. Schemes of progression of paraffin sections from de-waxing xylene to staining and dehydration and clearing prior to mounting.

Treatment with descending grades of alcohol

To avoid the possibility of diffusion currents causing damage and perhaps detachment of the section, it is standard practice to follow absolute alcohol by treatment for a minute or two with 90 per cent and sometimes, 70 per cent alcohol. (For extremely delicate objects such as films of protozoa, treatment with 50 per cent or even 30 per cent alcohol may be desirable.)

Water

It is desirable to pass sections from a reagent in the sequence which is the same as, or similar to, the solvent of the stain to be used first. This is commonly distilled water; in the case of alcoholic stains (e.g. Weigert's elastic stain, page 193), transfer from the grade nearest to that of the stain solvent, in this case, absolute alcohol.

NOTE

It is after the absolute alcohol stage in the sequence that the removal of the artifact pigments found after fixation in formalin and mercuric chloride is carried out. The methods are given on pages 50 and 45.

Staining

This may involve treatment with a single (simple or compound) stain solution, or the use of two or more separate stains, with washing and differentiation between. The method may take a few minutes, or several hours and may include a mordanting stage (sometimes in fixing agents) after de-waxing, but before proceeding with staining.

Dehydration

In the great majority of cases, paraffin sections are mounted in media miscible with xylene. It is necessary therefore, for sections to be dehydrated in alcohol before passing to xylene. Furthermore, xylene will not clear, or render sections transparent unless completely dehydrated and opaque areas in the section or droplets of water around the section indicate lack of dehydration. Some stains, however, are soluble in alcohol (particularly low-grade alcohol) and judgement must be exercised in obtaining dehydration without excessive extraction of stain. To assist in this, fluffless blotting paper may be used on sections to take off most of the water, after which the slide may be passed directly to absolute alcohol. Usually, a minute or less is sufficient for dehydration of paraffin sections.

Clearing

It is desirable (particularly when dealing with batches of sections in racks) to pass to an equal parts mixture of absolute alcohol and xylene before proceeding to pure xylene and, as indicated in FIGURE 7.1, a container of clean xylene should be reserved for receiving sections prior to mounting.

One minute in xylene is usually sufficient to achieve transparency of the section and the removal of alcohol. If prolonged treatment appears necessary it is likely that the section is not dehydrated and it should be returned to absolute alcohol. It should be noted that eosin, and some other stains, are slightly soluble in xylene although this is not apparent until after immersion for some hours.

Mounting

A coverslip is applied to protect and preserve the section. Surplus xylene is carefully wiped from around the section with a fluff-free cloth when, without allowing the section to dry, mounting medium is applied as a drop or streak, the size of which will be governed by the shape and size of the section and will be readily determined with experience. The slide is quickly inverted and carefully lowered, to make contact with a cleaned coverslip of suitable dimensions. Firm adhesion of the coverslip to the section will take some hours at room temperature but is hastened by heat.

OUTLINE OF PROCEDURE FOR STAINING FROZEN SECTIONS

Frozen sections mounted on slides may be handled in the same way as paraffin sections, the point of entry to the scheme of preliminary treatment depending on the stain to be used. The duration of staining, in most methods, is generally shorter for frozen sections than with comparable paraffin sections. Sections may be mounted in an aqueous medium directly from water where necessary.

Some procedures, particularly neurological staining methods, are carried out with unmounted frozen sections and in this case, sections are carefully transferred from one reagent to another by means of a bent glass rod or by pipetting off one solution from the dish before replacement with another. For the transfer of multiple frozen sections Albrecht (1956) has described a sieve-like device made from a piece of nylon stocking stretched over a ring of glass or plastic, the size according to the size and number of the sections.

Loose frozen sections to be mounted in resinous media will be shrunken and possibly distorted during dehydration and clearing with absolute alcohol and xylene. This may be lessened by use of either of the following methods of mounting:

1. a. Partially dehydrate in 95 per cent alcohol.
   b. Complete dehydration and clear in carbol-xylene (phenol crystals, 25 g, xylene, 75 cm^3).
   c. Mount in a synthetic resin medium. (Some basic stains, but not haematoxylin, are decolorized by carbol-xylene.)

or

2. a. Partially dehydrate in 95 per cent alcohol.
   b. Treat with 95 per cent alcohol, two parts, terpineol, one part for 1–2 minutes.
   c. Mount in Euparal.

OUTLINE OF PROCEDURE FOR STAINING CELLULOSE NITRATE SECTIONS

Cellulose nitrate sections are stored in 70–80 per cent alcohol until required for staining. Several methods (Williams 1957; Lundy 1958, 1963; and Lee's albumen method) have been described for attaching cellulose nitrate sections to slides prior to staining. None is entirely satisfactory and the standard method consists of staining either single or multiple sections before mounting on a slide and covering.

The transfer of sections from one solution to another may be done with a bent glass rod as with loose frozen sections, but since cellulose nitrate sections are generally thicker and more robust, they may be manipulated with the aid of forceps.

The same general principles of dehydration and clearing are applicable to both cellulose nitrate and paraffin sections, except that cellulose nitrate is soluble in absolute alcohol. For this reason, clearing procedures are designed to avoid the use of this reagent alone, and very many dehydrating and clearing mixtures have been advocated. A selection of four of these is given below; trial of each will indicate the best individual or combined method for the tissue and thickness of section. In each case, sections are arranged on slides after treatment with 95 per cent alcohol and because the embedding medium is still present and the sections thick, the duration of treatment with the various solutions will be appreciably longer than in the dehydration and clearing of paraffin sections.

Sheets of smooth toilet paper, cut slightly larger than the sections, and dropping bottles of the solutions should be available.

Method 1

1. Remove section from 95 per cent alcohol and arrange on the slide.
2. Cover with a piece of smooth toilet paper and flatten by gently rolling a piece of glass rod across the paper. Remove the paper and replace with a clean piece.
3. Pour on carbol-xylene [p. 135] and rub gently. Repeat with fresh paper and more carbol-xylene, two or three times over several minutes.
4. Replace paper and treat with xylene, several changes, until the section is clear.
5. Mount in Canada balsam.

Method 2

1.
2. } As in Method 1.
3. Treat with an equal parts mixture of chloroform, absolute alcohol, and xylene (CAX).
4. Treat with xylene.
5. Mount in Canada balsam.

Method 3

1.
2. } As in Method 2.
3.
4. Treat with pure beechwood creosote (not longer than 7 minutes).
5. Treat with xylene.
6. Mount in Canada balsam.

Method 4 (Slidders 1964)

1.
2. } As in Method 1.
3. Treat with 95 per cent alcohol two parts, terpineol one part.
4. Mount in Euparal.

NOTES

1. Because of the presence of the embedding medium and the thickness of the preparation, cellulose nitrate sections may stain deeply and unevenly. Better results may be obtained with diluted stains and Ehrlich's haematoxylin [p. 138] may be diluted with distilled water or alum and staining prolonged by several hours. Eosin of 1 per cent or less should be used for the same reason.

2. Because of the above, it is unrewarding to attempt stains such as Heidenhain's iron haematoxylin [p. 143] for cell structure or, for example, methods for the demonstration of mitochondria on cellulose nitrate sections since these methods depend in part on thin (3–6 μm) sections.

3. When mounting cellulose nitrate sections it is advisable to use a liberal quantity of a not too thin mounting medium. This is because the section will continue to soak up mounting medium for a little time after application of the coverslip and pressure on this (to express air bubbles) or wiping the edges of the coverslip with a xylene soaked cloth, thus diluting the medium, will make retraction of the medium and the formation of airspaces between section and coverslip inevitable.

SERIAL SECTIONS

The manipulation and staining of serial sections of cellulose nitrate embedded tissue is tedious and time consuming; several methods have been suggested for staining such sections in bulk, and in a way that will preserve the correct sequence. A method adapted from the collodion film method Lundy (1958) is as follows.

Sections are attached in sequence, about 5 mm apart, by means of an office stapling machine, through one margin of the cellulose nitrate, along a strip of polythene film (500-gauge), cut slightly wider than the width of the sections. The length of the strips will be determined by the size of the sections and the staining dishes available (developing dishes are suitable). Staining is carried out by transferring the strip of polythene with attached sections, from one dish to another. The sections are detached from the film with scissors and arranged in the correct order on numbered slides prior to mounting.

Strips of polythene film holding sections not immediately required for staining may be rolled up and stored in 70 per cent alcohol.

HAEMATOXYLIN

Haematoxylin is the most widely used and versatile dye in histological technique and is used in stains for the demonstration of cell nuclei, myelin, elastic fibres, fibrin, neuroglia, and muscle striations. For all these purposes, however, haematoxylin must be converted to haematein by oxidation and must be used in conjunction with a mordant such as the salts of aluminium, iron, or tungsten. Haematein is available commercially and is used in some stains.

Haematoxylin is most commonly used as a nuclear stain preceding staining of cytoplasm and connective tissue with eosin and examples of these solutions and a standard haematoxylin and eosin (HE) method are given below. In 1973 there was a general shortage of haematoxylin and this led to a renewal of interest in dyes that might act as substitutes, particularly as nuclear stains (Llewellyn 1974; Lillie 1974; Lillie, Pizzolato, and Donaldson 1974, 1975a, b,

1976). The reason for the shortage was never clearly established but it did not last long and supplies are now normal.

For a full account of haematoxylin stains see Cole (1943) and Lillie (1965).

ALUM HAEMATOXYLIN AND EOSIN

Regardless of the formula and whether the haematoxylin is oxidized slowly and spontaneously, or by chemical oxidizing agents, *all* alum haematoxylins will vary in staining power during their period of usefulness. This means that the optimum duration of staining with for example, Ehrlich's haematoxylin, may vary from 5 to 30 minutes depending on the amount of haematein present in the solution at the moment of use, as well as on the temperature at which staining takes place, and the fixative and previous treatment of the tissue. Furthermore, because of variation in actual dye content in samples of haematoxylin, it may be necessary to modify the amount of haematoxylin in the solutions given below. For these reasons, it is not possible to give reliable, precise directions for the duration of staining in alum haematoxylin stains although indications will be given.

Alum haematoxylin solutions do not retain their full powers of staining for as long as is sometimes supposed and the use of test sections, kept especially for checking new or doubtful samples is recommended. Sections of formalin fixed appendix would suit the purpose well and if stained with over-oxidized, or effete haematoxylin would show weak, non-selective staining of nuclei with greyish coloration of cytoplasm (even after acid differentiation) and possibly, intense staining of epithelial mucin.

Stock solutions should be stored in a cool place in tightly stoppered, dark glass bottles and the regular replacement of stain kept in jars with loose-fitting lids is a wise precaution in busy laboratories where several hundred sections may pass through the jar of stain in the course of a week.

Ehrlich's (1886) haematoxylin

This is probably the most commonly used alum haematoxylin in both normal and morbid histology.

PREPARATION

Haematoxylin	2 g
Absolute alcohol	100 cm³
Glycerol	100 cm³
Distilled water	100 cm³
Glacial acetic acid	10 cm³

Aluminium potassium sulphate (potassium alum) in excess (10–14 g)

Dissolve the haematoxylin in the alcohol before adding the other ingredients. The stain may be ripened naturally by allowing to stand in a large flask, loosely stoppered with cotton wool, in a warm place and exposed to sunlight. The flask should be shaken frequently and ripening takes some weeks. When good staining is attained on the test slide, the solution is bottled. Filter before use.

The haematoxylin may be partially oxidized and the stain used immediately, by the addition of 0.3 g sodium iodate ($NaIO_3$) to the above.

The glycerol acts as a stabilizer and retards evaporation, and as the haematoxylin becomes oxidized, the colour of the solution changes from purplish to deep red, while the pungent odour of the acetic acid is replaced by a pleasant vinous aroma.

Aluminium ammonium sulphate (ammonium alum) may be substituted for the potassium alum of the original formula and is equally satisfactory.

Ehrlich's haematoxylin is generally used regressively and after staining for about 20 minutes (see above), sections are differentiated in 1 per cent hydrochloric acid in 70 per cent alcohol (acid alcohol) until nuclei are selectively stained. It should be noted, however, that Ehrlich's haematoxylin also stains some mucopolysaccharide substances such as cartilage and the 'cement lines' of bone. Areas of calcification will also be stained intensely blue.

Mayer's (1903) haemalum (cited from Lendrum and McFarlane 1940)

Another widely used haematoxylin stain, Mayer's, is more vigorous in action than Ehrlich's haematoxylin and gives little or no staining of mucopolysaccharide material. It is used in the celestine blue-haemalum method of nuclear staining [p. 145]. Stain for 5–10 minutes.

PREPARATION

Haematoxylin	1 g
Sodium iodate	0.2 g
Potassium alum	50 g
Citric acid	1 g
Chloral hydrate	50 g
Distilled water	1000 cm³

Allow the haematoxylin, alum, and sodium iodate to dissolve overnight. Add chloral hydrate and citric acid and bring to the boil. Continue boiling for five minutes after which the solution is cooled and is ready for use.

If not required for immediate use, the boiling may be omitted, allowing further ripening to take place at room temperature, optimum oxidation then requiring up to three months. The chloral hydrate acts as a preservative, the citric acid sharpens nuclear staining.

Harris' (1900) haematoxylin

A powerful and selective nuclear stain giving sharp delineation of nuclear structure. For this reason, Harris' haematoxylin is used widely as a nuclear stain in exfoliative cytology and when staining sex chromatin with haematoxylin. Stain for 2—5 minutes.

PREPARATION

Haematoxylin	1 g
Absolute alcohol	10 cm³
Ammonium or potassium alum	20 g
Distilled water	200 cm³
Mercuric oxide	0.5 g

Dissolve the haematoxylin in the alcohol and add to the alum, previously dissolved in hot water. Bring quickly to the boil and add the mercuric oxide, when the solution will turn dark purple. Cool rapidly under the tap, filter before use. Mallory (1938) recommended the addition of 8 cm³ glacial acetic acid to the above, after cooling, to sharpen nuclear staining. The stain should be prepared in a flask of ample size on account of the frothing that takes place on addition of the mercuric oxide.

Cole's (1943) haematoxylin

A satisfactory alum haematoxylin for routine purposes, Cole's solution has good keeping qualities and is suitable for use in sequence with celestine blue, unlike Ehrlich's haematoxylin. Stain for ten minutes.

PREPARATION

Haematoxylin	1.5 g
1 per cent iodine in 95 per cent alcohol	50 cm³
Saturated aqueous ammonium alum	700 cm³
Distilled water	250 cm³

Dissolve the haematoxylin in the warmed distilled water before adding and mixing with the iodine. Add the alum solution and bring to the boil. Cool immediately and filter before use.

EOSIN

Eosin, a red dye, properly used on well fixed material, stains connective tissue and cytoplasm in varying intensity and shades of the primary colour giving a most useful differential stain. With haematoxylin, it is the routine stain in histopathology and much of the present knowledge of morbid histology has been gained from the study of HE stained sections.

One of the xanthene group of dyes, eosin is derived from fluorescein and is available in two main shades—as yellowish or as bluish (a deeper red). Eosin Y (yellowish) is most commonly used and is readily soluble in water, less so in alcohol.

A 5 per cent stock solution is convenient, using either tap water or distilled water as solvent, the alkalinity of the former being considered to give superior staining. In either case, moulds will grow in the solution. To help prevent this, a crystal of thymol or a few drops of formalin may be added, or moulds may be removed by filtration. They do not affect the stain. One per cent eosin is commonly used as a working solution although the exact concentration is not critical.

Haematoxylin and eosin staining method

As pointed out on page 116 it is now standard practice to stain sections with haematoxylin regressively; that is, with a stain of sufficient power and for long enough to ensure some over-staining of nuclei, the superfluous and obscurative coloration of structures being removed by treatment with acid (differentiation). This method is, in fact quicker, especially with multiple sections, than progressive staining, where it may be necessary to interrupt staining and examine microscopically on two or three occasions before satisfactory staining is achieved.

TECHNIQUE (MANUAL)

1. De-wax sections as outlined in the general scheme on page 133, removing artifact pigments en route [see pp. 45 and 50].
2. Stain in haematoxylin, in a jar, for 2–20 minutes depending on which of the above stains are used, the strength of the stain, and the fixative used.

3. Wash well in running tap water for 2–3 minutes. The section may be examined microscopically at this stage to confirm a sufficient degree of staining. If insufficient, return to the stain.
4. Remove excess stain by decolorizing (differentiating) in 0.5–1 per cent hydrochloric acid in 70 per cent alcohol for a few seconds. The blue staining of the haematoxylin is changed to red by the action of the acid.
5. Regain the blue colour and stop decolorization by washing in alkaline, running tap water for at least five minutes. The stain should again be checked microscopically until proficiency in naked-eye control of decolorization has been gained by experience with stain and tissues.
6. Stain in 1 per cent aqueous eosin for 1–3 minutes.
7. Wash off surplus stain in water.
8. Examine microscopically. Cytoplasm and muscle fibres should be deep pink, collagen a lighter pink. Red blood cells and eosinophil granules should be a bright orange-red.
9. Dehydrate in alcohol and clear in xylene as outlined in the general scheme, bearing in mind that aqueous eosin is removed from tissues by water and low grade alcohol, less readily by absolute alcohol. The degree of staining of eosin is thus easily controllable and a slight overstaining when sections are examined prior to dehydration will be remedied during the passage through alcohol.
10. Mount in a synthetic resin medium.

TECHNIQUE (AUTOMATIC STAINING MACHINE)

1.	Xylene I	3 min
2.	Xylene II	3 min
3.	Absolute alcohol I	3 min
4.	Absolute alcohol II	2 min
5.	70 per cent alcohol	3 min
6.	Distilled water	3 min
7.	Cole's haematoxylin	10 min
8.	Tap water	5 min
9.	0.25 per cent HCl in 70 per cent alcohol	1 min
10.	2 per cent sodium hydrogen carbonate	2 min
11.	Tap water	5 min
12.	0.5 per cent eosin	5 min
13.	Tap water	90 sec
14.	Absolute alcohol III	2 min
15.	Absolute alcohol IV	2 min
16.	Absolute alcohol–xylene	2 min
17.	Xylene III	3 min

Transfer sections to a final bath of xylene prior to mounting.

RESULTS

Nuclei—blue to blue–black.
Nucleoli—red or purple or blue depending on type.
Cartilage—pink or light blue to dark blue depending on type and the stain used, being darkest with Ehrlich's haematoxylin.
Cement line of bone—blue with Ehrlich's haematoxylin.
Calcium and calcified bone—purplish blue.
Basiphil cytoplasm (plasma cells and osteoblasts)—purplish.

Red blood cells, plasmasomes, eosinophil granules, Paneth cell granules, zymogen granules, keratin—bright orange–red.

Cytoplasm—shades of pink.

Muscle fibres, thyroid colloid, thick elastic fibres, decalcified bone matrix— deep pink.

Collagen and osteoid tissue—light pink.

NOTES

1. *Structures stained.* Useful as it is, many structures are not clearly demonstrated or are not stained by the HE method. Thus, neuroglia fibres, axons, nerve endings, much reticulin and cell constituents such as Golgi bodies and mitochondria are not demonstrated, even when preserved by the fixative. Occasionally, bacteria are stained purple or pink although this staining does not indicate that the organisms are Gram positive or Gram negative respectively. Special stains are necessary to demonstrate all of the above.

2. *Duration of staining with haematoxylin.* Staining with hamatoxylin may have to be prolonged with tissues given long treatment with chrome salts and following chrome–osmium fixatives such as Flemming. Material subjected to long acid decalcification, prolonged storage in acid formalin or in 70 per cent alcohol will require forced staining and iron haematoxylin or celestine blue-haemalum might be used with advantage. Warming greatly accelerates, while low temperatures retard staining with haematoxylin.

3. *Blueing of haematoxylin.* In some places, the tap water is not sufficiently alkaline, or is even acid, and unsatisfactory for blueing haematoxylin, in which case a tap water substitute (TWS) modified from Scott (1912) is used for the purpose. It is made by dissolving 3.5 g sodium hydrogen carbonate (sodium bicarbonate) and 20 g magnesium sulphate in 1000 cm³ of water with thymol added to inhibit mould formation. This acts quickly and thin paraffin sections are fully blued in 15–30 seconds. Equally effective and simpler is the 2 per cent aqueous solution of sodium hydrogen carbonate recommended by Cook (1974).

   The temperature of the tap water used for blueing also plays a part in the process and when very cold (below 10 °C) blueing will be slow and may be hastened by the use of warm water.

4. *Staining with eosin.* Fixing agents greatly influence subsequent staining with eosin and tissues fixed in chromates and in picric acid take up eosin strongly, as does acid decalcified material. Satisfactory staining with eosin however, does not depend solely on depth of staining but on the differentiation of the stain. For example, quite light eosin staining may be perfectly differential and therefore satisfactory, while an intensely stained section may show little or no differentiation of eosin and be unacceptable.

IRON HAEMATOXYLIN

Iron haematoxylin is so called because ferric chloride, or ferric ammonium sulphate (iron alum) are here used as mordants. These substances also act on haematoxylin as oxidizing agents, converting it to haematein and it is for this reason that iron haematoxylin stains do not generally keep well as prepared mixtures. An exception is the iron haematoxylin method solution of Slidders (1969) which has a working life of about two months. In two classical methods, mordant and stain are kept separately and either mixed immediately before use (Weigert's haematoxylin) or are kept and used separately (Heidenhain's haematoxylin). Because mordant and stain are kept separately, however, it has become established that a 'well-ripened' haematoxylin solution be used for mixing with the iron salt, although this may cause *over-oxidation* of the haematoxylin and an unsatisfactory stain. To avoid this, a not too aged (a few weeks old) solution of haematoxylin is advisable and some iron haematoxylin solutions are perfectly satisfactory with freshly prepared stain.

Heidenhain's (1896) iron haematoxylin

First described in 1892 and modified in 1896, Heidenhain's iron haematoxylin is a cytological stain. It is applicable after several fixatives and stains many structures. It is used regressively and requires careful differentiation, for which reason it is only completely successful on thin sections. It may be used to demonstrate chromatin, chromosomes, nucleoli, centrosomes, mitochondria, yolk, muscle striations, and myelin.

PREPARATION

Mordant and differentiator
Ferric ammonium sulphate   5 g
Distilled water   100 cm³

Use only the clear, violet crystals of alum, not those that have become opaque and yellowish-green. Dissolve without heat.

Haematoxylin stain
Haematoxylin   0.5 g
Absolute alcohol   10 cm³
Distilled water   90 cm³

Dissolve the haematoxylin in the alcohol and then add the water. Allow to ripen for a few weeks and store in a tightly-stoppered bottle.

TECHNIQUE

1. De-wax sections and take to water.
2. Place in iron alum mordant for 30 minutes to 24 hours (see notes).
3. Rinse in distilled water.
4. Place sections in the haematoxylin stain for a time equal to the duration of the mordanting. Sections are adequately stained when they are homogeneous jet-black, showing no cellular detail. This applies after all fixatives.
5. Rinse well in tap water.
6. Differentiate in the iron alum solution, controlling microscopically by removing the slide from the alum and washing briefly in tap water to halt the process during examination. Continue differentiation and examination until sections are suitably de-stained, noting that red blood cells, keratin, and bone take up and retain the stain strongly. Diluted (2.5 per cent) mordant may be found more easily controllable for differentiation until completely familiar with the stain.
7. Wash for at least ten minutes in running tap water to remove all traces of iron alum.
8. Dehydrate in alcohol, clear in xylene, and mount in synthetic resin or Euparal.

RESULTS

Tissues structures in tones of black and grey, or colourless, according to the extent of differentiation. Red blood cells usually remain black.

NOTES

1. *Duration of mordanting and staining.* This is largely dependent on the fixative used. After Susa, formalin, mercuric chloride-formalin, Bouin, and Carnoy, 30–60 minutes in mordant and stain is sufficient. After Zenker, Helly, and Orth, 3–12 hours is necessary, using the 12 hour period for the staining of mitochondria. After Flemming and other chrome–osmium fixatives, 12–24 hours treatment with mordant and stain is necessary.

2. *Differentiation.* The stain is given up first from ground substance and connective tissue, then from cytoplasmic constituents such as mitochondria and lastly from nuclear chromatin and nucleoli, red blood cells usually remaining black. No precise times can be given for the duration of differentiation, the only guide being the use of the staining microscope.

3. *Advantages of the method.* (1) Its application to tissues fixed in virtually any fixative and the number of structures that may be demonstrated. (2) Its permanency, for providing all iron alum is washed out, the stain is free from fading. (3) Its ability to stain tissues that fail to stain with other methods, such as tissue stored for some years in alcohol. (4) The stained section being in tones of black and grey, eye-strain is minimal, the picture is suitable for photomicrography and accurate reproduction of projected images may be made. (5) While a large number of counterstains could be applied after Heidenhain's iron haematoxylin, in practice a contrast stain is not necessary and rarely adds to the value of the preparation.

4. *Shorter method.* When time is not available for the optimum duration of mordanting and staining, useful results may be obtained by carrying out the sequence at 60 °C (in the wax oven) allowing 10–15 minutes in each solution. Jars should be tightly covered and the stain used in this procedure should be discarded and not returned to the stock bottle. Hot iron alum may be used for differentiation but with great care owing to the rapid extraction of the stain by this method.

Weigert's (1904) iron haematoxylin

This solution is the standard iron haematoxylin for staining nuclei and is used particularly when preceding stains containing acid, such as van Gieson [p. 182] where one of the constituents (picric acid) has a marked decolorizing action on nuclei stained with the alum haematoxylin stains described above. The stain is applicable after most fixatives.

PREPARATION

Solutions A (stain)

Haematoxylin	1 g
Absolute alcohol	100 cm³

The solution need not be ripened and may be used immediately.

Solution B (mordant)

30 per cent aqueous ferric chloride (anhyd.)	4 cm³
Concentrated hydrochloric acid	1 cm³
Distilled water	95 cm³

Solutions A and B are stored separately and mixed immediately before use, the prepared stain keeping only for a few hours.

With fresh, or recently prepared haematoxylin (A), add an equal amount of mordant (B). With aged solutions of haematoxylin (months or years old) less than an equal volume should be used. The colour of the mixture should be a deep purplish black. If muddy-brown, it is unsatisfactory.

TECHNIQUE

1. De-wax sections and take to water.
2. Stain with iron haematoxylin mixture for 5–15 minutes.
3. Wash in tap water.
4. Examine microscopically. Differentiation may not be necessary, especially if preceding van Gieson's stain. If required, use 0.5–1 per cent hydrochloric acid in 70 per cent alcohol for a few seconds.
5. Wash thoroughly in running tap water, or in tap water substitute.
6. Counter-stain as desired.
7. Dehydrate, clear, and mount.

RESULT

Nuclei, brownish black to black.

CELESTINE BLUE–HAEMALUM SEQUENCE STAINING

As an alternative to iron haematoxylin nuclear stains, Lendrum and McFarlane (1940) described the use of two stains, celestine blue (an oxazine dye) and alum haematoxylin, in sequence, to provide a powerful and precise nuclear stain resistant to decolorization by succeeding acid stains and solutions. The celestine blue is dissolved in iron alum which has an additional mordanting effect on the haematoxylin stain. Mayer's or Cole's haematoxylin solutions are equally suitable for use with celestine blue and the combination has proved effective and reliable; in some laboratories it has replaced Weigert's iron haematoxylin in most methods where the latter was formerly used. Note however, that celestine blue stains cellulose nitrate more or less strongly and irremovably and for these sections, an iron haematoxylin should be used.

PREPARATION

Celestine blue B	0.5 g
Ferric ammonium sulphate	5 g
Glycerol	14 cm^3
Distilled water	100 cm^3

Dissolve the iron alum in the water without heat. Add the celestine blue and boil for three minutes. Filter when cool and add the glycerol. The stain should keep for at least six months.

TECHNIQUE

1. De-wax sections and take to water.
2. Stain in celestine blue for five minutes.
3. Rinse in water.
4. Stain in Mayer's or Cole's haematoxylin for five minutes.
5. Wash well in running tap water.

Whether de-staining in acid alcohol is carried out will depend on the method in which the sequence is used. Instructions will be given where appropriate.

PHOSPHOTUNGSTIC ACID HAEMATOXYLIN (PTAH)

Mallory (1897, 1900)

This stain was originally propounded for the demonstration of neuroglia. It is now widely used for other purposes and is unique among haematoxylin stains in the number of structures that may be demonstrated, together with the two-colour staining (shades of blue and red) from the single solution.

The composition of the stain is simple (haematoxylin, phosphotungstic acid, and water) but variation in the proportions of dye and mordant have a profound effect on the efficiency of the stain. Mallory first advocated a 1 : 10 ratio of haematoxylin to mordant but later (1900) suggested, somewhat curiously, that because the phosphotungstic acid used earlier was impure, a 1 : 20 ratio should be used with the pure mordant. This latter formula is the one most widely quoted in texts on histological technique but there is increasing evidence (Lendrum 1947; Terner *et al.* 1964; Shum and Hon 1969) that this proportion of phosphotungstic acid is too high and does not give the most satisfactory staining.

Natural ripening of phosphotungstic acid haematoxylin (PTAH) is slow and several chemical oxidizing agents have been used to hasten the conversion of haematoxylin to haematein, particularly, potassium permanganate, hydrogen peroxide, mercuric oxide, sodium iodate, or combinations of these. Each have their advocates, but it is noteworthy that peak efficiency of the stain may not be achieved until some days or even weeks after the addition of these oxidizers. As an alternative to spontaneous or chemical oxidation, haematein may be used initially, instead of haematoxylin and provides a stain that is usable 24 hours after preparation.

The colour of the solution, which may range from reddish brown to purple, is not a reliable guide to the quality of the stain.

As with other haematoxylin solutions, staining with PTAH is affected by the fixative used but not as greatly as is generally accepted and a wide range of fixatives are suitable. Zenker's fluid was especially recommended by Mallory (1938) but while mercuric chloride and chrome fixatives are suitable and beneficial, their use is by no means obligatory and 10 per cent formalin is adequate for general purpose. However, several mordants have been recommended for the treatment of sections in lieu of the recommended Zenker fixation, the most important of these being strong iodine solutions, saturated mercuric chloride, chrome salts and iron alum. Of these, 4 per cent iron alum (Lieb 1948) is widely used and enhances the blue staining of structures.

Traditionally an integral part of the method, the so-called 'Mallory bleach', consisting of pre-treatment with potassium permanganate and oxalic acid, was originally incorporated to suppress the staining of myelin when using the solution for the demonstration of neuroglia. For the staining of nuclei, fibrin, muscle striations, and collagen however, its use is unnecessary and may be detrimental (Bulmer 1962).

Staining with PTAH is essentially progressive and the duration of staining may vary from 1–16 hours (overnight). It is doubtful whether longer treatment is ever effective, but heat accelerates staining and 1–2 hours at 60 °C is often adequate.

The stain is applicable to frozen sections as well as to paraffin and cellulose nitrate embedded material.

PREPARATION

Haematein   1 g
Phosphotungstic acid   10 g
Distilled water   1000 cm³

Dissolve the haematein in one half of the water, the phosphotungstic acid in the other, and then mix. Store in a tightly stoppered bottle and use after 24 hours.

TECHNIQUE

1. Take sections to water.
2. Mordant in 4 per cent iron alum for 20 minutes to one hour.
3. Wash well in distilled water.
4. Stain in PTAH for 1–16 hours.
5. Rinse briefly in 95 per cent alcohol.
6. Dehydrate in absolute alcohol, clear in xylene, and mount in synthetic resin medium.

RESULTS

Nuclei, fibrin (if freshly formed), striations of muscle, myofibrils, astrocytes and their processes, and fibroglia—blue.
Collagen, matrix of bone and cartilage—orange–red or brownish-red to deep brick red.

NOTES

1. Mordanting in iron alum is not always necessary.
2. The staining being progressive, microscopical examination at intervals of one hour is recommended.
3. Treatment with 95 per cent alcohol rapidly extracts the red component of the stain and should therefore be brief.
4. For observations on the use of PTAH for the staining of fibrin see page 228; muscle striations, page 192; mitochondria, page 179; and neuroglia, page 373.

COMMON COUNTERSTAINS

The term is used to denote the application of a different colour to provide contrast and background to the staining of the component or structure that the technique is designed to demonstrate. They may therefore be nuclear or cytoplasmic, single or multiple, and of several colours. They may give a flat, general background colour (as with light green after the Feulgen reaction, page 160) or a degree of tissue differentiation (as with iron haematoxylin and orange G or tartrazine, following the staining of elastic tissue, page 195).

It is important to bear in mind that the purpose of counterstains is supplementary. They should be used discreetly, never dominating, obscuring or causing change of colour of the primary stain, as may occur if too heavily applied.

The following is a list of some of the more important dyes that may be used as counterstains; some of them are also used as primary stains. Details of their use will be found in appropriate methods.

CYTOPLASMIC STAINS

Red	*Yellow*	*Green*
Eosin Y	Picric acid	Light green SF
Eosin B	Tartrazine	Fast green FCF
Erythrosin B	Metanil yellow	Lissamine green
Phloxine B	Orange G	
Biebrich scarlet		
Rose bengal		

NUCLEAR STAINS

Red	*Blue*
Neutral red	Methylene blue
Safranin O	Toluidine blue
Carmine	Celestine blue
	Haematoxylin

METALLIC IMPREGNATION METHODS

An outline of the theory underlying the demonstration of tissue components by metallic impregnation has been given on page 110 and details of methods are given in the following pages. Certain basic procedures are applicable to the use of metallic impregnation methods however, and are considered below.

First, the duration of treatment with the reagents used in these methods is often short and critical and freedom from interruption or distraction is essential.

Second, metallic impregnation methods are somewhat capricious and unhelpful results often inexplicable. Meticulous attention to detail is necessary and inadvertent modification, at any stage, may have a detrimental effect.

Third, the adventitious deposition of metallic silver on sections is a common failing and to help prevent this, all reagents should be chemically pure, glassware scrupulously clean, and a formalin-laden atmosphere avoided. Metal instruments should not be used to handle sections.

Finally, all users should be made aware of the potentially explosive properties of ammoniacal silver solutions. Serious accidents have occurred from the misuse of this reagent, although receiving little publicity. Stewart Smith (1943) described such as accident, Nauta and Gygax (1951) warned of the dangers, and Wallington (1965) gave accounts of several accidents, explained the probable cause of the explosions and offered advice on safety. This is as follows:

1. All ammoniacal silver solutions should be prepared immediately before use, in clean vessels and not in 'silvered glassware' which is especially dangerous. Flexible plastic containers offer greater safety. The recommendation of Lendrum (1947) to coat staining jars with black paper, bound with strong tape (for storage of solutions) might lessen the effect of an explosion but would not prevent (at least) subsequent blackening of person and surroundings.
2. Solutions should never be exposed to sunlight.
3. Any unused reagent should be immediately inactivated by the addition of

excess dilute hydrochloric acid or a solution of sodium chloride, and discarded. Refrigeration does not prevent formation of the explosive compound.

4. All new staff and students should be instructed in the above.

REFERENCES

ALBRECHT, M. H. (1956). *Stain Technol.* **31**, 231.
APATHY, S. VON (1892). *Z. wiss. Mikr.* **9**, 15.
BULMER, D. (1962). *Quart. J. micr. Sci.* **103**, 311.
CHAFFEY, N. J., and SPAIN, L. G. (1962). *J. med. Lab. Technol.* **19**, 180.
CLAYDEN, E. C. (1948). *Practical section cutting and staining.* Churchill, London.
COLE, E. C. (1943). *Stain Technol.* **18**, 125.
COOK, H. C. (1974). *Manual of histological demonstration techniques.* Butterworths, London.
CRAWFORD, R. A. (1952). *J. med. Lab. Technol.* **10**, 194.
EHRLICH, P. (1886). *Z. wiss. Mikr.* **3**, 150.
FURSE, H. (1955). *J. med Lab. Technol.* **13**, 3.
GRECO, J. F. (1950). *Stain Technol.* **25**, 11.
HAMPERL, H. (1961). *Virchows Arch. path Anat.* **334**, 79.
HARRIS, H. F. (1900). *J. appl Micr.* **3**, 777.
HEIDENHAIN, M. (1892). *Festschrift für Koelliker.* Leipzig.
—— (1896). *Z. wiss. Mikr.* **13**, 186.
HIGHMAN, B. (1946). *Arch. Path.* **41**, 559.
KAISER, E. (1880). *Bot. Zbl.* **1**, 25.
KIRKPATRICK, J., and LENDRUM, A. C. (1939). *J. Path. Bact.* **49**, 592.
—— (1941). *J. Path. Bact.* **53**, 441.
KRÖNIG. (1886). *Arch. mikr. Anat.* **27**, 657.
LENDRUM, A. C. (1947). In *Recent advances in clinical pathology* (ed. S. C. Dyke). Churchill, London.
—— and McFARLANE, D. (1940). *J. Path. Bact.* **50**, 381.
LIEB, E. (1948). *Arch. Path.* **45**, 559.
LILLIE, R. D. (1965). *Histopathologic technic and practical histochemistry*, 3rd edn. McGraw-Hill, New York.
—— (1974). *Am. J. med. Technol.* **40**, 355.
—— and ASHBURN, L. L. (1943). *Arch. Path.* **36**, 432.
—— PIZZOLATO, P., and DONALDSON, P. T. (1974). *Stain Technol.* **49**, 339.
—— —— —— (1975a). *Stain Technol.* **50**, 127.
—— —— —— (1975b). *Am. J. clin. Path.* **65**, 876.
—— —— —— (1976). *Stain Technol.* **51**, 25.
—— WINDLE, W. F., and ZIRKLE, C. (1950). *Stain Technol.* **25**, 1.
—— ZIRKLE, C., DEMPSEY, E., and GRECO, J. F. (1953). *Stain Technol.* **28**, 57.
LLEWELLYN, B. D. (1974). *Stain Technol.* **49**, 347.
LUNDY, J. (1958). *Stain Technol.* **33**, 188.
—— (1963). *Stain Technol.* **38**, 251.
MALLORY, F. B. (1897). *J. exp. Med.* **2**, 529.
—— (1900). *J. exp. Med.* **5**, 15.
—— (1938). *Pathological technique.* W. B. Saunders, Philadelphia.
MAYER, P. (1903). *Z. wiss. Mikr.* **20**, 409.
NAUTA, W. J. H., and GYGAX, P. A. (1951). *Stain Technol.* **26**, 5.
NEDZEL, G. A. (1951). *Quart. J. micr. Sci.* **92**, 343.
SCOTT, S. G. (1912). *J. Path. Bact.* **16**, 390.
SHUM, M. W. K., and HON, J. K. Y. (1969). *J. med. Lab. Technol.* **26**, 38.
SLIDDERS, W. S. (1964). Personal communication.
—— (1969). *J. Micros.* **90**, 61.
STEWART SMITH, G. (1943). *J. Path. Bact.* **55**, 227.

TERNER, J. Y., GURLAND, J., and GAER, F. (1964). *Stain Technol.* **39**, 141.
VLACHOS, J. D. (1968). *Stain Technol.* **43**, 89.
WALLINGTON, E. A. (1965). *J. med. Lab. Technol.* **22**, 220.
WEIGERT, C. (1904). *Z. wiss. Mikr.* **21**, 1.
WILLIAMS, T. D. (1957). *Stain Technol.* **32**, 97.

8 | Proteins, nucleic acids, and nucleoproteins

Proteins

Proteins, carbohydrates, and lipids are the basic constituents of animal tissues. Proteins are the most widely distributed and important and are found either as pure proteins or combined with carbohydrates or lipids. Table 8.1 shows that proteins can be *simple* (unconjugated) or *conjugated*.

Table 8.1. Main types of proteins in animal tissues

PROTEINS		
SIMPLE		CONJUGATED
GLOBULAR	FIBROUS	
Albumins, Globulins, Histones	Collagen, Reticulin, Elastin, Keratin, Fibrin	Nucleoproteins, Glycoproteins, Lipoproteins

The simple proteins are *globular* proteins such as albumins, globulins, or histones, or *fibrous* proteins which we recognize in tissues as reticulin, collagen, fibrin, keratin, etc. All simple proteins can be broken down by hydrolysis into amino-acids only, whilst the conjugated proteins are composed of amino-acids combined with carbohydrates (glycoproteins), lipid (lipoproteins), or nucleic acids (nucleoproteins).

Proteins are present in nuclei, and nucleoproteins will be described later in this chapter. The commonest proteins in tissues are in the cytoplasm and the fibrous proteins such as collagen, reticulin, elastin, and keratin are easily preserved and shown in sections. These are insoluble in water, but the simple proteins albumin and globulin are soluble and are more difficult to demonstrate.

THE STAINING AND IDENTIFICATION OF PROTEINS

The staining reactions of proteins and protein-containing compounds will depend upon the amino-acid composition and the pH of the staining solution. If the protein is composed of a large number of amino-acids with acidic groups, such as carboxyl ($-COOH$), it will be an acid protein combining with basic dyes. On the other hand, if there are many amino-groups ($-NH_2$) it will be a basic protein which will have an affinity with acid dyes. Some amino-acids contain one amino- and one carboxyl group and are neutral. Similarly proteins with approximately equal numbers of acidic and basic amino-acids will also be neutral. The ability of proteins to ionize as acid or basic substances may depend upon the pH of their environment; it is necessary for the pH of the stain solution to be appropriate to allow the protein to ionize strongly so that it can combine with the stain. Many tissue components can be destained by acids or alkalis (e.g. nuclei by acid-alcohol after haematoxylin) and amphoteric dyes or tissue constituents are basic or acidic according to their pH. These factors are significant in dye staining of proteins, but it must be appreciated that the staining reactions of conjugated proteins may be dependent upon the structure of the carbohydrate or lipid or nucleic acid component if this overshadows that of the protein.

The precise histochemical reactions of proteins are due to their reactive groups, and these are not peculiar to one amino-acid or one type of protein. Amino-groups are present in almost all amino-acids, but reactive carboxyl groups are characteristic of the acid amino-acids aspartic and glutamic acids and disulphide and sulphydryl groups are present in cystine, cysteine, and methionine. Histochemical methods for amino-acid reactive end-groups give some indication of the structure of a protein compound and Table 8.2 shows the reactive end groups and their amino-acids that can be demonstrated by the histochemical techniques which will be described. It is important to remember that proteins are highly complex structures with a huge number of components and these methods only give small pieces of information about their structure. In addition, fixation can affect the ability to preserve and demonstrate reactive end-groups and fixation must be appropriate for the method; many fixatives can be used for protein histochemical methods but formalin fixation should be brief and osmium tetroxide is contra-indicated.

Enzymes are proteins which react upon substrates and can be demonstrated by their specific activity. They will not be discussed in this chapter, but enzyme histochemistry is described in Chapter 16, page 298.

Table 8.2. Histochemical methods for reactive groups of amino-acids in proteins

Reactive group	Amino-acids	Histochemical methods
Amino— —NH$_2$	All except imino-acids	Ninhydrin–Schiff Blocking techniques
Disulphide —S—S	Cystine	Performic Alcian blue
Sulphydryl —S—H	Cysteine	DDD Ferric ferricyanide reaction
Guanidyl NH ‖ H$_2$N—C—N $\dot{\text{C}}$	Arginine	Sakaguchi
Phenyl OH—⬡	Tyrosine	Millon
Indole	Tryptophan	DMAB—nitrite

Immunoglobulins can be indentified with precision in tissue sections and can be localized with precision despite their small size. The immunofluorescent and immunoenzyme methods for antibodies and antigens are described in Chapter 17, page 323 and a large number of proteins can be shown in sections by immunological techniques.

The Ninhydrin–Schiff method for amino-groups (Yasuma and Ichikawa 1953)

Ninhydrin will react with amino-groups at neutral pH to form aldehydes. The aldehydes are demonstrated by Schiff's reagent. Not all protein-bound amino-groups are oxidized by ninhydrin but lysine, hydroxylysine, glutamic, and aspartic acids will give positive results. Neutral formalin fixation is satisfactory.

FIXATION

Neutral formal-saline, Zenker, absolute ethyl alcohol, and other fixatives.

SECTIONS

Paraffin, unfixed cryostat sections, or freeze-dried tissue.

TECHNIQUE

1. Bring sections to alcohol.
2. Treat with preheated 0.5 per cent ninhydrin in absolute ethyl alcohol at 37 °C for 16–20 hours.
3. Wash in running tap water for five minutes.
4. Place sections in Schiff's reagent [p. 239] for 30 minutes.
5. Wash in running tap water.
6. Counterstain with haematoxylin. Differentiate and wash in tap water.
7. Dehydrate in alcohol, clear in xylene, and mount in a synthetic resin medium.

RESULTS

Amino-groups—pinkish-red or magenta.

NOTES

1. PAS-positive compounds will be stained and control sections are needed.
2. 1.0 per cent Alloxan in absolute ethyl alcohol can be used instead of ninhydrin.

Blocking method for amino-groups by deamination (Stoward 1963)

TECHNIQUE

1. Bring sections to water.
2. Immerse in fresh pre-cooled nitrous acid solution (1 g of sodium nitrite in 30 cm^3 of 3 per cent sulphuric acid) for 48 hours in the refrigerator at 0.4 °C in the dark.
3. Wash in distilled water.
4. Treat for four hours in water or absolute ethyl alcohol at 60 °C.
5. Stain sections by the ninhydrin–Schiff method (see above) with an unblocked section back-to-back for comparative purposes.

RESULTS

The absence of staining compound with the unblocked section is a reliable indication of amino-groups before treatment.

Performic acid—Alcian blue method for disulphide (SS) groups (Adams and Sloper 1956)

Cystine is oxidized by performic acid to cysteic acid which can be stained by Alcian blue at pH 0.2. The method is specific but not highly sensitive.

FIXATION

Formalin-fixed tissues are satisfactory.

SECTIONS

Paraffin, cryostat, or freeze-dried sections. Sections should be well fixed to the slides to prevent loss.

PREPARATION

Performic acid

98 per cent formic acid	40 cm³
30 per cent (100 vol.) hydrogen peroxide	4 cm³
Conc. sulphuric acid	0.5 cm³

Add the hydrogen peroxide and the sulphuric acid to the formic acid. Allow to stand for an hour and use fresh.

Alcian blue (pH 0.2)

Alcian blue	2 g
Conc. sulphuric acid	5.4 cm³
Distilled water	94.6 cm³

Heat to 70 °C to dissolve the dye and filter when cool.

TECHNIQUE

1. Bring sections to water.
2. Stir the performic acid to remove dissolved gas and immerse the sections for five minutes.
3. Wash gently in tap water.
4. Dry at 60 °C until just dry. This helps the section to adhere to the slide.
5. Rinse section in tap water.
6. Stain in Alcian blue solution for one hour at room temperature.
7. Wash in tap water.
8. Counterstain in neutral red if required.
9. Dehydrate, clear, and mount in a synthetic resin medium.

RESULTS

Disulphides—light blue, or dark blue in higher concentrations.

NOTE

Keratin and the mucoid basiphilic cells of the anterior pituitary contain disulphide amino-acids; skin and pituitary can be used as positive control sections.

The DDD reaction for sulphydryl (SH) groups (Barrnett and Seligman 1952)

The reagent, dihydroxy-dinaphthyl-disulphide (DDD), combines with SH groups to form a naphthyl-disulphide compound. Free naphthols are removed by washing in alcohol and ether, and the naphthyl-disulphide is then demonstrated with the diazonium salt Fast blue B.

FIXATION

Formalin-fixed tissue can be used; avoid over fixation.

SECTIONS

Paraffin sections or unfixed cryostat sections.

PREPARATION

Dissolve 25 mg of DDD in 15 cm^3 of absolute alcohol. Add this to 35 cm^3 of 0.1 M veronal-acetate buffer [p. 499].

TECHNIQUE

1. Bring sections to water.
2. Incubate in preheated DDD reagent at 50 °C for one hour.
3. Cool to room temperature and rinse in distilled water.
4. Wash for ten minutes each in two changes of distilled water acidified to pH 4 with acetic acid. This converts the reagent and unwanted reaction products to free naphthols.
5. Wash out the free naphthols in four graded alcohols (70, 80, and 95 per cent and absolute) followed by absolute ether twice for five minutes.
6. Rinse in distilled water.
7. Stain for two minutes in freshly prepared solution of 50 mg of Fast blue B salt in 50 cm^3 phosphate buffer at pH 7.4 [p. 495].
8. Wash in running tap water.
9. Dehydrate in alcohol, clear in xylene, and mount in a synthetic resin medium.

RESULTS

Sulphydryl groups in high concentration—blue; in lower concentration—red.

The ferric-ferricyanide method for sulphydryl groups (Adams 1956)

Sulphydryl groups reduce ferricyanide to ferrocyanide at pH 2.4, and this is precipitated as insoluble Prussian blue with ferric chloride. Formal-saline fixed tissue can be used if fixation has been short. The method is described on page 273, but the reaction time should not be more than five minutes. This method is sensitive, but is not specific and control sections using a blocking technique for SH groups should be taken through the method with the test sections. Treatment with 1.24 per cent N-ethylmaleimide in phosphate buffer at pH 7.4 for four hours at 37 °C will block SH groups. Blue coloration that is present in the test sections and absent in the blocked sections indicates sulphydryl groups.

The Sakaguchi method for arginine
(Sakaguchi 1925, modified by Baker 1947)

This is the classical technique for proteins which demonstrates guanidyl groups in arginine. It suffers from the disadvantage of being a transient reaction that fades quickly and the sections cannot be mounted in conventional mounting media. Arginine reacts by its guanidyl groups with α-naphthol and an orange–red colour develops in the presence of alkaline hypochlorite.

FIXATION

Most fixatives can be used, including formalin.

SECTIONS

Paraffin, cryostat, or freeze-dried sections.

PREPARATION

Mix 2 cm^3 of 1 per cent sodium hydroxide, two drops of 1 per cent α-naphthol in 20 per cent alcohol and four drops of 1 per cent 'Milton' in distilled water. 'Milton' (and 'Chlorox') are stable sodium hypochlorite solutions.

TECHNIQUE

1. Bring sections to water. Testis can be used as tissue for positive control sections.
2. Rinse in 70 per cent alcohol.
3. Cover the section with alkaline α-naphthol solution for 15 minutes.
4. Drain and blot dry.
5. Immerse in a mixture of pyridine, 30 cm^3, and chloroform, 10 cm^3.
6. Mount in pyridine–chloroform and ring the coverslip. Examine the preparation immediately.

RESULTS

Arginine—orange–red.

The Millon reaction for tyrosine (Millon 1849; Baker 1956)

This is another classic method for proteins which indicates the presence of hydroxy-phenyl groups. Tyrosine is the only amino-acid that contains these groups. First a nitrosophenol is produced and this is converted into a coloured compound by the incorporation of a mercuric radicle.

FIXATION

Formalin, alcohol, and other fixatives.

SECTIONS

Paraffin or freeze-dried sections.

PREPARATION

1. Heat 10 g of mercuric sulphate in 10 per cent sulphuric acid until it is dissolved. Cool and make up to 200 cm^3.
2. Make a 0.25 per cent aqueous solution of sodium nitrite.

Take 30 cm^3 of solution 1 and mix with 3 cm^3 of solution 2.

TECHNIQUE

1. Bring sections to water.
2. Place the sections in a small beaker of the working solution (see above) and boil gently for two minutes.
3. Allow to cool to room temperature and wash in three changes of distilled water, two minutes in each.
4. Dehydrate in alcohol, clear in xylene, and mount in a synthetic resin medium.

RESULTS

Proteins that contain tyrosine—red or pink.

NOTE

This method can be used as a general staining method for proteins.

The DMAB–nitrite method for tryptophan (Adams 1957)

Indole groups in tryptophan combine with dimethylaminobenzaldehyde (DMAB) to produce β-carboline which is oxidized to a blue pigment, carboline blue, by sodium nitrite.

FIXATION

Formalin, preferably short duration (6-12 hours), alcohol, and other fixatives.

SECTIONS

Paraffin and freeze-dried sections.

PREPARATION

1. Dissolve 5 g of *p*-dimethylaminobenzaldehyde in 100 cm³ of conc. sulphuric acid.
2. Dissolve 1 g of sodium nitrite in 100 cm³ of conc. hydrochloric acid.

TECHNIQUE

1. Bring sections to alcohol.
2. If required, cover with a thin film of celloidin [p. 186].
3. Place sections in the DMAB solution for one minute.
4. Transfer to the sodium nitrite solution for one minute.
5. Wash in water for 30 seconds.
6. Rinse in acid-alcohol [p. 141] for about 15 seconds.
7. Dehydrate in alcohol, clear in xylene, and mount in a synthetic resin medium.

RESULTS

Tryptophan-containing proteins—deep blue.

NOTE

Fibrin, Paneth cell granules, and zymogen granules of pancreas all give strong reactions and can be used as positive control sections.

Nucleic acids and nucleoproteins

Nucleoproteins are combinations of nucleic acids and basic protein. *Deoxyribonucleic acid* (thymonucleic acid) is the main nuclear component, and is usually known as DNA. The other nucleic acid found in animal and plant tissues *ribonucleic acid* (plasmonucleic acid) is known as RNA and is present in the cytoplasm and to a lesser extent in the nucleus. In a HE stained section the darkly stained part of the nucleus is chromatin, made up of nucleoprotein that is largely DNA; as the nucleus is the directing force of the cell it can be appreciated that DNA is the most important part of the cellular structure. DNA is self-replicating, and determines the genetic characteritics that are passed on to each newly formed cell during cellular division. In the resting cell the chromosomes are spread out and cannot be seen separately, but during cellular division the chromosomes condense into individual components and it is then that the DNA is reproduced and passed on by the dividing chromosomes when they split along their lengths. RNA is present to a small extent in chromosomes, and to a greater extent in the nucleolus and in the ribosomes of the endoplasmic reticulum of the cytoplasm. In histological sections using dye staining and light microscopy the cytoplasmic RNA may be visible as basophilic granules; the cytoplasm of most cells is usually strongly acidophilic but plasma cells contain such a large amount of RNA in their cytoplasm that this is amphophilic (both basiphilic and acidophilic), staining purplish with a routine basic and acidic staining technique such as haematoxylin and eosin. RNA is especially concerned with the synthesis of protein and this is seen in plasma cells which produce globulins in the process of antibody formation; Russell bodies are hyaline inclusion bodies with a high RNA content that can be demonstrated in the cytoplasm of plasma cells.

THE STRUCTURE AND FUNCTION OF DEOXYRIBONUCLEIC ACID AND RIBONUCLEIC ACID

Nucleic acids are made up of nucleotide units, in the same way as proteins are built up from amino-acids. One of the components is a pentose or deoxypentose sugar, and as their names indicate, the pentose in DNA is deoxyribose and the pentose in RNA is ribose. Therefore DNA is a deoxyribose polynucleotide and RNA a ribose polynucleotide.

DNA has four nitrogenous bases, two purines (adenine and guanine) and two pyrimidines (thymine and cytosine). The nucleic acids are phosphorylated, and each nucleotide is a phosphate-pentose sugar-nitrogenous base compound. The DNA nucleotides are made up of phosphate and deoxyribose together with adenine, cytosine, guanine or thymine. DNA is a highly complex polymerized substance composed of many thousands of nucleotides which has been shown by Watson and Crick (1953) to be arranged in a double helix coiled in a spiral around a single axis with phosphate and sugar in the peripheral helices joined together by two nitrogenous bases, one a purine, the other a pyrimidine [FIG. 8.1]. RNA is a smaller compound of low molecular weight, with ribose instead of deoxyribose. Like DNA, it has four nitrogenous bases, three of which are common to both (adenine, cytosine, and guanine), but with uracil in place of thymine.

Nuclear chromosomes have two main functions: (1) the preservation and transmission of hereditary material; and (2) the production of substances that promote cell metabolism and carry it out according to characteristic inherited traits. DNA can reproduce itself synthetically if given a substrate containing the four nucleotides, and this reproduction is exact and would appear to be similar to that which occurs when DNA is replicated during the natural process of cellular division. In this way inherited DNA is passed from cell to cell and transferred to the next generation in the germ cells during reproduction. Chromosomes pass on genetic information by their genes, which are composed of DNA, and genetic characteristics are determined by the structure of the DNA in the gene. The sequence in which the four nucleotides are repeated along the length of the DNA molecule is the basis of genetic structure. The enormous number of permutations of the four nucleotides that can be produced allows vast numbers of genetic characteristics to be chemically coded in the form of 'words' in which four 'letters' are repeated

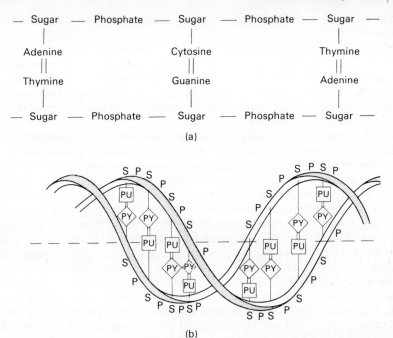

Fig. 8.1. The structure of DNA. (a) The constituents of a part of the molecule. (b) The double helical structure around a central axis. P = phosphate; S = sugar; PU = purine; PY = pyrimidine.

over and over again. Genes never leave their chromosomes but exert their influence in cytoplasmic activity by producing RNA that is modelled upon their own structure, and this RNA migrates into the cytoplasm. For each sequence of three nucleotides in the RNA molecule there is a corresponding amino-acid, and sequences of nucleotides in the DNA of the gene induce the synthesis of specific proteins through the intermediary of RNA. Most of the proteins synthesized according to the RNA pattern are enzymes that control metabolism and thus determine the physiological and morphological characteristics of the cell on a genetically induced basis.

STAINING METHODS FOR NUCLEIC ACIDS

It has been shown that the nucleic acids are phosphate–pentose–purine/pyramidine base compounds, and each of these constituents should be demonstrable by histological methods. The acidic phosphate radicle is the reason for their basiphilia, and basic dyes are widely used for the routine staining of nucleic acids, but as these combine with other substances in addition to nucleic acids they will not be specific. Methyl green has a special affinity for DNA and its use will be described in the methyl green–pyronin technique. For the demonstration of purines and pyramidines in the chromatin of chromosomes Danielli (1947) developed a tetrazonium reaction, but this has been shown to be non-specific for nucleoproteins. The sugar component of DNA is identified by the aldehyde–Schiff reaction after acid hydrolysis, and the Feulgen reaction is a precise and specific test for DNA. The results of the Feulgen reaction can be confirmed by the naphthoic acid hydrazide–Feulgen method which demonstrates aldehydes in a different manner.

RNA can be well shown by pyronin, and the pyronin–methyl green technique, despite some technical difficulties, remains a standard method for RNA and for DNA. When controlled with ribonuclease it may be regarded to be specific. In order to ensure valid and specific results enzyme controls and other chemical extraction procedures for nucleic acids can be performed, and these will be briefly described.

Nucleic acids have a strong affinity for basic dyes such as haematoxylin. Regressive haematoxylin staining methods, especially Heidenhain's iron haematoxylin, have been widely used and are still perfectly satisfactory for the routine demonstration of *nuclei* and *chromosomes*. The phosphate groups of DNA and RNA are acidic and combine with haematoxylin and other basic dyes by salt linkages; this is the most important mechanism of routine nuclear staining, though other factors may be involved. Basic dyes such as toluidine blue—which has a special affinity for RNA at pH 5 (Hermann *et al.* 1950)— safranin and neutral red can be used for the general staining of nucleic acids, but do not give such precise results as well differentiated haematoxylin. *Nucleoli* are basiphilic or acidophilic. Basiphilia is due to their high nucleic acid content, acidophilia to their protein constituents. The staining reaction with acidic and basic dyes will depend upon the relative proportions of nucleic acids and protein and will be influenced by fixation and by the pH of the staining solutions. Nucleoli can be stained by basic dyes such as haematoxylin or toluidine blue, but are Feulgen negative and are coloured green by the counterstain. They are pyroninophilic, being stained red with the methyl green–pyronin (Unna–Pappenheim) technique. They are not always stained by the methods for nuclear sex chromatin. Nucleoli fluoresce red with acridine orange, but the detail may be poor. Nucleoli are best demonstrated by general basic staining or by the modifications of the Feulgen reaction for nucleoli described by Semmens and Bhaduri (1939, 1941) which differentiates nucleoli from chromosomes. *Chromosomes* can be seen in histological sections but are usually studied in smears [p. 351]. *Nuclear sex chromatin*, present in normal females, is also easier to see in smears [p. 348].

THE FEULGEN REACTION FOR DEOXYRIBONUCLEIC ACID

The Feulgen reaction was described by Feulgen and Rossenbeck (1924) and is the most reliable and specific histochemical method for DNA. The original authors recommended the term 'nucleal test', which indicates that it is dependent upon the production of aldehydes and distinguishes it from the other Feulgen reaction, the plasmal test of Feulgen and Voit (1924).

The reaction is based upon the liberation of active aldehyde groups by breaking the purine-deoxyribose bond with acid hydrolysis. The aldehydes recolour Schiff's reagent (leucofuchsin, fuchsin sulphurous acid), giving a purple colour to nuclear chromatin. The method is analogous to the periodic acid–Schiff reaction for carbohydrates which is described on page 237. Doubts have been raised about specificity, but Pearse (1968) accepts the Feulgen reaction as specific for DNA. The plasmal reaction for acetal phospholipids, whose aldehydes can be freed by mild hydrolysis or oxidation, may interfere with the Feulgen reaction, but this is only of importance in frozen sections and can be ignored in paraffin sections.

In practice the Feulgen reaction will determine whether a basiphilic cellular component contains DNA. It is applicable, though not very widely used, to nuclear sex determination and general morphological studies. Quantitative histochemical estimation of DNA can be carried out by the Feulgen reaction; Stowell's (1942) photometric method is a reasonably simple one, and measures the amount of colour that is developed in the nuclei of the stained section.

Certain factors influence the performance of the Feulgen reaction.

FIXATION

Bouin is not recommended as it causes excessive hydrolysis during fixation. Most other fixatives can be used, but the optimum duration of acid hydrolysis varies with the fixative (Bauer 1932). Moreover, some fixatives, especially acetic-ethanol and acetic-sublimate, are associated with a short optimal hydrolysis time, lasting about one minute; others containing chromic acid, have long (10–20 minute) optima which give more latitude to the technique (Di Stefano 1948a and b). The speed of penetration of the fixative can affect the intensity of the Feulgen reaction; Swift (1953) found that there can be 30 per cent more staining of the nuclei at the edge of the block than in the centre with neutral formalin or acetic-ethanol.

HYDROLYSIS

This is usually carried out with N hydrochloric acid at 60 °C. Many alternative hydrolysing agents have been used, but these have no real advantages. Hydrolysis causes two different changes in the nucleic acids. The purine bases are rapidly removed and the aldehyde groups of the deoxyribose are exposed. This is the action that is required, but at the same time basic protein and nucleic acids are being removed from the chromosomes. Therefore an optimal time for hydrolysis exists for each fixative, and this time is a compromise between these two actions, giving maximum aldehyde liberation and hence greatest intensity of the Feulgen reaction. These optimal times are given in Table 8.3.

Table 8.3. Optimal hydrolysis times after various fixatives, using N HCl at 60 °C (after Bauer 1932; Lison 1953)

Fixative	Time (mins)	Fixative	Time (mins)
Acetic-sublimate	5	Flemming	16
Bouin—*not recommended*	—	Formalin	8
Carnoy	6–8	Formal-sublimate	8
Chrome-acetic	14	Helly	8
Absolute ethanol	5	Susa	18
Ethanol:formal:acetic (85:10:5)	7	Zenker	5

Insufficient hydrolysis will produce a weak Feulgen reaction, and excessive hydrolysis is associated with a negative result. In practice it may be desirable to put through a number of sections, giving each a different duration of hydrolysis, in order to determine the optimal time.

SCHIFF'S REAGENT

This was originally used for the demonstration of the aldehydes freed by the hydrolysis, and is still the reagent of choice. Alternatives such as naphthoic acid hydrazide, NAH (Pearse 1951), which combines with aldehydes and can be shown by coupling with a diazo-compound, can be used to confirm the findings with Schiff's reagent.

The Feulgen reaction for DNA (Feulgen and Rossenbeck 1924)

FIXATION

Various; not Bouin (see above).   *Sugar.*

SECTIONS

Paraffin sections. These must be well dried on the slides and should be attached with adhesive to avoid section loss.

PREPARATION

1. Schiff's reagent, see page 239. This may be purchased commercially.
2. Sulphite rinse. Mix equal volumes of 1 per cent potassium sulphite and 0.1 N HCl.

TECHNIQUE

1. Bring sections to distilled water.
2. Rinse briefly in cold N HCl and transfer to preheated N HCl at 60 °C for the optimal time (see Table 8.3). Place control section in distilled water at 60 °C for the same time.
3. Wash sections in distilled water.
4. Transfer to Schiff's reagent for $\frac{1}{2}$–1 hour.
5. Rinse in three changes of freshly prepared sulphite rinse.
6. Rinse in water.
7. Counterstain in 1 per cent aqueous light green for one minute. (Do *not* use haematoxylin.)
8. Dehydrate in alcohol, clear in xylene, and mount in a synthetic resin medium.

RESULTS

DNA, magenta.
Cytoplasm, green.

NOTES

1. The control section should be negative. Any positive reaction in this indicates free aldehydes present before hydrolysis.
2. Specificity can be determined by enzyme or chemical extraction controls [see p. 167].   *+ can be confirmed*

The naphthoic acid hydrazide–Feulgen reaction for DNA (Pearse 1951)

As Schiff's reagent will be recoloured by aldehydes in tissues (e.g. acetal phospholipids in frozen sections) in addition to those produced by acid hydrolysis it is an advantage to be able to use a different reagent. Naphthoic acid hydrazide combines with aldehydes to form a yellow compound which becomes purplish-blue when coupled with the diazonium salt Fast blue B. The results of DNA staining are similar to those using the classical Feulgen–Schiff reaction.

PREPARATION

1. 2-hydroxy-3-naphthoic acid hydrazide   50 mg
   Absolute alcohol   47.5 cm^3
   Acetic acid (conc.)   2.5 cm^3

2. Make a fresh solution of
   Fast blue B   50 mg
   Veronal-acetate buffer solution, pH 7.4 [p. 499]   50 cm^3

FIXATION

Various—not Bouin [p. 161].

SECTIONS

Paraffin sections, fixed to slides with adhesive and well dried.

TECHNIQUE

1. Bring sections to water.
2. Rinse briefly in cold N HCl.
3. Hydrolyse in preheated N HCl at 60 °C for the optimum time (Table 8.3).
4. Rinse in cold N HCl.
5. Wash in distilled water.
6. Rinse in 50 per cent ethyl alcohol.
7. Place sections in the naphthoic acid hydrazide solution for 3–6 hours at room temperature.
8. Wash in three changes of 50 per cent alcohol for ten minutes in each.
9. Rinse in distilled water.
10. Place sections in the freshly prepared Fast blue B solution for three minutes.
11. Wash in water.
12. Dehydrate in alcohol, clear in xylene and mount in a synthetic resin medium.

RESULT

DNA—bluish-purple.
Cytoplasm and other proteins may be pinkish-red.

THE METHYL GREEN–PYRONIN METHOD FOR NUCLEIC ACIDS

Pappenheim (1899, 1901) originally described the use of a mixture of the basic dyes methyl green and pyronin for staining chromatin green and basiphilic inclusion bodies (usually RNA) red. This was improved by the use of phenol by Unna (1902, 1913), and has been widely known as the Unna–Pappenheim technique.

The use of two basic dyes for the differential staining of DNA and RNA may seem illogical, but small differences in the chemical affinities of the two dyes can be made to produce considerable differences in their staining of tissues. It has been mentioned in Chapter 6 [p. 121] that basic dyes may combine with certain tissue constituents at one pH level and with others at a different pH. By the use of two basic dyes with these capacities a differential staining reaction can be obtained at a certain intermediate pH. This is seen with methyl green and pyronin; at low pH (1.5) there is total pyronin (red) staining, and with a high pH (9.0) the methyl green staining predominates. Between these two levels, usually pH 4.8, both dyes act, but in a differential manner. Unna's use of phenol gave the slight acidity that is necessary for this to take place. Kurnick (1950a, b) suggested that the degree of polymerization of DNA and RNA accounted for the differences in staining, and if DNA is depolymerized it looses its methyl green staining and stains red like the naturally less highly polymerized RNA.

Neither methyl green nor pyronin are specific for DNA or RNA, but in practice methyl green is highly selective for DNA. Pyronin can be regarded to be specific for RNA if it is controlled by ribonuclease (Brachet 1940) or by other extraction methods that are described on page 167. Alternative dyes have been used, such as malachite green and acridine red (Hitchcock and Ehrich 1930), and although these give similar green–red differential staining they have not superseded the use of methyl green and pyronin.

Difficulties have been encountered with the methyl green–pyronin technique. These have been due to a number of factors. Fixation has been regarded as critical, but satisfactory results can be obtained with neutral or buffered formal-saline; Ahlquist and Andersson (1972) have recommended staining at pH 3.8 after formalin fixation. Numerous modifications of the staining solution have been described, and variations between individual samples of dyes have been stressed. Other important practical points include the use of pyronin Y rather than pyronin B, and it is necessary to extract the methyl green and pyronin solutions with chloroform to remove impurities. Difficulties due to impurities in post-war samples of pyronin have been reported (Kasten 1962; Kasten *et al.* 1962).

The methyl green–pyronin stain for DNA and RNA
(Pappenheim 1899, 1901; Unna 1902, 1913)

The following modification (Trevan and Sharrock 1951) is suitable for material fixed in neutral formalin.

FIXATION

Neutral formalin and other fixatives, including alcohol, Carnoy and alcoholic formalin.

SECTIONS

Paraffin sections.

PREPARATION

Solution A
Make a 2 per cent aqueous solution of methyl green and extract all the methyl violet with chloroform. Wash the solution with several changes of chloroform in a separating funnel until the chloroform remains colourless. This washed solution is stable and can be used as a stock solution from which the following is prepared fresh.

2 per cent aqueous methyl green (chloroform washed)	10 cm^3
5 per cent aqueous pyronin Y	17.5 cm^3
Distilled water	250 cm^3

Solution B
Acetate buffer solution, pH 4.8. Mix 119 cm^3 of 0.1 M sodium acetate with 81 cm^3 0.1 M acetic acid. The original method also used orange G (31 cm^3 of 1

per cent aqueous orange G in 200 cm³ of the buffer solution) but this is not essential.

The *working solution* is prepared by mixing equal volumes of solutions A and B in a Coplin jar.

TECHNIQUE

1. Take paraffin sections to water.
2. Rinse in distilled water and blot dry.
3. Stain for 20–30 minutes in the working solution of methyl green and pyronin.
4. Rinse in distilled water for a few seconds and blot lightly until almost dry. Some pyronin is removed during this washing and the correct time should be determined by trial and error.
5. Dehydrate in acetone for not more than one minute.
6. Rinse in equal parts of acetone and xylene, and clear in pure xylene.
7. Mount in a synthetic resin medium.

RESULTS

DNA (chromatin), green or blue–green.
RNA (nucleoli), rose red; (granules), dark rose red; (plasma cell cytoplasm), purple.

NOTES

1. Full details of fixation, stains, and technique are given in Trevan and Sharrock's (1951) original paper; this should be consulted in case of difficulty.
2. Tissues which were not fresh when fixed, or fixed in acid formalin, will show too much red (pyronin) coloration.
3. Tissues that have been decalcified in acid are unsuitable, but after EDTA are satisfactory.
4. For specific control of RNA staining a control section from which the RNA has been extracted should be used. Ribonuclease is recommended (for details see Extraction Methods, page 167).
5. Similar control of DNA staining can be carried out with deoxyribonuclease, but this is not usually necessary due to the selectivity of methyl green for DNA.
6. Jordan and Baker's (1955) modification of Brachet's (1953) method is slightly different from the technique described above. Prepare the following solution fresh:

0.5 per cent aqueous methyl green (chloroform washed)	13 cm³
0.5 per cent aqueous pyronin Y	37 cm³
M/5 acetate buffer, pH 4.8	50 cm³

   Staining times and technique are otherwise similar.
7. After Zenker fixation (with acetic acid) the following malachite green–acridine red stain (Hitchcock and Ehrich 1930) may give good results.

Malachite green 0.3 g in 15 cm³ distilled water.	
Acridine red 0.9 g in 45 cm³ distilled water.	

   Mix immediately before use and stain for about half a minute. Other fixatives may be used if the pH of the staining solution is adjusted to a correct mild acidity; staining times should be prolonged to two or three minutes.

The gallocyanin–chrome alum method for RNA and DNA (Einarson 1932, 1951)

This method can be used with a wider range of fixatives than the methyl green–pyronin technique, is easier to perform and requires no differentiation. Specificity may not be as good, but this can be controlled with enzymes or extraction techniques [p. 167]. Gallocyanin combines with the phosphoric acid groups of nucleic acids at acid pH.

FIXATION

Most fixatives can be used.

SECTIONS

All sections.

PREPARATION

Chrome alum	5 g
Gallocyanin	150 mg
Distilled water	100 cm³

Dissolve the chrome alum in the distilled water. Then add the gallocyanin and slowly heat to boiling; boil for five minutes. Cool to room temperature and add distilled water to make up volume to 100 cm³. Filter before use.

TECHNIQUE

1. Bring sections to water.
2. Stain in the gallocyanin–chrome alum solution for 18–48 hours.
3. Wash in tap water.
4. Dehydrate in alcohol, clear in xylene, and mount in a synthetic resin medium.

RESULTS

DNA and RNA—blue.

NOTES

1. The pH of the staining solution should be 1.64. Nucleic acids will stain at a higher pH level, but this may be associated with non-specific staining in addition.
2. Berube *et al.* (1966) recommend purification of the chelate and using this as a 3 per cent solution in N sulphuric acid. Details are quoted by Pearse (1968).

FLUORESCENT STAINING OF NUCLEIC ACIDS

The fluorochrome acridine orange can be used to demonstrate DNA and RNA in sections of fresh tissue and in fresh or fixed smears. Acridine orange combines with nucleic acids in cells by salt linkages and by other cohesive forces, and when examined with a fluorescence microscope (blue light is adequate, see page 24) DNA fluoresces green and RNA fluoresces red. The most widely used application of this has been the screening of cervical smears for carcinoma cells, which is described on page 348). The method of Bertalanffy and Bickis (1956), using fresh unfixed cryostat sections, will give green DNA and specific red RNA fluorescence, and can be recommended for the routine demonstration of RNA, though permanent preparations cannot be obtained. Hicks and Matthaei (1955) found practically no RNA fluorescence with acridine orange in fixed tissues.

Acridine orange method for nucleic acids
(Bertalanffy and Bickis 1956)

FIXATION

Use fresh unfixed tissue. Mounted sections may be post-fixed in 5 per cent acetic acid in absolute ethyl alcohol. Fresh smears can be stained immediately.

SECTIONS

Cut cryostat sections of fresh unfixed tissue and mount on coverslips or slides.

PREPARATION

Take one part of 0.1 per cent acridine orange in distilled water and dilute with nine parts of Krebs–Ringer solution that has been adjusted to pH 6.2 with phosphate buffer.

TECHNIQUE

1. Place sections or smears in the above staining solution for at least 15 minutes at room temperature.
2. Remove staining solution with filter paper.
3. Mount in a drop of the buffered Krebs–Ringer solution and examine by fluorescence microscopy [p. 24].

RESULTS

DNA (nuclei), green.
RNA (nucleoli and cytoplasmic nucleic acids), red.
Fibrous tissue also green.
Background, black.

EXTRACTION METHODS FOR NUCLEIC ACIDS

The specific control of staining techniques for DNA and RNA can be carried out by extraction methods which remove or denature the nucleic acids, leaving other basiphilic substances such as mucopolysaccharides unaffected. There are two types of procedure, enzymatic, using deoxyribonuclease and ribonuclease, and chemical, using strong acids. The chemical methods extract both types of nucleic acids, but at different rates, thus enabling some degree of selective removal to be obtained. The use of specific enzymes is, of course, more satisfactory. The extraction methods that have been most widely used are shown in Table 8.4.

RIBONUCLEASE

This is a heat-resistant enzyme that splits RNA into its component nucleotides. It can be isolated from fresh beef pancreas by acidic extraction (Brachet 1940) and a crude ribonuclease is obtainable from saliva (Bradbury 1956). These are suitable for routine purposes, but pure commercial ribonuclease is recommended for more critical work. The optimum temperature for ribonuclease is 65 °C, but as some RNA is extracted by salt solutions or distilled water above 60 °C it is advisable to use ribonuclease at

Table 8.4. The extraction of nucleic acids

Agent	Temp.	Time	RNA	DNA
Ribonuclease	37 °C	1 hour	Extracted	Unaffected
Deoxyribonuclease	37 °C	1–24 hours	Unaffected	Extracted
5% perchloric acid	4 °C	4–18 hours	Extracted	Feulgen reaction positive. May polymerize and stain red with methyl green–pyronin
5% perchloric acid	70 °C	20 minutes	Extracted	Extracted
5% trichloracetic acid	90 °C	15 minutes	Extracted	Extracted

37 °C. Ribonuclease is specific for RNA and all cytoplasmic basiphilia that is destroyed can be assumed to have been due to RNA. Mucopolysaccharide basiphilia remains unchanged and the Feulgen reaction for DNA is also unaffected.

Ribonuclease extraction techniques

Use one of the following ribonuclease solutions.

1. Commercial crystalline ribonuclease, 8 mg in 10 cm³ distilled water.
2. Saliva (Bradbury 1956). Collect human saliva and place in a cold water bath. Heat to 80 °C and maintain for ten minutes at this temperature. Cool and centrifuge; use the supernatant fluid.
3. Extract of beef pancreas (Brachet 1940). Pulp fresh beef pancreas and suspend in 1–2 volumes of 0.1 N acetic acid at 37 °C for 24 hours. Boil for ten minutes and filter. Use at pH 7.0–7.5.

FIXATION

Neutral formal-saline, formal-sublimate, Carnoy, and Susa are satisfactory. Dichromate interferes with the removal of RNA and is best avoided. The type of fixation affects the rate of removal of RNA from the section.

TECHNIQUE

1. Bring paraffin sections to water.
2. Incubate for one hour at 37 °C in the enzyme solution. Place a control section in distilled water at 37 °C for the same time.
3. Wash in running water.
4. Stain with methyl green–pyronin (or toluidine blue).

RESULTS

RNA, extracted.
DNA, unaffected.

DEOXYRIBONUCLEASE

This is not heat-resistant and is activated by magnesium ions. Though available commercially it is expensive and has not been used widely in histological techniques. The enzyme acts only on fixed nuclei and like ribonuclease the extraction rate may vary with the fixative. It is specific for DNA and cytoplasmic basiphilia is not altered. Use 2–10 mg of the enzyme in 10 cm^3 of Gomori's Tris buffer [p. 498] at pH 7.6, diluted with 50 cm^3 distilled water. Kurnick (1952) suggests two hours at 37 °C or 24 hours at room temperature. A control section is placed in distilled water at 37 °C for the same time. The Feulgen reaction is then performed; positive staining in the control section that is abolished by the enzyme is due to DNA.

Acidic extraction methods

Perchloric acid (HClO$_4$) will extract both DNA and RNA, but RNA is removed more quickly. Use 5 per cent perchloric acid for 4–18 hours at 4 °C for the differential extraction of RNA; this removes all RNA but leaves the Feulgen reaction unchanged. Perchloric acid will depolymerize DNA and this may make the nuclei stain red (instead of green) with methyl green–pyronin. Both nucleic acids are removed by hot perchloric acid [see Table 8.4]. Perchloric acid is useful for the complete extraction of all nucleic acids, but ribonuclease is preferable for the extraction of RNA.

Trichloracetic acid (CCl$_3$COOH) will remove both DNA and RNA, but it is not suitable for differential extraction. DNA can be extracted by hydrolysis with Bouin's fluid and treatment with aniline (Tandler 1974); RNA is well preserved.

Other extraction methods

Bile salts have been shown to remove RNA (Foster and Wilson 1952). Sections are treated in 2 per cent sodium cholate for 2–3 hours at 60 °C. Continuous oxygenation is required during this time by means of a pressure system or a small pump.

REFERENCES

ADAMS, C. W. M. (1956). *J. Histochem. Cytochem.* **4**, 23.
—— (1957). *J. clin. Path.* **10**, 56.
—— and SLOPER, J. C. (1956). *J. Endocrinol.* **13**, 321.
AHLQUIST, J. and ANDERSSON, L. (1972). *Stain Technol.* **47**, 17.
BAKER, J. R. (1947). *Quart. J. micr. Sci.* **88**, 115.
—— (1956). *Quart. J. micr. Sci.* **97**, 161.
BARRNETT, R. J. and SELIGMAN, A. M. (1952). *J. nat. Cancer Inst.* **13**, 215.
BAUER, H. (1932). *Z. Zellforsch.* **15**, 225.
BERTALANFFY, L. VON and BICKIS, I. (1956). *J. Histochem. Cytochem.* **4**, 481.
BERUBE, G. R., POWERS, M. M., KERKAY, J., and CLARK, G. (1966). *Stain Technol.* **41**, 73.
BRACHET, J. (1940). *C. R. Soc. Biol.* (*Paris*) **133**, 88.
—— (1953). *Quart. J. micr. Sci.* **94**, 1.
BRADBURY, S. (1956). *Quart. J. micr. Sci.* **97**, 323.
DANIELLI, J. F. (1947). *Symp. Soc. exp. Biol.* **1**, 101.
DI STEFANO, H. S. (1948a). *Proc. nat. Acad. Sci.* (*Wash.*) **34**, 75.
—— (1948b). *Chromosoma* (*Berl.*) **3**, 282.
EINARSON, L. (1932). *Am. J. Path.* **8**, 295.
—— (1951). *Acta path. Scand.* **28**, 82.
FEULGEN, R. and ROSSENBECK, H. (1924). *Z. phys. Chem.* **135**, 203.
—— and VOIT, K. (1924). *Pflügers Arch. ges. Physiol.* **206**, 389.
FOSTER, C. L. and WILSON, R. R. (1952). *Quart. J. micr. Sci.* **93**, 147.
HERMANN, H., NICHOLAS, J. S., and BORICIOUS, J. K. (1950). *J. biol. Chem.* **184**, 321.

HICKS, J. D. and MATTHAEI, E. (1955). *J. Path. Bact.* **70**, 1.
HITCHCOCK, C. H. and EHRICH, W. (1930). *Arch. Path.* **9**, 625.
JORDAN, B. M. and BAKER, J. R. (1955). *Quart. J. micr. Sci.* **96**, 177.
KASTEN, F. H. (1962). *Stain Technol.* **37**, 265.
—— BURTON, V., and LOFLAND, S. (1962). *Stain Technol.* **37**, 277.
KURNICK, N. B. (1950a). *Exp. Cell Res.* **1**, 151.
—— (1950b). *J. gen. Physiol.* **33**, 243.
—— (1952). *Stain Technol.* **27**, 233.
LISON, J. (1953). *Histochimie et cytochimie animales*, 2nd edn. Gauthier-Villars, Paris.
MILLON, A. N. E. (1849). *C. R. Soc. Biol. (Paris)* **28**, 40.
PAPPENHEIM, A. (1899). *Virchows Arch. path. Anat.* **157**, 19.
—— (1901). *Virchows Arch. path. Anat.* **166**, 424.
PEARSE, A. G. E. (1951). *J. clin. Path.* **4**, 1.
—— (1968). *Histochemistry, theoretical and applied*, 3rd edn., Vol. 1. Churchill, London.
SAKAGUCHI, S. (1925). *J. Biochem. (Tokyo)* **5**, 25.
SEMMENS, C. S. and BHADURI, P. N. (1939). *Stain Technol.* **14**, 1.
—— (1941). *Stain Technol.* **16**, 119.
STOWARD, P. J. (1963). D. Phil. Thesis, University of Oxford.
STOWELL, R. E. (1942). *J. nat. Cancer Inst.* **3**, 111.
SWIFT, H. (1953). *Int. Rev. Cytol.* **2**, 1.
TANDLER, C. J. (1974). *Stain Technol.* **49**, 147.
TREVAN, D. J. and SHARROCK, A. (1951). *J. Path. Bact.* **63**, 326.
UNNA, P. G. (1902). *Mh. prakt. Derm.* **35**, 76.
—— (1913). *Virchows Arch. path. Anat.* **214**, 320.
WATSON, J. D. and CRICK, F. H. C. (1953). *Nature (Lond.)* **171**, 737.
YASUMA, A. and ICHIKAWA, T. (1953). *J. Lab. clin. Med.* **41**, 296.

9 | Cytoplasmic granules

EOSINOPHIL LEUCOCYTES

The demonstration of the cytoplasmic granules of eosinophil leucocytes in tissues presents no special problems. As the name implies, the granules are well shown in haematoxylin and eosin stained sections, especially if the washing out of eosin is extended until connective tissue is a very pale pink, affording good contrast to the brilliant orange–red staining of the granules.

The Romanowsky blood stains [p. 215] may be applied to sections for the demonstration of eosinophil cells and the carbol-chromotrope method of Lendrum (1944) stains the granules strongly and selectively.

Lendrum's (1944) method for eosinophils

FIXATION
Not critical: any routine fixative.

SECTIONS
Paraffin or frozen sections.

PREPARATION
Melt 1 g phenol crystals by warming the flask under a hot water tap. Add 0.5 g Chromotrope 2R and mix with phenol. Dissolve the mixture in 100 cm^3 distilled water. The stain keeps for three months.

TECHNIQUE
1. Take sections to water.
2. Stain nuclei in Mayer's or Cole's haematoxylin.
3. Wash well in tap water.
4. Differentiate nuclei in acid-alcohol.
5. Blue nuclei in running tap water.
6. Stain in carbol-chromotrope for 30 minutes.
7. Rinse in water.
8. Dehydrate, clear, and mount in a synthetic resin medium.

RESULTS
Eosinophil granules—red.
Nuclei—blue.
Red blood cells and Paneth cell granules—a distinctive pale rust colour.
Enterochromaffin cell granules—brown.

MAST CELLS

Mast cells are found normally in connective tissue, particularly in relation to blood vessels and nerves. They may be increased in number in certain pathological conditions (mastocytosis and mastocytoma).

The cytoplasm of mast cells contains abundant granules and while these are inconspicuous in haematoxylin and eosin stained sections, their high content of heparin (a sulphated acid mucopolysaccharide) allows their demonstration by the staining of this substance.

The distribution and character of mast cells varies somewhat from species to species and according to their functional state (Eady 1976) and numerous methods have been described for the demonstration of the granules. In human tissues, the metachromatic staining of the granules is well shown by the uranyl nitrate method of Hughesdon [p. 250]. Mast cells are also clearly demonstrated with the Romanowsky stains [p. 215] and while the granules are variably PAS positive, they are stained a deep purple–violet with Gomori's aldehyde–fuschin stain [p. 196].

For a general account of the staining characteristics and histochemistry of mast cells see Montagna et al. (1954) and the 29 articles on mast cells and basiphils (including electron microscopy) in Padawer, Whipple, and Silver-zweig (1963).

PANETH CELLS

Paneth cells are situated at the base of the crypts of Lieberkuhn in the small intestine and their cytoplasm contains strongly acidophil, coarse granules. Their precise function is not known, but they contain zinc (Gardner and Dodds 1976) and are thought to be exocrine cells of zymogenic nature (Lewin 1969). Immunoglobulins IgA and IgG have been demonstrated in Paneth cells and it is postulated that the cells may have capability for phagocytosing and degrading micro-organisms (Rodning, Wilson, and Erlandsen 1976).

Prompt fixation is essential to preserve the granules but they are dissolved by primary treatment with acid fixatives such as Zenker, Bouin, and Susa. Preliminary treatment for a few hours with neutral formal-saline however, renders the granules resistant to the solvent action of these fixatives if used secondarily (Wallington 1955).

Paneth cell granules are strongly acidophil and are well shown in haematoxylin and eosin stained sections, with Romanowsky stains, the phloxine-tartrazine method [p. 400] of Lendrum (1947), the fuchsin-miller method of Slidders [p. 230] and the MSB method [p. 229].

THE CELLS OF THE PANCREAS

The pancreas is a gland with both exocrine and endocrine functions, the main bulk of the organ being concerned with the exocrine (zymogenic) activity. The cells of this part, whose arrangement resembles that of salivary glands, contains eosinophil (zymogen) granules in the apical part of the cytoplasm while the basal part contains RNA and stains purplish with haematoxylin. Zymogen granules are concerned with the formation of enzymes involved in digestive processes.

Formalin, Helly's fluid, and formal-sublimate are satisfactory fixatives for zymogen granules but acetic acid-containing fixatives may dissolve the granules (in human material) and should be avoided.

Zymogen granules are well shown with haematoxylin and eosin, trichrome stains [p. 183] and the phloxine–tartrazine method [p. 400]. Results with the PAS method are variable.

The endocrine function of the pancreas is performed by the cells of the islets of Langerhans which are distributed throughout the organ but are more abundant in the tail.

The two main cell types found in the islets are alpha (A) cells and beta (B) cells with the latter predominating. The A cells produce glucagon and are normally found at the periphery of the islets while the B cells produce insulin and occupy the interior. Two other and less numerous cell types have been identified in the islets. These are C cells which are thought to be undifferentiated precursors of A and B cells (Rhodin 1974) and D cells which produce somatostatin and are located among A cells at the periphery of the islets (Orci and Unger 1975).

The specific granules of the islet cells of the pancreas cannot be distinguished in haematoxylin and eosin stained sections and the special methods used for the purpose are not invariably successful. The prompt fixation of fresh material is a prerequisite. Two of the more reliable methods for demonstrating islet cells are given below. Trichrome stains of the Masson type are not generally satisfactory for this purpose.

Gomori's (1941) chrome alum haematoxylin–phloxine stain

FIXATION

Thin slices of tissue are fixed in Bouin or Helly, preferably primarily, although good results may be obtained by secondary treatment with these reagents after initial fixation in formal-saline.

SECTIONS

Thin paraffin sections.

PREPARATION

Chrome alum haematoxylin.

Haematoxylin	0.5 g
Chromium alum	1.5 g
5 per cent potassium dichromate	2 cm³
0.5 N sulphuric acid	2 cm³
Distilled water	100 cm³

The mixture is ripe in about 48 hours and may be used as long as a film with a metallic lustre continues to form on the surface of the mixture that has stood in a Coplin jar for 24 hours. This is about 4–8 weeks. Filter before use.

TECHNIQUE

1. Take sections to water.
2. Mordant in Bouin's fluid for 16–24 hours.
3. Wash sections thoroughly in tap water to remove picric acid.
4. Treat sections for one minute with an equal parts mixture of 0.3 per cent potassium permanganate and 0.3 per cent sulphuric acid.
5. Decolorize with a 2–5 per cent solution of sodium bisulphite.
6. Wash well in running water.
7. Stain in the haematoxylin solution for 10–15 minutes until microscopical examination shows the beta cells to be deep blue.
8. Rinse in water and differentiate in 1 per cent hydrochloric acid in 70 per cent alcohol for about one minute to remove background staining.

9. Wash in running tap water until the section is a clear blue.
10. Stain in 0.5 per cent aqueous phloxine for five minutes.
11. Rinse in water and treat with 5 per cent phosphotungstic acid for one minute.
12. Wash in running tap water for five minutes when the section should regain its red colour.
13. Differentiate in 95 per cent alcohol. If the section is too red and the alpha cells are not clear, rinse for 10–20 seconds in 80 per cent alcohol.
14. Dehydrate with absolute alcohol, clear in xylene, and mount in a synthetic resin medium.

RESULTS

Beta cells—blue.
Alpha cells—red (D cells are also pink to red).

Modified aldehyde–fuchsin stain (Halmi 1952)

FIXATION

Ten per cent formal-saline or Bouin's fluid.

SECTIONS

Thin paraffin section.

PREPARATION

Aldehyde-fuchsin (*Gomori*) see page 196.

Counterstain

Light green	0.2 g
Orange G	1 g
Phosphotungstic acid	0.5 g
Glacial acetic acid	1 cm^3
Distilled water	100 cm^3

This solution keeps well.

TECHNIQUE

1. Take sections to water.
2. Oxidize with Lugol's iodine for ten minutes.
3. Rinse in tap water and bleach with 2.5 per cent sodium thiosulphate.
4. Wash well in tap water followed by 70 per cent alcohol.
5. Stain in a jar of aldehyde-fuchsin stain for 15–30 minutes.
6. Wash in 95 per cent alcohol followed by water.
7. Stain nuclei with celestine blue and haemalum.
8. Wash in water, differentiate briefly in acid-alcohol, and wash well in tap water.
9. Rinse with distilled water and counterstain with orange G—light green for 45 seconds.
10. Rinse briefly with 0.2 per cent acetic acid followed by 95 per cent alcohol.
11. Dehydrate in absolute alcohol, clear in xylene and mount in a synthetic resin medium.

RESULTS

Beta cells—deep purple–violet; alpha cells—yellow; D cells—green; nuclei—blue–black; collagen—green; mast cells, elastic tissue and some mucopolysaccharide—purple–violet.

NOTE

Scott (1952) has described a modification of the above method which considerably reduces the duration of oxidation and staining. He oxidizes in an equal parts mixture of 0.5 per cent potassium permanganate and 0.5 per cent sulphuric acid (instead of iodine) for two minutes, bleaches in 2 per cent sodium bisulphite, washes, and stains in aldehyde fuchsin for 30 seconds to two minutes.

CELLS OF THE ANTERIOR LOBE OF THE PITUITARY

The cells of the anterior lobe of the pituitary (adenohypohysis) are of two main types, chromophil and chromophobe, according to the staining or lack of staining of their cytoplasm. The two types of cell are present in approximately equal numbers. Chromophil cells are also of two types according to their staining and are acidophil (40 per cent) and basiphil (10 per cent).

All these cells are in some way involved in the production of hormones and go through cycles of storage, secretion, and exhaustion and so their staining reaction and histological appearance will vary according to their functional state.

Characteristics of cell types (Rhodin 1974).

Chromophobes. These cells have small nuclei and little cytoplasm. Some of them (corticotrophs) secrete adrenocorticotrophic hormone (ACTH) while others are thought to be precursors of other cell types.

Acidophils (alpha cells). Among these cells are somatotrophs which secrete growth hormone (STH) and have abundant cytoplasmic granules, and mammotrophs which secrete a lactogenic hormone (LTH).

Basiphils (beta cells). These are generally larger than acidophils and have PAS positive (mucoprotein) granules in their cytoplasm. They include gonadotrophs which secrete two hormones, the follicle stimulating hormone (FSH) and the luteinizing hormone (LH), and thyrotrophs which are large polygonal cells secreting thyrotrophic hormone (TSH).

Tumours arising from the cells of the anterior lobe of the pituitary are usually benign adenomas which may stem from any of the cell types above with chromophobe adenomas being the most common.

DEMONSTRATION TECHNIQUES

Instructions for the selection of blocks from the pituitary are given on page 40.

Formal-saline, formal sublimate, and Helly's fluid are recommended as fixatives and paraffin sections are satisfactory. Thin, 3–4 µm sections are essential.

Fairly good distinction between the main types of cells is given by thin paraffin sections stained with haematoxylin and eosin, the cytoplasm of acidophils being bright red, basiphils a more purplish red, and chromophobes a pale greyish pink. Better distinction is given by the following simple methods.

Kerenyi and Taylor's (1961) pontamine sky blue method

FIXATION

Ten per cent formal-saline or formal-sublimate are suitable.

SECTIONS

Thin paraffin sections.

TECHNIQUE

1. Take sections to water.
2. Stain in 1 per cent aqueous pontamine sky blue 5BX for two minutes or longer.
3. Wash in running water for one minute.
4. Stain nuclei in Cole's, Mayer's, or Harris' haematoxylin.
5. Rinse in tap water and differentiate nuclei in 1 per cent hydrochloric acid in 70 per cent alcohol.
6. 'Blue' nuclei in running tap water for at least five minutes.
7. Stain in 0.5 per cent aqueous eosin for two minutes.
8. Differentiate eosin in water, dehydrate in alcohol, clear in xylene, and mount in a synthetic resin medium.

RESULTS

Nuclei—blue to blue-black.
Basiphils—bluish purple.
Acidophils—bright red.
Chromophobes—pale pink.

PAS–orange G stain (Pearse 1953)

The basiphils contain mucoprotein and are PAS positive, the acidophils are stained by orange G.

FIXATION

Routine fixatives are suitable.

SECTIONS

Thin paraffin sections.

TECHNIQUE

Stages 1–6 of the PAS method given on page 237, but after washing in water.
7. Stain briefly in 2 per cent orange G in 5 per cent phosphotungstic acid.
8. Wash in water until the section is microscopically a pale yellow.
9. Dehydrate in alcohol, clear in xylene, and mount in a synthetic resin medium.

RESULTS

Nuclei—black.
Mucoid cells—magenta.
Acidophils—orange.
Chromophobes—pale grey.

OFG (orange–fuchsin green) method of Slidders (1961)

Numerous trichrome stains of the Masson and Mallory type have been evolved for the differential staining of the cells of the anterior lobe of the pituitary and of these, one of the most reliable and rewarding is the method given below.

FIXATION

Not critical; formal-saline, formal-sublimate, and Helly's fluid are satisfactory.

SECTIONS

Thin paraffin sections.

TECHNIQUES

1. Sections are taken to water.
2. Stain nuclei with celestine blue–haemalum sequence.
3. Wash in water and differentiate nuclei in 0.25 per cent hydrochloric acid in 70 per cent alcohol.
4. Wash well in running water.
5. Rinse with 95 per cent alcohol and stain in a saturated solution of orange G in 95 per cent alcohol with 2 per cent phosphotungstic acid for two minutes.
6. Rinse in distilled water.
7. Stain in 0.5 per cent acid fuchsin in 0.5 per cent acetic acid for 2–5 minutes. Staining is progressive and should be continued until the basiphils are prominent.
8. Rinse in distilled water.
9. Treat with 1 per cent aqueous phosphotungstic acid for five minutes.
10. Rinse in distilled water.
11. Stain in 1.5 per cent light green in 1.5 per cent acetic acid for 1–2 minutes.
12. Rinse in distilled water.
13. Dehydrate in absolute alcohol, clear in xylene, mount in a synthetic resin medium.

RESULTS

Nuclei—black.
Acidophils—orange-yellow.
Basiphils—reddish-purple.
Chromophobes—greyish.
Erythrocytes—yellow.
Connective tissue—green.

Slidders' Br–AB–OFG (bromine, Alcian blue, orange, fuchsin green) method (1961)

This is a development and improvement of the performic acid–Alcian blue–PAS–orange G method of Adams and Swettenham (1958) whose method distinguishes two types of basiphil cells. These have been called S cells and R cells. The S cells because the Alcian blue demonstrates sulphur-containing amino-acids and R cells because these are resistant to oxidation and subsequent staining with Alcian blue. Slidders substituted bromine water for performic acid and also modified the Alcian blue stain.

FIXATION

Not critical; formal-sublimate is recommended.

SECTIONS

Thin paraffin sections.

PREPARATION

Bromine oxidizer: add 5 cm³ of 2.5 per cent potassium permanganate to 45 cm³ of 10 per cent hydrobromic acid.

Alcian blue: place 0.1 g Alcian blue in a beaker and add 1 cm³ concentrated sulphuric acid. Mix with a glass rod and then add 9 cm³ glacial acetic acid. Mix again to dissolve the dye sludge and make up to 100 cm³ with distilled water. Filter.

TECHNIQUE

1. Sections are taken to water.
2. Rinse in distilled water.
3. Treat with bromine for 30–60 min.
4. Wash well in running tap water followed by distilled water.
5. Stain in Alcian blue for 30–60 min.
6. Wash in water and proceed with the OFG method above.

RESULTS

Nuclei—black.
S type basiphils—blue.
R type basiphils—magenta.
Acidophils—orange–yellow.
Chromophobes—greyish green.
Erythrocytes—yellow.
Stroma—green.

NOTES

1. Slidders states that acid-alcohol differentiation of the celestine blue–haemalum nuclear stain may slightly weaken staining of S cells with Alcian blue but that this may be avoided by differentiating with half saturated picric acid in 70 per cent alcohol. The picric acid must be thoroughly washed out of the section before proceeding with the method.
2. The Alcian blue will stain neurosecretory substance in the posterior pituitary as well as mast cell granules and keratin.

**One-stage MSB technique for the anterior pituitary
(Dawes and Hillier 1964)**

This is a modification of the martius-scarlet-blue method of Lendrum *et al.* (1962); the full method is described as a staining method for fibrin on page 229. A balanced staining solution containing the three stains makes this a reliable and rapid technique that requires no microscopical control; it may be used for fibrin and as a trichrome method for general purposes, but gives good differential staining of the acidophil and basiphil cells of the anterior pituitary.

FIXATION

Ten per cent formal-saline.

SECTIONS

Paraffin sections.

PREPARATION

Stock solutions.

1. 0.1 per cent martius yellow in 95 per cent alcohol containing 2 per cent phosphotungstic acid.
2. 1 per cent brilliant crystal scarlet 6R in 2.5 per cent acetic acid.
3. 0.5 per cent aniline blue in 1 per cent acetic acid.

Filter, through separate filter papers, into a Coplin jar in the following order:

3 parts of yellow stock solution No. 1.
2 part of red stock solution No. 2.
3 parts of blue stock solution No. 3.

This staining solution is ready for use after a few days at room temperature and will keep for about three months.

TECHNIQUE

1. Take sections to water.
2. Stain nuclei using the celestine blue–Mayer's haemalum sequence [p. 145].
3. Differentiate in acid alcohol and blue in tap water.
4. Stain in combined staining solution in Coplin jar for eight minutes.
5. Rinse quickly in water and blot dry.
6. Dehydrate in absolute alcohol and clear in xylene.
7. Mount in a synthetic resin medium.

RESULTS

Acidophils—cherry red; basiphils—blue; erythrocytes—yellow; collagen—pale blue; colloid—orange-red; nuclei—blue–black.

MITOCHONDRIA

Mitochondria are rounded or rod-shaped cytoplasmic structures which vary in size and number but are found in all animal cells. They are sources of cellular energy and are concerned with protein synthesis and lipid metabolism.

Mitochondria are not visible in routine haematoxylin and eosin stained sections and special fixation and staining methods are necessary for their demonstration: information on the fine structure of these bodies has been gained by use of the electron microscope. They may be seen in fresh, unstained preparations examined with dark-ground illumination or phase contrast microscopy [p. 28]. Supravital staining of dissociated cells may be carried out with a 1:10 000 (or weaker) solution of Janus green B in isotonic saline in which cells are examined. Specific staining is only obtainable before the onset of autolysis and the bluish green staining of mitochondria is transient, the dye being reduced to its leuco-base. Heidenhain's iron haematoxylin [p. 143] and Mallory's phosphotungstic acid haematoxylin [p. 146] may be used for staining mitochondria after fixation in a chrome salt but most of the special methods stem from Altmann (1894) who fixed in chrome–osmium, stained with hot, strong acid fuchsin and differentiated with picric acid.

Thin (2–3 mm) pieces of tissue should be fixed immediately after removal from the body and post-mortem tissue is rarely satisfactory. The obligatory long treatment with chrome salts makes tissue brittle but thin (2–4 μm) sections are essential for good results. Slow cutting with a very sharp knife is necessary, ester wax [p. 68] may be better than paraffin wax for embedding and with either, the use of a section adhesive is recommended.

Modified Altmann method

FIXATION

Helly's fluid [p. 52] for 24–48 hours. Transfer to 3 per cent potassium dichromate for 3–7 days, changing the fluid daily during this period. Wash in running water for 8–16 hours.

SECTIONS

2–4 μm paraffin or ester wax sections.

PREPARATION

Aniline-fuchsin (after Gray 1954).
Add 5 cm³ aniline oil to 100 cm³ distilled water and shake vigorously for a short time. Add 20 g acid fuchsin and shake vigorously again. Leave in a warm place for 24 hours shaking the bottle at intervals, or, place the bottle in a mechanical shaker. The highest possible concentration of acid fuchsin is a prerequisite for the success of the method.

Picric acid A.
Saturated solution of picric acid in absolute alcohol	1 volume
20 per cent alcohol	4 volumes

Pictric acid B.
Saturated solution of picric acid in absolute alcohol	1 volume
20 per cent alcohol	7 volumes

TECHNIQUE

1. Take sections to absolute alcohol.
2. Dry the underneath of the slide and wipe round the section.
3. Place the slide on a tripod and without allowing the section to dry, flood with aniline-fuchsin.
4. Gently heat the stain by passing a small flame to and fro under the slide until steam rises.
5. Remove the flame and allow the stain to cool (about five minutes).
6. Rinse briefly with distilled water and transfer to picric acid A for one minute.
7. Transfer directly to picric acid B for one minute (see Note 1).
8. Dehydrate quickly in two changes of absolute alcohol, clear in xylene, and mount in a synthetic resin medium.

RESULTS

Mitchrondria, nucleoli, and erythrocytes—red.
Nuclei, cytoplasm, and connective tissue—yellow.

NOTES

1. Differentiation in stage 6 and 7 is critical. Sections may be examined microscopically before mounting and given further treatment with picric acid if necessary. Over-decolorized sections cannot be satisfactorily re-stained; another section should be taken and given shorter treatment with picric acid.
2. If an osmium tetroxide-containing fixative has been used the blackened fat may obscure mitochondria. To prevent this, sections should be dewaxed in xylene and then treated with turpentine. This re-oxidizes and dissolves the fat.

KERATOHYALIN GRANULES

The cells of the stratum granulosum of the epidermis contain cytoplasmic granules and flakes of varying size. These stain strongly with alum haematoxylin and with basic dyes generally. They are acid-alcohol-fast with the Ziehl–Neelsen method and retain the violet in Gram's stain. They are believed to be involved in the production of keratin. For the demonstration of keratin see page 230.

REFERENCES

ADAMS, C. W. M. and SWETTENHAM, K. V. (1958). *J. Path. Bact.* **75**, 95.
ALTMANN, R. (1894). *Die Elementarorganismen*, 2nd edn. Veit, Liepzig.
DAWES, R. E. and HILLIER, M. H. (1964). *J. med. Lab. Technol.* **21**, 62.
EADY, R. A. J. (1976). *Clinical Exp. Dermatol.* **1**, 313.
GARDNER, D. L. and DODDS, T. C. (1976). *Human Histology*, 3rd edn. Churchill Livingstone, Edinburgh.
GOMORI, G. (1941). *Am. J. Path.* **17**, 395.
GRAY, P. (1954). *The microtomist's formulary and guide*. Constable, London.
HALMI, N. S. (1952). *Stain Technol.* **27**, 61.
KERENYI, N. and TAYLOR, W. A. (1961). *Stain Technol.* **36**, 169.
LENDRUM, A. C. (1944). *J. Path. Bact.* **56**, 441.
—— (1947). *J. Path. Bact.* **59**, 399.
—— FRASER, D. S., SLIDDERS, W., and HENDERSON, R. (1962). *J. clin. Path.* **15**, 401.
LEWIN, K. (1969). *J. Anat.* **105**, 171.
MONTAGNA, W., EISEN, A. Z., and GOLDMAN, A. S. (1954). *Quart. J. micr. Sci.* **95**, 1.
ORCI, L. and UNGER, R. H. (1975). *Lancet* **ii**, 1243.
PADAWER, J., WHIPPLE, H. E., and SILVERZWEIG, S. (1963). *Ann. N.Y. Acad. Sci.* **103**, 1.
PEARSE, A. G. E. (1953). *Histochemistry, theoretical and applied*. Churchill, London.
RHODIN, J. A. G. (1974). *Histology. A text and atlas*. Oxford University Press, New York.
RODNING, C. B., WILSON, I. D., and ERLANDSEN, S. L. (1976). *Lancet* **i**, 984.
SCOTT, H. R. (1952). *Stain Technol.* **27**, 267.
SLIDDERS, W. (1961). *J. Path. Bact.* **82**, 532.
WALLINGTON, E. A. (1955). *J. med. Lab. Technol.*, **13**, 53.

10 | Connective tissue fibres

Procedures for the differential staining of connective tissue fibres and muscle are an important part of histological technique and their use is often helpful in the diagnosis of pathological changes in tissues. Because of this, many methods have been described for the demonstration of these components, some of them selectively staining different types of fibres by the use of several dyes, in combination or in sequence. Metallic impregnation methods however, are necessary for the complete demonstration of reticulin fibres.

Whatever method is used, it is necessary to be aware of its limitations and exact requirements for successful employment. For example, the fixative used will greatly influence the take-up and retention of many of the dyes used in these methods and the duration of staining may require amendment in the absence of the recommended fixative. Moreover, few of these methods are automatic, and most require careful microscopical control to ensure satisfactory sequence staining of the different structures.

Sections thicker than 5–6 µm are not generally satisfactory for the demonstration of connective tissue fibres and muscle with any of the 'trichrome stains' and paraffin sections of 3–5 µm should be used. Van Gieson's stain (see below) is satisfactory for the demonstration of collagen in thicker sections and cellulose nitrate embedded material may be used successfully with this method.

COLLAGEN

Collagen is derived from fibroblasts, is acellular and occurs as wavy fibrils, either singly or fused together in dense bundles. It is quite resistant to autolytic changes but is susceptible to damage before fixation and Craik and McNeil (1965) described the reorientation of fibres and altered staining reaction with Masson's trichrome method in skin that had been stretched and subsequently sectioned. Collagen is birefringent and the examination of an unstained section with a polarizing microscope and a powerful light source is useful, particularly with bone.

Being dense in texture, tissue rich in collagen requires longer rather than shorter processing schedules to ensure thorough impregnation with the embedding medium.

Van Gieson's (1889) stain

Van Gieson's mixture of picric acid and acid fuchsin is the simplest method for the differential staining of collagen. Its main disadvantages are its inability to stain young fibrils the deep red that is imparted to mature collagen and the tendency for the red colour to fade, whatever mounting medium is used. To avoid this fading, Curtis (1905) suggested the use of ponceau S as a substitute for acid fuchsin but this dye, unfortunately, stains young collagen fibres even less well than does acid fuchsin.

FIXATION

Van Gieson's stain gives good results after a wide range of fixatives.

SECTIONS

Paraffin, frozen or cellulose nitrate sections.

PREPARATION

Saturated aqueous picric acid	100 cm³
1 per cent acid fuchsin in distilled water	5–10 cm³

The optimum concentration of acid fuchsin may vary with different batches of dye but will be readily determined by test staining of control material. One of the best of the many variants of van Gieson's solution is that of Unna who used acid fuchsin, 0.25 g, nitric acid 0.5 cm³, glycerol 10 cm³, distilled water 90 cm³, and picric acid to saturation.

TECHNIQUE

1. Take sections to water.
2. Stain nuclei either with Weigert's iron haematoxylin [p. 144] or with celestine blue–haemalum [p. 145].
3. Wash well in tap water followed by a rinse in distilled water.
4. Stain in van Gieson's solution for 2–5 minutes.
5. Rinse in distilled water or proceed directly to 95 per cent alcohol. Do not wash in alkaline tap water which extracts the red stain.
6. Dehydrate in absolute alcohol, clear in xylene, and mount in a synthetic resin medium.

RESULTS

Nuclei—brown–black to black.
Collagen—deep red.
Muscle, cytoplasm, red blood cells, fibrin—yellow.

NOTES

1. Nuclei stained with alum haematoxylin are readily decolorized by the picric acid in the stain. To avoid this, iron haematoxylin or the celestine blue–haemalum sequence are used and subsequent differentiation with acid alcohol is not generally necessary.
2. To enhance the yellow staining of structures, some workers treat sections briefly with alcoholic picric acid during dehydration.

Masson's trichrome stain (modified from Masson 1929)

FIXATION

Zenker, Helly, Bouin, and formal-sublimate are especially recommended. Ten per cent formalin is adequate but unembedded formalin material will benefit from appropriate secondary fixation [p. 54]. Formalin fixed sections may be mordanted for up to three hours in saturated alcoholic picric acid containing 3 per cent mercuric chloride (Lendrum *et al.* 1962) followed by thorough washing to remove picric acid staining.

SECTIONS

Thin paraffin sections.

PREPARATION

Cytoplasmic (plasma) stain

1 per cent ponceau de xylidine (ponceau 2R) in 1 per cent acetic acid	2 parts
1 per cent acid fuchsin in 1 per cent acetic acid	1 part

Differentiator and Mordant
1 per cent phosphomolybdic acid in distilled water.

Fibre stain
Either, 2 per cent light green (or fast green) in 1 per cent acetic acid
    or, 2 per cent methyl blue in 2 per cent acetic acid (see Note 3).

TECHNIQUE

1. Take sections to water.
2. Stain nuclei either with Weigert's iron haematoxylin [p. 144] or with celestine blue–haemalum [p. 145].
3. Wash well in water.
4. Differentiate nuclear stain with 0.5 per cent hydrochloric acid in 70 per cent alcohol.
5. Wash well in tap water, rinse in distilled water.
6. Stain in the red cytoplasmic stain 5–10 minutes.
7. Rinse in distilled water.
8. Differentiate in 1 per cent phosphomolybdic acid until collagen is decolorized, muscle, red blood cells, and fibrin remaining red.
9. Rinse in distilled water.
10. Counterstain in aniline blue or light green for 2–5 minutes.
11. Wash well in 1 per cent acetic acid for at least one minute.
12. Blot, dehydrate in absolute alcohol, clear in xylene, mount in a synthetic resin medium.

RESULTS

Nuclei—black.
Muscle, red blood cells, fibrin and some cytoplasmic granules—red.
Collagen, some reticulin, amyloid, and mucin—green or blue, according to counterstain.

NOTES

1. The optimum duration of staining in step 6 will largely depend on the fixative used, being shortest after mercuric, chromic, or picric acid fixation, longer being required with formalin-fixed material. Masson recommended diluting the ponceau-fuchsin mixture 1 in 10 with 1 per cent acetic acid and prolonging the staining time to one hour or more to obtain best results.
2. The duration of treatment with phosphomolybic acid will also vary according to the fixative used, five minutes or longer being required after mercuric, chromic, and picric acid fixatives, appreciably less after plain formalin. Microscopical control is essential.
3. The use of a blue or green fibre stain is a matter of individual preference. In either case, the longer the previous treatment with phosphomolybdic acid, the longer the time required for satisfactory staining with the fibre stain.

Aniline blue was formerly used in this and similar staining methods but because of its variable composition has now been generally replaced by methyl blue.

4. The treatment with 1 per cent acetic acid in step 11 is intended to remove overlying green or blue from cytoplasmic structures.
5. Collagen fibres that have been stretched prior to fixation (see above) may retain the red cytoplasmic stain in spite of prolonged treatment with sphophomolybdic acid.

The Masson trichrome procedure given above was developed from Mallory's (1900) acid fuchsin-aniline blue-orange G method and these may be taken as standards from which numerous polychrome combination staining methods have been evolved. All use dyes in acid solutions and most involve a haematoxylin nuclear stain followed by staining of cytoplasm with a red dye, treatment (differentiation and 'fixing') of the red dye with phosphomolybdic acid, phosphotungstic acid or mixtures of both, followed finally by a blue or green fibre stain. Some methods include a stain for elastic fibres in the sequence.

For a detailed account of the principle of these methods and the dyes that may be used in them, see Lillie (1945, 1965), Lendrum (1949), and Lendrum *et al.* (1962), the latter especially in relation to the staining of fibrin [p. 228].

One channel of development of the Mallory and Masson methods has been the introduction of 'one step' trichrome stains. These combine the various dyes in one solution and so reduce the number of steps required in the procedure. They are generally more applicable to duplicate (class) sections, fixed and prepared in the same way than to a variety of tissues fixed in a variety of fixatives. One of the most effective of these methods is given below.

Gomori's (1950a) Rapid one step trichrome stain

FIXATION

As for Masson's trichrome [p. 183].

SECTIONS

Thin paraffin sections.

PREPARATION

Chromotrope 2R	0.6 g
Fast green FCF	0.3 g
Phosphotungstic acid	0.6 g
Glacial acetic acid	1 cm^3
Distilled water	100 cm^3

The stain keeps well.

TECHNIQUE

1. Take sections to water.
2. Stain nuclei with Cole's, Harris', or Mayer's haemalum.
3. Wash well in tap water, rinse in distilled water.
4. Stain in chromotrope-green mixture for 5–20 minutes.
5. Rinse well in 0.2 per cent acetic acid.
6. Blot, dehydrate in absolute alcohol, clear in xylene, mount in a synthetic resin medium.

RESULTS

Nuclei—grey-blue
Collagen—green
Muscle, cytoplasm, red blood cells and fibrin—red.

RETICULIN

Reticular connective tissue or recticulin, consists of fine branching fibres which give a supporting framework to the richly cellular tissues of the lymphoreticular system and to other solid organs. They are largely invisible in haematoxylin and eosin stained sections though some may be demonstrated by Masson's trichrome and similar methods. They are argyrophilic and silver impregnation methods are necessary for their complete demonstration.

Like collagen, reticulin fibres are resistant to autolytic changes and silver impregnation methods may be useful with autolysed or infarcted tissue where routine staining methods may fail to show any details of structure. [Figs. 10.1 and 10.2].

Fig. 10.1.   Infarcted testis. HE. × 30.

As with other silver impregnation methods, those for the demonstration of reticulin are not entirely reliable which accounts for the many procedures described for the purpose. Nearly all of these stem from Bielschowsky's (1904) silver method for neurofibrils the first modification being that of Maresch (1905) cited by Mallory (1938) which was followed by many other versions in succeeding years. For a review of these methods see Lille (1965). Three methods of proven reliability are given below.

The alkalinity of the impregnating solutions used in these methods has a marked loosening effect on paraffin sections and the use of an adhesive is desirable [p. 92]. An alternative, or additional precaution is to cover the section with a film of celloidin. This is done by de-waxing the section in xylene, rinsing in absolute alcohol, immersion in 1 per cent celloidin in equal parts ether and absolute alcohol for five minutes, draining, and immersion in 80 per cent alcohol for a few minutes to harden the celloidin film.

Attention to detail is important with silver impregnation methods. All glassware should be chemically clean and the reagents pure. The ammonia solution should be fresh, low in lead content and the 35 per cent solution (weight per cm³ about 0.88 g) should be used. This will be referred to as 'strong ammonia' in the following methods. The explosive properties of ammoniacal silver solutions [p. 148] and the precautions to be taken in their disposal should be kept in mind.

Gordon and Sweets' (1936) reticulin method

FIXATION

Not critical; formalin is recommended.

SECTIONS

Thin paraffin sections. An adhesive is advisable.

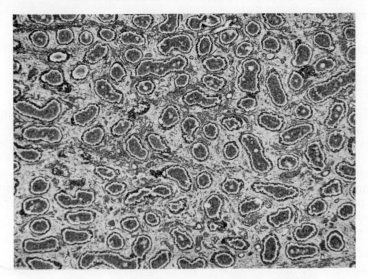

FIG. 10.2.   Infarcted testis. Reticulin. × 30.

PREPARATION

Silver solution
To 5 cm³ of 10.2 per cent silver nitrate, add strong ammonia drop by drop until the resulting precipitate is just dissolved. Add 5 cm³ of 3.1 per cent sodium hydroxide and re-dissolve the precipitate with a few more drops of ammonia. Dilute to 50 cm³ with distilled water.

TECHNIQUE

1. Take sections to water.
2. Oxidize for 1–5 minutes in 0.5 per cent potassium permanganate. 47.5 cm³, 3 per cent sulphuric acid, 2.5 cm³.
3. Wash briefly in water.
4. Bleach in 1 per cent oxalic acid.
5. Rinse in distilled water followed by thorough washing in tap water.

6. Sensitize in 2.5 per cent iron alum for 15 minutes to two hours. (The shorter time is generally suitable and the iron alum may be used repeatedly.)
7. Wash thoroughly with two or three applications of distilled water.
8. Cover with the silver solution for 10–30 seconds, until sections become transparent.
9. Wash well with distilled water.
10. Reduce with 10 per cent neutral formalin for 1–2 minutes.
11. Wash in tap water followed by distilled water.
12. Tone in 0.2 per cent gold chloride for 1–2 minutes (the sections turn a purplish colour). (See Note 2.)
13. Wash briefly with distilled water.
14. Fix in 5 per cent sodium thiosulphate ('hypo') for five minutes.
15. Wash well in water.
16. Counterstain nuclei in 1 per cent neutral red or 0.5 per cent safranin, wash in water.
17. Dehydrate, clear, and mount in a synthetic resin medium.

RESULTS

Reticulin fibres—black.
Collagen and cytoplasm—brown to yellow–brown if untoned, purplish-grey if toned.
Nuclei—as counterstain.

NOTES

1. Elastic fibres may also be black whether the preparation be toned or untoned.
2. Toning may be omitted and is, in the words of the original authors, 'merely a refinement'.
3. Sections overstained by prolonged treatment with silver solution may be completely de-stained after reduction in formalin (but not after toning and 'hypo' treatment) by replacing in the iron alum solution when, after a brief wash, they may be re-impregnated and again reduced.
4. This method is reliable and is recommended for routine purposes.

Gomori's (1937) reticulin method

FIXATION

Not critical; formalin gives best results.

SECTIONS

Thin paraffin sections. An adhesive is advisable.

PREPARATION

Silver solution
Add 4 cm³ of 10 per cent potassium hydroxide to 20 cm³ of 10 per cent silver nitrate. A precipitate is formed and is dissolved by the addition of strong ammonia drop by drop. Add more 10 per cent silver nitrate drop by drop until the resulting precipitate dissolves on shaking. Dilute with an equal volume of distilled water. The solution should be freshly prepared.

TECHNIQUE

1. Take sections to water.
2. Oxidize with 1 per cent potassium permanganate for 1–2 minutes.

3. Rinse in tap water and bleach with 3 per cent potassium metabisulphite.
4. Wash well in tap water.
5. Treat with 2 per cent iron alum for one minute.
6. Wash well with tap water and two changes of distilled water.
7. Treat with ammoniacal silver solution for one minute.
8. Rinse briefly with distilled water.
9. Reduce with 10 per cent neutral formalin for three minutes.
10. Wash well with tap water.
11. Tone with 0.2 per cent gold chloride for up to ten minutes.
12. Rinse with distilled water and treat with 3 per cent potassium bisulphite for one minute.
13. Rinse with distilled water and fix with 2.5 per cent sodium thiosulphate ('hypo') for 1–2 minutes.
14. Wash in tap water, dehydrate, clear, and mount in a synthetic resin medium.

RESULTS

Reticulin fibres—black.
Nuclei—greyish.
Collagen—dark greyish-purple.

Nassar and Shanklin's (1961) reticulin method

FIXATION

Formalin is recommended.

SECTIONS

Paraffin sections with an adhesive.

PREPARATION

Silver solution
Place 1 cm^3 strong ammonia in a flask and rapidly add 7 cm^3 10 per cent silver nitrate. Continue to add 10 per cent silver nitrate drop by drop, shaking between each addition, until a faint permanent turbidity remains after the last drop added. Dilute with an equal volume of distilled water.

TECHNIQUE

1. Take sections to distilled water.
2. Oxidize in an equal parts mixture of 0.5 per cent potassium permanganate and 0.5 per cent sulphuric acid for 1–2 minutes, until sections are brown.
3. Rinse with distilled water and decolorize with 2 per cent oxalic acid (1–2 minutes).
4. Rinse with distilled water followed by tap water for five minutes and a rinse in 95 per cent alcohol.
5. Treat with 2 per cent silver nitrate to which is added three drops pyridine per 10 cm^3 silver nitrate for 30–60 minutes at 50 °C or longer at room temperature (see Note).
6. Rinse quickly in 95 per cent alcohol and impregnate in the silver hydroxide solution to which has been added three drops pyridine per 10 cm^3 silver solution for five minutes at 50 °C.
7. Rinse quickly in 95 per cent alcohol and reduce for two minutes in an equal parts mixture of 2 per cent neutral formalin and absolute alcohol.

8. Wash well in distilled water and tone in 2 per cent gold chloride until sections turn greyish.
9. Rinse in distilled water and fix in 5 per cent sodium thiosulphate for two minutes.
10. Wash in tap water and stain nuclei with alum haematoxylin; blue in tap water.
11. Dehydrate, clear in xylene, and mount in a synthetic resin medium.

RESULTS

Reticulin fibres—black.
Collagen—greyish.
Nuclei—blue.

NOTE

The shorter (30 minute) period in 2 per cent silver nitrate facilitates impregnation of finer fibres. After 60 minutes, relatively few fine fibres are seen but there is an increase in the number of coarse fibres impregnated.

GENERAL NOTES ON RETICULIN METHODS

1. The directions given above relate to paraffin sections. If frozen or cellulose nitrate sections are used, some alteration of the duration of impregnation and washings may be necessary.
2. Formalin is the preferred fixative for reticulin methods though mercuric chloride and chromate fixatives do not preclude successful impregnation of fibres.
3. Raising the temperature will accelerate impregnation.
4. In all methods, toning in gold chloride is an optional procedure and many histologists prefer the yellow to yellow–brown staining of collagen and muscle given with untoned preparations.
5. The fine characteristically arranged reticulin fibres of human spleen provide excellent test material for trials of reticulin methods.

BASEMENT MEMBRANES

Basement membranes are thin layers of intercellular substance situated between epithelial surfaces or glandular epithelium and their supporting connective tissue. They are composed of mucopolysaccharide and protein and are associated with fine connective tissue fibres. They are not clearly discernible in haematoxylin and eosin stained sections and trichrome stains [p. 183] the PAS method [p. 237] and silver impregnation methods are used for their demonstration.

The demonstration of glomerular basement membranes is important in the diagnosis of some kidney diseases and the following periodic acid–silver nitrate method was designed for this purpose.

Periodic acid–silver nitrate method for basement membranes (after Jones 1957)

FIXATION

Bouin's fluid is recommended; 10 per cent formal saline is satisfactory.

SECTIONS

Paraffin sections not thicker than 3 μm.

PREPARATION

Gomori's methenamine–silver nitrate solution

3 per cent hexamethylenetetramine (commonly, methenamine or hexamine)	100 cm³
5 per cent silver nitrate	5 cm³

The silver nitrate is added to the methenamine solution and a precipitate is formed which is dissolved by shaking the mixture. This should be freshly prepared.

Methenamine silver working solution (prepare immediately before use)

Methenamine silver nitrate solution	50 cm³
5 per cent sodium tetraborate (borax)	5 cm³

TECHNIQUE

1. Take sections to water.
2. Place in 0.5 per cent periodic acid for 15 minutes.
3. Wash well in distilled water.
4. Place in hexamine silver nitrate solution pre-heated to 50 °C, in the dark, for 1½ to 3 hours (see Note 3).
5. Wash well in distilled water.
6. Tone in 0.2 per cent gold chloride for two minutes.
7. Rinse in distilled water and treat with 2.5 per cent sodium thiosulphate for three minutes.
8. Wash in running tap water for five minutes.
9. Counterstain, either with a light haematoxylin and eosin stain, or with 0.2 per cent light green in 0.2 per cent acetic acid for one minute to provide a general background stain.
10. Dehydrate, clear, and mount in a synthetic resin medium.

RESULTS

Basement membranes and some connective tissue fibres—black.
Other structures according to counterstain.

NOTES

1. Impregnation is progressive and sections should be examined microscopically at frequent intervals.
2. Basement membranes of tubular epithelium are blackened before those of glomeruli.
3. It is essential that the methenamine silver solution be at 50 °C throughout the impregnation period. This is best achieved by the use of a water bath and Disbrey and Rack (1970) point out that solutions in thick glass containers such as Coplin jars may require two hours or more to reach this temperature if an incubator is used.

MUSCLE

Muscle is very susceptible to damage during preparation and this applies particularly to skeletal muscle in which contraction artifacts can severely distort the morphology of the fibres. In biopsy specimens, this can be largely avoided by inserting sutures into each end of the muscle *in situ* and attaching these to a wooden applicator thus 'splinting' the specimen which after removal should be kept in a moist atmosphere for about 30 minutes before being placed in fixative. This short delay and early 'post mortem change' reduces the cytoplasmic staining artifacts that are seen in specimens placed in fixative immediately after removal. Ten per cent formal-saline, formal-sublimate, and Helly's fluid are suitable fixatives.

Paraffin wax embedding is generally suitable for muscle but the cellulose nitrate–paraffin wax double embedding method [p. 71] is preferable for maintaining the cohesion of the muscle bundles in larger pieces of skeletal and cardiac muscle.

Muscle is strongly acidophil and is well stained with haematoxylin and eosin and with Masson's trichrome method and its variants. Muscle striations of normal tissue are also often well shown by these stains but when the identification of striations in tumours of voluntary muscle (rhabdomyosarcoma) is required, use is made of Heidenhain's iron haematoxylin [p. 143] which requires particularly careful differentiation, or Mallory's phosphotungstic acid haematoxylin [p. 146]. Thin, not thicker than 5 μm sections are essential for this purpose.

For the demonstration of mitochondria see page 179; for the demonstration of nerve fibres and nerve endings in muscle see pages 387–8.

If strong, high contrast staining of muscle is required perhaps for photography, the following variant of the Masson principle is recommended.

Lissamine fast red–tartrazine method for muscle (Lendrum 1947)

FIXATION
Formal-sublimate is particularly recommended.

SECTIONS
Thin paraffin sections.

TECHNIQUE
1. Take sections to water.
2. Stain nuclei with celestine blue–haemalum.
3. Wash in water.
4. Differentiate nuclei in 0.5 per cent hydrochloric acid in 70 per cent alcohol.
5. Wash well in tap water for five minutes.
6. Stain in 1 per cent lissamine fast red B in 1 per cent acetic acid for 5–10 minutes.
7. Rinse in distilled water.
8. Differentiate in 1 per cent phosphomolybdic acid until red stain is removed from collagen.
9. Rinse in 1 per cent acetic acid.
10. Counterstain in 1.5 per cent tartrazine N.S. in 1.5 per cent acetic acid for 2–5 minutes.
11. Rinse briefly in 70 per cent alcohol. (Some of the yellow stain will be extracted.)
12. Dehydrate in absolute alcohol, clear in xylene, mount in a synthetic resin medium.

RESULTS

Nuclei—black.

Muscle, erythrocytes and neurokeratin of myelinated nerve fibres—red.

Collagen—yellow.

NOTE

A similar method to the above has been used by Ralis, Gadsdon, and Ralis (1977) who recommended their brilliant crystal scarlet–phosphotungstic acid–tartrazine method for staining muscle sections for use in quantitative and automated morphometric studies.

ELASTIC TISSUE

Elastic tissue is widely distributed in animal tissues and occurs as fine, sometimes branching fibres (in the dermis) or in laminated sheets, as in blood vessels. It is subject to alteration and possibly calcification with advancing age and in disease.

Elastic fibres are not swollen by acetic acid and their presence may be recognized in acid treated fresh preparation by a refractile appearance, which contrasts with the swollen and glassy form of associated collagen.

Elastic tissue is markedly resistant to autolytic changes and fibres have been successfully stained in Egyptian mummies (Sandison 1963). Choice of a fixative is not critical although Weigert's elastic tissue stain gives poor results following Susa fixation.

Elastic fibres are autofluorescent (greenish yellow) and are stained by both acid and basic dyes. Several methods are available for their selective staining, some being virtually automatic, while others require careful differentiation to obtain selective staining. They may be combined with a simple nuclear or plasma stain to give contrast, or with a trichrome connective tissue or fibrin stain.

Weigert's (1898) elastic tissue stain

FIXATION

Ten per cent formalin, formal-sublimate, or Helly.

SECTIONS

Thin paraffin sections.

PREPARATION

Add 2 g basic fuchsin and 4 g resorcin to 200 cm³ distilled water in a beaker. Bring to the boil and when both ingredients have dissolved and while still boiling, add 25 cm³ of 30 per cent ferric chloride, stirring the while. Continue stirring and boiling for a further 2–5 minutes until the coarse precipitate ceases to form. Cool and filter, discarding the filtrate. Dry the precipitate on the filter paper by leaving overnight in the incubator. Next day, return the filter paper and contents to the original vessel which will contain small amounts of residual precipitate. Add 200 cm³ of 95 per cent alcohol and dissolve the precipitate by gently heating in a water bath or on an electric hotplate. When dissolved, cool and filter, restoring the volume to 200 cm³ with 95 per cent alcohol. Add 4 cm³ concentrated hydrochloric acid and bottle with a tightly fitting stopper. The stain keeps for a few months, but batches vary.

TECHNIQUE

1. Take sections to 95 per cent alcohol.
2. Place in a closed container of the stain for 1–3 hours at room temperature or for 30 minutes to one hour at 60 °C.
3. Wash well in 95 per cent alcohol. (If there is staining of collagen, this may be removed by treatment with 1 per cent hydrochloric acid in 70 per cent alcohol.)
4. Wash well in tap water.
5. Counterstain as desired. This may be with neutral red, haematoxylin and eosin, or haematoxylin and van Gieson.
6. Dehydrate, clear, and mount in a synthetic resin medium.

RESULTS

Elastic fibres—blue–black; other structures according to the counterstain.

NOTES

1. No doubt because of the method of preparation, there is some variation in performance from batch to batch of Weigert's elastic tissue stain. The basic fuchsin dye should not be the variety prepared especially for the Schiff reagent, this having been found to give inferior results.
2. The staining of fibres is fast to prolonged treatment with alcohol, acid-alcohol, or counterstain.
3. Of the many variants of Weigert's elastic tissue stain, that of Hart (1908) is one of the most useful. This is simply a dilution of Weigert's stain with 1 per cent acid-alcohol in the proportion of 10–30 parts of stain to 90–70 parts of diluent, staining being extended to overnight at room temperature. Furthermore, even unsatisfactory samples of Weigert's stain (staining of collagen) may give very selective staining of elastic fibres after dilution as above.
4. Effete and non-selective stains may sometimes be rejuvenated by the addition of a further 1 per cent or 2 per cent hydrochloric acid.
5. To simplify preparation, the dry precipitate may be purchased from suppliers of biological stains and requires only solution in alcohol and the addition of acid.
6. Sheridan (1929) used crystal violet instead of basic fuchsin to give green staining of fibres while French (1929) combined these dyes, giving dark bluish-green staining. Moore (1943) used these dyes in a solution of excellent keeping qualities, while Miller (1971) combined Victoria blue 4R, crystal violet, and new fuchsin with resorcin and ferric chloride to give a highly selective black staining of elastic tissue.

ORCEIN

It is not clear whether the use of orcein for the staining of elastic fibres was first described by Taenzer, or Unna, or both. However, orcein is an excellent stain for elastic fibres and is much favoured by histopathologists with an interest in dermatology because of its ability to demonstrate the finest and most delicate fibres found in the skin.

Formerly, natural orcein (obtained from certain lichens) was used, but for some years, synthetic orcein has been prepared and is generally superior to the natural variety, giving stronger and more precise staining.

Modified Taenzer–Unna orcein method (Unna 1891)

FIXATION

Not critical.

SECTIONS

Thin paraffin sections.

PREPARATION

Orcein (synthetic)	1 g
80 per cent alcohol	100 cm³
Concentrated hydrochloric acid	1 cm³

TECHNIQUE

1. Take sections to 70 per cent alcohol.
2. Place in a closed jar of the stain for 30 minutes to two hours at room temperature or for a shorter time at 37 °C.
3. Wash well in 70 per cent alcohol; staining of collagen may be removed by treatment with 1 per cent acid alcohol.
4. Wash well in tap water.
5. Counterstain nuclei lightly with methylene blue or alum haematoxylin (see Notes).
6. Dehydrate, clear, and mount in a synthetic resin medium.

RESULTS

Elastic fibres—dark brown.
Nuclei—blue.

NOTES

1. With some samples of orcein, improved staining may be obtained by diluting the above solution with 1 per cent acid alcohol though such diluted solutions do not keep.
2. A heavy, dark collagen counterstain is likely to obscure or obliterate staining of the finest fibres and for this reason, van Gieson is less useful after orcein than following Weigert or Vehoeff's stain. The yellowsolve methods of Lendrum *et al.* (1962) and the fuchsin-miller method of Sidders (1961) [p. 230] however, may be usefully applied after orcein staining of elastic fibres.
3. Sections of normal human skin are useful test objects for use with samples of orcein.

Verhoeff's (1908) haematoxylin elastic tissue stain

FIXATION

Not critical.

SECTIONS

Thin paraffin sections.

PREPARATION

Haematoxylin	1 g
Absolute alcohol	20 cm³

Dissolve the haematoxylin in the alcohol and add in order, 10 per cent ferric chloride, 8 cm³, and strong iodine (iodine, 2 g, potassium iodide, 4 g, distilled water, 100 cm³) 8 cm³.

TECHNIQUE

1. Take sections to water. (It is not necessary to remove mercuric chloride pigment as this is dissolved by the stain.)
2. Stain in a jar for 15–60 minutes until sections are uniformly black.
3. Rinse in tap water and differentiate in 2 per cent ferric chloride. Control the differentiation by alternating brief applications of ferric chloride with washing in tap water and microscopical examination. As stain is removed from collagen and muscle, elastic fibres will remain black; nuclei will also remain stained though not so deeply. If elastic fibres are accidently decolorized, sections may be immediately returned to the stain (see Notes).
4. Wash well in tap water.
5. Treat either with 95 per cent alcohol for five minutes or with 2.5 per cent sodium thiosulphate for 1–2 minutes to remove iodine staining of background.
6. Wash for five minutes in running tap water.
7. Counterstain with 1 per cent eosin or with van Gieson.
8. Dehydrate, clear, and mount in a synthetic resin medium.

RESULTS

Elastic fibres—black.
Nuclei (and sometimes, myelin)—brown.
Cytoplasm and connective tissue—according to counterstain.

NOTES

1. The stain solution does not keep and should be freshly prepared. The use of a (possibly aged) stock solution of haematoxylin is not recommended and it is advisable to keep the appropriate amounts of haematoxylin in small tubes ready for mixing.
2. An alternative formula, which avoids the use of potassium iodide is haematoxylin, 1.5 g, 70 per cent alcohol, 30 cm³, 10 per cent ferric chloride, 12 cm³, and 2 per cent iodine in 80 per cent alcohol, 12 cm³.
3. Differentiation is a critical part of the technique and even in experienced hands it is possible to unwittingly decolorize fine fibres and thus partially invalidate the preparation. For this reason, Verhoeff's stain is of greatest value for the demonstration of the coarser elastic fibres of large blood vessels when combined with van Gieson's stain.

Gomori's (1950b) aldehyde fuchsin stain for elastic fibres

FIXATION

Not critical, but 10 per cent formalin and Bouin's fluid give a colourless background, mercuric chloride a pale lilac colour, and chrome fixatives a somewhat darker background.

SECTIONS

Thin paraffin sections.

PREPARATION

Basic fuchsin (see Notes)   0.5 g
70 per cent alcohol   100 cm³

Concentrated hydrochloric acid	1 cm^3
Paraldehyde	1cm^3

Dissolve the dye in the alcohol and then add the acid and paraldehyde. Leave at room temperature for 24–72 hours until the stain has assumed the deep purple colour which indicates fitness for use. The stain should be stored in the refrigerator at 4 °C but should be replaced after 2–3 months.

TECHNIQUE

1. Take sections to water.
2. Treat with Lugol's iodine [p. 243] for ten minutes.
3. Rinse in tap water and decolorize in 2.5 per cent sodium thiosulphate for two minutes.
4. Wash in tap water followed by 70 per cent alcohol.
5. Stain in a jar of aldehyde fuchsin for ten minutes.
6. Wash well in 95 per cent alcohol.
7. Countertain as desired. Celestine blue–haemalum staining of nuclei followed by orange G [p. 145] is suitable, or, for full differentiation of connective tissue, Masson's trichrome with a green collagen stain may be used.
8. Dehydrate, clear, and mount in a synthetic resin medium.

RESULTS

Elastic fibres and some mucopolysaccharides and mast cell granules—deep purple–violet. Other structures according to counterstain.

NOTES

1. The basic fuchsin should be pure and of the kind especially prepared for use with this and Schiff's reagent.
2. This is an automatic stain and demonstrates the finest fibres.
3. For the application of this stain to the demonstration of the cells of the pancreas, see page 174.

REFERENCES

BIELSCHOWSKY, M. (1904). *J. Psychol. Neurol. (Lpz.)* **3**, 169.

CRAIK, J. E. and MCNEIL, I. R. R. (1965). In *Biomechanics and related bioengineering topics* (ed. R. M. Kenedi). Pergamon Press, Oxford.

CURTIS, F. (1905). *Arch. Méd. exp.* **17**, 603.

DISBREY, B. D. and RACK, J. H. (1970). *Histological laboratory methods.* Livingstone, Edinburgh.

FRENCH, R. W. (1929). *Stain Technol.* **4**, 11.

GOMORI, G. (1937). *Am. J. Path.* **13**, 993.

—— (1950a). *Am. J. clin. Path.* **20**, 661.

—— (1950b). *Am. J. clin. Path.* **20**, 665.

GORDON, H. and SWEETS, H. H. (1936). *Am. J. Path.* **12**, 545.

HART, K. (1908). *Zbl. allg. Path. path. Anat.* **19**, 1.

JONES, D. B. (1957). *Am. J. Path.* **33**, 313.

LENDRUM, A. C. (1947). In *Recent advances in clinical pathology* (ed. S. C. Dyke). Churchill, London.

—— (1949). *J. Path. Bact.* **61**, 443.

——, FRASER, D. S., SLIDDERS, W., and HENDERSON, R. (1962). *J. clin. Path.* **15**, 401.

LILLIE, R. D. (1945). *J. techn. Meth.* **25**, 1.

—— (1965). *Histopathological technic and practical histochemistry.* McGraw-Hill, New York.

MALLORY, F. B. (1900). *J. exp. Med.* **5**, 15.
—— (1938). *Pathological technique.* Saunders, Philadelphia.
MASSON, P. (1929). *J. techn. Meth.* **12**, 75.
MILLER, P. J. (1971). *Med. Lab. Technol.* **28**, 148.
MOORE, G. W. (1943). *Bull. Inst. med. Lab. Technol.* **9**, 9.
NASSAR, T. K. and SHANKLIN, W. M. (1961). *Arch. Path.* **71**, 611.
RALIS, H. M., GADSDON, D. R., and RALIS, Z. A. (1977). *Stain Technol.* **52**, 31.
SANDISON, A. T. (1963). *Nature (Lond.)* **198**, 597.
SHERIDAN, W. F. (1929). *J. techn. Meth.* **12**, 123.
SLIDDERS, W. (1961). *J. med. Lab. Technol.* **18**, 36.
UNNA, P. (1891). *Mschr. prakt. Dermatol.* **12**, 394.
VAN GIESON, I. (1889). *N.Y. St. J. Med.* **50**, 57.
VERHOEFF, F. H. (1908). *J. Am. med. Ass.* **50**, 876.
WEIGERT, C. (1898). *Zbl. allg. Path. path. Anat.* **9**, 289.

11 | Bone and decalcification

Because of the mineral content of bone, some modification of the methods used for the preparation of sections of soft tissue is necessary and, as with any other material, the most suitable technique will vary according to the size and nature of the specimen, the purpose of the investigation (whether research or diagnostic) and the time and equipment available.

Bone and pathologically calcified soft tissues generally require the removal of calcium salts before sectioning although the preparation of sections of undecalcified bones and teeth is possible with special methods and equipment.

FIXATION

Before commencing decalcification, by any method, it is essential that the tissue be thoroughly fixed and acid-fixative mixtures that are supposed to decalcify and fix tissue simultaneously are not satisfactory, save for minute foci of calcification. It is also essential that bone selected for histological examination should be promptly sawn into thin slices. This is necessary for two reasons: (1) to allow penetration of the fixative into this dense tissue; and (2) to reduce the time required for decalcification, since prolonged immersion in acid solutions will seriously impair subsequent staining of sections.

Slices of bone, 3–5 mm in thickness may be obtained with a fine-tooth fretsaw or, more easily, with a power driven band-saw. These are available in a variety of sizes and are invaluable where much bone is examined. Whatever method is used for obtaining blocks of bone, sawdust will be produced and small fragments of bone, cartilage, and soft tissue may be deposited on the cut surfaces or more deeply in the specimen. Microscopically, bone dust is seen in two main forms. The first is easily recognized as splinters of bone or cartilage and these are commonly seen at the edges of the section. The second form is less obvious as an artifact and is seen as rounded masses of debris 200–700 μm in diameter [FIG. 11.1].

While it is impossible to completely avoid the production of sawdust and its deposition in blocks selected for sectioning its extent may be minimized by the use of sharp saws and drills and by gently feeding the bone specimen through the blade of the bandsaw without the use of force (Wallington 1972). Brushing of the cut surfaces of bone to remove sawdust is not recommended since this is likely to damage or dislodge marrow cells.

Neutral 10 per cent formal-saline is satisfactory as a fixative before decalcification and slabs of dense bone should receive at least 48 hours' fixation, preferably longer. Formal-sublimate is also recommended as a primary fixative although causing tissues to become radiopaque and thus preventing the use of X-rays as a test for decalcification. It may sometimes be used with advantage however, as a secondary fixative *after* decalcification. When a

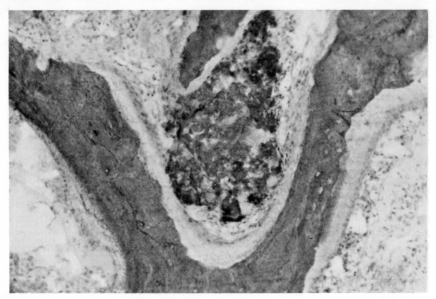

FIG. 11.1.   Bone sawdust. HE. × 100.

section is required urgently, fixation must be brief and very thin slices of bone (2–3 mm) are *adequately* fixed after two hours in 10 per cent formal-saline at 60 °C (Clayden 1952).

If it is intended to demonstrate calcium salts in bone or other tissue then all acid solutions must be avoided and fixation should be carried out in neutral formalin or alcohol.

Blocks of bone should be segregated from other blocks during fixation to avoid the possibility of loose fragments of bone becoming lodged in a piece of soft tissue causing unexpected difficulty during section cutting.

DECALCIFICATION

There are many decalcifying fluids; probably as many as there are fixatives and for the same reason. No single solution is ideal in every respect and as with fixatives, a choice has to be made between those methods of general utility and those of more limited application.

A satisfactory decalcifying procedure should ensure:

1. Complete removal of calcium salts.
2. Lack of distortion of cells and connective tissue.
3. Lack of harmful effect on staining reactions.

In addition to these criteria, the speed of decalcification is of importance in histopathology where the treatment of a patient may await a report on a section. Fortunately, however, a diagnosis may often be made from a less densely bony area of a tumour.

There is some doubt as to whether agitation of tissues during decalcification makes any significant difference to the rate of removal of calcium salt. Clayden (1952) concluded that there is no worthwhile increase in the rate of decalcification with agitation, while Lillie (1948) stated that 'periodic manual or even mechanical agitation materially speeds the decalcification process'. In 1965, however, Lillie observed that 'mechanical agitation appears to have no great effect on the speed of decalcification'. Similarly, while Russell (1963) reported a greatly increased rate of decalcification by rotation of blocks in the decalcifying fluid at 1 rev/min, these results were not obtained by one of us (EAW) who repeated the experiments.

While continuous agitation may not materially increase the rate of decalcification, it seems that a complete lack of movement combined with an inadequate volume of decalcifying fluid may favour production of the decalcification (reprecipitation) artifact described by Webb (1952), Browne and Rowles (1975), and Rowles and Browne (1975). This is seen as often rounded, granular, or crystalline masses lying mainly in the soft tissue and marrow adjacent to bone. Browne and Rowles have shown this material to be secondary calcium phosphate. It is birefringent, generally stains strongly with alum haematoxylin and gives a positive von Kossa reaction. It may be removed from sections by treatment with 10 per cent formic acid for 10–30 minutes. An ample volume of decalcifying fluid and occasional agitation of the specimen should minimize the incidence of this artifact.

The use of heat to speed up decalcification should be used with discretion and temperatures above 37 °C only in an emergency, for while a raised temperature will hasten decalcification, with acid solutions this will be attended by impaired preservation of tissue structure through maceration and seriously affected staining reactions. Smith (1962b) however, drew attention to the wide variation in room temperature that may occur and which, at lower levels, may even retard decalcification. He suggests that containers should be placed in a water-bath at 25 °C during decalcification.

An ample volume of decalcifying solution should always be used, at least 50–100 times the volume of the tissue. The concentration of the solution used will influence the frequency of its renewal.

Blocks should be removed from the decalcifying fluid immediately on completion of the process. Treatment beyond this point will not improve cutting qualities and will adversely affect staining. An exception to this is with the use of EDTA (see below) where treatment appreciably beyond the time of complete decalcification causes no apparent harm to the tissue or its staining. The best means of determining the progress or completion of decalcification is by X-ray examination and the use of this method may occasionally reveal objects such as metal implants not suspected of being present in the specimen. Where X-ray facilities are not available, a chemical test for the presence of calcium in the decalcifying fluid is sometimes useful, Without doubt, the practice of prodding with a needle, 'feeling', scraping, or bending the block as a test for decalcification is unreliable and damaging to tissue structure. In an emergency, however, it is not necessary to completely decalcify a block of dense bone before cutting a few sections to permit an early diagnosis. It is desirable though, that the only partial decalcification of the block be recorded when it is stored, for the benefit of any other microtomist called upon to deal with the block in the future.

With some calcified soft tissue such as inactive tuberculous lymph glands, immersion of the unsupported tissue in decalcifying solutions may result in loss of contents or severe disruption of the structure of the tissue. This may be avoided by embedding the tissue in wax without prior decalcification but with the subsequent use of surface decalcification of the block [p. 208].

ACID DECALCIFYING FLUIDS

The commonest method of decalcification is by dissolving the calcium salts in an acid solution.

A substantial number would result from a count of acid decalcifying mixtures that have been published since the latter half of the nineteenth century, but in practice a comparatively few mixtures using nitric acid, formic acid, and trichloracetic acid will meet most needs as acid decalcifying solutions.

Nitric acid (SG 1.4)

Nitric acid decalcifies quickly but causes damage to tissue and inhibits nuclear staining if its application be prolonged. Because of this, it is used mainly for the rapid decalcification of small pieces of bone.

Thin slices of fixed tissue are placed in a freshly prepared 5–10 per cent solution of nitric acid in distilled water. Test for completion of decalcification after four hours and thereafter at short intervals. Decalcification should not extend beyond 48 hours. Formalin is sometimes added to nitric acid to protect the tissue against maceration and swelling but there is little evidence that this is particularly beneficial.

Transfer tissues directly to 70 per cent alcohol for paraffin wax or cellulose nitrate embedding. Washing for long periods in water is not necessary, excess acid being removed during dehydration.

A less vigorous, but useful decalcifying solution for routine purposes is the nitric acid, chromic acid, and alcohol mixture of Perenyi (1882).

Perenyi's fluid

10 per cent nitric acid	40 cm^3
Absolute alcohol	30 cm^3
0.5 per cent chromic acid	30 cm^3

Prepare freshly for use and transfer directly to 70 per cent alcohol after decalcification.

Crawford (1957) modified the chemical test for decalcification to make it usable with the above solution (see below).

Formic Acid (SG 1.2)

Formic acid is widely used as a decalcifying agent in a variety of mixtures. It is much slower than nitric acid but considerably less damaging to tissue structures and staining.

Gooding and Stewart (1932) added formalin to protect the tissue against the harmful effects of the acid but as with nitric acid, there is little, if any advantage in this. It should be noted, incidentally, that these authors used frozen sections and not embedded material in their studies.

For routine use, 10 per cent formic acid in distilled water is recommended for while higher concentrations (up to 30 per cent) give more rapid decalcification, impairment of staining may follow. Furthermore, solutions of greater concentration than 10 per cent formic acid possess an inherent cloudiness which prevents reliable assessment of the chemical test for completion of decalcification (Clayden 1952).

A large volume of fluid should be used and renewed every 48 hours. Decalcification will take from two days for small pieces of cancellous bone to 20 days for larger pieces of dense, compact bone.

Transfer formic acid decalcified material directly to 70 per cent alcohol for paraffin wax or cellulose nitrate embedding.

Another efficient formic acid decalcifying solution for routine use is that of Evans and Krajian (1930). It is slightly quicker than 8 per cent formic acid in water and preserves the stainability of tissues equally well. A slightly modified formula is given below.

Formic acid–sodium citrate

Formic acid (SG 1.2)   35 cm³
20 per cent sodium citrate   65 cm³

Transfer tissue directly to 70 per cent alcohol after decalcification.

Trichloracetic Acid
Trichloracetic acid has been used as a decalcifying agent for many years and Smith (1962b) recommends this acid for the decalcification of teeth. A 5 per cent aqueous solution of trichloracetic acid is freshly prepared and is rather quicker in action than the same concentration of formic acid. Staining results are good and the tissue may be transferred directly to 70 per cent alcohol, although Smith advocates a preliminary washing in water.

ION EXCHANGE RESINS WITH ACID DECALCIFYING FLUIDS

Dotti, Paparo, and Clarke (1951) recommended the use of ion exchange resins in conjunction with formic acid, the rationale of the method being that the removal of calcium ions from the decalcifying fluid by the resin leads to quicker and more efficient decalcification. The method was reviewed by Lillie (1951), Morris and Benton (1956), and Inwood (1958) who all concluded that no improvement in staining results from the use of the method and that equally rapid decalcification may be effected by acid solutions without the use of the resins. The chemical test for completeness of decalcification is not possible when using ion exchange resins.

ELECTROLYTIC DECALCIFICATION

Richman, Gelfand, and Hill (1947) were the first to describe an electrolytic bath with solutions of hydrochloric and formic acids as the electrolytic medium for the decalcification of bone. They claimed speedier decalcification without damage to cytological detail or staining. It has been shown by several workers however, that the heat produced by the method is largely responsible for the increased rate of decalcification and that there is a risk of charring the specimen in the process (Clayden 1952).

CHELATING AGENTS

EDTA
Ethylenediamine-tetra-acetic acid (EDTA), a chelating agent, is a white, crystalline powder soluble in distilled water to about 20 per cent. As a decalcifying solution it combines with calcium ions to form soluble, non-ionized compounds. Deposits of iron and other metals may also be removed by EDTA but because the solution is effective at neutral pH, staining generally is excellent and superior to that obtained after any other decalcifying agent.

Tissue is not hardened after decalcification in EDTA; on the contrary, some microtomists believe that bone is easier to cut after this than after acid decalcifying solutions. Hilleman and Lee (1953) advocated the use of EDTA for dental tissues and the reagent may be used with success for bone, teeth, or any calcified tissue.

The exact concentration of EDTA used is relatively unimportant so long as uncombined reagent is available to the tissue at all times. In practice, using a volume of 150 times that of the tissue, the following solution has been found satisfactory and is renewed every 5–7 days during decalcification. A weaker solution should be changed more frequently.

Neutral EDTA decalcifying solution

EDTA (di-sodium salt)	250 g
Distilled water	1750 cm^3

The solution is adjusted to pH 7 by the addition of about 26 g sodium hydroxide.

Decalcification will take from 4 to 40 days depending on the composition of the specimen but prolonged exposure to EDTA is without detriment to the subsequent staining of tissues.

Chemical tests for determining the progress of decalcification are particularly unreliable with EDTA and X-ray examination should be used. No special after-treatment is required and tissues may be transferred directly to 70 per cent alcohol except when frozen sections are required when the specimen should be washed thoroughly in water to prevent damage to the microtome knife.

Where speed can be secondary to quality of tissue preservation and staining there is no doubt that EDTA is the best decalcifying agent currently available.

TESTS FOR COMPLETION OF DECALCIFICATION

As noted above, the only completely reliable method for determining the completion or progress of decalcification is by means of X-ray examination and while it is appreciated that all laboratories do not have such facilities, many pathology laboratories do not use the method only because of lack of liaison with the hospital X-ray department.

In the absence of X-ray examination, the chemical test is designed to detect calcium salt in the decalcifying fluid, a negative result indicating completion of decalcification. Described by Arnim (1935), Morse (1945), and Clayden (1952) the general method is as follows:

To about 5 cm^3 of decalcifying fluid add strong ammonia, drop by drop until alkaline to litmus. Add 0.5 cm^3 saturated ammonium oxalate.

Cloudiness indicates the presence of calcium. (If the solution goes cloudy after adding the ammonia, this indicates the presence of calcium and there is no point in proceeding with the rest of the test.) The specimen is then placed in a fresh (calcium-free) solution of decalcifying fluid and the test is repeated after a suitable interval. If the fluid remains clear for 30 minutes after the addition of both ammonia and ammonium oxalate, it may be assumed that decalcification is complete.

With strongly acidic decalcifying fluids gas bubbles form on the surface of the bone as decalcification takes place. If the container is shaken occasionally the bubbles are removed and will not reform when decalcification is complete. This is a rough guide to the completion of decalcification but is inferior to the radiological or chemical tests.

POST-DECALCIFICATION PROCEDURES

Some recommended procedures for the treatment of tissues immediately following acid decalcification are complicated and time-consuming. After decalcification in the solutions given above, tissues may with advantage be transferred directly to 70 per cent alcohol in the first stage of the paraffin wax or cellulose nitrate dehydration schedule. If it is intended to prepare frozen sections, a wash in water is desirable and 10 per cent formal-saline may be used for the temporary storage of decalcified tissues.

PREPARATION OF SECTIONS OF BONE AND BONE MARROW

Frozen sections are useful in the examination of bone and bone tumours. Small pieces of decalcified, compact bone cut well on the simple freezing microtome without any supporting medium but cancellous bone may require embedding to prevent loss of fine bone trabeculae and marrow cells during subsequent manipulation of sections. Cryostats, with a heavier microtome than the Cambridge rocker, and thermo-electrically cooled stages and knives on heavy microtomes, offer scope for the preparation of frozen sections from large masses of unsupported decalcified bone. Such sections lack the shrinkage and distortion associated with paraffin embedding and are very much quicker to prepare than either wax or cellulose nitrate embedded material.

Paraffin wax embedding, in spite of its faults, is the routine method of preparation in bone pathology. A combination of paraffin wax and cellulose nitrate (double-embedding, page 71) is undoubtedly advantageous in promoting a superior consistency for cutting and for maintaining the cohesion of mixed soft and hard tissues such as cancellous bone. The so-called 'plastic waxes' [p. 61] offer similar advantages to double embedding.

Whatever embedding mixture is chosen, a slow and thorough dehydration and impregnation schedule is essential, for while bone is certainly shrunken and hardened by wax embedding, hardness does not in itself prevent the preparation of good sections as does incomplete dehydration or permeation with embedding medium. The short (16–24 hours) schedules used with automatic tissue processing machines in routine histopathology are not suitable for the processing of bone save for small fragments of cancellous bone and bone marrow biopsies. The use of the vacuum oven for wax impregnation is strongly recommended.

A very sharp knife is essential and a heavy microtome desirable for cutting sections of wax embedded bone. The slant of the knife in relation to the block will affect the cutting and it is easier to cut in the same direction, rather than across the lamellae of compact bone in longitudinal section. The knife should be the heaviest that the microtome will accommodate, of wedge or tool-edge profile and very securely clamped. A thickness of 6–8 µm is satisfactory for most bone sections embedded in wax and attempts to cut thinner sections often result in a 'moth-eaten' appearance of the bone matrix. Prliminary soaking of the exposed surface of the tissue in running cold water or in a dish of water plus a drop or two of wetting agent often improves cutting and ice treatment may be necessary in warm conditions. Sections should be attached to the slide with an adhesive [p. 92] and carefully dried.

Cellulose nitrate (celloidin or LVN) is of value as an embedding medium for the microtomy of bone for two main purposes. The first is the facility of preparation of large masses of tissue of variable consistency such as vertebrae, and of dense, cortical bone such as mid-shaft of femur. The second is the important reduction in shrinkage and distortion caused to more delicate bony structures such as the inner ear. Against these advantages must be set the slowness of the process and the thickness of the sections (15–20 μm).

BONE MARROW

More information can be obtained from bone marrow films or smears than from sections. It is not so easy to stain sections as films; cells are smaller in sections and are less easy to identify and it is difficult to obtain the full range of Romanowsky colours. The advantages of sections are that it is possible to assess the cellularity of the marrow with more accuracy, and the architectural arrangement of the cells is preserved. Bone marrow trephine biopsy may be performed if aspiration is unsuccessful or fails to give a definite diagnosis. Bone taken at post-mortem, even many hours after death, often shows a well preserved bone marrow structure, and carefully decalcified sections give good preparations that have been underestimated in the past.

ASPIRATED MARROW

Occasionally only the examination of sections of marrow will confirm the diagnosis of diseases such as myelofibrosis, aplastic anaemia, or secondary carcinoma. The following technique of Smith and Signy (1966) is a development of the earlier methods of Cappell *et al.* (1947) and Hutchison (1953). It is advisable in all cases to place the excess bone marrow into oxalate mixture and to preserve this in fixative whilst the smears are stained and examined. If the smears do not give clear-cut results the fixed bone marrow particles are processed and sections cut and stained; the fixed material is discarded if sections are not required. Marrow that has been mixed with blood and allowed to clot is of little value for histological sections; aspirated specimens must be kept liquid until placed in fixative, and are then processed as follows.

TECHNIQUE

1. 1–2 cm³ of marrow is obtained in the usual way by rapid aspiration and smears and squashes are made directly on to clean slides. The remainder of the marrow is placed in a watch glass containing six drops of Wintrobe's oxalate mixture. (Sequestrene and heparin are less satisfactory for this purpose.) The marrow particles are transferred with a Pasteur pipette to a bijou bottle containing approximately 3 cm³ of acetic acid–formalin.

Formalin	10 cm³
Glacial acetic acid	5 cm³
Distilled water	35 cm³

The specimen can be transferred to the laboratory in this bottle. Allow to fix for 2–4 hours.

2. On receipt in the laboratory, transfer the whole contents of the bijou

bottle to a universal bottle, containing 10 cm³ of 70 per cent alcohol and mix. The marrow fragments sink to the bottom and fat particles float to the top. After a few minutes, using a very fine Pasteur pipette, draw off the fluid between the lower fragments and the top fatty layer, taking great care to avoid aspirating any particles.

3. Transfer the fragments on to piece of cigarette paper and fold to make a small envelope.
4. Place the envelope in a cassette or biopsy basket for processing; this is conveniently done on a machine. If only one or two tiny fragments are available processing should be done by the replacement technique in the tube, removing each reagent in turn by means of a fine Pasteur pipette. In each case the following schedule is recommended:

70 per cent alcohol	60 min
95 per cent alcohol	30 min
74 OP or 100 per cent alcohol (four changes each)	30 min
Toluene (three changes each)	15–30 min
Molten paraffin wax (three changes each)	30 min

5. Transfer the specimen to a fresh change of molten paraffin wax in 7.5 × 1.25 cm test-tube which has previously been rinsed with glycerol. Place the tube in a wax oven for a few minutes to allow the particles to settle.
6. Remove the tube from the oven and cool the wax as rapidly as possible, taking care to keep the tube upright so that the particles are embedded at the bottom of the tube.
7. Carefully break the tube.
8. Remove the cast.
9. Trim if necessary.
10. Attach to a microtome chuck.
11. Cut a serial ribbon of nine sections.
12. Stain as described below.

NOTE

When searching for malignant cells in bone marrow, an alternative technique (Kuper 1965) can be used, whereby the marrow fragments are placed into a plastic precipitin tube, which is centrifuged, the supernatant plasma is removed, fixative is added, and the tube again centrifuged. After fixation, the tube is dissolved off the compact fragment with chloroform, and the tissue then prepared in the ordinary way in an envelope as before.

BONE MARROW BIOPSIES

Neutral formalin or acetic acid–formalin fixation is satisfactory and suitable for most staining methods. Over-decalcification in strong acids is a frequent cause of poor staining with routine methods and make Romanowsky techniques unreliable or impossible. Careful control of decalcification by radiology or chemical tests [p. 204] is required as there are wide variations in the decalcification times between thin trabecular bone from a child and dense sclerotic bone from an adult. Paraffin embedding is generally satisfactory.

SURFACE DECALCIFICATION

Sometimes, often during initial trimming of the block, unsuspected areas of calcification become apparent through tears in the sections and resistance against the knife. Under no circumstances (at any rate in diagnostic histology) should such areas be excavated with knife or needle but rather, the block should be removed from the microtome and immersed for an hour or more in either 10 per cent formic acid in distilled water or in 5 per cent nitric acid. Progressive decalcification will occur, with little or no adverse effect on subsequent staining. The block should be washed briefly in water, dried, and replaced in the microtome for cutting.

PREPARATION OF UNDECALCIFIED SECTIONS

Sections of undecalcified bone are required for two main purposes. One is for the study of normal bone structure and the distribution of bone mineral, the latter by examination of microradiographs prepared from these sections. The other is in the diagnosis of metabolic bone diseases such as osteomalacia and rickets where there is impairment of the normal process of calcification resulting in an increase of osteoid tissue (non-mineralized bone matrix). The differential staining of osteoid in routinely decalcified, paraffin embedded sections of bone is not sufficiently reliable or accurate for diagnostic purposes though Ralis and Ralis (1975) claim consistently valid results with their staining methods. Sections of undecalcified bone are also required in techniques based on the discovery that tetracycline and related antibiotics administered to man and animals are localized in areas of bone growth and can be seen in sections with fluorescence microscopy (Frost and Villaneuva 1960; Frost 1969).

The technical difficulties inherent in the preparation of undamaged sections of undecalcified bone have not yet been fully overcome although many methods have been described for the purpose. These may be considered in three groups: (1) sawing and grinding of unembedded or resin-embedded bone; (2) sectioning of cellulose nitrate–paraffin wax double-embedded material, with or without the use of adhesive tape; (3) sectioning of resin embedded bone with a heavy microtome and knife. The last two groups of methods are only applicable to small pieces of cancellous bone.

SAWING AND GRINDING

A combination of these procedures is necessary for the preparation of sections of dense cortical bone such as a transverse section through an adult long bone, or of a tooth. In its simplest form, the method consists of cutting a thin slice of the bone with a fine saw followed by manual grinding on a flat abrasive surface such as a hone, or between sheets of plate glass previously 'sharpened' with silicon carbide abrasive, using 70 per cent alcohol or water as a lubricant. The section is finally washed, dried, and mounted on a glass slide (Sissons 1968; Page 1977).

In more elaborate procedures (Jowsey 1955; Saxby 1959; Friend and Smith 1962, 1964; Gore and Abbott 1964) sections of teeth and bone are prepared with an engineer's lathe, milling machine, or a mechanical grinding device, with or without prior embedding in a synthetic resin. More serious than the special equipment required is the wastage of tissue, for ten times (and often much more) of the final thickness of the section is lost during preparation.

Nevertheless, the employment of such a method is (at present) obligatory for the preparation of thin sections of undecalcified compact bone and mature teeth.

ADHESIVE TAPE METHOD

This method is more readily applicable to the general laboratory and does not require any special apparatus. It is only suitable for small pieces ($10 \times 5 \times 3$ mm) of cancellous bone and is frequently used in histopathology for biopsies of the iliac crest.

First described by Duthie (1954), and modified by Ball (1957) and Albert and Linder (1960) the method consists of the application of a strip of transparent adhesive tape (Sellotape) to the surface of a paraffin block to prevent breakage or disintegration of the undecalcified bone. The tape is removed from the section after mounting on a slide and before staining. Hart (1962) has described a similar method but using gummed paper instead of plastic tape.

Plastic tape method (modified from Ball 1957)

FIXATION

10 per cent neutral formal-saline for 12–24 hours.

PROCESSING

1. Dehydrate in 70 per cent, 90 per cent, and three changes of absolute alcohol.
2. Impregnate with two changes of 3 per cent LVN in methyl benzoate, four hours each change.
3. Transfer to 20 per cent LVN in methyl benzoate overnight.
4. Remove excess cellulose nitrate from around tissue and place in three changes of toluene, two hours each change.
5. Transfer to paraffin wax (m.p. 56 °C). Give two changes of one hour each and leave in third wax overnight. Embed in fresh wax on the following morning.

CUTTING

Secure the block in a heavy microtome and expose the surface of the tissue with a trimming knife.

Replace the trimming knife with a very sharp, wedge or D-profile knife. Set the thickness regulator at 8 μm.

Apply the adhesive side of a narrow strip of tape firmly to the surface of the block with about 25 mm of tape forward of the specimen. Holding this free end of the tape clear of the knife edge, a section is cut with a steady but forceful action.

The tape is re-applied to the block and a further section taken and so on, until the requisite number of sections has been obtained.

MOUNTING OF SECTIONS

A portion of the tape with attached sections is cut from the strip with scissors and firmly applied, section downwards, to an albumenized slide. The slide is placed on the hot plate for 20–30 minutes to secure adhesion of the section to the slide.

The backing of the tape is water soluble and is removed after covering for a short time with strips of wet blotting paper. The adhesive of the tape is less easily removed and requires soaking of the slide in warm benzene or toluene or a mixture of these with chloroform at 60 °C in a sealed container. When the adhesive has been dissolved the section is ready for staining but may with advantage be covered with a thin film of cellulose nitrate [p. 186] as a precaution against detachment.

NOTES

1. Woods (1969) considered that the use of tape is not particularly advantageous with double-embedded material but emphasized that where its use is contemplated, preliminary tests should be undertaken with different tapes to find a variety with a soluble adhesive.
2. Three preparations are particularly useful for the examination of sections of undecalcified bone. These are: (1) an unstained section for examination with polarized light; (2) a haematoxylin and eosin stained section; and (3) a von Kossa stain to demonstrate calcium [see p. 217].

Sectioning resin-embedded undecalcified bone (Wallington 1972)

A number of synthetic resins and resin mixtures have been described for embedding undecalcified bone prior to sectioning. With all of these, support and tissue preservation are good and superior to paraffin wax although some cracking of bone trabeculae may still occur. The following simple methyl methacrylate embedding method is reliable and has been widely used with success. The method is applicable to tissues for sawing and grinding as well as microtomy.

FIXATION

Fix for at least 24 hours, preferably 48 hours, in neutral 10 per cent formal-saline.

PREPARATION OF METHYL METHACRYLATE

Methyl methacrylate monomer as supplied by the manufacturer contains hydroquinone (quinol) as an inhibitor and this is removed before use by shaking an equal volume of monomer and 5 per cent sodium hydroxide for a few minutes in a separating funnel. Repeat this twice and follow with three washes with distilled water. Filter the washed monomer through anhydrous calcium chloride and store over a layer of this material in a tightly stoppered bottle in the refrigerator at 4 °C.

To partially polymerize the methacrylate for embedding, 1 g dried benzoyl peroxide is added to 100 cm³ monomer and this is carefully heated in a large flask placed in a water bath with constant stirring until it has the consistency of thick syrup. On no account should the temperature of the methacrylate be allowed to rise above 85 °C. When the methacrylate has thickened, it is immediately cooled by placing the flask in cold water. It is then bottled and stored in the refrigerator.

Difford (1974) modified the above procedure and avoided the critical heating stage by adding 40 g poly-(methylmethacrylate) low molecular weight, natural beads [p. 503] to 100 cm³ catalysed monomer, dissolved by mixing on a rotary mixer for 24 hours.

PROCESSING

The following schedule is suitable for small pieces of cancellous bone up to 20 × 10 × 5 mm. Larger specimens will require proportionally longer processing.

1. 70 per cent alcohol—eight hours.
2. 90 per cent alcohol—overnight.
3. Three changes of absolute alcohol during the day.
4. Methyl methacrylate monomer and absolute alcohol, equal parts—overnight.
5. Methyl methacrylate monomer—during day.
6. Transfer tissue to thickened monomer in a thin-walled, stoppered glass tube. Place the tube in a small dish of water and polymerize in the incubator at 35–40 °C for 2–3 days.
7. When the methacrylate is hard, remove from the incubator, break the glass tube, and trim the block with a saw.

CUTTING

A sharp, stout knife and a heavy, vibration-free microtome are essential. The Jung KM microtome [FIG. 5.5] and No. 4 knife are especially suitable. With conventional microtomes, a wedge or D-profile (tool edge) knife should be used.

1. The block is clamped directly into the chuck of the microtome.
2. Sections are cut with a slow, steady cutting action at 6–8 μm.
3. Use 70 per cent alcohol as a lubricant for both block and knife. Sections should slide up the knife in the same way as celloidin sections.
4. Sections are received and stored in 70 per cent alcohol prior to staining.
5. The block is stored dry.

For the staining of resin embedded sections of bone see page 212.

DEMONSTRATION OF OSTEOID IN DECALCIFIED TISSUE

The possibility of applying the von Kossa method [p. 217] to blocks of tissue followed by decalcification, paraffin embedding, and sectioning for the demonstration of mineralized bone was recognized by Lillie (1928) and a similar method for the demonstration of 'insoluble lime salts' was described by Gomori (1933). Neither of these procedures seems to have had much application for the demonstration of osteoid but the modification described by Tripp and MacKay (1972) overcomes the lack of reliablity of the earlier methods and provides a useful method for the demonstration of osteoid. No special equipment is necessary and conventional methods of embedding and sectioning are used.

Tripp and MacKay (1972) method for osteoid

FIXATION

Absolute alcohol is recommended but neutral formal saline may be used provided that all traces of free formaldehyde are removed by very thorough washing in distilled water before placing the tissue in the silver nitrate solution. Thin, 1–2 mm slices of bone are essential.

TECHNIQUE

1. Wash tissue in several changes of distilled water for four hours.
2. Place in 2 per cent aqueous silver nitrate for 48 hours in complete darkness.
3. Rinse in three changes of distilled water, 15–20 seconds each.
4. Wash in running tap water for four hours.
5. Place in reducing solution for 48 hours; (sodium hypophosphite 5 g, 0.1N sodium hydroxide 0.2 cm³, distilled water 100 cm³).
6. Wash in running tap water for one hour.
7. Place in 5 per cent sodium thiosulphate (anhydrous) for 24 hours.
8. Wash in running tap water for one hour.
9. Decalcify in 10 per cent formic acid.
10. Dehydrate and embed using a routine paraffin wax processing schedule.
11. Cut sections at 5 μm and mount on slides with an adhesive.
12. Take sections to water and stain for two minutes in van Gieson's stain.
13. Dehydrate, clear, and mount in a synthetic resin medium.

RESULTS

Osteoid—red.
Boundaries of mineralized areas—black.
Bone matrix—variably yellow to brown to black.

STAINING BONE AND BONE MARROW

Ehrlich's haematoxylin stains the mucopolysaccharide content of cartilage and the cement-lines of bone as well as nuclei and with an eosin counterstain is the routine method in bone histology. However, while this property of Ehrlich's haematoxylin is, for example, of special value in demonstrating the characteristic pattern of cement-lines in Paget's disease, the strong staining of basiphil material in cartilage-forming tumours may sometimes obscure nuclear detail and the use of a more precisely nuclear haematoxylin stain such as Cole's, Mayer's, or Harris' may be preferable in such cases.

Bone decalcified in EDTA does not require prolonged staining with haematoxylin but material subjected to long periods of decalcification in strong acid solutions may fail to stain in the usual time. In such cases, a longer duration of staining (16–24 hours in haematoxylin diluted 1 : 5 with distilled water), the use of an iron haematoxylin or the celestine blue-haemalum sequence may be helpful.

Acid decalcified tissue takes up eosin avidly and dilution of the usual solution or longer washing may be necessary to achieve differential staining of collagen, mature bone and osteoid.

Haematoxylin and eosin staining of methacrylate sections

TECHNIQUE

1. Transfer sections from 70 per cent alcohol to distilled water.
2. Stain in Cole's haematoxylin for 60 minutes.
3. Wash well in tap water.
4. Stain in 1 per cent aqueous eosin for 30 minutes.
5. Differentiate in tap water until osteoid is pink and calcified bone a deep purplish brown.

6. Dehydrate sections in 70 per cent followed by 90 per cent and absolute alcohol.
7. Transfer section to Euparal essence.
8. Place section on a slide, apply a strip of smooth hard paper over the section, and remove wrinkles by rolling a glass rod over the paper. Peel off the paper.
9. Mount in Euparal. A small weight applied to the cover glass helps flattening of the section.

RESULTS

Osteoid tissue—pink.
Calcified bone—purplish brown.
Nuclei—blue.
Erythrocytes—generally remain unstained.

The solochrome cyanin method of Matrajt and Hioco (1966) has been used for the demonstration of osteoid tissue which is stained orange–red, calcified bone being bright blue.

Masson's trichrome stain gives interesting results with undecalcified plastic embedded bone sections, giving bright red osteoid tissue and blue or green bone matrix according to the fibre stain employed. This is a reversal of the staining results usually obtained on decalcified paraffin sections of bone. The reason for this is not known.

Connective tissue stains are useful with bone and the collagen matrix of mature bone being birefringent is also well shown in unstained sections examined with polarized light [FIG. 11.2].

In cellulose nitrate and frozen sections, van Gieson's picro-fuchsin stains bone bright red, while the Masson trichrome method gives blue or green

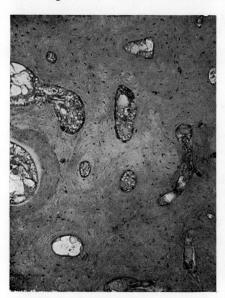
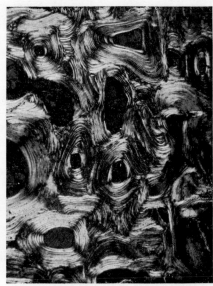

(a)   (b)

FIG. 11.2. Section of compact bone photographed (a) with ordinary light and (b) with crossed polaroids showing the lamellar arrangement of the bone matrix.

staining according to the fibre stain employed. Unfortunately, however, with paraffin sections the Masson and similar procedures are of less value, bone matrix staining variably with either plasma stain or fibre stain, or an unhelpful mixture of both. This may be due to the inability of the dyes and reagents used in these methods to gain proper access to the dense bone tissue when this is affixed to a glass slide or to the heat involved in the flattening and drying of sections (Smith 1962a). It is likely that both factors are implicated. In practice, van Gieson's stain is more useful and it is often possible to distinguish the bright red staining of osteoid and woven bone from the yellowish-pink staining of mature lamellar bone although this method lacks the precision required for diagnosis and accurate assessment of amounts of osteoid tissue.

Silver impregnation methods for reticulin fibres [p. 186] may be applied to sections of bone without modification. Cement-lines are not impregnated and are seen negatively against the brown staining of bone matrix in untoned preparations.

The PAS method [p. 237] is of some value in bone pathology; woven bone is always strongly positive, osteoid and lamellar bone, negative (Curran and Collins 1957). With a diastase control [p. 241] the method will aid the identification of glycogen-bearing osteosarcomata. Hughesdon's procedure [p. 250] stains the acid mucopolysaccharide of cartilage metachromatically and permanently.

Lacunae and canaliculi of bone may be demonstrated by the method of Schmorl (1934). Best results are obtained with cellulose nitrate or frozen sections, probably because the principle of the method is the precipitation of a basic dye (thionin) by picric acid in the narrow channels and spaces, these sections being less shrunken and allowing more ready access of the granules of precipitate than paraffin sections on slides.

FIXATION

This is not critical although Schmorl advised against the use of mercuric chloride. Ten per cent formal-saline is satisfactory.

SECTIONS

Cellulose nitrate or frozen sections.

TECHNIQUE

1. Cellulose nitrate or frozen sections are washed for ten minutes in several changes of distilled water.
2. Stain in half-saturated (0.125 per cent) aqueous solution of thionin for 5–10 minutes.
3. Wash in distilled water.
4. Place in saturated aqueous picric acid for 30–60 seconds.
5. Wash in distilled water.
6. Differentiate in 70 per cent alcohol until stain ceases to pour out from the section. This will take five minutes or longer according to the thickness of the section.
7. Rinse in distilled water.
8. Return to saturated picric acid for 30–60 seconds.
9. Rinse in distilled water.
10. Dehydrate in 95 per cent alcohol.
11. Mount section on slide, clear in 95 per cent alcohol–terpineol mixture [p. 136].
12. Mount in Euparal.

RESULTS

Lacunae and canaliculi—dark brown to black.
Bone matrix—yellow or yellowish-brown.
Nuclei—red.
Cartilage—purplish.

NOTES

1. Samples of thionin vary considerably in their suitability for this method. If a test section (TS cortical bone) stains unsatisfactorily, add one drop of strong ammonia to each 25 cm³ of stain, filter, and use immediately.
2. The second treatment with picric acid (stage 8) is an addition to the original method. It serves to restore the desirable coloration of bone matrix sometimes lost during alcohol and water treatment.
3. Cellulose nitrate sections stored for some time in 70 per cent alcohol may fail to stain satisfactorily. The reason is not known; freshly cut sections of the same material stain successfully.
4. Other dyes than thionin may be used in this method and Azur A has given good results.

STAINING OF BONE MARROW SECTIONS

Stained bone marrow sections are ideally examined in conjunction with stained smears. Cellular detail should be studied in the smears stained by the Romanowsky methods. The sections show changes in cellularity and architecture, and well differentiated H and E staining is often sufficient for their interpretation. Smith and Signy (1966) recommended that a serial ribbon of nine sections of aspirated bone marrow fragment should be stained as follows: 1 and 2, spares; 3, H and E; 4, Perls' reaction for iron; 5, Wolbach's modification of Giemsa's technique (see below); 6, reticulin; 7, H and E; 8 and 9, spares.

Leishman's stain

1. Take thin paraffin sections to water and leave in buffered water at pH 6.8 for 30 minutes.
2. Immerse in Leishman's stain diluted with two parts of buffered water at pH 6.8 to one part of stain. Leave for 10–15 minutes.
3. Wash and differentiate in 50 per cent methyl alcohol in buffered water at pH 5.0.
4. When the nuclei are purple and the granules of polymorphs are clearly seen the section is blotted until completely dry, cleared in xylene, and mounted in green Euparal.

RESULTS

Nuclei—purple.
Leucocyte granules—red (eosinophils) to dark purple (basiphils).
Red blood corpuscles—pink.

Wolbach's Giemsa stain (Lillie 1965)

FIXATION

Zenker or Möller's (Regaud's) fluid [p. 280]. Can be used after other fixatives.

SECTIONS

Thin paraffin sections.

TECHNIQUE

1. Take sections to distilled water.
2. Stain one hour in Giemsa's stain 1 cm³, methyl alcohol 1.25 cm³, 0.5 per cent sodium carbonate solution 0.1 cm³ (two drops), distilled water 40 cm³.
3. Pour off and replace with two further changes of the same mixture during the first hour and leave in the third change overnight.
4. Differentiate in 95 per cent alcohol containing a few drops of 10 per cent colophonium alcohol.
5. Dehydrate with 100 per cent alcohol, clear in xylene, and mount in cedar wood oil.

RESULTS

Nuclei—dark blue to violet.
Red blood corpuscles—yellow to pink.
Cytoplasm of haemopoietic cells—varying shades of light blue, with granules stained differentially.

Bayley's acid Giemsa method (Bayley 1949)

This was described for tissues fixed in acetic formalin and decalcified in nitric acid. Satisfactory results can be obtained after other fixatives and with tissues like spleen that do not require decalcification.

TECHNIQUE

Take sections to distilled water and stain as follows:

1. Ehrlich's haematoxylin. Differentiate rather more than usual.
2. Blue in tap water.
3. Rinse in distilled water.
4. Stain on the slide for ten minutes with:
   Giemsa stock solution   15 vols.
   1 per cent acetic acid   10 vols.
5. Rinse in distilled water and blot.
6. Differentiate and complete dehydration in absolute alcohol.
7. Xylene.
8. Mount in a synthetic resin medium.

RESULTS

Bone trabeculae—pink; cartilage ground-substance—purple; eosinophil and basiphil granules of myelocytes well shown; red blood corpuscles—pink; nuclei—blue.

NOTES

1. The counterstain can be controlled by the proportion of acetic acid, more acid producing stronger eosin staining.
2. The speed of final dehydration controls the blue stain, which is extracted by absolute alcohol.
3. The method works well through a coating of celloidin [p. 186].
4. Any Romanowsky-type stain may be substituted for Giemsa, but the latter is less liable to precipitate.

DEMONSTRATION OF CALCIUM SALTS

More effort is devoted to the decalcification of tissues than to the identification of calcium. This is critically discussed by Cameron (1930) in which the technique of making artificial 'tissue' blocks containing metallic compounds for sectioning and staining is described. The sections are useful when testing a new method and can be used as controls when stained back-to-back with the test section.

FRESH PREPARATIONS

Teased preparations (in 40 per cent alcohol) or fresh frozen sections are treated with 3 per cent sulphuric acid. If present in sufficient quantity, rhombic crystals of gypsum ($CaSO_4$) will be formed. This test is not suitable for the precise localization of deposits.

SECTIONS

Acid fixatives should not be used and buffered neutral formalin or formalin-alcohol mixtures are recommended. Calcium salts stain a deep purplish blue in routine haematoxylin and eosin stained sections and the treatment of an adjacent section with 5 per cent acetic acid or 0.25 per cent nitric acid for two minutes should dissolve the salts and act as a control; but these are not reliable tests for calcium salts.

Histochemical methods for the demonstration of calcium have been reviewed by McGee-Russell (1958). They fall into two main groups: (1) *metal substitution*; and (2) *dye-lake reactions.*

In the first group, one of the oldest and still most widely used methods is that of von Kossa (1901). This substitutes silver for calcium in the calcium salts found in animal tissues; the silver salt is then reduced to black metallic silver by light or a photographic developer (Gomori 1952). While not specific for calcium, and applicable to histological rather than cytological investigations, the method is valuable for the demonstration of pathological calcification and calcified bone.

Modified von Kossa method

FIXATION

Neutral formalin or formalin-alcohol.

SECTIONS

Paraffin, frozen or synthetic resin.

TECHNIQUE

1. Remove wax from paraffin sections.
2. Wash sections in several changes of distilled water.
3. Place in 2 per cent silver nitrate in a thin walled, clear glass staining tube and expose to bright daylight or a high intensity artificial light source for 20–60 minutes. Short wavelength blue light from a halogen lamp or ultraviolet light will produce reduction and blackening of deposits in the shortest time. Completion of the reaction may be confirmed by microscopical examination.
4. Wash in several changes of distilled water.
5. Treat with 2.5 per cent sodium thiosulphate ('hypo') for five minutes.

6. Wash well in tap water.
7. Counterstain as desired. A light, neutral red nuclear stain may be used or, with sections of undecalcified bone, brief staining with van Gieson's picro-fuchsin will colour osteoid tissue red.
8. Dehydrate, clear, and mount in a synthetic resin medium.

RESULTS

Calcium deposits—black. Other tissues according to counterstain.

NOTE

Urates may also be blackened by this method. To distinguish from calcium, a control section should be treated with saturated aqueous lithium carbonate in which urates are readily soluble (see below).

Cobalt, lead, iron, and copper substitution methods have also been described. None is wholly satisfactory for the specific demonstration of all the calcium salts occurring in animal tissues and McGee-Russell stresses the need for meticulous attention to the details of the techniques and the use of appropriate controls.

Of the *dye-lake reactions* for calcium, the anthraquinone dyes, alizarin and pupurin have been extensively used, the former especially for the staining of the skeletal system in embryos and foetuses [p. 479]. Recent work has shown that the pH of the stain is critical for the precise identification of calcium salts in sections.

Alizarin red S method for calcium (McGee-Russell 1958)

FIXATION

Neutral formalin or formalin-alcohol.

SECTIONS

Paraffin or frozen sections.

PREPARATION

A 2 per cent aqueous solution of alizarin red S is adjusted to pH 4.1–4.3 with dilute ammonium hydroxide using a glass electrode pH-meter. The solution should be a deep iodine colour and keeps well.

TECHNIQUE

1. Remove wax from sections and bring to 50 per cent alcohol.
2. Rinse briefly with distilled water and cover with stain.
3. Examine with the staining microscope. Development of the orange–red staining takes from 30 seconds to five minutes.
4. When the staining is strong but not too diffuse, shake off excess stain and blot the section with filter paper.
5. Treat immediately with acetone for 20 seconds, then with equal parts of acetone and xylene for a similar time and finally, with pure xylene. Mount in a synthetic resin medium.

RESULTS

Sites of calcium will be covered and surrounded by a heavy orange–red pre-cipitate which is birefringent. Background is faint pink.

DEMONSTRATION OF URIC ACID

Uric acid occurs in tissues as acid sodium urate and the typical crystals of this substance are seen in the lesions associated with gout (gouty tophi).

Urates are slightly soluble in dilute alkalies but insoluble in concentrated ammonia and alcohol. The crystals are birefringent. It is one of the few argentaffin substances found in human tissues.

Methenamine silver method for urates (modified from Gomori 1952)

FIXATION

95 per cent or absolute alcohol.

SECTIONS

Paraffin sections, which should be floated out very briefly on warm water or, preferably, on alcohol.

PREPARATION

Add 5 cm³ of 5 per cent silver nitrate to 100 cm³ of 3 per cent methenamine. Shake until the whole precipitate that forms disappears. This solution keeps well in the refrigerator. For use, add 8 cm³ of pH 7.8 boric acid-borate buffer [p. 498] to 30 cm³ of methenamine silver solution.

TECHNIQUE

1. Remove wax with xylene and wash with absolute alcohol.
2. Transfer directly from alcohol to the methenamine silver solution pre-warmed to 37 °C. Allow to act at 37 °C for 30 minutes or longer, until deposits of urates are black.
3. Rinse in distilled water.
4. Treat with 2.5 per cent sodium thiosulphate for five minutes. Wash in tap water.
5. Counterstain as desired. Dehydrate, clear, and mount in synthetic resin medium.

RESULTS

Deposits of urates are black, other structures according to the counterstain.

NOTES

1. Large masses of calcium salts are a potential source of false positive results but silver phosphate and carbonate are soluble in methenamine and should be washed out.
2. Control sections may be pre-treated for 1–2 minutes with 0.5 per cent hydrochloric or nitric acid in absolute alcohol followed by a wash in absolute alcohol to exclude calcium salts.
3. Urates are readily soluble in aqueous lithium carbonate. Calcium salts are not affected by this treatment.

REFERENCES

ALBERT, D. L. and LINDER, J. E. (1960). *Stain Technol.* **35**, 277.
ARNIM, S. S. (1935). *Anat. Rec.* **62**, 321.
BALL, J. (1957). *J. clin. Path.* **10**, 281.
BAYLEY, J. H. (1949). *J. Path. Bact.* **61**, 448.
BROWNE, R. M. and ROWLES, S. L. (1975). *Stain Technol.* **50**, 179.

CAMERON, G. R. (1930). *J. Path. Bact.* **33**, 329.
CAPPELL, D. F., HUTCHISON, H. E., and SMITH, G. H. (1947). *Br. med. J.* i, 403.
CLAYDEN, E. C. (1952). *J. med. Lab. Technol.* **10**, 103.
CRAWFORD, R. A. (1957). *J. med. Lab. Technol.* **14**, 111.
CURRAN, R. C. and COLLINS, D. H. (1957). *J. Path. Bact.* **74**, 207.
DIFFORD, J. (1974). *Med. Lab. Technol.* **31**, 79.
DOTTI, L. B., PAPARO, G. P., and CLARKE, E. (1951). *Am. J. clin. Path.* **21**, 475.
DUTHIE, R. B. (1954). *J. Path. Bact.* **68**, 296.
EVANS, N. and KRAJIAN, A. (1930). *Arch. Path.* **10**, 447.
FRIEND, J. V. and SMITH, G. S. (1962). *J. med. Lab. Technol.* **19**, 255.
—— —— (1964). *J. med. Lab. Technol.* **21**, 51.
FROST, H. M. (1969). *Calcif. Tissue Res.* **3**, 211.
—— and VILLANEUVA, A. R. (1960). *Stain Technol.* **35**, 135.
GOMORI, G. (1933). *Am. J. Path.* **9**, 253.
—— (1952). *Microscopic histochemistry.* Chicago University Press.
GOODING, H. and STEWART, D. (1932). *Lab. J.* **7**, 55.
GORE, L. F. and ABBOTT, J. J. (1964). *J. med. Lab. Technol.* **21**, 293.
HART, P. (1962). *J. med. Lab. Technol.* **19**, 115.
HILLEMAN, H. H. and LEE, C. H. (1953). *Stain Technol.* **28**, 285.
HUTCHISON, H. E. (1953). *Blood* **8**, 236.
INWOOD, J. M. (1958). *J. med. Lab. Technol.* **15**, 253.
JOWSEY, J. (1955). *J. sci. Instrum.* **32**, 159.
KOSSA, J. VON (1901). *Beitr. path. Anat.* **29**, 163.
KUPER, S. W. A. (1965). *J. clin. Path.* **18**, 255.
LILLIE, R. D. (1928). *Z. Wiss. Mikr.* **45**, 380.
—— (1948). *Histopathologic technic.* McGraw-Hill, Philadelphia.
—— (1951). *Stain Technol.* **26**, 276.
—— (1965). *Histopathologic technic and practical histochemistry*, 3rd. edn. McGraw-Hill, New York.
McGEE-RUSSELL, S. M. (1958). *J. Histochem. Cytochem.* **6**, 22.
MATRAJT, H. and HIOCO, D. (1966). *Stain Technol.* **41**, 97.
MORRIS, R. E. and BENTON, R. S. (1956). *Am. J. clin. Path.* **26**, 771.
MORSE, A. (1945). *J. dent. Res.* **24**, 143.
PAGE, K. M. (1977). In *Theory and practice of histological techniques* (eds. J. D. Bancroft and A. Stevens). Churchill-Livingstone, Edinburgh.
PERENYI, J. (1882). *Zool. Anzeig.* **5**, 459.
RALIS, Z. A. and RALIS, H. M. (1975). *Med. Lab. Technol.* **32**, 203.
RICHMAN, I. M., GELFAND, M., and HILL, J. M. (1947). *Arch. Path.* **44**, 92.
ROWLES, S. L. and BROWNE, R. M. (1975). *Stain Technol.* **50**, 187.
RUSSELL, N. L. (1963). *J. med. Lab. Technol.* **20**, 299.
SAXBY, P. M. (1959). *J. med. Lab. Technol.* **16**, 2.
SCHMORL, G. (1934). *Die pathologisch-histologischen Untersuchungmethoden*, 16th edn. Vogel, Berlin.
SISSONS, H. A. (1968). *Preparation of undecalcified bone sections.* Broadsheet No. 62, Association of Clinical Pathologists.
SMITH, A. (1962a). *Stain Technol.* **37**, 339.
—— (1962b). *J. med. Lab. Technol.* **19**, 1.
SMITH, D. R. and SIGNY, A. G. (1966). *Preparation of sections from bone marrow biopsies.* Broadsheet No. 53, Association of Clinical Pathologists.
TRIPP, E. J. and MACKAY, E. H. (1972). *Stain Technol.* **47**, 129.
WALLINGTON, E. A. (1972). *Histological methods for bone.* Butterworths, London.
WEBB, D. V. (1952). *J. med. Lab. Technol.* **10**, 23.
WOODS, C. G. (1972). *Diagnostic orthopaedic pathology.* Blackwell, Oxford.

12 | Extracellular substances

Tissue constituents can rarely be said to be entirely intracellular or extracellular and some substances such as mucopolysaccharide may be found both in the cell cytoplasm and in ground-substance, e.g. cartilage. Similarly, while amyloid, fibrin, and keratin are considered here as extracellular substances, all three may be found within cells in certain conditions.

AMYLOID

Amyloid, which means starch-like, is the name given by Virchow more than 100 years ago to describe the firm, amorphous, translucent substance that may be deposited in virtually any tissue of the body though often being first seen in the walls of blood vessels.

The precise composition of amyloid has been the subject of speculation and investigation for some years but it is now apparent that it is predominantly protein in nature with a small (about 5 per cent) carbohydrate fraction. This latter includes a proportion of heparan sulphate but amyloid may vary somewhat in its chemical composition, this accounting for variation in staining results (see below). Fortunately, amyloid has a unique fibrillary ultrastructure and its unequivocal recognition is now possible with the electron microscope.

It is customary to categorize depositions of amyloid in the body as being either primary or secondary, according to the presence or absence of some predisposing disease and the organs affected.

Primary amyloidosis most commonly affects muscle, skin, the tongue, alimentary tract, and the heart and Pomerance (1965) showed that 10 per cent of hearts from subjects aged 75 years or more showed deposits of amyloid. Primary amyloidosis may also be hereditary and one form of this disease affects peripheral nerves and sympathetic ganglia.

Secondary amyloidosis (the most common form of the disease) is associated with chronic inflammatory conditions such as tuberculosis, rheumatoid arthritis, and ulcerative colitis. In these cases, the organs most frequently affected are the liver, spleen, kidney, and adrenal. Amyloidosis may also be associated with multiple myeloma (when the distribution is more like that seen in primary amyloidosis) and with carcinoma of the thyroid and Hodgkin's disease.

DEMONSTRATION METHODS FOR AMYLOID

Amyloid may be demonstrated in fresh tissues by the avidity with which it takes up Gram's iodine, being stained a deep mahogany-brown. This procedure is commonly used in the post-mortem room to confirm a macroscopic appearance of amyloidosis. Tissues are washed briefly in 1 per cent acetic acid and treated with Gram's iodine solution for 3–5 minutes. Amyloid is stained dark brown and may be changed to blue–violet by further treatment with 10 per cent sulphuric acid.

Although the brown iodine staining of amyloid is soon lost after immersion of the tissue in formalin, slices of tissues may be so stored for some years without loss of ability to be re-stained with iodine for demonstration purposes.

The variable composition of amyloid has been noted and results with staining methods may be inconsistent. Negative results may be obtained with material stored for months or years in formalin prior to embedding and Culling (1963) noted that unstained paraffin sections of amyloid material will fail to stain if kept for longer than 3–4 months. This is not invariably so, but failure or alteration in staining reaction in sections kept for some time is a possibility with the following and other techniques.

Amyloid is variably eosinophilic in haematoxylin and eosin stained sections is moderately PAS positive and generally, but not always, takes the blue or green fibre stain in trichrome methods of the Masson type. Results with van Gieson's stain are also variable and amyloid may be yellow or pale pink, while some deposits of primary amyloid may stain a distinctive khaki colour (Symmers 1956).

Four groups of methods are in general use for the demonstration of amyloid in tissue sections. These are: (1) metachromatic staining with methyl violet and related dyes; (2) staining with Congo red; (3) induced fluorescence with thioflavine T; and (4) staining with Alcian blue.

METACHROMATIC METHOD

The acid polysaccharide component of amyloid is stained metachromatically by methyl violet, crystal violet, and dahlia (Hoffmann's violet).

New samples of dye should be tested on a control section.

Methyl violet–crystal violet method (after Jurgens 1875)

FIXATION

Not critical. Carnoy, formal-sublimate, and 10 per cent formal-saline are suitable but long immersion in the latter may cause failure of the stain.

SECTIONS

Paraffin or frozen sections are suitable, the latter giving superior results. Cryostat sections of fresh tissue are particularly recommended.

TECHNIQUE

1. Take sections to water.
2. Stain in 1 per cent aqueous methyl or crystal violet for 2–5 minutes.
3. Wash in water and examine with the microscope (see Note 1).
4. Differentiate in 0.5–1 per cent acetic acid until amyloid is purplish-red or red in good contrast with the blue–violet staining of nuclei and normal tissue.
5. Wash in running tap water for at least five minutes.
6. Drain the slide and while the section is still moist, mount with modified Apathy's gum syrup [p. 129]. Ring coverslip with nail varnish.

RESULTS

Amyloid—purplish-red to red.
Nuclei, cytoplasm, and connective tissue—shades of blue–violet.

NOTES

1. It is necessary to examine sections microscopically at stage 3 because in some cases, little or no differentiation in acid is required, amyloid showing bright and sharp metachromatic staining at this point.
2. It is not possible to dehydrate sections and mount in resinous media because the stain is readily soluble in alcohol. Mallory (1938) however, quotes Mayer's method whereby paraffin sections are floated on the surface of the stain, differentiator, and water, before being affixed to slides, de-waxed in xylene, and mounted in a resinous medium.
3. Numerous modifications of the above basic method have been devised. All aim at avoiding fading by preventing 'bleeding' of the stain in the aqueous mounting media. With the mounting medium recommended above and protection of the slide from strong light, there should be little fading for some years.
4. Blue glass filters should be removed from microscope or light source when examining metachromatic staining.

CONGO RED METHODS

The affinity of amyloid for Congo red has been known for many years and absorption of the dye by amyloid was formerly used as a clinical diagnostic test.

Amyloid stained with Congo red exhibits a yellow–green birefringence in polarized light and this feature was formerly thought to be confined to amyloid deposits. That this is not so has been demonstrated by several workers including Klatskin (1969) who found non-specific green birefringence in a variety of tissues, especially when fixed in Carnoy, Zenker, alcohol, or Bouin's fluid. Reissenweber and Decaro (1969) described the green birefringence of prostatic, pulmonary, and sometimes cerebral corpora amylacea when stained with Congo red and Wolman (1975) in supporting these findings refers to 'prostatic amyloid bodies' and 'amyloid bodies of pulmonary alveoli' [see p. 227].

Heptinstall (1974) observed that green birefringence may be lacking in Congo red stained sections of amyloid tissue if the sections are too thin and recommended 6 µm sections for the purpose.

Bennhold (1922) described a Congo red stain for amyloid in sections and several modifications of his method have been published. Two of the most reliable of these are given below. While highly selective for amyloid, neither are specific, since other tissue components may be stained pink or red, especially elastic tissue.

Highman's (1946) Congo red method for amyloid

FIXATION

Not critical, formalin is satisfactory.

SECTIONS

Paraffin or frozen sections.

TECHNIQUE

1. Take sections to 70 per cent alcohol.
2. Stain in 0.5 per cent Congo red in 50 per cent alcohol for five minutes.

3. Differentiate in 0.2 per cent potassium hydroxide in 80 per cent alcohol for 1–3 minutes, controlling microscopically.
4. Wash in water.
5. Counterstain nuclei in alum haematoxylin.
6. Wash in water.
7. Dehydrate, clear in xylene, and mount in a synthetic resin medium.

RESULTS

Amyloid—deep pink to red.
Nuclei—blue.

NOTES

1. Although involving a critical differentiation step (3) this method sometimes gives a stronger staining of amyloid than the (automatic) method below.
2. The reagents are stable.

Alkaline Congo red method for amyloid (Puchtler, Sweat, and Levine 1962)

FIXATION

Carnoy's fluid or ethanol are recommended but results are adequate after formalin and mercuric chloride fixatives.

SECTIONS

Paraffin or frozen sections.

PREPARATION

Alkaline solution
Stock solution: 80 per cent alcohol saturated with sodium chloride.
Working solution: Add 0.5 cm³ 1 per cent aqueous sodium hydroxide to 50 cm³ of the stock solution. Filter and use within 15 minutes.

Congo red stain
Stock solution: 80 per cent alcohol saturated with Congo red and sodium chloride.

Working solution: Add 0.5 cm³ 1 per cent aqueous sodium hydroxide to 50 cm³ of the stock solution. Filter and use within 15 minutes.

TECHNIQUE

1. Take sections to water.
2. Stain nuclei in alum haematoxylin.
3. Wash, differentiate, and wash in water.
4. Treat with alkaline solution for 20 minutes.
5. Stain in Congo red for 20 minutes.
6. Dehydrate with three brief rinses with absolute alcohol.
7. Clear in xylene and mount in a synthetic resin medium.

RESULTS

Nuclei—blue.
Amyloid—deep pink to red.
Elastic fibres and some cytoplasmic granules may be stained pink to red.

NOTES

1. This method is highly selective and requires no differentiation.
2. Both stock solutions will keep several months.
3. Freshly prepared Congo red solution should be allowed to stand for 24 hours before use. It must be saturated with the dye.
4. The working solutions are not stable.

FLUORESCENCE OF AMYLOID

Vassar and Culling (1959) showed that fluorescence may be imparted to amyloid with an appropriate fluorochrome and selected thioflavine T from the many others tested. An ultraviolet or short wavelength blue light source is required [p. 24].

The method is highly sensitive but not specific for amyloid.

Thioflavine T method for amyloid (Vassar and Culling 1959)

FIXATION

Ten per cent formal-saline is suitable. Fixatives containing salts of heavy metals are less satisfactory.

SECTIONS

Paraffin or frozen sections may be used.

TECHNIQUE

1. Sections are taken to water.
2. Stain with alum haematoxylin for two minutes to quench fluorescence of nuclei. Differentiation is not necessary.
3. Wash briefly in water.
4. Stain in freshly filtered 1 per cent aqueous thioflavine T for three minutes.
5. Rinse in water.
6. Treat with 1 per cent acetic acid for 20 minutes (this is to reduce background fluorescence).
7. Wash well in running water.
8. Mount in Apathy's gum syrup [p. 129].

RESULTS

Amyloid and mast cells fluoresce bright yellow against an olive-green background.

NOTES

1. Solutions of thioflavine T do not keep indefinitely and a control section should always be used.
2. Sections should be thin; with thick sections, bone may fluoresce strongly and extension of treatment with acetic acid and water may be required.
3. Hobbs and Morgan (1963) have favourably compared results using this technique with those of the other methods for amyloid but McKinney and Grubb (1965) stated that false positive results may be given by hyaline substances due to the persistence after staining of their strong autofluorescence.
4. See page 26 for details of appropriate filters for use with light source.

ALCIAN BLUE METHOD

Sodium sulphate–Alcian blue (SAB) method for amyloid (Lendrum, Slidders, and Fraser 1972)

The advantage of this method lies in the combined demonstration of amyloid with differential staining of connective tissue. The authors suggest that amyloid (like fibrin, page 228) undergoes an aging process with concomitant alteration in staining reaction.

FIXATION

10 per cent neutral formalin is adequate. The authors recommend secondary fixation in 5 per cent aqueous mercuric chloride for post mortem material.

SECTIONS

6 μm paraffin sections.

PREPARATION

Stock solutions
A. 1 per cent Alcian blue in 95 per cent alcohol.
B. 1 per cent sodium sulphate hydrate in distilled water.

SAB working solution

Stock solution A	45 cm³
Stock solution B	45 cm³
Glacial acetic acid	10 cm³

Mix; stand 30 minutes before use; prepare freshly each day.

Acetic–alcohol rinse

95 per cent alcohol	45 cm³
Distilled water	45 cm³
Glacial acetic acid	10 cm³

Mix; ready for use; prepare freshly each day.

TECHNIQUE

1. Take sections to water removing mercury pigment if necessary; wash ten minutes.
2. Transfer to acetic-alcohol for one to two minutes.
3. Stain in SAB solution for two hours.
4. Transfer to acetic-alcohol for one to two minutes.
5. Wash in water.
6. Alkalinize in 80 per cent alcohol saturated with borax for 30 minutes.
7. Wash in water.
8. Stain nuclei in celestine blue–haemalum or in iron haematoxylin.
9. Wash well in water.
10. Take each slide individually and differentiate by dipping in 80 per cent alcohol saturated with picric acid, 20 to 30 seconds. Rinse briefly in water to remove the alcohol.
11. Stain in van Gieson for two to three minutes.
12. Rinse rapidly with 95 per cent alcohol, dehydrate in absolute alcohol, clear in xylene, and mount in a synthetic resin mountant.

Amyloid—green.
Nuclei—black.
Collagen—red.
Muscle, cytoplasm, and erythrocytes—yellow.

NOTES

1. Epithelial and stromal mucins, mast cell granules, and some colloids may stain green with this method.
2. The shade and brightness of the green staining amyloid varies, tending to be a more brilliant, pure green in newer, smaller deposits and a dull grey-green in larger, older deposits.

CORPORA AMYLACEA

Corpora amylacea are irregular or rounded, or oval bodies of varying size and may be found in the prostate, lungs, brain, pineal, spinal cord, and other tissues, particularly in elderly subjects.

Prostatic corpora amylacea are concentrically laminated, generally rounded but often irregular bodies formed from inspissated secretion of the gland. They stain pink with eosin, brown with iodine, and are usually PAS positive. They may attain a size of several millimetres in diameter and sometimes become calcified, causing difficulty in sectioning. Prostatic corpora amylacea are discussed by Marx, Gueft, and Moskal (1965).

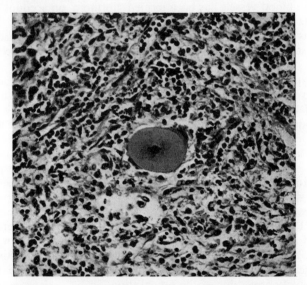

FIG. 12.1   Pulmonary corpora amylacea. One of the oval bodies with a central fragment of carbon. HE. × 200.

Pulmonary corpora amylacea are round or oval bodies about 200 μm in diameter [FIG. 12.1]. They stain with eosin and are PAS negative or weakly positive. Serial sectioning of these bodies shows them to be concentrically laminated, sometimes, showing radial cracking and usually containing a speck of black insoluble material (possibly carbon) at the centre (Michaels and

Levine 1957). Foreign-body giant cells are often seen closely adjacent to pulmonary corpora amylacea.

Corpora amylacea of nervous tissues are generally smaller than the above varieties although similar bodies (psammoma bodies) are sometimes found in meningiomata. Corpora amylacea of brain and spinal cord (brain sand) are often basiphilic, may stain metachromatically with toluidine blue and are frequently calcified, especially in the pineal gland. Their presence is associated with degenerative processes in these tissues.

As noted above, corpora amylacea, although most commonly seen in the prostate, brain, and lungs may be found in other situations and Averback and Langevin (1978) described intra-axonal corpora amylacea in peripheral nerve biopsies, David and Buchner (1978) described corpora amylacea in an adenolymphoma while David and Hiss (1978) found similar bodies in a case of mesothelioma of the atrioventricular node.

It is noteworthy that any type of corpora amylacea, in any situation, may give (false) positive staining reactions for amyloid, including green birefringence in Congo red stained sections.

FIBRIN

Fibrin is formed from the fibrinogen of blood plasma and is seen in the earliest stages of development as a network of fine threads, progressing to coarser threads and eventually, as amorphous, sometimes laminated masses. The similar, amorphous, hyaline material seen, for example, in rheumatic lesions and in blood vessels has been termed 'fibrinoid' on account of its staining reactions being the same as, or similar to, those of fibrin. The precise nature of this material has not been determined but Lendrum, Fraser, Slidders, and Henderson (1962) believe that fibrin undergoes an aging process and that 'fibrinoid' is old fibrin.

The principle of the methods described by Lendrum and his colleagues is the use of dyes of different molecular size in accordance with the alteration in structure of fibrin at different stages of development. Complete validity of these methods depends on prolonged fixation in formal-sublimate and meticulous attention to the details of the methods.

Fibrin is acidophil and stains strongly with eosin; it is yellow after van Gieson and weakly to moderately PAS positive. Mallory's phosphotungstic acid haematoxylin [p. 146] stains fibrin threads readily but denser masses of older fibrin stain red, as does collagen.

The earliest method designed for the differential staining of fibrin was that of Weigert (1887) who modified Gram's stain for bacteria by differentiating in a mixture of aniline oil and xylene, nuclei being stained with carmine. In this method [p. 394], apart from the staining of fibrin and Gram positive bacteria, dense collagen is difficult and sometimes impossible to decolorize, thus reducing the selectivity and value of the preparation.

Since fibrin is often intimately associated with erythrocytes in tissues, the staining of these in contrasting colours is a desirable feature of methods for the demonstration of fibrin and this distinction was given with the acid fuchsin–aniline blue–orange G method of Mallory (1938). This method has been modified by many workers, however, with the selective and differential staining of fibrin in view. In Britain, development of the method has proceeded mainly from Lendrum and McFarlane (1940), McFarlane (1944), and

Lendrum (1949), (the picro-Mallory methods) to the more recent work of Lendrum and colleagues cited above. In every case, contrast staining of erythrocytes has been obtained by the use of one or more yellow dyes followed by the fibrin stain, phosphotungstic acid treatment, and a collagen stain. In contemporary methods, the trend is towards stains that are more automatic in action and less dependent on skilful differentiation.

MSB (martius, scarlet, blue) method for fibrin (after Lendrum *et al*. 1962)

FIXATION

Primary or secondary formal-sublimate, up to eight weeks.

SECTIONS

Thin paraffin sections.

TECHNIQUE

1. Sections are taken to water.
2. Stain nuclei with celestine blue–haemalum.
3. Rinse in tap water.
4. Differentiate nuclei in 0.25 per cent hydrochloric acid in 70 per cent alcohol.
5. Wash well in tap water.
6. Rinse in 95 per cent alcohol and stain with 0.5 per cent martius yellow in 95 per cent alcohol containing 2 per cent phosphotungstic acid for two minutes.
7. Rinse in distilled water and stain in 1 per cent brilliant crystal scarlet 6R in 2.5 per cent acetic acid for ten minutes (see Note 4).
8. Rinse in distilled water and treat with 1 per cent phosphotungstic acid to fix and differentiate the red stain for up to five minutes.
9. Rinse with distilled water and stain in 0.5 per cent soluble blue in 1 per cent acetic acid for up to ten minutes.
10. Rinse in 1 per cent acetic acid, blot, dehydrate in absolute alcohol, clear in xylene, and mount in a synthetic resin medium.

RESULTS

Nuclei—black; erythrocytes—yellow; fibrin—red; connective tissue—blue.

NOTES

1. In the absence of mercuric chloride fixation Lendrum *et al*. recommend treatment of sections as follows. After removal of wax with xylene, leave in a closed jar of trichloroethylene for 48 hours. Rinse in absolute alcohol and place in 3 per cent mercuric chloride in saturated alcoholic picric acid for 24 hours. Wash in water followed by treatment with iodine and 'hypo' [p. 45] and further washing.
2. Thin, flat sections are essential, it being difficult to remove the red stain from dense collagen in thick sections.
3. The method is highly selective for fibrin though not specific; Paneth cell granules and other cytoplasmic inclusions may stain red. Bone may also retain the red stain.
4. Brilliant crystal scarlet 6R has several synonyms. These are given on page 499.

Fuchsin–miller method for fibrin (Slidders 1961)

This method stains fibrin red and connective tissue yellow and is suitable for use after the staining of elastic fibres with Weigert's elastic tissue stain [p. 193] or after orcein [p. 194]. It follows the same general principle of the staining of fibrin with a red sulphonated dye in acid solution followed by differentiation and mordanting in phosphotungstic acid, but with simultaneous further differentiation and replacement of the red dye in collagen by a yellow dye dissolved in Cellosolve (2-ethoxyethanol). Both dye and solvent influence the process of differentiation.

FIXATION

Formal-sublimate or secondary formal-sublimate for 2–3 weeks after primary fixation in formal-saline. The use of the degreasing procedure given above is recommended for poorly fixed material.

SECTIONS

Thin paraffin sections.

TECHNIQUE

1. Sections are taken to water.
2. Stain nuclei with the celestine blue–haemalum sequence.
3. Differentiate nuclei in 0.25 per cent hydrochloric acid in 70 per cent alcohol.
4. Wash well in running tap water.
5. Stain in 1 per cent acid fuchsin in 2.5 per cent acetic acid for ten minutes.
6. Rinse in distilled water.
7. Treat with 1 per cent aqueous phosphotungstic acid for five minutes.
8. Rinse with distilled water, blot, rinse thoroughly with Cellosolve, and transfer to a closed dish of Cellosolve containing 2.5 per cent Milling yellow 3G.
9. Satisfactory differentiation may take from ½–4 hours and Slidders observes that it is generally possible to extract the red dye from erythrocytes and muscle before fibrin is destained.
10. Rinse with Cellosolve, clear in xylene, and mount in a synthetic resin medium.

RESULTS

Nuclei—black.
Fibrin—magenta-red.
Other tissue constituents—yellow.

NOTES

1. In addition to fibrin, various intracellular inclusions will retain the red stain.
2. The action of the differentiating solution is impaired by contamination with solvents other than Cellosolve, its selectivity being reduced even by breathing on the slide during microscopical control and, presumably, in a very humid atmosphere.

KERATIN

Keratin is a fibrous protein derived from the superficial layers of the epidermis. It is relatively insoluble and contains a variable though high percentage of sulphur, greater in hard keratin (hairs, nails, and feathers) than in soft keratin (skin). This may explain the variation in staining reactions of keratin in different situations, normal and abnormal.

Keratin is birefringent, takes up picric acid strongly, is Gram positive and retains the phloxine in the phloxine–tartrazine method [p. 400]. It is variably PAS positive and soft keratin stains with oil soluble dyes when containing lipid derived from sebaceous glands.

The high sulphur content of keratin is the rationale of its demonstration with the performic acid–Alcian blue method for disulphide groups [p. 154] and the DDD reaction and ferric–ferricyanide reaction for sulphydryl [p. 273].

REFERENCES

AVERBACK, P. and LANGEVIN, H. (1978). *Arch. Neurol.* **35**, 95.
BENNHOLD, H. (1922). *Münch. med. Wschr.* **2**, 1537.
CULLING, C. F. A. (1963). *Handbook of histopathological technique*, 2nd edn. Butterworths, London.
DAVID, R. and BUCHNER, A. (1978). *Am. J. clin. Path.* **69**, 173.
—— and HISS, Y. (1978). *J. Path.* **124**, 111.
HEPTINSTALL, R. H. (1974). *Pathology of the kidney*, 2nd edn, Vol. 2, p. 737. Little and Brown, Boston.
HIGHMAN, B. (1946). *Arch. Path.* **41**, 559.
HOBBS, J. R. and MORGAN, A. D. (1963). *J. Path. Bact.* **86**, 437.
JURGENS, R. (1875). *Virchows Arch. path. Anat.* **65**, 189.
KLATSKIN, G. (1969). *Am. J. Path.* **56**, 1.
LENDRUM, A. C. (1949). *J. Path. Bact.* **61**, 443.
—— and MCFARLANE, D. (1940). *J. Path. Bact.* **50**, 381.
——, SLIDDERS, W., and FRASER, D. S. (1972). *J. clin. Path.* **25**, 373.
——, FRASER, D. S., SLIDDERS, W., and HENDERSON, R. (1962). *J. clin. Path.* **15**, 401.
MCFARLANE, D. (1944). *Stain Technol.* **19**, 29.
MCKINNEY, B. and GRUBB, C. (1965). *Nature (Lond.)* **205**, 1023.
MALLORY, F. B. (1938). *Pathological technique.* W. B. Saunders, Philadelphia.
MARX, A. J., GUEFT, B., and MOSKAL, S. F. (1965), *Arch. Path.* **80**, 487.
MICHAELS, L. and LEVINE, C. (1957). *J. Path. Bact.* **74**, 49.
POMERANCE, A. (1965). *Br. Heart J.* **27**, 711.
PUCHTLER, H., SWEAT, F., and LEVINE, M. (1962). *J. Histochem. Cytochem.* **10**, 355.
REISSENWEBER, N. J. and DECARO, J. (1969). *Virchows Arch. path. Anat.* **347**, 254.
SLIDDERS, W. (1961). *J. med. Lab. Technol.* **18**, 36.
SYMMERS, W. St. C. (1956). *J. clin. Path.* **9**, 187.
VASSAR, P. S. and CULLING, C. F. A. (1959). *Arch. Path.* **68**, 487.
WEIGERT, C. (1887). *Fortschr. Med.* **5**, 228
WOLMAN, M. (1975). *J. Histochem. Cytochem.* **23**, 21.

13 | Carbohydrates and mucosubstances

A large number of compounds that contain carbohydrates are present in tissues. They can be divided into *polysaccharides* and a larger group of mucoid tissue components that are collectively called *mucosubstances*. These can be classified in several different ways; the histologist will describe their location, the histochemist will categorize some of their chemical structure, and the biochemist may be able to determine their complete chemical identity.

Glycogens are the only *polysaccharides* that are widely distributed in animal tissues, and can be preserved in paraffin sections of fixed tissues. Starch and cellulose are polysaccharides that are present in plants. Glycogens are composed of chains of glucose units [FIG. 13.1A] and are labile, being converted

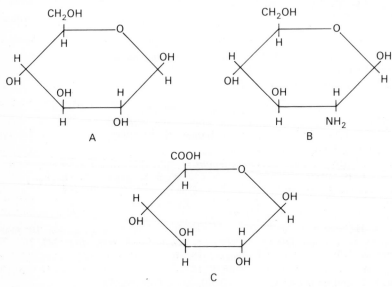

FIG. 13.1. Basic structure of carbohydrates. (A) d-glucose. (B) d-glucosamine. (C) d-glucuronic acid.

into sugar quickly after tissue death; they are soluble in water before fixation. Ever since Best's (1906) carmine method for the demonstration of glycogen it has been believed that glycogens can only be retained in tissue blocks by immediate fixation in absolute alcohol; tissues removed more than an hour or so after death, or fixed in aqueous fixatives, have been thought to contain little or no glycogen. These traditional beliefs are now realized to be exaggerated. Formalin fixes proteins in conjunction with glycogen, rendering it insoluble (Baker 1945) and glycogen is as well preserved in thin blocks of tissue fixed in formalin as it is by fixation in absolute alcohol or picric acid

(Vallance-Owen 1948). The movement of a fixative through the cytoplasm often causes streaming of glycogen towards one side of the cell, and for exact localization of glycogen cryostat sections or freeze-drying should be employed. In addition, whilst it is true that glycogen progressively disappears by glycogenolysis from tissues after death (Murgatroyd 1971) glycogen may persist in human post-mortem material for many hours, especially in some pathological tissues. Histologists should not be deterred from staining formalin-fixed tissues for glycogen, or assume that post-mortem tissues will be free from glycogen; it may well be present if thin slices have been fixed, and surgical specimens, especially small biopsies and curettings, fixed immediately in formalin, may show almost perfect preservation of glycogen. Staining of glycogen can be carried out by the two classical methods—iodine or Best's carmine—though these have been superseded by the periodic acid–Schiff technique in conjunction with diastase control; silver impregnation methods also demonstrate other substances and are not recommended for routine purposes.

The *mucosubstances* are a much larger group of different compounds which are often found as mixtures. They include the 'mucins', an imprecise term that has in the past been used to describe substances in tissues, or secretions from glands, that were slimy, were precipitated with alcohol and acetic acid, and stained with mucicarmine. Mucosubstances include the mucins and are mucoid carbohydrates which can be divided into three main types (Stacey and Barker 1962).

1. Mucopolysaccharides—polysaccharide–protein complexes that are predominantly carbohydrate.
2. Mucoproteins—polysaccharide–protein complexes that are predominantly protein.
3. Mucolipids—polysaccharide–fat compounds.

These three groups contain an enormous number of mucosubstances that are widely distributed throughout connective tissues and epithelia. Spicer, Leppi, and Stoward (1965) has recommended that they should be described by their localization in tissues and also by broad subdivision by histochemical tests for the presence of sialic acid, sulphate, and glycol groups. Connective tissue 'mucins' have now been characterized in detail and are acid mucopolysaccharides; epithelial 'mucins' are less well understood, but are neutral and acid mucoproteins and glycoproteins. The main types of mucosubstances that are found in animal tissues are listed in Table 13.1, together with the location in which they are found.

The *mucopolysaccharides* may be neutral or acid. A neutral mucopolysaccharide contains carbohydrate made up of hexose units, usually acetylated, such as glucosamine [FIG. 13.1B]; chitin is an example, being composed of a glucosamine polysaccharide in combination with protein and calcium. The acid mucopolysaccharides contain carboxylated glucose units (glucuronic acid, FIG. 13.1C); hyaluronic acid is a simple acid mucopolysaccharide composed of chains of glucosamine and glucuronic acid. Complex acid mucopolysaccharides contain, in addition to glucuronic acid, sulphated glucosamine units. Chondroitin sulphuric acid, widely distributed in cartilage and connective tissues, is a complex acid mucopolysaccharide made up of sulphated galactosamine and glucuronic acid; heparin is another example, in this case sulphated glucosamine and glucuronic acid.

Table 13.1 Classification and sites of carbohydrates and mucosubstances

Carbohydrate mucosubstance	Chemical character	Tissue compounds	Tissue locality	
			Epithelium	Connective tissue
POLY-SACCHARIDE	GLUCOSE containing (1:2 glycol)	GLYCOGEN	LIVER	
ACID MUCOPOLY-SACCHARIDE connective tissue 'mucins'	CARBOXY-LATED (COOH)	HYALURONIC ACID		UMBILICAL CORD SKIN
	SULPHATED (COOH and SO₄)	CHONDROITIN SULPHATE A and C		CARTILAGE HEART VALVES
		CHONDROITIN SULPHATE B HEPARIN		AORTA MAST CELLS
	SULPHATED (SO₄)	KERATO-SULPHATE		CARTILAGE INTERVER-TEBRAL DISC
MUCO-PROTEINS and GLYCO-PROTEINS Epithelial 'mucins'	NEUTRAL (1:2 glycol)	GASTRIC MUCIN	STOMACH PROSTATE	
	CARBOXY-LATED (1:2 glycol and COOH)	SIALO-MUCINS	SMALL INTESTINE SALIVARY GLANDS	
	SULPHATED (1:2 glycol and COOH and SO₄)	SULPHATED SIALOMUCINS	COLON	
GLYCOLIPIDS	LIPID containing (1:2 glycol and lipid)	CEREBROSIDE	CENTRAL NERVOUS SYSTEM	

The *mucoproteins*, though predominently protein, are usually considered to contain more than 4 per cent of a hexosamine-containing polysaccharide. When the polysaccharide content is high (over 20 per cent) sialic acid is usually present, and these sialic acid-containing mucins are known as sialomucins. The glycoproteins, which contain less than 4 per cent poly-saccharide, are classified with the mucoproteins and cannot be readily distinguished from them by histological techniques.

The third group, the *mucolipids*, are made up of fatty acids combined with carbohydrate, usually galactose. The cerebrosides are the most important glycolipids, and includes kerasin of Gaucher's disease, which is a glucose cerebroside.

The staining reactions of carbohydrates, polysaccharides, and mucosubstances

A considerable number of different types of reactions are involved in the methods used for the demonstration of carbohydrate-containing compounds.

These techniques include two that are the most important, the periodic acid–Schiff reaction and the basic-dye methods, or combinations of both. The most widely used basic dye is Alcian blue, but metachromatic dyes such as Azur A and thionin are valuable, as is aldehyde fuchsin. Colloidal iron and high iron diamine act in the same way as Alcian blue by combining with acidic groups, and their results tend to be similar. The long-established techniques for glycogen, such as Best's carmine and iodine, and the traditional mucicarmine stain for 'mucins' have been overtaken by the more modern methods but they still give excellent results under certain circumstances and their rationale has become more clearly understood; they are now scientifically more respectable and have not been completely superseded. Silver solutions are reduced by aldehydes produced by the oxidation of glycogen and this method has some similarity to that of the periodic acid–Schiff reaction, which will be described in detail. Less commonly used techniques include fluorescent microscopy using fluorochrome dyes or fluorescent antibodies and auto-radiography of tissues that have been labelled with radioactive sulphur (^{35}S) *in vivo*. The main types of reaction are shown in Table 13.2.

Table 13.2 Types of staining reaction for carbohydrates, polysaccharides and mucosubstances

1. Demonstration of aldehydes by periodic acid oxidation of 1:2 glycols (PAS reaction)

2. Demonstration of acid groups by basic dyes (Alcian blue, aldehyde fuchsin, high iron diamine, colloidal iron)

3. Combinations of 1 and 2 (Alcian blue–PAS, colloidal iron–PAS)

4. Demonstration of acid groups by metachromatic dyes

5. Traditional methods (iodine, Best's carmine, mucicarmine)

6. Reduction of silver solutions (methenamine–silver method)

7. Fluorochrome dye method (acridine orange)

8. Immunofluorescent technique using fluorescent antibodies

9. Autoradiography, using ^{35}SO$_4$ or tritiated sugars

10. Blocking techniques, enzyme methods, pH extinction, critical electrolyte concentration

Many of these techniques can be used in conjunction with blocking methods such as methylation and saponification or with enzyme digestion reactions using diastase or hyaluronidase. In this way specificity may be obtained, but this is not always possible and the characteristics of mucosubstances can be determined in more detail by using staining solutions at different pH levels or in critical electrolyte concentrations.

The periodic acid–Schiff (PAS) reaction is a true histochemical method, and is a development of the Feulgen reaction for the demonstration of deoxyribonucleic acid [p. 160]. In the Feulgen reaction hydrolysis with hydrochloric acid liberates aldehydes and these recolour Schiff's reagent. McManus (1946) described the use of periodic acid in the PAS reaction (in place of the acid hydrolysis of the Feulgen reaction) for the staining of mucins; this oxidizing agent produces the aldehydes that are required for the recoloration of Schiff's reagent but does not hydrolyse nucleic acids. This was further developed by Hotchkiss (1948) into a histochemical technique for polysaccharides, as it acts by breaking the carbon bonds (C−C) of various structures when they are present in the form of adjacent 1:2 glycol groups (CHOH−CHOH), turning them into aldehydes (CHO). This configuration is present in carbohydrates, and the changes are shown in FIGURE 13.2. Many different oxidizing agents have been used, but periodic acid is the most satisfactory as it does not continue to oxidize the aldehydes to carboxyl (COOH) after they have been produced.

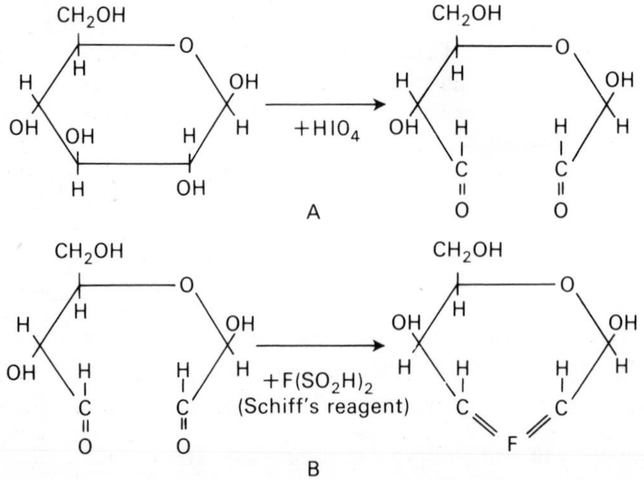

FIG. 13.2. The chemical changes in the periodic acid–Schiff reaction (A) Periodic acid oxidation. (B) Recoloration of Schiff's reagent by aldehyde groups.

Certain derivatives of 1:2 glycol groups (amino-, alkylamino-, and the oxidation product CHOH − CO) are also converted into aldehydes by periodic acid and will give a positive PAS reaction. The aldehydes recolour the colourless Schiff's reagent and the sites of PAS reactive groupings are shown by a red colour. It has already been seen that carbohydrates in tissues may be soluble or unstable, so the PAS reaction as an accurate histochemical technique is dependent upon satisfactory fixation or freshly prepared cryostat sections. With this proviso the method will demonstrate substances that possess the 1:2 glycol group, or its equivalent, if these are present in sufficient quantity to give a final red colour, and if the oxidation product is not diffusible. The PAS reaction is histochemically specific, but since many different components of tissues give a positive reaction it is not diagnostic of any single tissue component or group of substances. To improve the value of the PAS reaction for identification of tissue structures it is used in conjunction with enzymic or chemical controls, blocking techniques, or with additional staining methods. A simple example is the use of diastase control in the identification of glycogen. The PAS reaction will demonstrate the sites of glycogen and many other substances in sections, and by the removal of glycogen from a control section with diastase it is possible to determine the site and approximate quantity of glycogen in the tissue by comparison of the two sections.

Using *basic dyes*, simple acid and complex sulphated mucopolysaccharides give: (1) positive reactions with metachromatic dyes; (2) positive Alcian blue staining; and (3) a positive reaction with Hale's dialysed iron. Sialic acid-containing compounds also give similar staining reactions, and as many mucoproteins and glycoproteins contain sialic acid they will behave in the same way. These three methods depend upon the presence of acidic groups, and the strongly sulphated compounds give the most intense colour reactions. Like the PAS reaction, these three ways of staining carbohydrates are not specific for tissue components; they stain a wide group of compounds, among them the acidic mucins, but in order to identify the type of carbohydrate that is demonstrated blocking techniques and enzyme controls are needed. Methylation will block subsequent staining of carboxylated acid mucopolysaccharides by esterification of carboxyl groups and will block complex sulphated mucopolysaccharides by desulphation. The staining of carboxylated acid mucopolysaccharides can be restored by treatment with potassium hydroxide after methylation (methylation-saponification); sulphated mucopolysaccharides remain blocked. Carboxylated sialomucins, but not sulphated sialomucins, can be identified by loss of staining after sialidase digestion. Hyaluronic acid and chondroitin sulphate A and C are removable from sections by testicular hyaluronidase; streptococcal hyaluronidase only digests hyaluronic acid.

The histological methods for the demonstration of carbohydrates have been shown to fall into two main groups—the PAS reaction and the methods for the acidic polysaccharides. Table 13.3 gives the staining reactions of the main groups of carbohydrate compounds found in tissue sections, and with these methods it is often possible to identify the composition of a carbohydrate with some precision, but it must always be remembered that individual staining methods are not specific, and that carbohydrates are usually present in tissues in mixtures. A carbohydrate that is present in small concentration may, by a strong colour reaction, give a misleading impression of its importance, and may mask other less reactive compounds. Technical methods for carbo-hydrates will now be described, followed by practical notes on the identification of carbohydrate-containing compounds.

METHODS FOR CARBOHYDRATES, POLYSACCHARIDES, AND MUCOSUBSTANCES

The periodic acid–Schiff (PAS) reaction
(after McManus 1946)

The theoretical basis of the PAS reaction has been described in the previous section [p. 235]. Adjacent 1:2 glycol groups (CHOH – CHOH) are broken by periodic acid and converted into aldehydes (two CHO groups); these are demonstrated with Schiff's reagent.

FIXATION

Most fixatives may be used. For labile polysaccharides fixation must be immediate, and thin pieces of tissue are required [p. 232].

SECTIONS

Paraffin, frozen, freeze-dried, or cryostat sections.

Table 13.3 Staining reactions of carbohydrates and mucosubstances

			PAS [p. 237]	Diastase PAS [p. 241]	Alcian blue pH 2.5 [p. 246]	Alcian blue pH 1.0 [p. 247]	Meth. Alcian blue pH 2.5 [p. 254]	Meth./sap. Alcian blue pH 2.5 [p. 254]	Test. hyal. Alcian blue pH 2.5 [p. 256]	Sialidase Alcian blue pH 2.5 [p. 255]	Metachromatic dyes [p. 249]	Hale's colloidal iron [p. 252]	Aldehyde-fuchsin [p. 196]	Sudan black [p. 291]
POLYSACCHARIDE	GLUCOSE containing (1:2 glycol)	GLYCOGEN	+	−	−	−	−	−	−	−	−	−	−	−
	CARBOXYLATED (COOH)	HYALURONIC ACID	−	−	+	−	−	+	−	+	+	+	−	−
ACID MUCOPOLYSACCHARIDES	SULPHATED (COOH and SO₄)	CHONDROITIN SULPHATE A and C	−	−	+	+	−	± or +	−	+	+	+	+	−
		CHONDROITIN SULPHATE B HEPARIN	−	−	+	+	−	± or +	+	+	+	+	+	−
Connective tissue 'mucins'	SULPHATED (SO₄)	KERATOSULPHATE	−	−	+	+	−	± or +	+	+	+	+	+	−
MUCOPROTEINS and GLYCOPROTEINS Epithelial 'mucins'	NEUTRAL (1:2 GLYCOL)	GASTRIC MUCIN	+	+	+	−	−	−	−	−	−	+	−	−
	CARBOXYLATED (1:2 GLYCOL and COOH)	SIALOMUCIN	+	+	+	−	−	+	+	− or +	+	+	−	−
	SULPHATED (1:2 GLYCOL and COOH and SO₄)	SULPHATED SIALOMUCINS	+	+	+	−	−	+	+	+	+	+	+	−
GLYCOLIPIDS	LIPID containing (1:2 GLYCOL and LIPID)	CEREBROSIDE	+	+	−	−	−	−	−	−	−	−	−	+

PREPARATION

Schiff's reagent

Boil 200 cm^3 of distilled water and add 1 g of basic fuchsin. When dissolved, cool and filter. Bubble SO$_2$ gas slowly through the solution from a syphon (see Note 8, below), shaking occasionally, until it becomes a clear transparent red colour. Stand the stoppered flask in a dark cupboard overnight. If the solution is pale straw-coloured or colourless next morning it is ready for use. If some residual red colour remains decolorize with 1 g of activated charcoal; shake and filter. Store in the refrigerator in a dark bottle and discard if a pink colour develops.

Alternatively decolorize with sodium metabisulphite as follows. Dissolve 1 g basic fuchsin and 1.9 g sodium metabisulphite to 100 cm^3 0.15 N hydrochloric acid. Do not heat, but shake at intervals, or agitate with a mechanical shaker for two hours. The solution should be clear and yellow. Add 500 mg activated charcoal and shake for 1–2 minutes. Filter and make up to 100 cm^3 with distilled water. It should now be clear and colourless. Store at 4 °C in the dark.

TECHNIQUE

1. Bring sections to water.
2. Oxidize for five minutes in 1 per cent aqueous periodic acid.
3. Wash in running water for five minutes and rinse in distilled water.
4. Place in Schiff's reagent for 10–20 minutes.
5. Wash for ten minutes in running water.
6. Stain nuclei with Harris' haematoxylin or an iron haematoxylin. Do not use Ehrlich's haematoxylin which will also stain some PAS positive compounds.
7. Dehydrate in alcohol, clear in xylene, and mount in a synthetic resin medium.

RESULTS

PAS positive substances—red or magenta.
Nuclei—blue.

The most important PAS positive carbohydrates in tissues are polysaccharides (glycogen), neutral mucopolysaccharides, mucoproteins, glycoproteins, and glycolipids. Acid mucopolysaccharides are only weakly positive or negative. The PAS reaction can be used to demonstrate many other normal and pathological tissue constituents, the most important of which are:

Amyloid.
Basement membranes.
Cartilage.
Cellulose.
Cerebrosides.
Epithelial mucins.
Fungi.
Hyaline membrane of neonatal lung.
Lipochrome pigments.
Mucoid cells of the anterior lobe of the pituitary.
Pancreatic zymogen granules.
Starch.
Thyroid colloid.

NOTES

1. The method described above is the watery PAS reaction. This gives maximum staining, but may be associated with a little background coloration. The alcoholic PAS reaction (Hotchkiss 1948) uses a buffered alcoholic solution of periodic acid and reducing sulphite rinses.
2. Many oxidizing agents break the $C-C$ bonds, but permanganate, chromic acid, and hydrogen peroxide continue to oxidize the aldehydes to carboxyl groups, giving a weaker PAS reaction.
3. A control section, which has not been treated with periodic acid but is otherwise carried through with the section under investigation, should be negative.
4. For the specific demonstration of glycogen a diastase control should be used [p. 241].
5. Schiff's reagent may vary from batch to batch, and new solutions should be tested with control sections before they are taken into use. It has a limited life, up to three months in the refrigerator, and should be discarded if it becomes pink.
6. Orange G or tartrazine in Cellosolve may be used as cytological counterstains, but usually only a nuclear counterstain, as described, or simple haematoxylin staining is desirable. Omit counterstains if critical observation is necessary.
7. Some batches of basic fuchsin are unsuitable for Schiff's reagent. Satisfactory basic fuchsin for Schiff's reagent is obtainable from many laboratory suppliers. A dye which gives good results should be reserved for the preparation of Schiff's reagent.
8. Syphon SO_2 gas can be obtained from BDH Chemicals Ltd. [p. 503]. A syphon will last for several years.
9. Colourless solutions of ready-made Schiff's reagent can be obtained from laboratory suppliers; these appear to have a similar life to those made up in the laboratory.

METHODS FOR GLYCOGEN

Traditional beliefs about the fixation of glycogen have already been mentioned. It is no longer held necessary to fix in absolute alcohol or picric acid, but it is important to fix immediately, and to use thin slices of tissue. Neutral 10 per cent formal-alcohol was recommended by Lillie (1947), though Vallance-Owen (1948) found that formal-saline could preserve glycogen without loss. After both these fixatives glycogen is insoluble and is not lost in subsequent washing or staining in aqueous solutions. One of the difficulties associated with the fixation of glycogen is its tendency to stream through the cell with the fixative towards one pole (polarization). Lison and Vokaer (1949) claim to have overcome this with cold acetic acid–formalin in 95 per cent alcohol saturated with picric acid. In practice, it is most important to fix immediately, and whilst aqueous fixatives may be satisfactory, formal/alcohol or 10 per cent formalin in saturated alcoholic picric acid at 4 °C are recommended.

Most laboratories now use the PAS reaction in conjunction with a diastase control for the demonstration of glycogen. This has the disadvantage that other tissue components are also demonstrated, and the glycogen can only be assessed by its disappearance from the control section. For this reason there still remains a place for the older empirical Best's carmine method; the iodine technique is now mainly of historical interest.

PAS reaction for glycogen with diastase control

Glycogen is removed from sections by diastase, which is present in saliva. Malt diastase, available commercially, is reliable; but it is advisable to use a known positive control section in addition to the one under test. Glycogen is the only important PAS positive tissue component that is removed by diastase, so that for practical purposes diastase digestion converts the PAS reaction into a specific test for glycogen.

FIXATION

See above.

SECTIONS

Paraffin and other sections. It is not necessary to cover sections with a thin layer of celloidin [p. 242], but if this is done to preserve small quantities of glycogen diastase digestion must be completed first. Celloidin may prevent the complete removal of glycogen from the section by diastase.

TECHNIQUE

Two sections are required. *One* is treated as follows:

1. Bring to water.
2. Treat with 0.1 per cent malt diastase in distilled water, freshly prepared, for 30 minutes at 37 °C. Human saliva may be used in place of diastase.
3. Wash in running water for five minutes.

For exact comparison, the *other* section is left in distilled water for a similar time in place of step 2; *both* sections are then stained by the PAS reaction [p. 237].

RESULTS

PAS positive material that is present in the untreated section and absent in the digested section may be assumed to be glycogen.

NOTE

Human saliva can be used in place of diastase, but diastase is recommended and is essential for large numbers of sections.

Best's carmine method for glycogen (Best 1906)

The mechanism of staining of Best's carmine has been studied by Murgatroyd (1970). Hydrogen bonding of the dye appears to take place with OH groups on glycogen and can be blocked by urea, which is a powerful hydrogen bonding agent which competes for hydrogen bonding sites on the tissue.

FIXATION

See above [p. 240].

SECTIONS

Paraffin sections are suitable, but should be covered with a thin layer of celloidin to prevent loss of slides due to the ammoniacal staining solutions and to preserve small quantities of glycogen.

PREPARATION

1. Best's carmine.

Stock solution

Carmine	2 g
Potassium carbonate	1 g
Potassium chloride	5 g
Distilled water	60 cm³

Carefully boil for five minutes. This should be done in a large flask on account of the marked frothing. Cool and add 20 cm³ of concentrated ammonia. Keep in a dark bottle at 4 °C.

Working solution

Best's carmine (stock solution)	2 parts
Ammonia (conc)	2 parts
Absolute methyl alcohol	3 parts

2. Best's differentiator.

Absolute methyl alcohol	40 cm³
Absolute ethyl alcohol	80 cm³
Distilled water	100 cm³

CELLOIDINIZATION OF SLIDES

1. Remove wax from mounted paraffin sections with xylene and take to absolute alcohol.
2. Place sections in 1 per cent celloidin in equal parts of absolute ethyl alcohol and ether for five minutes.
3. Wipe the back of the slide and, without allowing the celloidin to dry, transfer the slide to 80 per cent ethyl alcohol for five minutes.

TECHNIQUE

1. Rinse celloidinized slides very briefly in water.
2. Stain with alum haematoxylin and differentiate in acid alcohol. Blueing in tap water is unnecessary as the ammoniacal stain will do this. Quickly rinse in water.
3. Stain in the working solution of Best's carmine in a small closed jar for 10–20 minutes.
4. Differentiate in Best's differentiating fluid for 1–5 minutes.
5. When the stain stops diffusing from the section transfer to absolute alcohol. The celloidin film will slowly dissolve (this is faster in a mixture of equal parts of absolute alcohol and ether).
6. Clear in xylene.
7. Mount in a synthetic resin medium.

RESULTS

Glycogen—bright red granules.
Nuclei—blue.

NOTES

1. Sometimes staining is improved by altering the amounts of ammonia and/or methyl alcohol. Occasionally it has been found advantageous to use the undiluted stock solution.

2. The stock solution keeps for some months at 4 °C. The efficacy of the stock solution should be tested on known positive material. Rabbit liver (that has been fed on carrots for two or three days) is suitable, and early secretory endometrial curettings can also be used.
3. Diastase control for specificity is described on page 241. This must be carried out before celloidinization of the section on the slide as celloidin may prevent the complete removal of glycogen by diastase.
4. The celloidin film may become insoluble after Best's carmine and it may be impossible to remove the film completely. The section is examined through the lightly stained film.

The Langhans iodine method for glycogen (modified from Langhans 1890)

This was used by Claude Bernard (1877) and Ehrlich (1883) in their classical researches on the liver. The difficulty is to produce permanent preparations, but the following method may give good results. Iodine is not specific for glycogen; it stains, among other compounds, amyloid [p. 221]. Diastase control may be used to ensure specificity.

FIXATION

See above [p. 240].

SECTIONS

Paraffin sections can be used.

TECHNIQUE

1. Bring sections to water, but wash only briefly in water.
2. Stain sections in Lugol's iodine (iodine 1 g, potassium iodide 2 g, distilled water 100 cm³) for ten minutes. Pour off and blot dry.
3. Dehydrate in a saturated solution of iodine in absolute alcohol. This also improves the staining. Blot dry.
4. Clear rapidly in origanum oil.
5. Mount in origanum oil and ring the coverslip. Or mount in origanum oil balsam.

RESULTS

Glycogen—mahogany brown.
Tissue constituents—yellow.

NOTES

1. It is possible to stain nuclei with Ehrlich's haematoxylin after stage 1.
2. The origanum oil decolorizes the tissues, leaving glycogen stained brown. After some months the preparation tends to fade.

Methenamine (hexamine) silver method for glycogen (Gomori 1946; Grocott 1955)

The blackening of glycogen by this technique is due to the reduction of the silver solution by aldehydes produced by oxidation of the glycogen by chromic acid. It is not specific, as it stains some mucosubstances (Cook 1972), but can be used with diastase control [p. 241]. In addition to glycogen, this method blackens some mucins, melanin, and fungi. Details of the technique are given on page 270.

METHODS FOR MUCOSUBSTANCES (MUCINS)

It has already been seen [p. 233] that mucins are mucopolysaccharides or mucoproteins with differing degrees of acidification, whose staining reactions are shown in TABLE 13.3 [p. 238]. General staining methods for mucins, including the PAS reaction and the mucicarmine technique, will first be given. Connective tissue mucins and some epithelial mucins can only be demonstrated satisfactorily by techniques for acid mucopolysaccharides, and these will be described in a subsequent section. There is often considerable overlap in the results of the staining methods for mucins, due to the fact that mucins commonly occur as mixtures of mucopolysaccharides and mucoproteins which are stained by a number of techniques with variable specificity.

In practice epithelial mucins can be stained by Alcian blue and/or the PAS reaction, and TABLE 13.3 shows that together these two techniques will demonstrate all mucopolysaccharides and mucoproteins. Connective tissue mucins are best demonstrated by Alcian blue, colloidal iron, aldehyde fuchsin, or metachromatic dyes.

GENERAL STAINING METHODS FOR MUCINS

The adaptation of the PAS reaction as a method for mucin has become widely used, but it must be remembered that whilst neutral mucopolysaccharides and mucoproteins are well stained, acid mucopolysaccharides are usually PAS negative. The PAS reaction should be used for mucins in parallel with other methods such as the Alcian blue technique; results should be interpreted with caution as it is non-specific and stains many tissue components. The classical mucicarmine stain for mucin will be described as this still gives good results with some of the epithelial and connective tissue mucins.

The PAS reaction for mucin

Glycogen must be removed from the section by diastase digestion. Proceed as described on page 241. Mucins are some of the commonest tissue components that remain positive after diastase digestion, but the results must be interpreted critically.

Southgate's mucicarmine method (modified from Mayer 1896)

Despite its great age, this method is not completely understood. The aluminium/carmine compound appears to be positively charged and combines with the negatively charged acid mucosubstances. Goldstein (1962) has also suggested that its large molecular size is able to penetrate and combine with low-density acidic compounds. Neutral mucopolysaccharides and strongly-acidic sulphated mucins are negative or weakly staining, carboxylated or weakly acidic compounds give positive results.

FIXATION

Formal-saline or most other fixatives.

SECTIONS

Paraffin sections.

PREPARATION

Place 1 g of powdered carmine and 1 g of dry aluminium hydroxide in a 500 cm³ flask. Add 100 cm³ of 50 per cent alcohol, then 0.5 g of anhydrous aluminium chloride whilst shaking. Place on boiling water-bath and boil for 2½ minutes. Cool and filter. Store at 4 °C.

TECHNIQUE

1. Bring sections to water.
2. Stain nuclei with haematoxylin (avoid Ehrlich's); differentiate in acid-alcohol and blue in tap water.
3. Stain for 30–45 minutes in the staining solution.
4. Rinse in distilled water.
5. Dehydrate in alcohol, clear in xylene, and mount in a synthetic resin medium.

RESULTS

Mucins—red.
Nuclei—blue.

NOTES

1. The chief difficulty is the preparation of an avid staining solution. This seems to depend upon the carmine, and some batches give very poor results. Cheap, impure, commercial carmine may be satisfactory. The staining solution keeps fairly well, and once a good specimen has been prepared it should be used sparingly as it may not be easy to repeat the preparation. Satisfactory carmine should be reserved for mucicarmine. It is possible to buy mucicarmine commercially, but these staining solutions do not usually give such good results as one that has been successfully prepared in the laboratory.
2. Southgate's mucicarmine may be improved if the stain is diluted with distilled water.
3. Mucicarmine may demonstrate cryptococci (*Cryptococcus neoformans*) better than any other method.

METHODS FOR ACID MUCOPOLYSACCHARIDES AND MUCOPROTEINS

Acid mucopolysaccharides are a large group of mucosubstances that are not PAS positive, and the sialomucins and sulphated sialomucins may not always be positive despite the fact that they contain 1:2 glycol groups and are theoretically positive. Thus the PAS reaction has limitations for the demonstration of mucosubstances. Acid mucopolysaccharides and acid mucoproteins are well stained by Alcian blue, Hale's colloidal iron, and metachromatic dyes. The complex sulphated mucoproteins (sulphated sialomucins) can also be demonstrated with aldehyde–fuchsin. Acridine orange can be used as a fluorochrome dye for acid mucopolysaccharides. Additional information about the nature of mucosubstances is obtained by using some of these methods at different pH levels or by carefully controlled critical electrolyte concentration. Methylation will destroy the staining reactions of carboxylated and sulphated compounds, but subsequent saponification will restore that of carboxylated mucopolysaccharides. Sialic acid-containing compounds stain with Alcian blue, colloidal iron, and metachromatic dyes. It might be anticipated that sialidase digestion would categorize the sialic acid compounds, but this is not invariable as there are some sialic acids which are completely resistant. Connective tissue acid mucopolysaccharides and epithelial mucoproteins can be demonstrated by many of these methods but the neutral mucosubstances may only stain with the PAS reaction.

The effects of fixation on the subsequent demonstration of acid mucopolysaccharides by these staining methods has been investigated by Allison (1973) who found that 10 per cent neutral formal-saline performed better than other fixative solutions. The techniques will now be described, together with modifications of the basic methods such as pH control or critical electrolyte concentration, which make the results more precise.

THE ALCIAN BLUE METHODS

Alcian blue is a copper phthalocyanin basic dye, and at low pH will stain acid (including sulphated) mucosubstances by salt linkage with acid groups in the tissue. It is almost specific, insoluble, and permanent.

The usual method is with a staining solution at pH 2.5, but if used at pH 1.0 it will distinguish between acid and sulphated mucoproteins (Lev and Spicer 1964) as carboxyl groups are not ionized and will not stain. The critical electrolyte concentration of an electrolyte, such as magnesium, can prevent staining by Alcian blue and may also be used to distinguish the main types of Alcian blue-positive mucosubstances. Alcian blue staining methods combined with other techniques will also be briefly described.

The Alcian blue method (pH 2.5) for acid mucosubstances (Steedman 1950; Lison 1954)

FIXATION

Formalin is recommended (Allison 1973).

SECTIONS

Paraffin sections; other sections can be used.

PREPARATION

Alcian blue	0.5 g
Glacial acetic acid	3 cm^3
Distilled water to	100 cm^3

This gives a staining solution of pH 2.5.

TECHNIQUE

1. Take sections to water.
2. Stain in Alcian blue solution for 10–30 minutes.
3. Rinse in distilled water and wash in running water for five minutes.
4. Counterstain (see Note 1, below).
5. Dehydrate in alcohol, clear in xylene, and mount in a synthetic resin medium.

RESULTS

Acid mucopolysaccharides—blue.
Nuclei—red.

NOTES

1. Lison (1954) recommended counterstaining with 0.5 per cent aqueous

chlorantine fast red 5B for 15 minutes, after mordanting with 1 per cent aqueous phosphomolybdic acid for ten minutes. This gave good coloration of collagen fibres, and satisfactory colour contrast with connective tissue mucins. Alternatively, counterstaining may be carried out with 1 per cent aqueous neutral red.

2. Alcian blue staining can be carried out after blocking techniques and enzyme controls in order to distinguish between simple acid mucopolysaccharides, complex sulphated mucopolysaccharides, and sialic acid-containing compounds. These methods are described on page 254.

3. Alcian green 2GX may be used in place of Alcian blue. The following method (Putt and Hukill 1962) gives good results.

   1. Bring sections to water.
   2. Stain in 1 per cent Alcian green in 2 per cent acetic acid for 5–10 minutes.
   3. Rinse in distilled water.
   4. Stain in 0.1 per cent nuclear fast red in 5 per cent aluminium sulphate for 5–10 minutes.
   5. Rinse in distilled water.
   6. Stain in 0.25 per cent aqueous metanil yellow, to which two drops of glacial acetic acid per 100 cm³ have been added, for 30–60 seconds.
   7. Dehydrate in alcohol, clear in xylene, and mount in a synthetic resin medium.

   RESULTS

   Acid mucopolysaccharides—green.
   Cell nuclei—red.
   Background—yellow.

Alcian blue method (pH 1.0) for sulphated mucosubstances (Lev and Spicer 1964)

At pH 1.0 carboxylated mucopolysaccharides and mucoproteins will not stain with Alcian blue but strongly sulphated compounds continue to do so. N/10 hydrochloric acid gives a pH of 1.0.

PREPARATION

Alcian blue 1.0 g in 100 cm³ 0.1 N hydrochloric acid.

TECHNIQUE

1. Bring sections to water.
2. Stain in the Alcian blue solution for 10–30 minutes.
3. Briefly rinse in 0.1 N hydrochloric acid.
4. Blot dry and dehydrate in alcohol.
5. Clear in xylene and mount in a synthetic resin medium.

RESULTS

Sulphated mucopolysaccharides and mucoproteins—blue.

Alcian blue method using critical electrolyte concentration

It is believed that electrolytes like magnesium chloride can compete with Alcian blue for tissue anions if the electrolyte is present in a sufficient quantity above a critical level of concentration. Increasing the concentration of magnesium chloride has the same effect as lowering the pH of an Alcian blue-staining solution; if the magnesium is present in high molarity only the most strongly sulphated mucopolysaccharides will stain. Scott and Dorling (1965) recommend staining in buffered Alcian blue solution containing increasing concentrations of magnesium chloride.

PREPARATION

Make a fresh solution of

Alcian blue	0.2 g
M/5 acetate buffer pH 5.8	400 cm³

Make four staining solutions with increasing molarities of magnesium chloride by adding the required quantity of $MgCl_2$ $6H_2O$ to 100 cm³ of the Alcian blue solution (Table 13.4).

Table 13.4 Critical electrolyte concentrations (CEC) of mucopolysaccharides with appropriate staining solutions of magnesium chloride (after Dorling 1969)

	Mucopolysaccharide	CEC (M)	Staining solution	
			M	$MgCl_2$ $6H_2O$
1	Hyaluronic acid	0.05	0.04	0.8 g/100 cm³
2	Chondroitin sulphate	0.45	0.3	6.1 g/100 cm³
3	Heparin	0.65	0.5	10.1 g/100 cm³
4	Keratan sulphate	1.0	0.9	18.3 g/100 cm³

TECHNIQUE

1. Bring four sections to water.
2. Stain one section in each of the four Alcian blue solutions containing 0.04 M, 0.3 M, 0.5 M, and 0.9 M magnesium chloride.
3. Wash in water and counterstain with 0.5 per cent aqueous neutral red.
4. Dehydrate quickly in alcohol, clear in xylene, and mount in a synthetic resin medium.

RESULTS

See Table 13.4.
Only keratan sulphate will stain blue in solution 4.
Only keratan sulphate and heparin will stain blue in solution 3.
Chondroitin sulphate, heparin and keratan sulphate will stain blue in solution 2.
Hyaluronic acid and all others will stain blue in solution 1.
Nuclei—red.

NOTES

1. There may be background staining in the low molarity solution.
2. Keep magnesium chloride dry as it is deliquescent.

COMBINED ALCIAN BLUE METHODS

The combined Alcian blue–PAS reaction (Mowry 1956)

This can be used for the demonstration of all mucosubstances and it distinguishes neutral and acid compounds. The section is first stained with

Alcian blue and Alcian blue-positive acid mucosubstances that are also PAS positive will not react with PAS. Only neutral compounds will be PAS positive. When mixtures are present there will be a combination of the blue and red colours.

TECHNIQUE

1. Bring sections to water and stain with Alcian blue at pH 2.5 [p. 246].
2. Wash in water and then wash again in distilled water.
3. Carry out the PAS reaction [p. 237].
4. Dehydrate, clear, and mount.

RESULTS

Acid mucosubstances—blue.
Neutral mucosubstances—magenta red.
Mixtures of both will produce a mixed colour depending upon the predominant type.

NOTES

1. Haematoxylin counterstaining should be light or may be omitted as it may resemble Alcian blue staining.
2. The effect of decalcification on the subsequent staining of acid mucopolysaccharides by combined Alcian blue–PAS and other methods has been investigated by Charman and Reid (1972), who found that satisfactory staining was obtained after EDTA or formic acid.

Combined Alcian blue–Alcian yellow technique for differentiating acid mucosubstances (Ravetto 1964)

This method uses Alcian blue at low pH (0.5) to stain sulphated compounds and Alcian yellow at pH 2.5 to stain carboxylated mucosubstances.

PREPARATION

1. 1 g Alcian blue 8 GX in 100 cm^3 of N/5 hydrochloric acid.
2. 1 g Alcian yellow in 100 cm^3 of 3 per cent acetic acid.

TECHNIQUE

1. Bring sections to water and rinse in N/5 hydrochloric acid.
2. Stain in Alcian blue solution for five minutes.
3. Rinse in N/5 HCl and wash in water.
4. Stain in Alcian yellow solution for five minutes.
5. Wash in water.
6. Counterstain in 0.5 per cent neutral red.
7. Wash in water, dehydrate in alcohol, clear in xylene, and mount in a synthetic resin medium.

RESULTS

Sulphated mucosubstances—blue.
Carboxylated mucosubstances—yellow.
Mixtures of the two—shades of green.
Nuclei—red.

METACHROMATIC STAINING METHODS

Acid mucosubstances can be demonstrated by a number of metachromatic dyes. Carboxylated and sulphated compounds are metachromatic, neutral mucins are orthochromatic. The techniques stain epithelial and connective tissue mucins but in practice the metachromatic dyes have been used mainly for connective tissue acid mucopolysaccharides. It is possible to distinguish between the carboxylated and sulphated types by varying the pH of the staining solution. At pH 2 sulphated mucins are metachromatic whilst at pH 5 the carboxylated compounds are metachromatic but the results with Alcian blue using controlled pH are usually easier to interpret than are those with metachromatic dyes. The techniques are quick and simple, but suffer from the disadvantages that metachromasia may be variable and is usually not alcohol-fast, making permanent preparations difficult to prepare. The uranyl nitrate–Azur A method of Hughesdon (1949) gives excellent results with connective tissue mucins and is alcohol-fast, allowing permanent preparations to be made without difficulty.

Uranyl nitrate metachromatic method (Hughesdon 1949)

FIXATION

Formalin; other fixatives can be used.

SECTIONS

Paraffin sections.

TECHNIQUE

1. Take sections to water.
2. Oxidize with 1 per cent aqueous potassium permanganate for five minutes; rinse in tap water.
3. Treat with 5 per cent aqueous oxalic acid until colourless; wash well in running tap water.
4. Stain for five minutes in 0.2 per cent aqueous Azur A; rinse in tap water.
5. Rinse in 0.2 per cent aqueous uranyl nitrate for ten seconds or longer until sufficient dye is extracted to give a good colour contrast. Rinse in tap water.
6. Blot and complete dehydration with absolute alcohol, clear in xylene, and mount in a synthetic resin medium.

RESULTS

Acid mucopolysaccharides and mucoproteins—red or purple.
Other tissue components—blue.

NOTES

1. When staining young connective tissue the initial oxidation with potassium permanganate should not exceed one minute. For epithelial mucins a full five minutes in the permanganate solution is an advantage.
2. If, after short initial oxidation, staining is weak the section can be destained in acid–alcohol and the whole sequence repeated with further oxidation. The section must not be returned to stage 4, as uranyl nitrate–dye–uranyl nitrate gives a diffuse metachromatic stain, especially of collagen.
3. Mast cell granules are well stained.

Toluidine blue method (Vassar and Culling 1959)

FIXATION

Formalin and other fixatives.

SECTIONS

Paraffin or frozen sections.

PREPARATION

The metachromasia of toluidine blue is variable and it is important to select and retain a suitable sample of dye. For permanent preparations Vassar and Culling (1959) used a 0.25 per cent solution of toluidine blue made up in Michaelis' veronal acetate–hydrochloric acid buffer solution at pH 4.5 [p. 499].

TECHNIQUE

1. Bring sections to water.
2. Stain in toluidine blue solution for 10 seconds.
3. Rinse in distilled water.
4. Examine in watery mount, or mount in glycerin jelly; *or* blot with hard filter paper, allow to dry, and clear in xylene. If the section does not clear completely blot again and wash with fresh xylene from a dropping bottle. Mount in a synthetic resin medium.

RESULTS

Metachromatic substances—red, pink, or purple.
Nuclei and other components—blue.

NOTE

All metachromatic staining reactions are modified by the colour of the light by which the stained section is examined. During staining the differentiation may be checked by the staining microscope using daylight. Daylight is desirable for examination of the final preparation, though this may be impossible with microscopes with built-in artificial illumination. The colour value of the light of these systems is very variable, and they may have blue filters; the colour value of the light should be adjusted to approximate to daylight and for comparative work the same quantity and quality of light should always be used when examining metachromatic preparations.

Schmorl's thionin method

FIXATION

Formalin and other fixatives.

SECTIONS

Paraffin or frozen sections.

PREPARATION

Prepare a hot aqueous saturated solution of thionin and allow to cool. A working solution is made of two drops of this stock solution added to 5 cm^3 distilled water.

TECHNIQUE

1. Bring sections to water.
2. Treat with saturated aqueous mercuric chloride, 30 seconds.
3. Wash briefly in water.
4. Stain in the diluted thionin solution for 5–15 minutes.

5. Wash in distilled water.
6. Mount in glycerol jelly.

RESULTS

Metachromatic substances—red.
Nuclei—blue.

OTHER STAINING METHODS

Other techniques that may be used for acid mucosubstances include Hale's colloidal iron, aldehyde-fuchsin, and the fluorescent acridine orange method.

Hale's colloidal iron method (Hale 1946)

This technique depends upon the interaction of colloidal iron with acidic groups at low pH. The iron forms a chelate with the acidic groups of carboxylated and sulphated acid mucopolysaccharides and mucoproteins; this is demonstrated by the Prussian blue reaction (Perls' method, page 264).

The technique stains the same types of mucosubstances as Alcian blue and the metachromatic dyes. Although it takes longer, it may give stronger coloration than these methods but non-specific linkages between protein and iron may take place, giving false positive staining reactions.

FIXATION

Formalin or other fixatives.

SECTIONS

Paraffin sections or fresh frozen sections. Sections should be mounted without adhesive.

PREPARATION

Dialysed iron solution.
Dialysed iron   1 vol.
2 M acetic acid   1 vol.

The colloidal iron reagent may be made according to the method of Rinehart and Abul-Haj (1951), but this requires three days' dialysis against regularly changed distilled water and most histological laboratories will prefer to buy a commercial preparation of dialysed iron (British Drug Houses, Ltd., page 503).

TECHNIQUE

1. Bring sections to water.
2. Flood with the dialysed iron solution for ten minutes.
3. Wash well with several changes of distilled water.
4. Flood with equal parts of 2 per cent aqueous potassium ferrocyanide and 2 per cent hydrochloric acid, made up in distilled water. Leave for ten minutes.
5. Rinse in distilled water and wash in running water.
6. Counterstain lightly with neutral red.
7. Wash in water, and dehydrate rapidly in alcohol.
8. Clear in xylene and mount in a synthetic resin medium.

RESULTS

Acidic mucosubstances—blue.

Nuclei—red.

NOTE

A false positive result due to the presence of haemosiderin in the tissue should be excluded by using a duplicate section as a control by staining with the Prussian blue reaction (steps 4–8 only).

Aldehyde–fuchsin method (Gomori 1950)

Paraldehyde and basic fuchsin, when combined in strongly acid solution, have an affinity for certain mucins, mast cell granules, etc. This is dependent upon the presence of sulphate groups, and staining is lost by previous methylation and is not restored by saponification. Substances which react in this way, and are Alcian blue-positive, can be regarded to be complex sulphated mucopoly-saccharides. The mode of action is not completely understood, but Abul-Haj and Rinehart (1952) have suggested a similarity to the PAS reaction in which Schiff's reagent, which is basic fuchsin + sulphur, becomes coloured by aldehydes (basic fuchsin + sulphur + aldehyde = coloured compound). With aldehyde–fuchsin the combination with sulphate groups forms a colour reaction (aldehyde + fuchsin + sulphur = coloured compound).

The method is a simple automatic technique and is described on page 196. It can also be used with subsequent Alcian blue staining as the combined aldehyde fuchsin–Alcian blue method of Spicer and Meyer (1960) to demonstrate sulphated and carboxylated mucosubstances.

The fluorescent acridine orange technique (Hicks and Matthaei 1958)

It was discovered accidentally that mucin in a section stained with iron haematoxylin and acridine orange gave a selective brilliant orange fluorescence. The iron in the haematoxylin quenched other fluorescence in the tissue, leaving mucin—shown to be acid mucopolysaccharides—unaffected. Iron alum can be used to convert acridine orange into a useful fluorescent stain for acid mucopolysaccharides.

FIXATION

Formalin or other fixatives. Avoid heavy metals.

SECTIONS

Frozen or paraffin sections.

TECHNIQUE

1. Bring sections to water.
2. Place in 4 per cent aqueous iron alum for 5–10 minutes.
3. Wash briefly in running tap water.
4. Stain in 0.1 per cent aqueous acridine orange for $1\frac{1}{2}$ minutes.
5. Wash briefly and mount in glycerol.
6. Examine immediately with a fluorescence microscope [see page 22].

RESULTS

Acid mucosubstances fluoresce reddish orange.

Fungi also fluoresce green–red.
Background—dark green or black.

BLOCKING TECHNIQUES AND ENZYME CONTROLS

It has already been shown that the methods for mucopolysaccharides and mucoproteins are not specific. It is sometimes possible to improve specificity by removing a particular tissue component by enzyme action or by blocking its staining reaction by chemical methods; sections treated in these ways are stained back-to-back with untreated sections and the results compared. The loss of positive staining after enzyme treatment can be taken as reliable evidence of the presence of the substance attacked by that enzyme, and blocking techniques, though less precise, will enable a carbohydrate-containing compound to be classified with more exactness.

Methylation

For blocking the staining reactions of carboxylated mucosubstances by esterification of carboxyl groups and for blocking sulphated compounds by desulphation. This is carried out with hydrochloric acid in methyl alcohol at 37 °C (mild methylation) or at 60 °C (active methylation). Mild methylation will block the subsequent staining of carboxylated mucosubstances and also some connective tissue sulphated acid mucopolysaccharides.

TECHNIQUE

1. Bring sections to water.
2. Methylate in preheated 1 per cent hydrochloric acid in methanol, *either* for four hours at 37 °C (mild methylation) *or* for five hours at 60 °C (active methylation).
   In either case a control section should be treated with distilled water at the same temperature for the same time.
3. Rinse in alcohol and stain both sections with Alcian blue at pH 2.5 [p. 246].
4. Dehydrate, clear, and mount.

RESULTS

After methylation at 37 °C carboxylated mucosubstances unstained, sulphated mucosubstances—blue.
After methylation at 60 °C Alcian blue staining of carboxylated and sulphated mucosubstances is lost.

Methylation and saponification

After methylation, saponification with potassium hydroxide in ethyl alcohol will restore the staining of carboxyl groups, but will leave sulphate groups still blocked. There is a risk of loss of sections in the potassium hydroxide of the saponification reagent; sections should be mounted on the slides with adhesive [p. 92] or covered with a thin layer of celloidin [p. 242].

TECHNIQUE

1. Methylate two sections with 0.85 per cent hydrochloric acid in methyl alcohol by the active methylation technique at 60 °C (see above).
2. Wash in water.

3. Saponify one section with N/10 potassium hydroxide in 70 per cent ethyl alcohol (0.5 g KOH in 100 cm³) for 30 minutes at room temperature. The other section should be placed in 70 per cent ethyl alcohol at the same temperature for the same time.
4. Wash and stain with Alcian blue at pH 2.5 [p. 246].
5. Dehydrate, clear, and mount.

RESULTS

In the methylated and saponified section carboxylated mucosubstances will stain blue; in the methylated section without saponification carboxylated and sulphated mucosubstances will be blocked.

NOTE

A duplicate control section without methylation or saponification should also be stained with Alcian blue.

Diastase digestion of glycogen

This enzyme control method converts the PAS reaction and other methods for glycogen into techniques that are specific. It is described on page 241.

Sialidase digestion of sialic acid
(Spicer, Neubecker, Warren, and Henson 1962)

Sialidase (neuraminidase) is an enzyme obtained from *Vibrio cholerae* organisms. It splits the sialic acid from sialomucins converting Alcian blue-positive mucoproteins into Alcian blue-negative and PAS positive compounds. It is not specific, as there are sialidase resistant sialomucins; these can be made sialidase labile by prior deacetylation with alkaline aqueous alcohol (conc. ammonia 20 cm³, ethyl alcohol 70 cm³, distilled water 10 cm³) for 24 hours at 37 °C (Ravetto 1968). Alternatively, Lamb and Reid (1969) have described a quicker and cheaper method of hydrolysing both sialidase labile and sialidase resistant sialomucins with N/10 sulphuric acid.

PREPARATION

Dilute *V. cholerae* sialidase (Koch-Light Laboratories Ltd., page 503) to 100 units/cm³ in M/5 acetate buffer pH 5.5 to which 1 per cent calcium chloride has been added.

TECHNIQUE

1. Use positive control sections as well as the sections under investigation.
2. Bring to water and rinse in buffer solution.
3. Treat positive control and test sections with the sialidase solution overnight (16 hours or more) at 37 °C. Treat duplicate sections with buffer solution for the same time and at the same temperature.
4. Wash all sections in running water.
5. Stain all sections with Alcian blue at pH 2.5 [p. 246].
6. Dehydrate, clear, and mount.

RESULTS

Enzyme treated tissues that show loss of staining in comparison with the untreated controls contain sialidase-labile sialomucins.

NOTE

The enzyme is expensive and in order to reduce cost a small amount of sialidase solution is placed over the tissue on the slide in a closed Petri dish containing damp cotton wool.

Sulphuric acid hydrolysis method for sialomucins (Lamb and Reid 1969)

TECHNIQUE

1. Use positive control sections and use blank untreated control sections as well as the test sections. Cover sections with a thin film of celloidin.
2. Teat positive control and test sections with N/10 sulphuric acid at 60 °C for 2–4 hours. Duplicate sections are treated with distilled water.
3. Wash in running water and remove celloidin with equal parts of ethyl alcohol and ether.
4. Stain with Alcian blue at pH 5.5 [p. 246].
5. Dehydrate, clear, and mount.

RESULTS

Sialidase-labile and sialidase-resistant sialomucins will lose their Alcian blue-positive staining in comparison with the controls.

Testicular hyaluronidase digestion method for acid mucopolysaccharides

Hyaluronidase can be used for the removal of hyaluronic acid and chondroitin sulphate from sections. Testicular hyaluronidase will digest hyaluronic acid and chondroitin sulphates A and C. Streptococcal hyaluronidase is only active with hyaluronic acid (Zugibe 1962).

TECHNIQUE

1. Use a test section, a duplicate control section, and known positive control sections such as umbilical cord.
2. Take all sections to water.
3. Treat test and positive control sections with 10 mg bovine testicular hyaluronidase (Sigma Chemical Company) in 10 ml phosphate buffer at pH 6.7 for three hours at 37 °C. Place the negative control sections in buffer solution at the same temperature for the same time.
4. Wash in water and stain with Alcian blue at pH 2.5 [p. 246].
5. Dehydrate, clear, and mount.

RESULTS

Hyaluronic acid, chondroitin sulphates A and C, unstained and identified by comparison with the negative control section.

NOTES

1. It may be possible to distinguish between hyaluronic acid and chondroitin sulphates A and C by treating with streptococcal hyaluronidase (1500 units/100 cm³) in acetate buffer at pH 5.0 for 24 hours at 37 °C.
2. Hyaluronidase is of value in the diagnosis of pleural mesotheliomas. Wagner, Munday, and Harington (1962) showed that hyaluronic acid was produced by diffuse pleural mesotheliomas and that this was preserved in tissues fixed in formal-sublimate, alcohol, or acetic acid or their mixtures (not formal-saline).

IDENTIFICATION OF CARBOHYDRATE MUCOSUBSTANCES

The PAS reaction and Alcian blue staining, either separately or as the combined Alcian blue–PAS reaction, will give a considerable amount of information. Only *glycogen*, *neutral mucopolysaccharides*, and *glycolipids* will be PAS positive and Alcian blue (pH 2.5) negative. Glycogen is digested by diastase and glycolipids will be stained by Sudan black, leaving neutral mucopolysaccharides identified by exclusion and by their localization in the tissue.

Table 13.5 Identification of carbohydrates and mucosubstances by PAS reaction and Alcian blue (pH 2.5) staining

	PAS reaction	Alcian blue pH 2.5	Identify by
Glycogen	+	−	diastase
Neutral mucopolysaccharides	+	−	exclusion
Acid mucopolysaccharides	−	+	see below
Carboxylated sialomucins	+ or ±	+	see below
Sulphated sialomucins	+ or ±	+	see below
Glycolipids	+	−	Sudan black

The next problem is the separation of the Alcian blue-positive mucosubstances. Carboxylated acid mucopolysaccharides, such as *hyaluronic acid*, lose their capacity to stain with Alcian blue after treatment with testicular and streptococcal hyaluronidase and they do not stain with Alcian blue at pH 1.0. *Chondroitin sulphates A and C* will be negative after testicular hyaluronidase, but will be unaffected by streptococcal hyaluronidase. Methylation will result in carboxylated and sulphated MPS losing their Alcian blue staining, but saponification will restore the staining reaction of the simple carboxylated compounds; sulphated MPS like *keratosulphate* will be negative, and carboxylated and sulphated compounds (chondroitin sulphates, heparin) may show reduced staining (Table 13.6).

We are now left with sulphated mucopolysaccharides (*chondroitin sulphate B* and *heparin*) and carboxylated and sulphated *sialomucins*, all with the same staining results. Carboxylated sialomucins will not stain with aldehyde–fuchsin, but the strongly acidic sulphated sialomucins will give a positive reaction, as will the sulphated mucopolysaccharides. Sialidase/Alcian blue will give similar reactions. These methods will have given a considerable amount of information about the nature of a mucosubstance and although connective tissue sulphated MPS and epithelial sulphated sialomucins have the same results after these simple staining reactions it may be possible to exclude

Table 13.6 Identification of Alcian blue (pH 2.5) positive acid mucosubstances by Alcian blue (pH 1.0), hyaluronidase digestion, and methylation/ saponification. (V = variable result.)

	Alcian Blue (pH 1.0)	Hyaluronidase Alcian Blue (pH 2.5)		Meth/SAP Alcian Blue (pH 2.5)
		Testicular	Streptococcal	
Hyaluronic acid	−	−	−	+
Chondroitin sulphates A and C	+.	−	+	+ or ±
Chondroitin sulphate B	+	+	+	+ or ±
Heparin	+	+	+	+ or ±
Keratosulphate	+	+	+	−
Sialomucins	−	+	+	+ or V
Sulphated sialomucins	+	+	+	+ or V

chondroitin sulphate B and heparin by digestion with *Flavobacterium heparinum* hyaluronidase (Zugibe 1962, 1970). The connective tissue mucopolysaccharides are found in different types of tissue from the epithelial sialomucins and Alcian blue staining with pH control or critical electrolyte concentration or Azur A staining with careful pH control (Lillie and Fullmer 1976; Highman 1945) are techniques for distinguishing them. Finally it must be emphasized that mucosubstances are usually present in mixtures and the positive identification of one type in a tissue may only be part of the investigation.

The growth of knowledge of the histochemistry of mucosubstances in normal tissues has been applied to the diagnostic histopathology of tumours. Unfortunately, tumours do not always produce the same mucosubstances as the tissues from which they arise but a limited number of carcinomas contain mucosubstances with histochemical features which are of diagnostic value, even in metastatic deposits (Cook 1973). By the use of the PAS reaction following treatment with potassium hydroxide and with subsequent reduction with sodium borohydride Culling *et al.* (1975) were able to demonstrate epithelial mucosubstances peculiar to the large intestine. In this way metastases of lower intestinal origin were identified and primary tumours of the lung could be distinguished. A new method for demonstrating potassium hydroxide PAS positive and negative mucosubstances in contrasting colours has been described by Culling *et al.* (1977) and indicates that malignant change in the colon is associated with a reduction in side chain O-acylation of the sialic acid components of the mucosubstances that are secreted.

REFERENCES

ABUL-HAJ, S. K. and RINEHART, J. F. (1952). *J. nat. Cancer Inst.* **13**, 232.
ALLISON, R. T. (1973). *Med. Lab. Technol.* **30**, 27.
BAKER, J. R. (1945). *Cytological technique*, 2nd edn. Methuen, London.
BERNARD, C. (1877). *Leçons sur le diabète*. Paris.
BEST, F. (1906). *Z. wiss. Mikr.* **23**, 319.
CHARMAN, J. and REID, L. (1972). *Stain Technol.* **47**, 173.
COOK, H. C. (1972). *Human tissue mucins*. Butterworths, London.
—— (1973). *Med. Lab. Technol.* **30**, 217.
CULLING, C. F. A., REID, P. E., BURTON, J. D., and DUNN, W. L. (1975). *J. clin. Path.* **28**, 656.
—— —— WORTH, A. J., and DUNN, W. L. (1977). *J. clin. Path.* **30**, 1056.
DORLING, J. (1969). *J. med. Lab. Technol.* **26**, 124.
EHRLICH, P. (1883). *Z. klin. Med.* **6**, 33.
GOLDSTEIN, D. J. (1962). *Stain Technol.* **37**, 79.
GOMORI, G. (1946). *Am. J. clin. Path. (Technical Bulletin, Vol. 10)*. **16**, 177.
—— (1950). *Am. J. clin. Path.* **20**, 665.
GROCOTT, R. G. (1955). *Am. J. clin. Path.* **25**, 975.
HALE, C. W. (1946). *Nature (Lond.)* **157**, 802.
HICKS, J. D. and MATTHAEI, E. (1958). *J. Path. Bact.* **75**, 473.
HIGHMAN, B. (1945). *Stain Technol.* **20**, 85.
HOTCHKISS, R. D. (1948). *Arch. Biochem.* **16**, 131.
HUGHESDON, P. E. (1949). *J. roy. micr. Soc.* **69**, 1.
LAMB, D. and REID, L. (1969). *J. Path.* **100**, 127.
LANGHANS, C. (1890). *Virchows Arch. path. Anat.* **120**, 28.
LEV, R. and SPICER, S. S. (1964). *J. Histochem. Cytochem.* **12**, 309.
LILLIE, R. D. (1947). *Bull. int. Ass. med. Mus.* **27**, 23.
—— and FULMER, H. M. (1976). *Histopathologic technic and practical histochemistry*, 4th edn. McGraw-Hill, New York.
LISON, L. (1954). *Stain Technol.* **29**, 131.
—— and VOKAER, R. (1949). *Ann. Endocr. (Paris)* **10**, 66.
McMANUS, J. F. A. (1946). *Nature (Lond.)* **158**, 202.
MAYER, P. (1896). *Mitt. Zool. Stat. Neapel.* **12**, 303.
MOWRY, R. W. (1956). *J. Histochem. Cytochem.* **4**, 407.
MURGATROYD, L. B. (1970). *J. med. Lab. Technol.* **27**, 512.
—— (1971). *Med. Lab Technol.* **28**, 217.
PUTT, F. A. and HUKILL, P. B. (1962). *Arch. Path.* **74**, 169.
RAVETTO, C. (1964). *J. Histochem. Cytochem.* **12**, 44.
—— (1968). *J. Histochem. Cytochem.* **16**, 663.
RINEHART, J. F. and ABUL-HAJ, S. K. (1951). *Arch. Path.* **52**, 189.
SCOTT, J. E. and DORLING, J. (1965). *Histochemie* **5**, 221.
SPICER, S. S. and MEYER, D. B. (1960). *Am. J. clin. Path.* **33**, 453.
—— LEPPI, T. J., and STOWARD, P. J. (1965). *J. Histochem. Cytochem.* **13**, 599.
—— NEUBECKER, R. D., WARREN, L., and HENSON, J. G. (1962). *J. nat. Cancer Inst.* **29**, 963.
STACEY, M. and BARKER, S. A. (1962). *Carbohydrates of living tissues*. Van Nostrand, London.
STEEDMAN, H. F. (1950). *Quart. J. micr. Sci.* **91**, 477.
VALLANCE-OWEN, J. (1948). *J. Path. Bact.* **60**, 325.
VASSAR, P. S. and CULLING, C. F. A. (1959). *Arch. Path.* **67**, 128.
WAGNER, J. C., MUNDAY, D. E., and HARINGTON, J. S. (1962). *J. Path. Bact.* **84**, 73.
ZUGIBE, F. T. (1962). *Histochem. J.* **2**, 191.
—— (1970). *Diagnostic histochemistry*. Mosby, St. Louis.

14 | Pigments

Pigments are produced in normal and pathological tissues. They include haemoglobin derivatives, melanin, and lipofuscins which are *endogenous*. Pigmented, coloured, or opaque substances are also introduced into the body; organic lipochromes and inorganic substances such as carbon and metallic compounds are *exogenous*. Additional pigments can be deposited in tissues during the course of histological techniques; these are *artifacts*. These three groups of pigments, with their staining reactions and other characteristics whereby they can be recognized, will be described and it will be seen that some can be easily identified by colour reactions in sections (Table 14.1).

Table 14.1 Simple colour reactions of pigments

Pigment	Method	Colour reaction
Haemosiderin	Perls' reaction	Blue
Melanin Lipofuscins Argentaffin Chromaffin	Ammoniacal silver	Black
Melanin Lipofuscins Argentaffin Chromaffin	Schmorl's ferricyanide reaction	Blue
Melanin Argentaffin Chromaffin	Strong oxidizing agents	Natural colour is bleached

Other pigments are not easily identified by simple tests involving colour changes. These include haemoglobin and bile pigments, which may not be easy to recognize by the tests in Table 14.1, and certain artifact and exogenous pigments that are non-reactive and identifiable by exclusion or solubility (Table 14.2); some artifact and exogenous pigments have characteristic appearances or typical situations in tissues by which they may be recognized.

Artifact pigments

Formalin pigment (acid formaldehyde haematin) is produced by the fixation of tissues, especially post-mortem specimens, in acid solutions of formaldehyde. It is dark brown in colour, birefringent, maximal in and around blood vessels and congested tissues. It is best avoided by the use of neutral or buffered

Table 14.2 Characteristics of non-colour reactive pigments

Pigment	Soluble in	Identified by
Formalin pigment	Alcoholic picric acid	Birefringence Characteristic site
Mercury pigment	Alcoholic iodine	Appearance and distribution
Malaria pigment	Alcoholic picric acid	Birefringence Intracellular site
Haemoglobin	—	Peroxidase reaction, etc.
Bile pigments	—	Stein's iodine test
Carbon and other exogenous pigments	—	—

formalin [p. 49], but is soluble in a 1 per cent alcoholic solution of sodium hydroxide. Formalin pigment can be quickly removed from sections with a saturated alcoholic solution of picric acid; this avoids the main disadvantage of treatment with alkalies—the tendency of sections to come off the slide.

Removal of formalin pigment with alcoholic picric acid (Barrett 1944)

FIXATION

Acid solutions containing formalin are the usual cause of formalin pigment.

SECTIONS

Frozen or paraffin sections.

TECHNIQUE

1. Remove paraffin wax with xylene.
2. Transfer to absolute alcohol.
3. Treat section for two hours in a closed jar containing a saturated alcoholic solution of picric acid. Fine granules will be removed in less than two hours; occasionally very heavy precipitates may require longer.
4. Take sections to water and wash briefly. For some staining techniques the picric acid should be completely removed by prolonged washing, or by treatment with dilute lithium carbonate.

RESULTS

Formalin pigment is removed.
Most other pigments are unaffected, though malaria pigment is removed, and argentaffin granules may be partly dissolved.

NOTE

As malaria pigment is removed by this technique it may not be possible to distinguish *malaria pigment* from formalin pigment by picric acid solubility. Malaria pigment is intracellular, and this may be sufficient to separate it from formalin pigment, which is extracellular.

Mercury deposits are seen as dark brown granules in sections of tissues that have been fixed in solutions containing mercuric chloride. They are removed by iodine in alcohol, or iodine may be added to the alcohols during dehydration. However, the presence of mercury in paraffin blocks does no harm, and the mercury is easily removed from the sections on the slide with iodine–alcohol [p. 45].

Chrome deposits may occur as fine brown or black granules after dichromate fixation (e.g. Zenker). They can be removed from tissues by thorough washing, and from sections by the use of acid alcohol.

Stain precipitates are the result of faulty technique. They are highly coloured, usually amorphous, and granular in sections, sometimes crystalline (crystal violet). These may follow the over-oxidation of staining solutions and will occur if saturated solutions of stains (especially alcoholic) are allowed to evaporate in a warm, dry atmosphere. Stain precipitates may be a problem in automatic slide staining machines.

Some of the characteristics and staining reactions of pigments and related substances are shown in Table 14.2.

Endogenous pigments

HAEMATOGENOUS PIGMENTS

Haemoglobin can be demonstrated by the methods described below, but despite its presence in such large amounts in all tissues in the red corpuscles it may be difficult to stain; this is especially true of cells containing small amounts of ingested haemoglobin, of haemoglobinating cells in the bone marrow, and extravasated haemoglobin or haemoglobin casts in the tissues. The iron in haemoglobin is very firmly bound and cannot be readily liberated, though other iron-containing pigments such as haemosiderin easily give up their iron. Altered haemoglobins such as methaemoglobin or sulphmethaemoglobin can be distinguished by spectroscopy. Porphyrins in tissues give orange to red fluorescence with ultraviolet light (Lison 1953). Bile pigments in tissues have variable compositions and their staining methods cannot give specific results. Iron-containing pigments from which the iron can easily be mobilized (e.g. haemosiderin) are easily demonstrated, even in minute quantities, and contrast with the difficulties that may be encountered in staining other haematogenous pigments, and with the inconstancy of the methods for lipofuscins and some of the other endogenous pigments. The reason for these variable results is mainly due to the lack of a constant composition of many pigments, such as the lipofuscins and the haemoglobin derivatives. Malarial pigment (haemazoin) is a haematin and is generally intracellular; its properties are otherwise similar to those of formalin pigment [p. 261].

HAEMOGLOBIN

Haemoglobin is poorly preserved after some fixatives, such as 'Susa'. It is well stained by acid dyes such as eosin after formalin fixation. Red blood corpuscles are stained black by Heidenhain's iron haematoxylin [p. 143] and are usually stained blue by Mallory's phosphotungstic acid haematoxylin [p. 146]; they also stain well with the solochrome cyanine method (Page 1965) for myelin [p. 383] and the kiton red-almond green method of Lendrum (1949). The Dunn–Thompson modified van Gieson method stains haemoglobin green or greenish-black and is simple and usually satisfactory.

The Dunn–Thompson method for haemoglobin
(Dunn and Thompson 1945)

This is a modified van Gieson stain that gives quick and reliable results.

FIXATION

Neutral formalin is best, providing fixation has not been greatly prolonged. Zenker or Helly are satisfactory with fresh tissue; avoid Carnoy.

SECTIONS

Paraffin sections.

TECHNIQUE

1. Take sections to water.
2. Stain in a ripened aqueous solution of alum haematoxylin (0.25 per cent in 5 per cent alum) for 15 minutes. Any unacidified haematoxylin solution may be used.
3. Wash in tap water.
4. Mordant for one minute in an aqueous solution of 4 per cent ferric ammonium sulphate (iron alum).
5. Stain in the aqueous alum haematoxylin solution for ten minutes.
6. Rinse quickly in tap water.
7. Stain for 15 minutes in a van Gieson solution [p. 182].
8. Transfer directly to 95 per cent alcohol and differentiate for about three minutes.
9. Dehydrate, clear, and mount in a synthetic resin medium.

RESULTS

Red blood corpuscles—greenish-black.
Haemoglobin casts or phagocytosed haemoglobin—lighter shades of green.

NOTE

The double haematoxylin staining gives a stronger colour to haemoglobin than modifications using a single haematoxylin stain.

Haemoglobin is also well stained by methods for haemoglobin peroxidase. Dunn and Thompson's (1946) modification of Lison's (1938) leuco-Patent blue-technique or Dunn's (1946) cyanol variant are recommended.

The leuco-patent blue V method for haemoglobin peroxidase
(Dunn and Thompson 1946)

This is described on page 316.

In addition to haemoglobin the peroxidase granules of leucocytes are also stained dark blue.

Benzidine methods

A classical method for haemoglobin peroxidase has been the Lepehne (1919) and Pickworth (1934) benzidine technique. Modifications such as that of

Doherty, Suh, and Alexander (1938), using thick sections, give elegant preparations of capillaries filled with erythrocytes, but all the benzedine techniques have been overshadowed by the carcinogenicity of benzidine. Benzidine is not now widely available and its use demands rigorous safety precautions. The future of the benzidine methods is in doubt and they cannot be recommended but substitutes for benzidine, such as 3-amino-9-ethylcarbazole (Kaplow 1975), may take the place of benzidine and revive this otherwise valuable method for haemoglobin.

HAEMOSIDERIN AND INORGANIC IRON

Haemoglobin may be quickly broken down in tissues to an iron-containing pigment, haemosiderin; it takes a few days longer for iron-free bile pigments to be produced. The classical methods for haemosiderin and inorganic iron are the Prussian blue reaction for ferric iron and the Turnbull blue reaction for ferrous iron. Since almost all iron in tissues is in the ferric state, Perls' Prussian blue reaction is more valuable, but ferric iron may be converted into ferrous iron by ammonium sulphide, forming black ferrous sulphide (Quinke's reaction 1880); the ferrous sulphide may then be stained by the Turnbull blue reaction (Tirmann and Schmeltzer method, Schmeltzer 1933). Treatment with dilute acid is necessary before the Prussian blue reaction, in order to liberate ferric ions from non-reactive combinations with proteins.

Perls' Prussian blue method for haemosiderin (Perls 1867)

The ferric iron combines with potassium ferrocyanide to form the insoluble Prussian blue precipitate as follows:

$$4FeCl_3 + 3K_4Fe(CN)_6 = Fe_4[Fe(CN)_6]_3 + 12KCl.$$
(ferric   (potassium   (ferric
  iron)   ferrocyanide)   ferrocyanide)

This is a specific histochemical reaction in the section [see p. 110]. Avoid the treatment of tissues with acid or iron-containing fluids before or after fixation. Distilled water must be iron-free, and the hydrochloric acid must be of Analar grade, or it will contain iron.

FIXATION

Neutral formalin gives good results. Other fixatives may be used, but acid fixatives and potassium dichromate should be avoided.

SECTIONS

All sections.

TECHNIQUE

1. Take sections to tap water and rinse in distilled water.
2. Transfer to a mixture of equal parts of 2 per cent potassium ferrocyanide and 2 per cent hydrochloric acid in distilled water for 20–30 minutes.
3. Wash in distilled water.
4. Counterstain in eosin, safranin, or neutral red.
5. Dehydrate, clear and mount in a synthetic resin medium.

RESULTS

Haemosiderin and ferric salts—deep blue.

Other pigments retain their natural colours.
Tissues and nuclei—red (according to counterstain).

NOTES

1. More pronounced staining is obtained by heating the ferrocyanide solution to 55 °C. There may be a risk of producing artifacts, but no harm is done by preheating to 37 °C in the incubator.
2. The sharpest staining is given by Gomori's (1952) technique. Place sections in 10 per cent potassium ferrocyanide for ten minutes. Then add to this about $\frac{1}{2}$ volume of 10 per cent hydrochloric acid (iron-free analytical grade). Mix and leave the sections in this for 20–30 minutes. The reason for the improved results with this method is that potassium ferrocyanide diffuses more slowly than hydrochloric acid, and if mixed with the latter may arrive too late to react with the ferric ions in the correct part of the tissue. This modification gives the ferrocyanide a start, and is present in the tissues when the ferric salts are liberated.

Turnbull's blue reaction for ferrous salts

The basis of this is the formation of a blue precipitate (Turnbull's blue) by the interaction of ferrous salts with potassium ferricyanide as follows:

$$3FeCl_2 + 2K_3Fe(CN)_6 = Fe_3[Fe(CN)_6]_2 + 6KCl.$$
(ferrous   (potassium   (ferrous
  iron)   ferricyanide)   ferricyanide)

It is less useful than the Prussian blue reaction, since it only shows ferrous salts, which are less common in animal tissues than ferric salts.

FIXATION

As for the Prussian blue reaction of Perls [p. 264].

SECTIONS

As for the Prussian blue reaction of Perls.

TECHNIQUE

1. Take sections to tap water and rinse in distilled water.
2. Treat for 5–15 minutes in a freshly prepared solution of equal parts of 20 per cent potassium ferricyanide and 2 per cent hydrochloric acid in distilled water.
3. Transfer to 1 per cent hydrochloric acid for 5–15 minutes.
4. Rinse in distilled water.
5. Counterstain and mount as for the Perls reaction.

RESULTS

Ferrous salts are stained blue.
Other pigments are unstained.

Quincke's reaction and the Tirmann–Schmeltzer reaction
(Quincke 1880; Tirmann 1898; Schmeltzer 1933)

For both ferrous and ferric iron. Quincke's test is dependent upon the reduction of ferric iron to ferrous iron with ammonium sulphide, and the formation of green–black ferrous sulphide. The ferrous sulphide is converted into Turnbull's blue in the Tirmann–Schmeltzer reaction.

Table 14.3 Characteristics and staining reactions of pigments and related substances

	Usual situation	Colour	Soluble in	Birefringence	Perls' reaction	Masson–Fontana	Melanin bleach	Schmorl's reaction	Formalin-induced fluorescence	Additional staining reactions
FORMALIN ARTIFACT ACID HAEMATIN	Extracellular blood vessels	Brown-black	Alcoholic picric acid	+	–	–	–	–	–	Should not be present in sections
MERCURY ARTIFACT	Extracellular uniform	Brown	Alcoholic iodine	–	–	–	–	–	–	Should not be present in sections
MALARIA PIGMENT HAEMOZOIN	Intracellular RE system	Brown–Black	Alcoholic picric acid	+	–	–	–	–	–	
HAEMOGLOBIN	Red cells and other sites	Red, pale brown		–	–	–	–	–	–	Leuco-Patent blue [p. 316] Dunn–Thompson [p. 263]
HAEMOSIDERIN	Widespread	Brown	Strong acids	–	+	–	–	–	–	Tirmann–Schmeltzer [p. 265]
BILE PIGMENTS	Liver, old haemorrhages	Brown, orange, green		–	–	–	–	–	–	Gmelin reaction [p. 268] Stein's iodine [p. 268]
MELANIN	Skin, tumours	Brown	Strong alkali	–	–	+	+	+	+*	Dopa-oxidase [p. 315] *for precursors
LIPOFUSCINS	Widespread	Yellow to brown		–	+	+	+	+	–	PAS [p. 237] Variable results with other methods [p. 274]
ARGENTAFFIN E. C. GRANULES	Intestine, carcinoid tumours	Pale yellow granules	Alcohol	–	–	+	–	+	+	Diazo-reaction [p. 277] Gibbs method [p. 278]
CHROMAFFIN	Adrenal medulla phaeochromocytoma	Pale yellow granules		–	–	+	–	+	+	Chromaffin reaction [p. 280] Iodate method [p. 280]
CARBON	Lungs, lymph nodes	Black	Highly insoluble	–	–	–	–	–	–	Non-reactive Resists micro-incineration
ASBESTOS	Lungs	Brown	Insoluble	+ (if recent)	+	–	–	–	–	Resists micro-incineration

FIXATION

Formalin or alcohol. Avoid mercury, as minute traces of mercury in the sections will give a black precipitate with ammonium sulphide.

SECTIONS

All sections. Paraffin sections may come off the slide, and steps to prevent this are described below [see Note 1].

TECHNIQUE

1. Bring sections to distilled water.
2. Treat sections for 1–3 hours in 10 per cent ammonium sulphide.
3. Wash in distilled water.
4. Treat for 15 minutes with a freshly prepared solution of equal parts of 20 per cent potassium ferricyanide and 1 per cent hydrochloric acid (analytical grade) in distilled water. *OMIT THIS STEP* in the Quincke reaction.
5. Wash in distilled water.
6. Counterstain with neutral red, safranin, or eosin.
7. Dehydrate, clear, and mount in a synthetic resin medium.

RESULTS

Quincke's reaction: ferrous and ferric iron is greenish-brown or black.
Tirmann–Schmeltzer reaction: ferrous and ferric iron is dark blue.
Other pigments in natural colours.
Background red according to counterstain.

NOTES

1. Mallory (1938) used one part of strong yellow ammonium sulphide diluted with three parts of 95 per cent alcohol, in order to minimize loss of sections from the slide, and to protect celloidin sections from wrinkling. Paraffin sections may be celloidinized [p. 242] to prevent them coming off the slide.
2. The ferrous sulphide method has been suggested to be the most sensitive technique, but comparison with the Prussian blue reaction shows that the efficiency of the two methods is similar. Gomori (1936) did not recommend the Tirmann–Schmeltzer reaction, stating that the acid attacks the ferrous sulphide in an explosive way, causing solid granules to be converted into balloon-like artifacts.
3. Brownish iron sulphide is less readily distinguished from other brown pigments than the blue colour of the Prussian blue reaction. Silver, lead, mercury, and bismuth will give blackish precipitates with ammonium sulphide; these sulphides are resistant to dilute hydrochloric acid, whereas ferrous sulphide will be removed in a few minutes.

BILE PIGMENTS

In the process of breakdown of red blood cells the haemoglobin splits into haem and the protein globin. Iron is then removed from the haem leaving *biliverdin*, which is found in the spleen and bone marrow. In the liver biliverdin is reduced to *bilirubin*; this is insoluble in water but becomes soluble in its conjugated form when combined with glucuronic acid. Bile pigments may be biliverdin, unconjugated or conjugated bilirubin or mixtures of any of these three. Their normal situations may be guides to their identity—biliverdin being found in the cells of the reticuloendothelial system of lymph nodes, bone marrow, and spleen, unconjugated bilirubin in hepatic cells, and conjugated bilirubin in bile canaliculi and in the gall-bladder. Bile pigments in the liver may resemble haemosiderin [p. 264] and lipofuscins [p. 272], all of which may be present in hepatic cells and can be recognized by their histological staining reactions. Another bile pigment is *haematoidin*, a bright yellow or orange pigment which is usually found in old haemorrhagic dead tissues such as spleen or brain. This has usually been in the tissues for a long time and appears to be a haem breakdown product of variable composition that has similarities to biliverdin and bilirubin.

Bile pigments do not give primary fluorescence, and their solubilities in fixed tissues are not very helpful for identification. Most of the techniques for bile pigments are oxidation methods which progressively oxidize bilirubin to biliverdin and other compounds. The Gmelin reaction and the Stein method are established techniques which will be described; other methods include the classical Fouchet (1917) reaction, using ferric chloride, the Glenner (1957) technique with potassium dichromate and that of Lillie and Pizzalato (1967) in which bromine in carbon tetrachloride is the oxidizing agent.

The Gmelin reaction for bile pigments (Tiedemann and Gmelin 1826)

This is due to the progressive oxidation of bilirubin into different coloured compounds. It may be a variable test and is transient, but is diagnostic if positive. Negative reactions should be repeated.

FIXATION

All fixatives.

SECTIONS

All sections.

TECHNIQUE

1. Bring the sections to water.
2. Mount a section in water under a coverslip and find the pigment; leave firmly clamped on the microscope stage under high power magnification.
3. Apply a drop of strong nitric acid to one side of the coverslip with a Pasteur pipette.
4. Put a small piece of dry filter paper on the opposite side of the coverslip in order to draw the nitric acid through the section.
5. Immediately watch the pigment through the microscope for a change of colours.

RESULTS

Within a few seconds the yellowish-brown pigment will change to green, then to blue and purple.

NOTE

It is difficult to apply this test to small granules of pigment within cells, since it may be impossible to see these in the uncleared section mounted in water, and tiny amounts of pigment do not give satisfactory plays of colours.

Stein's iodine test for bile pigments (Stein 1935)

This is believed to depend upon the oxidation of the pigment to green biliverdin by iodine.

Formalin or alcohol; most other fixatives may be used.

SECTIONS

Paraffin sections.

TECHNIQUE

1. Bring sections to water.
2. Treat with a mixture of 2–3 parts of Lugol's iodine [p. 243] and one part of alcoholic tincture of iodine (potassium iodide, 2 g; iodine, 2 g; 90 per cent ethyl alcohol, 75 cm^3). Leave overnight for 12–18 hours.
3. Wash in running water for five minutes.
4. Decolorize with 5 per cent aqueous sodium thiosulphate for 30 seconds.
5. Wash in water and counterstain with Mayer's carmalum for several hours, or with 1 per cent neutral red for five minutes.
6. Dehydrate with absolute *acetone*, clear in xylene, and mount in a synthetic resin medium.

RESULTS

Bilirubin—green.
Other pigments in their natural colours.
Nuclei—red.

NOTE

Alcohol removes the green colour and dehydration must be in acetone.

MELANIN

Melanin is a brown or black pigment normally present in the skin and the eye. In pathological tissues it is found in variable quantities in benign and malignant melanomata and in some other tumours and diseases of the skin. Melanin is produced from tyrosine, which is converted into dihydroxy-phenylalanine (DOPA) by tyrosinase and then into melanin. Active sites of melanin formation can be demonstrated by the DOPA-oxidase (tyrosinase) reaction; tissues require special treatment before embedding and routine paraffin sections are not suitable (details are given on page 315).

Positive identification of melanin can be carried out by methods which use the reducing properties of melanin. As it combines with and reduces ammoniacal silver nitrate solutions to metallic silver without an additional reducing agent it is argentaffin, and the Masson–Fontana technique is usually used. It also reduces ferricyanide to ferrocyanide and gives a positive reaction with Schmorl's ferric-ferricyanide method [p. 273]. These are not specific techniques as argentaffin cell granules [p. 275] give positive reactions with both methods and lipofuscins [p. 272] will be positive with the Schmorl technique; a knowledge of the situations of the pigment in the tissue, its natural colour and other methods such as melanin bleaching and formaldehyde-induced fluorescence will usually prove identity. Melanin bleaches also remove other pigments but are especially valuable if large amounts of melanin obscure cellular details. A negative Prussian blue reaction, a positive argentaffin (silver) reaction, and a positive melanin bleach will usually be sufficient to identify a pigment as melanin, provided the situation of the pigment is also taken into account. Melanin is insoluble in all normal solvents, except normal sodium hydroxide solution. Counterstains will obscure small amounts of melanin, and eosin staining of routine sections must be very light. When searching for small quantities of melanin (or other brown pigment) a section lightly stained with haematoxylin only (no counterstain) will often reveal surprisingly large amounts of pigment that were previously invisible.

The Masson–Fontana method for melanin and the hexamine silver modification (Masson 1914; Fontana 1925; Gomori 1946)

These methods (argentaffin reactions) are dependent upon the ability of certain phenolic compounds or tyrosine derivatives to reduce silver solutions to metallic silver. The argentaffin method should be distinguished from the argyrophil reaction, in which a secondary reducing agent (hydroquinone, formalin) is also used [p. 275].

FIXATION

Most fixatives, especially formalin. Avoid dichromate.

SECTIONS

Paraffin sections.

PREPARATION

Silver solutions
Fontana
Add strong ammonia drop by drop to 20 cm^3 of 10 per cent silver nitrate until only a slight trace of the precipitate still remains. Add 20 cm^3 of distilled water. This is best prepared fresh, but will keep for a few days in a dark bottle.

Hexamine silver solution
Stock solution. Add 5 cm^3 of 5 per cent silver nitrate solution to 100 cm^3 of 3 per cent hexamine. Shake until the white precipitate dissolves. For use, add 25 cm^3 of boric acid–borate buffer (pH 7.8) to 100 cm^3 hexamine silver solution. The buffer solution [p. 498] is made up with 16 parts of one-fifth molar boric acid (M/5 H$_3$BO$_3$) and four parts of one-twentieth molar sodium tetraborate (M/20 Na$_2$B$_4$O$_7$10H$_2$O). The stock silver solution will keep in the refrigerator for several months.

TECHNIQUE

1. Bring paraffin sections to water.
2. Treat with Gram's iodine [p. 393] for ten minutes.
3. Transfer to 5 per cent sodium thiosulphate for two minutes.
4. Wash well in several changes of distilled water.
5. Leave overnight in one of the two silver solutions, described above, in the dark in a closed jar.
6. Rinse in several changes of distilled water.
7. Tone briefly (about three minutes) in 0.2 per cent gold chloride.
8. Rinse in distilled water.
9. Fix in 5 per cent sodium thiosulphate for two minutes.
10. Wash in running tap water for two minutes.
11. Counterstain with 0.1 per cent safranin or 1 per cent neutral red for two minutes.
12. Wash and differentiate the counterstain in water and 70 per cent alcohol; dehydrate in alcohol, clear, and mount in a synthetic resin medium.

RESULTS

Melanin—black.
Argentaffin cell granules—black [see Note 3].
Nuclei—red.

NOTES

1. The iodine serves to prevent false reactions due to sulphydryl groups, in addition to removing mercury from mercury-fixed tissues. Steps 2 and 3 are optional.
2. Fontana's solution may precipitate black granules of silver on to the section, and is more liable to give non-specific black background staining than the hexamine–silver solution.
3. In addition to argentaffin cell granules in intestinal epithelium, chromaffin granules and lipofuscins may give positive silver reactions of variable intensities.
4. The silver solution may become explosive; follow the safety precautions described on page 148.
5. Toning in gold chloride (step 7) is optional.

The DOPA-oxidase (tyrosinase) reaction

This method shows sites of DOPA-oxidase activity as dark brown granules. Fresh tissue is required and previously fixed tissues are not suitable. The technique is described on page 315.

Formaldehyde-induced fluorescence technique for melanin precursors (after Eränkö 1955)

Yellow fluorescence of basal cells of the epidermis and in tumour cells of melanomas was described by Baroni in 1933. This has been shown to be induced by formaldehyde and Pearse (1972) has reviewed formaldehyde-induced fluorescence of biogenic amines [p. 274] in detail. The fluorescent compound in melanin-forming tissues is thought to be a DOPA-like precursor which can easily be seen in formalin fixed tissues. Although the technique was first used with frozen or freeze-dried sections it is applicable to formalin-fixed, paraffin embedded sections; stored blocks can be recut and reviewed.

FIXATION

Formaldehyde (see technique, below).

SECTIONS

Frozen, freeze-dried, or paraffin.

TECHNIQUES

For *frozen sections* use fresh tissue and allow sections to thaw on the surface of a solution containing 1 vol. 40 per cent formaldehyde, 5 vols. 2 per cent calcium chloride, and 4 vols. distilled water. After 2–6 hours, rinse in distilled water and mount sections in glycerol.

For *freeze-dried sections* the blocks of freeze-dried tissue are fixed in hot formaldehyde vapour (for details see Pearse 1972).

Paraffin sections are dewaxed in xylene, rinsed in fresh xylene, and mounted in a synthetic resin medium.

Examine with a fluorescence microscope.

RESULTS

Cells with melanin-precursor activity—yellow fluorescence.

NOTE

A large number of amines, including 5-hydroxytryptamine, histamine, adrenalin, and noradrenalin also give formaldehyde-induced fluorescence.

BLEACHING METHODS FOR MELANIN

These are especially valuable for the examination of cellular detail in deeply pigmented tissues or tumours. Many endogenous pigments may be bleached by these techniques, and therefore they are not satisfactory for the identification of melanin. Various strong oxidizing agents can be used and permanganate is recommended. The times stated below are only a guide, as the time needed will depend on the amount of melanin; ocular melanin usually needs much longer than melanin from the skin. Sections should be examined with the staining microscope and returned to the bleaching solution if melanin is still present. Pearse (1972) prefers 40 per cent peracetic acid for 2–16 hours as a rapid bleaching agent, and states that other pigments such as lipofuscins tend to resist for longer than 16 hours.

Permanganate method

Treat sections with 0.1 per cent potassium permanganate for 12 hours, rinse in water, and treat with 1 per cent oxalic acid for one minute. Repeat if necessary.

Peroxide method

Place sections in 30 vols. (10 per cent) hydrogen peroxide for 24–48 hours.

Chlorate method

Place a small amount of potassium chlorate at the bottom of a Coplin jar. Fill with 50 per cent alcohol. Take the sections down to 50 per cent alcohol, and place in the jar. Add a few drops of concentrated hydrochloric acid to the bottom of the jar with a pipette. Leave sections for 24 hours.

LIPOFUSCINS

The lipochrome pigments are a group of substances of variable structure that are widely distributed throughout animal tissues. They appear to be produced by the progressive oxidation of lipid precursors (Pearse 1972), and as oxidation proceeds their capacity to reduce silver or ferricyanide solutions increases and fat staining decreases. The strongly basiphilic and deeply pigmented lipofuscins are highly oxidized. Ceroid pigment is at an early stage of oxidation, while 'pseudomelanin', the pigment found in the colon with melanosis coli, has characteristics of a lipofuscin that is sufficiently highly oxidized to give negative results with Sudan dyes. 'Pseudomelanin' should not be regarded as a true melanin.

Lipofuscins usually give strong positive reactions with Sudan black B but are less strongly stained with Sudan IV and other fat-soluble stains. The PAS reaction is generally positive, the Masson–Fontana and hexamine–silver solutions are slowly reduced, and Schmorl's ferricyanide is rapidly reduced. Some lipofuscins (especially ceroid) are acid-fast, especially if the long Ziehl–Neelsen method is used (stain for *three hours at 60 °C* with carbol fuchsin solution, page 398). Some of the characteristics and the staining reactions of lipofuscins are shown in Figure 14.1.

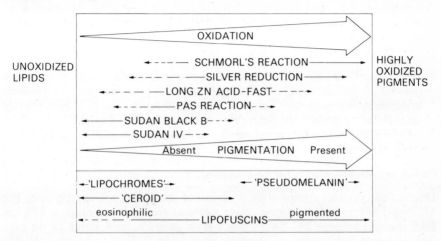

FIG. 14.1.   The characteristics and the spectrum of the staining reactions of lipofuscins (after Pearse 1972).

Schmorl's ferric-ferricyanide method for lipofuscins (Golodetz and Unna 1909)

This has been considered to be based upon the reduction of ferricyanide to ferrocyanide, which combines with ferric ions to form Prussian blue. Lillie and Donaldson (1974) have shown that at the pH of the reaction (2.5) ferric ions are reduced to ferrous in the presence of ferricyanide and Turnbull's blue is produced.

FIXATION

Formalin. Most other fixatives are satisfactory; avoid dichromate.

SECTIONS

All sections.

PREPARATION

Ferric ferricyanide solution. Lillie (1953) recommended the following as an improvement upon the original; it must be freshly prepared before use. To 4 cm³ fresh 1 per cent potassium ferricyanide solution in distilled water add 30 cm³ of 1 per cent ferric chloride in distilled water and an additional 6 cm³ distilled water.

TECHNIQUE

1. Bring sections to distilled water.
2. Treat with the ferric-ferricyanide solution for ten minutes at room temperature.
3. Wash briefly in 1 per cent aqueous acetic acid solution.
4. Wash in water.
5. Counterstain 1 per cent neutral red for three minutes (optional).

6. Dehydrate rapidly in alcohol, clear, and mount in a neutral synthetic medium.

RESULTS

Lipofuscins—dark blue.
Other reducing substances which will stain blue include melanin, intestinal argentaffin granules, and tissue components with active sulphydryl groups.

NOTES

1. The ferricyanide in the mixture will react with ferrous salts if these are present in the sections, and for critical work it is necessary to perform control stains with the Turnbull blue method [p. 265]. If the control sections are negative, the Schmorl reaction findings are valid.
2. This method demonstrates chromaffin in the adrenal medulla in dichromate-fixed material.

Other staining methods for lipofuscins

Due to their variable composition a variety of techniques are appropriate. The Masson–Fontana and hexamine–silver methods are described on page 270, the PAS reaction on page 237, Sudan black B on page 291, and Sudan IV on page 290. For acid-fast lipofuscins the long method [p. 273] must be used. Highly oxidized lipofuscins are strongly basiphilic and most show gold or brown fluorescence with ultraviolet light.

THE APUD SYSTEM

The APUD concept is important as it links together many cells, including the argentaffin, argyrophil, and chromaffin cells, whose staining reactions will be described. In a long series of papers Pearse (summarized 1975) has shown that many cells, of widely differing distribution in the body, produce polypeptide hormones or amines (Gould 1978). Many of these cells are argyrophilic [p. 278], and contain electron-dense, membrane-bound granules in their cytoplasm. In the APUD system are the intestinal argentaffin (Kultschitzky or enterochromaffin) cells, adrenal chromaffin cells, the islet B cells of the pancreas, and pituitary basiphils which produce ACTH. In addition there are the thyroid C cells, pancreatic islet A and D cells, and intestinal argyrophil cells, many of which are part of the gastro-intestinal endocrine system; these cells are present in normal tissues but tumours arising from them, with the same endocrine function and staining reactions, have been recognized (such as the gastrinoma of G cell origin and the glucagonoma of the pancreatic islets). APUD cells are able to take up and decarboxylate amine precursors, and the initial letters APUD stand for Amine and Amine Precursor Uptake and Decarboxylation.

Endocrine cell granules can be stained with lead haematoxylin, but their morphology is best shown by electron microscopy. Detailed knowledge of cells of the APUD system has been obtained by immunofluorescent and immunoenzyme techniques which are described in Chapter 17 [p. 323].

Lead haematoxylin method for APUD cell granules (Solcia, Capella, and Vassallo 1969)

This is a modification of MacConaill's (1947) lead haematoxylin and has been thought to depend on carboxyl linkage with the stain.

FIXATION

Helly's fluid [p. 52] has been recommended, but formal-calcium [p. 303] at 4 °C for 4–48 hours and other fixatives have been used.

SECTIONS

Paraffin sections.

PREPARATION

1. Stabilized lead solution.

5 per cent lead nitrate in distilled water	100 cm³
Saturated ammonium sulphate in distilled water	100 cm³

Mix, filter, and add 4 cm³ of 40 per cent commerical formaldehyde. This stock solution will keep for several weeks.
2. Lead haematoxylin solution.

Add 0.2 g of haematoxylin in 1.5 cm³ of 95 per cent alcohol to 10 cm³ of the stabilized lead solution (No. 1, see above). Dilute with 10 cm³ of distilled water, stirring continuously. Stand for half an hour, filter, make up to 75 cm³ with distilled water and use immediately.

TECHNIQUE

1. Bring paraffin sections to water.
2. Stain in the lead haematoxylin solution for 2–3 hours at 37 °C or for 1–2 hours at 45 °C. Formaldehyde-fixed sections need less time than Helly-fixed sections.
3. Wash in distilled water.
4. Dehydrate, clear, and mount in a synthetic resin medium.

RESULTS

APUD cell granules—blue–black.

NOTE

Endocrine cells producing polypeptides and monoamines are all shown by this technique, including pancreatic A and D cells, gastric G cells, thyroid C cells, and enterochromaffin (EC) cells. Adrenal medulla, carotid body, pituitary ACTH, and MSH cells are also positive.

THE ARGENTAFFIN AND ARGYROPHIL CELLS OF THE INTESTINE

These cells are distributed as individual cells scattered throughout the intestinal canal (and other organs), in contrast with endocrine organs which are made up of large compact collections of specialized cells. They comprise a main part of the 'diffuse' endocrine system of the gastro-intestinal canal and the cells which make up this system, and the tumours that arise from them, have been described by Dawson (1976). Endocrine cells of the gastro-intestinal system, their secretions and staining reactions, are shown in Table 14.4.

The *argentaffin reaction* is brought about by cells which can reduce silver solutions without the use of a reducing agent (a non-reducing silver technique). The *argyrophil reaction* also blackens cells with metallic silver, but it differs from the argentaffin reaction because argyrophilic cells combine with silver compounds but cannot reduce them without the use of an additional reducing agent such as hydroquinone or formalin (reducing silver technique).

Table 14.4 Histochemical reactions of gastro-intestinal endocrine cells (after Dawson 1976)

CELL	HORMOME	Argentaffin reaction [p. 276] / Diazo- [p. 277]	Argyrophil reaction [p. 278]	Metachromasia Toluidine blue [p. 250]	Lead haematoxylin [p. 274]	PTAH [p. 146]	
PANCREATIC							
A (α2)	Glucagon	−	+	±	+	+	
B (β)	Insulin	−	−	−	−	−	
D (α1)	?Gastrin ?Secretin	−	+	+	+	+	
INTESTINAL							
Enterochromaffin (EC)	5-Hydroxy-tryptamine	+	+	+	+		
Enteroglucagon (EG)	Enteroglucagon	−	+	±	+		
Gastrin (G)	Gastrin	−	− or ±	−	+		
Secretin (S)	Secretin	−	±		+	+	
Others, e.g. VIP*, GIP†	VIP, GIP	−	+ or ±		+ or ±		

* Vasoactive Intestinal Peptide.   † Gastric Inhibitory Polypeptide.

Argentaffin cells are argyrophil, but argyrophil cells are not argentaffin. Although the argyrophil cells are not so easily demonstrated they are more numerous than argentaffin cells.

Argentaffin granules in the Kultschitzky cells of the small intestine are soluble in alcohol and alcoholic fixatives must be avoided. The granules of carcinoid tumours are not preserved as easily as those of normal argentaffin cells and these tumours give weak or negative results, especially in post-mortem specimens. Argentaffin cells are well shown by the Masson–Fontana silver method, and are more specifically demonstrated by the diazo-technique and the Gibbs indophenol reaction. These, and the argyrophil reaction, will be described.

The Masson–Fontana method for argentaffin granules

Phenolic compounds have the capacity of reducing silver solutions to metallic silver. This direct reduction (argentaffin reaction) can only be achieved after non-alcoholic fixation. Any of the silver impregnation techniques using an additional reducing substance will blacken argentaffin *and* argyrophil cells.

FIXATION

Formal-saline, or formalin-containing fixatives. Alcohol or alcoholic fixatives should not be used.

Paraffin sections.

TECHNIQUE

See page 270.

RESULTS

Argentaffin granules—black. Other reducing substances such as melanin, chromaffin granules, and lipofuscins will also be blackened.
Nuclei—red.

The Diazo-reaction for argentaffin granules (Lison 1931; Gomori 1952)

This is a simple, rapid, and more specific method which demonstrates unsubstituted phenolic compounds by alkaline reduction of diazonium salts into diazo-dyes.

FIXATION

Formal-saline.

SECTIONS

Paraffin sections.

PREPARATION

Staining solution
Take 5 cm³ of a 1 per cent aqueous solution of fast red salt B (the stable diazotate of 5-nitroanisidine) and add a few drops of a saturated solution of borax or 2 cm³ of saturated aqueous lithium carbonate. Staining may be improved if the solution is cooled in the 4 °C refrigerator for 10–15 minutes before use.

TECHNIQUE

1. Take sections to distilled water.
2. Pour the staining solution on the slide and leave for one minute.
3. Rinse in distilled water and wash in running tap water.
4. Counterstain nuclei with haematoxylin (see Note, below).
5. Differentiate with acid alcohol and wash well in running water for 15 minutes.
6. Dehydrate in alcohol, clear with xylene, and mount in a synthetic resin mountant.

RESULTS

Argentaffin granules—a fiery orange–red.
Nuclei—blue.

NOTE

The argentaffin granules may stain lightly, especially in carcinoid tumours or in post-mortem material. Because of this it is important not to overstain with haematoxylin, which may obscure feebly positive results. The haematoxylin should be differentiated longer than usual, leaving a light nuclear stain and no cytoplasmic coloration. Ehrlich's haematoxylin, which stains cytoplasmic mucus, should be avoided.

Gibbs' method for argentaffin granules (Gibbs 1926; Gomori 1952)

This depends upon the formation of a brownish or black indophenol dye when a phenol in alkaline solution reacts with Gibbs' reagent (2:6-dichloro-quinone-chloroimide). The method gives good specificity and colour contrast.

FIXATION

Formal-saline.

SECTIONS

Paraffin sections.

PREPARATION

Staining solution
Dissolve 50 mg of 2:6-dichloroquinone-chloroimide in 5–10 cm^3 of alcohol; add 50 cm^3 of distilled water and a few drops of a saturated solution of borax. Pearse (1972) recommended warming a similar concentration of the compound in 0.1 M veronal acetate buffer solution pH 9.2 at 70 °C until dissolved. Cool before use and filter.

TECHNIQUE

1. Take sections to water.
2. Immerse in the staining solution at room temperature for 10–15 minutes.
3. Wash well in running water.
4. Counterstain nuclei with 1 per cent neutral red.
5. Dehydrate rapidly with alcohol and clear in xylene.
6. Mount in a synthetic resin mountant.

RESULTS

Argentaffin granules—grey–black. The granules of carcinoid tumours may be brownish.
Nuclei—red.

Reducing silver methods for argyrophil cells

Silver methods using a reducing agent (reticulin techniques, Bielschowsky's method) will blacken argyrophil and argentaffin cells. The Bodian (1936) method using protargol with hydroquinone reduction has been widely used and a number of silver techniques, such as that of Grimelius (1968) for argyrophil cells of pancreatic islets, have been developed for the identification of different argyrophil cells of the APUD system. The double silver impregnation modification of Pascual (1976) is a simple method which gives good contrast of the argyrophil cells without background impregnation. The basis of the argyrophil reaction has already been described [p. 275].

FIXATION

Formal-saline.

SECTIONS

Paraffin sections.

PREPARATION

1. Bodian's reducing solution.

Anhydrous sodium sulphite	5 g
Hydroquinone	1 g
Distilled water	100 cm³

2. Nuclear-fast red counterstain.

Nuclear-fast red (Kernechtrot)	0.1 g
Aluminium sulphate	5 g
Distilled water	100 cm³

TECHNIQUE

1. Bring paraffin sections to water.
2. Place in freshly prepared 0.5 per cent silver nitrate in distilled water for two hours at 60 °C or overnight at room temperature.
3. Rinse in distilled water.
4. Transfer sections to freshly prepared Bodian's reducing solution (solution 1, see above) previously heated to 60 °C for five minutes.
5. Wash in running tap water for three minutes and rinse in distilled water.
6. Reimpregnate in the same silver solution at 60 °C for ten minutes.
7. Rinse in distilled water.
8. Repeat the reducing solution as in steps 4 and 5.
9. Counterstain with nuclear-fast red (solution 2, see above) for three minutes.
10. Rinse in tap water, dehydrate, clear, and mount in a synthetic resin medium.

RESULTS

Argyrophil cells—black.
Nuclei—red.

NOTE

1. The staining can be monitored by examining the sections with the staining microscope during step 6, increasing the impregnation time if necessary.
2. Argentaffin cells are also stained and the non-reducing silver technique (argentaffin reaction, page 276) should also be carried out on sections from the same block.
3. Ten methods for pancreatic A, B, and D cells have been compared by Schweisthal, Frost, and Brinn (1975).

CHROMAFFIN CELLS

Cells of the adrenal medulla, and to a lesser extent other tissues such as paraganglia and the organs of Zuckerkandl, give the chromaffin reaction. This is the development of a brown colour following the treatment of fresh tissue with chromic acid or a chrome salt (and other mild oxidants such as iodates); it is given by adrenalin, noradrenalin, and other related compounds. Chromate oxidation rapidly produces the brown pigment in adrenalin and noradrenalin, but iodate oxidizes noradrenalin much more quickly than adrenalin and this can be used as a way of distinguishing between the two compounds. Chromaffin granules will reduce ammoniacal silver solutions and the ferricyanide of Schmorl's test [p. 273] is quickly reduced, giving a positive reaction.

Chromaffin reaction for adrenalin and noradrenalin

Fix fresh tissue in Muller's fluid, Orth's fluid or in Regaud's (Möller's) fluid. Prolonged fixation has been recommended but two days is usually sufficient. Cut frozen sections.

MULLER'S (1860) FLUID

Dissolve 2.5 g of potassium bichromate and 1 g of sodium sulphate in 100 cm^3 of distilled water.

ORTH'S (1896) FLUID

To 100 cm^3 of Muller's fluid add 10 cm^3 of 40 per cent formaldehyde immediately before use.

REGAUD'S (1910) (MÖLLER'S) FLUID

To 80 cm^3 of 3 per cent potassium dichromate add 20 cm^3 of 40 per cent formaldehyde immediately before use.

The chromaffin reaction will be weakly positive or negative if the tissue has been previously fixed in formalin or other fixatives.

The Vulpian reaction is seen as a green colour in medullary cells following the fixation of fresh adrenal tissue in 5 per cent ferric chloride solution.

The iodate method for noradrenalin
(Hillarp and Hökfelt 1955; Pearse 1972)

TECHNIQUE

This depends upon the more rapid oxidation by iodate of noradrenalin than adrenalin.

1. Place very thin (0.5 mm) blocks of fresh adrenal in 10 per cent aqueous potassium iodate and leave for 16 hours at room temperature. Do not exceed this time.
2. Transfer to 10 per cent formalin for two hours.
3. Cut frozen sections 10–20 μm thick.
4. Wash in distilled water.
5. Sections may be counterstained if required, and can be dehydrated, cleared, and mounted as permanent preparations.

RESULTS

Noradrenalin—brown.

Giemsa staining after dichromate fixation

This is a classical staining method for the adrenal. After dichromate fixation the chromaffin granules stain a greenish-yellow colour with the Romanowsky stains.

FIXATION

Any dichromate fixative—Orth, Regaud (Möller), Zenker, etc.

SECTIONS

Paraffin sections.

TECHNIQUE

1. Bring sections to water and leave in distilled water for at least 30 minutes.

2. Stain in dilute Giemsa (one drop of stain per cm^3 of distilled water). Leave for 24 hours at room temperature.
3. Rinse in distilled water.
4. Blot.
5. Differentiate in 90 per cent alcohol (rapidly) and then pass quickly through absolute alcohol *or* dehydrate and differentiate in pure acetone.
6. Clear in xylene and mount in a synthetic resin medium. Sections tend to fade in balsam.

RESULTS

Chromaffin granules—greenish-yellow.
Nuclei—blue.
Cytoplasm—red to violet.

OTHER ENDOGENOUS PIGMENTS

Copper is present in the liver and is increased in cirrhosis. It is especially abundant in Wilson's disease (hepatolenticular degeneration) and can be demonstrated in sections of liver and brain. Rubeanic acid forms a greenish-black precipitate of copper rubeanate in tissues containing excess copper; normal quantities cannot be stained. Other metals such as cobalt and nickel also produce rubeanates but Uzman (1956) blocked these by the use of sodium acetate in an acid-staining solution. Uzman also recommended that non-reactive, protein-bound copper in fixed tissues should be released by placing sections face downwards over a beaker of concentrated hydrochloric acid.

Rubeanic acid method for copper (Howell 1959)

FIXATION

Formal-saline or other fixatives.

SECTIONS

All sections.

PREPARATION

Make a stock solution of 0.1 per cent rubeanic acid in absolute alcohol. The staining solution is made up of 5 cm^3 of the stock solution to 100 cm^3 of 10 per cent aqueous sodium acetate.

TECHNIQUE

1. Bring sections to water.
2. Place sections in the staining solution at 37 °C overnight.
3. Transfer to 70 per cent ethyl alcohol for 15 minutes.
4. Place in absolute alcohol for six hours.
5. Clear in xylene and mount in a synthetic resin medium.

RESULTS

Copper—greenish-black, if present in excessive amounts.

Calcium is not a pigment, but may be deposited in an insoluble form in tissues, often combined with iron and other compounds. Methods for the demonstration of calcium are given on page 217.

Exogenous pigments

Extraneous materials found in tissues which are often coloured, opaque, or crystalline are traditionally described as exogenous pigments. They are completely different in origin and structure from the pigments that have been discussed, but are now considered because it may be necessary to distinguish these exogenous substances from naturally occurring pigments, and because some staining methods for both groups are similar.

CARBON

Carbon is present in the lungs and lymphoid tissue of human and other animals living in a dusty atmosphere. Coal-miners may show a widespread deposition of carbon throughout the lymphatic system, skin and viscera. It is seen as black particles, though fine granules may be brownish and resemble other pigments. It is not reactive, and all the methods for staining pigments are negative; it cannot be bleached. It is insoluble in strong alkalies and strong acids, and can usually be recognized easily by its site.

Silica is also found in the same sites as carbon in coal-miners; it causes fibrosis of the lungs, and may be recognized by the birefringence of silica compounds and their resistance to micro-incineration.

IRON ORE PIGMENTS

Iron-ore miners may show these variably coloured pigments in their lungs. They may give positive ferrocyanide (Prussian blue) or ferricyanide (Turnbull blue) reactions, or both. However, haematite (Fe_2O_3) usually fails to give a positive Perls' test; this may become positive if stronger (4N–10N) hydrochloric acid is used, and if the reactions are carried out at 60 °C. For the Quincke reaction it is necessary to substitute a 1–2 day exposure to saturated hydrogen sulphide water for the usual ammonium sulphide sequence [p. 265].

ASBESTOS

Asbestos fibres are found in the body as long, beaded rods which are birefringent and resistant to micro-inceration. They become coated with protein and haemosiderin, develop a yellow colour and lose their birefringence. They can be seen in routine sections and stain blue with Perls' Prussian blue reaction; if present in small numbers they are easier to find in 20 μm sections, examined unstained. The presence of asbestos fibres in the lungs can be demonstrated by making smears from the cut surfaces of fresh lungs taken at autopsy; these are examined unstained and the yellow or brown asbestos bodies are seen.

OTHER METALLIC COMPOUNDS

Methods for barium, bismuth, lead, beryllium, and other inorganic cations are specialized techniques which are not usually required in routine material. They have a variable sensitivity and specificity, and are described by Pearse (1972).

IDENTIFICATION OF AN UNKNOWN PIGMENT

Unknown pigments are usually identified by histologists by the results of certain specific and non-specific staining reactions, combined with a knowledge of their appearance and situation in the tissues in the routine sections. Usually the simple staining methods are carried out first, and in most instances these will give exact identification or a good indication of the type of pigment. If not, many pigments will have been excluded, and it is then possible to undertake specialized techniques for the most likely pigments that remain. The characteristics and staining reactions of pigments that are of help in their identification are shown in Table 14.4 [p. 276].

Brown pigments create the most difficulty in preliminary recognition but can usually be identified. Less pigmented substances have special characteristics—phagocytosed haemoglobin usually retains some red colour with eosin, calcium is blue with haematoxylin, argentaffin and chromaffin granules have special situations, as do the exogenous pigmented or opaque substances. The problem of the brown pigment in tissues can be caused by formalin and mercury artifacts, malaria pigment, bile, haemosiderin, melanin, and the lipofuscins. The fixation artifact pigments are extracellular, diffuse in the tissue and can be removed by their solubilities; malaria pigment is intracellular and birefringence may help, but is not always reliable. Once artifact pigments have been excluded sections should be stained for haemosiderin (Perls' reaction). This can be done quickly and if this is negative, sections should be put in a silver solution overnight (Masson–Fontana) and in a melanin bleaching solution. Next morning a positive silver reaction will indicate melanin, though less strong reactions will be produced by lipofuscins, and by chromaffin granules. Argentaffin cells from the small intestine will also be positive, but the site of the pigment or the morphology of the tumour will identify enterochromaffin pigment. The section in the melanin bleach can be examined wet, and if bleaching has taken place the section can be mounted; if not, the section is put back in the bleaching fluid. A pigment that is insoluble in everything except normal sodium hydroxide solution, which reduces silver but is bleached in 24 hours, is almost always melanin. Within 24 hours these steps will have identified formalin pigment, malarial pigment, haemosiderin, and pigments containing reactive ferric ions, melanin and argentaffin intestinal cell granules. Chromaffin granules and lipofuscins, suggested by the silver reaction or slow bleaching, can be identified more definitely by the appearance and site of the pigment, and by special methods, such as Schmorl's reaction. Of the common endogenous brownish pigments, only bile pigments remain, and these may give a positive Stein's test, be recognized by their situation, or be identified by exclusion.

REFERENCES

BARONI, B. (1933). *Arch. ital. Derm.* **9**, 543.

BARRETT, A. M. (1944). *J. Path. Bact.* **56**, 135.

BODIAN, D. (1936). *Anat. Rec.* **65**, 89.

DAWSON, I. M. P. (1976). In *Pathology of the gastro-intestinal tract* (ed. B. C. Morson). Springer-Verlag, Berlin.

DOHERTY, M. M., SUH, T. H., and ALEXANDER, L. (1938). *Arch. Neurol. Psychiat. (Chic.)* **40**, 158.

DUNN, R. C. (1946). *Arch. Path.* **41**, 676.

DUNN, R. C. and THOMPSON, E. C. (1945). *Arch. Path.* **39**, 49.

―――― ―――― (1946). *Stain Technol.* **21**, 65.

ERÄNKÖ, O. (1955). *Nature (Lond.)* **175**, 88.

FONTANA, A. (1925–6). *Derm. Z.* **46**, 291.

FOUCHET, A. (1917). *C.R. Soc. Biol. (Paris)* **80**, 826.

GIBBS, H. D. (1926). *Chem. Rev.* **3**, 291.

GLENNER, G. G. (1957). *Am. J. clin. Path.* **27**, 1.

GOULD, R. P. (1978). In *Recent advances in histopathology* (eds P. P. Anthony and N. Woolf). Churchill Livingstone, Edinburgh.

GOLODETZ, L. and UNNA, P. G. (1909). *Mh. prakt. Derm.* **48**, 149.

GOMORI, G. (1936). *Am. J. Path.* **12**, 655.

―――― (1946). *Am. J. clin. Path.* **10**, 177.

―――― (1952). *Microscopic histochemistry.* Chicago University Press.

GRIMELIUS, L. (1968). *Acta Soc. med. Upsal.* **73**, 243.

HILLARP, N. A. and HÖKFELT, B. (1955). *J. Histochem. Cytochem.* **3**, 1.

HOWELL, J. S. (1959). *J. Path. Bact.* **77**, 473.

KAPLOW, L. S. (1975). *Am. J. clin. Path.* **63**, 451.

LENDRUM, A. C. (1949). *J. Path. Bact.* **61**, 443.

LEPEHNE, G. (1919). *Beitr. path. Anat.* **65**, 163.

LILLIE, R. D. and BURTNER, H. J. (1953). *J. Histochem. Cytochem.* **1**, 87.

―――― and DONALDSON, P. T. (1974). *Histochem. J.* **6**, 679.

―――― and PIZZALATO, P. (1967). *J. Histochem. Cytochem.* **15**, 600.

LISON, L. (1931). *Arch. Biol. (Paris)* **41**, 343.

―――― (1938). *Beitr. path. Anat.* **101**, 94.

―――― (1953). *Histochimie et cytochimie animales.* 2nd edn. Gauthier-Villars, Paris.

MACCONAILL, M. A. (1947). *J. Anat. (Lond.)* **81**, 371.

MALLORY, F. B. (1938). *Pathological technique.* W. B. Saunders, Philadelphia.

MASSON, P. (1914). *C.R. Acad. Sci. (Paris)* **158**, 57.

MULLER, H. (1860). *Verh. phys.-med. Ges. Würzb.* **10**, 138.

ORTH, J. (1896). *Berl. klin. Wschr.* **33**, 273.

PAGE, K. M. (1965). *J. med. Lab. Technol.* **22**, 224.

PASCUAL, J. S. F. (1976). *Stain Technol.* **51**, 231.

PEARSE, A. G. E. (1972). *Histochemistry, theoretical and applied.* 3rd edn., Vol. 2. Churchill Livingstone, London.

―――― (1975). In *Pathology annual* (ed. S. C. Sommers), Vol. 10. Appleton–Century–Crofts, New York.

PERLS, N. (1867). *Virchows Arch. path. Anat.* **39**, 42.

PICKWORTH, F. A. (1934). *J. Anat. (Lond.)* **69**, 62.

QUINCKE, H. I. (1880). *Dtsch. Arch. klin. Med.* **25**, 567.

REGAUD, C. (1910). *Arch. Anat. micr.* **11**, 291.

SCHMELTZER, W. (1933). *Z. wiss. Mikr.* **50**, 99.

SCHWEISTHAL, M. R., FROST, C. C., and BRINN, J. E. (1975). *Stain Technol.* **50**, 161.

SOLCIA, E., CAPELLA, C., and VASSALLO, G. (1969). *Histochemie* **20**, 116.

STEIN, J. (1935). *C. R. Soc. Biol. (Paris)* **120**, 1136.

TIEDEMANN, F. and GMELIN, L. (1826). *Die Verdauung nach Versuchen.* Heidelberg.

TIRMANN, J. (1898). *Görbersdorfer veröffentl.* **2**, 101.

UZMAN, L. L. (1956). *Lab. Invest.* **5**, 299.

15 | Lipids

Although some disagreement still exists among histologists and biochemists regarding the terminology and classification of lipids, the word itself is now accepted as a generic term to denote any fatty or fat-like substance found naturally and capable of being utilized by animal and vegetable organisms. A more precise definition is difficult for while most lipids are insoluble in water and soluble in 'fat solvents' such as acetone, xylene, and chloroform, some compound lipids are slightly soluble in water but insoluble in acetone.

Classification of lipids

The following is intended as a general working guide to the different types of lipid.

Simple lipids are esters of fatty acids and alcohols.

Neutral fats, triple esters of fatty acids and glycerol (triglycerides).
Ester waxes, esters of fatty acids and higher alcohols.

Compound lipids possess a nitrogenous base and other compounds in addition to fatty acids and an alcohol.

Phospholipids, containing a phosphoric acid radical.
Sphingolipids, in which the nitrogenous base is sphingosine; these will be grouped with the *glycolipids* which contain a hexose sugar in addition to sphingosine.

Derived lipids are obtained from simple (or compound) lipids by hydrolysis.

Fatty acids are derived from triglycerides.
Sterols (cholesterol) obtained from hydrolysis of ester waxes.

SIMPLE LIPIDS

NEUTRAL FATS

The neutral fats are predominantly triglycerides of the saturated fatty acids, palmitic ($C_{15}H_{31}COOH$) or stearic acid ($C_{17}H_{35}COOH$), or of the unsaturated fatty acid, oleic acid ($C_{17}H_{33}COOH$) which has a double bond in the middle of its fatty acid chain. More often, triglycerides are mixtures of two or three fatty acids. Stearodiolein, an oleic-stearic-oleic acid triglyceride, is typical of human fat.

$$\text{CH}_2.\text{O.CO.C}_{17}\text{H}_{33}$$
$$|$$
$$\text{CH.O.CO.C}_{17}\text{H}_{35}$$
$$|$$
$$\text{CH}_2.\text{O.CO.C}_{17}\text{H}_{33}$$

Neutral fats are the most abundant lipid in nature and comprise more than 90 per cent of the stored lipids in humans.

WAXES

The most important members of this group are the cholesterol esters which are present in greatest amount in animal tissues in the adrenals. The cholesterol esters are usually considered in association with cholesterol which is a derived lipid.

Simple lipids are readily soluble in fat solvents and insoluble in water. They are demonstrated with oil soluble dyes. On exposure to air they tend to become oxidized and partially hydrolysed with the liberation of fatty acid.

COMPOUND LIPIDS

PHOSPHOLIPIDS

Phosphoric–fatty acid esters

These differ from the triglycerides in that two, not three, of the glycerol radicals are esterified by fatty acids, the third by a phosphoric acid–nitrogenous base. The lecithins and the cephalins are the most important members of this type of phospholipid. In the case of the lecithins, choline $(\text{CH}_2\text{OH.CH}_2.\text{N}(\text{CH}_3)_3)$ is the determinative base: lecithins are widespread in animal and plant tissues and disturbances of their metabolism result in far greater effects on the cell than do alterations in simple or derived lipids of the storage type. Cephalins are characterized by the presence of either ethanolamine $(\text{CH}_2\text{OH.CH}_2.\text{NH}_2)$ or serine $(\text{CH}_2\text{OH.CH.COOH.NH}_2)$ as the nitrogenous bases. They are invariably found in close association with lecithins and participate with them in the cellular metabolic cycle.

Plasmals

These comprise the acetal phospholipids and the plasmalogens. The acetal phosphatides differ from the phosphoric–fatty acid esters in that, instead of two hydroxyl groups of glycerol being each bound to a fatty acid they are together bound by acetal linkage to a single fatty acid, one by semi-acetal linkage to a fatty aldehyde, and the third, as in all the phospholipids, to the phosphoric acid–nitrogen complex.

SPHINGOLIPIDS

Sphingomyelins

A group of lipids previously classified with the phospholipids lecithin and cephalin, but differing from them chemically in the absence of glycerol and the presence of sphingosine as well as choline, and biologically in that they are associated particularly with the nervous system. In addition they possess a considerably greater degree of stability and resistance to oxidation and emulsification. Massive accumulations of sphingomyelin are found in the liver and spleen in the lipidosis known as Niemann–Pick disease.

Cerebrosides

These have many points in common with the sphingomyelins; as the name implies they also are primarily distributed in the tissues of the nervous system. They have some chemical properties in common with the sphingomyelins, but instead of the phosphoric acid–nitrogen complex the alcohol radical is attached to a hexose sugar, usually galactose, sometimes glucose. The existence of at least three cerebrosides is acknowledged: kerasin, phrenosin, and nervon, the identity of their respective fatty acids being variable. In Gaucher's disease large amounts of kerasin are found in the liver, spleen, bone marrow, and lymph nodes.

Gangliosides

This group of sphingolipids is of fairly recent recognition and although essentially similar to the cerebrosides differs from them in having in addition hexosamines and neuraminic acid, thus conferring on them markedly acidic qualities. Although these lipids are found predominantly in the neurones of the grey matter of the brain, they may be demonstrated in the ganglion cells of the rectal myenteric plexus and this is made use of in the diagnosis of Tay–Sachs disease, a familial lipidosis, where rectal biopsies are taken to show the characteristic distension of ganglion cells.

Sulphatide

Like the above, sulphatide or cerebroside sulphate, is a constituent of nervous tissue and accumulations of this substance in neurones, astrocytes, peripheral nerves, and elsewhere in the body are found in the disease known as metachromatic leucodystrophy; so-called because of the characteristic brown metachromasia given by staining with cresyl-fast violet (Hirsch and Peiffer 1955) or with toluidine blue (Bodian and Lake 1963).

DERIVED LIPIDS

FATTY ACIDS

These are produced by hydrolysis of simple lipids (triglycerides) and are straight-chain compounds possessing the carboxyl radical COOH. The saturated fatty acids have the general formula $C_nH_{(2n+1)}COOH$, e.g. palmitic acid $(C_{15}H_{31}COOH)$.

The unsaturated fatty acids have one or more double bonds and the general formula $C_nH_{(2n-x)}COOH$, x representing the number of double bonds. Oleic acid $(C_8H_{16}:C_9H_{17}COOH)$ is histologically far the most important.

STEROLS

Of the higher molecular weight compounds obtained from the hydrolysis of ester waxes the sterols containing the steroid nucleus are the most important and the basic structure is cholesterol. This has four fused rings (three

six-membered and one five-membered) and the identity of the sterol is dependent upon the side-chain in the C_{17} position in the five-membered ring.
Testosterone and its metabolites (androgens) have no C_{17} side-chain;
progesterone and the adrenocortical hormones have a two carbon atom side-
chain; bile acids have five carbon atoms at C_{17} and cholestrol and the
precusors of vitamin D have an eight carbon atom side-chain.

Demonstration of lipids

The amount of lipid that can be demonstrated by simple techniques is often
very much less than can be shown to be present by chemical analysis. Fat in
storage cells of adipose tissue and myelin in nerve fibres are easily stained, but
lipid may not be seen normally in sections of organs such as liver, kidney, or
heart in spite of chemical proof of its existence. Such lipid that is present but
not demonstrable by simple techniques is known as masked or bound lipid.
This is combined with other tissue constituents, particularly protein and in
this state may survive paraffin embedding. Unmasking or dissociation of this
lipid (after which it may be demonstrated with oil soluble dyes) may be
accomplished in a variety of ways including prolonged washing in water, heating, and by the action of proteolytic enzymes (Zugibe 1970).

The difference between masked and unmasked lipids will be better understood by consideration of their chemical and physical states. Lipid droplets
such as those in the storage cells exist as entirely separate entities in a continuous phase; the droplets consist solely of lipid, the surface of which is hydrophobic. This type of lipid structure was described as 'homophasic' by Lison
(1960). Where the lipid is combined with non-lipid elements such as water or
protein the phase is not continuous. In these cases the surface may be hydrophilic, this type of structure being called by Lison 'heterophasic'. The terms
hydrophobic and hydrophilic are of great value in understanding the effects of
the physical states of lipids on their demonstration by staining methods.
Droplets of continuous phase (Lison 'homophasic'), the surface of which is
hydrophobic, can be demonstrated by the use of oil soluble dyes, the principle
of which is the greater solubility of the dye in the lipid than in the dye solvent
(see below). In lipid structures where the phase is not continuous (Lison
'heterophasic') the lipid combination with water or protein may result in
hydrophilic properties that will prevent the dye from dissolving in the lipid.
In histopathology, the demonstration of lipid in tissues is of diagnostic
significance in a number of conditions. These include the demonstration of fat
emboli in various tissues, lipid in some tumours, in fatty degeneration of the
heart and liver, atheromatous plaques in blood vessels and in the lipidoses
referred to above.

Since most lipids are soluble in the reagents used in paraffin embedding, it is
perhaps prudent to retain a fragment of biopsy specimens in fixative against
the possibility of the demonstration of lipid being desirable as a result of the
examination of the paraffin sections.

FIXATION

Simple lipids such as in adipose tissue are not fixed or dissolved by the use of
formalin (its action being confined to the other tissue elements) but compound

lipids may be affected by its use in such a way that their solubility is changed. The reason for this effect is not clearly understood. A lipid may be insoluble in aqueous media yet loss of material may occur through emulsification. This led to the introduction of the formal-calcium and cobalt fixatives for the better preservation of phospholipids. As they may still be extracted by the use of solvents they are not fixed in the usual sense of the word. The term fixation, rather than preservation, can be used with regard to fixatives containing potassium dichromate or osmium tetroxide, as their use results in the oxidation of phospholipids which then become less soluble in fat solvents.

Buffered formalin [p. 49] or 10 per cent formalin in 1 per cent calcium chloride are recommended for general purposes.

CONTROL SECTIONS

The use of control sections is important in lipid demonstration methods and as a positive control, Bayliss High (1977) suggests the use of cryostat sections from a composite block comprising rat or human brain (phospholipids), fatty liver (triglycerides and fatty acids), and atheroma or adrenal (cholesterol and cholesterol esters).

As a negative control, Cook (1974) recommends treating sections at 56 °C for at least 30 minutes with the chloroform–methanol extraction mixture (see below).

EXTRACTION METHODS

One of the criteria of lipids and other naturally occurring fat-like substances is their solubility in fat-solvents and their insolubility in water (fats can also act as solvents for other fats) and use has been made of various extraction techniques, either for the removal of lipids or to demonstrate their differential solubility in such solvents. Examples are the use of pyridine in the Baker acid–haematin technique, and acetone, ether and chloroform–methanol used by Keilig in the differential extraction of lipid from unfixed material. Discretion is necessary in the use of solvents however, as the interpretation of the results obtained may also be affected by the chemical and physical states of the lipids in question.

Keilig's (1944) extraction method

Blocks of unfixed tissue 2–3 mm thick are extracted with the solvents shown in Table 15.1; three changes of solvents are used, the first and second for three hours, the third for 12 hours. A Soxhlet apparatus is used for the hot solvents.

Table 15.1

Lipid extracted	Solvent
Glycerides, cholesterol and its esters	Cold acetone
Cerebrosides	Hot acetone
Lecithins and cephalins	Hot ether
All lipids	Hot chloroform–methanol (equal parts)

After extraction, the blocks are taken down to water through descending grades of alcohol. Frozen sections are cut and stained and compared with untreated material stained in the same way.

NOTE

The results obtained are not as clear cut as Table 15.1 might suggest (Pearse 1968). Phospholipid dispersion occurs, for example, in cold acetone, and since one is dealing with unfixed tissue, or at least tissue that is inadequately fixed by the incidental action of the solvents, loss of both lipid and non-lipid material may well occur on rehydration.

Baker's (1946) pyridine extraction method

FIXATION

Weak Bouin

Saturated aqueous picric acid	50 cm³
Commercial formalin	10 cm³
Glacial acetic acid	5 cm³
Distilled water	35 cm³

SECTIONS

10 μm frozen sections.

TECHNIQUE

1. Fix small portions of tissue in weak Bouin for 20 hours.
2. Wash in alcohol to remove picric acid.
3. Extract in pyridine at room temperature for 30 minutes.
4. Extract in pyridine at 60 °C for 24 hours.
5. Wash in running water for two hours.
6. Treat with dichromate-calcium [p. 294] as in Baker's acid haematin method.

RESULTS

All lipids removed.

NOTE

This technique was devised to be used in conjunction with Baker's acid haematin method (below), but may be followed by Sudan black B or other stains.

OIL SOLUBLE DYES

These weakly acidic disazo dyes are virtually insoluble in water and only sparingly so in alcohol. They are soluble in most lipids however, and for this reason are widely used for the demonstration of lipids in tissues. Since they colour lipids by solubility they are called lysochromes. The first of these dyes was introduced by Daddi (1896) who used the orange–red Sudan III with 70 per cent alcohol as the solvent. Later, Michaelis (1901) advocated the use of Sudan IV because of its darker colour, French (1926) recommended oil red O as a further improvement, while Lison and Dagnelie (1935) introduced Sudan black B, the most sensitive of all oil soluble dyes (Casselman 1959). Superior solvents have also been discovered to replace the 70 per cent alcohol of Daddi and the equal parts 70 per cent alcohol and acetone mixture of Herxheimer

(1903) because of the tendency of alcohol and acetone to dissolve small droplets of lipid. Superior solvents which dissolve little or no lipid but more dye are propan-2-ol (isopropyl alcohol) (Lillie and Ashburn 1943), propane-1,2-diol (propylene glycol) (Chiffelle and Putt 1951), and triethyl ortho-phosphate (Gomori 1952). These and several other solvents for oil soluble dyes have been reviewed by Feldman and Dapson (1974) who concluded that triethyl orthophosphate was the solvent of choice. Marshall (1977) has described a rapid thin-layer chromatography system for the quality control of oil soluble dyes.

Oil red O-triethyl phosphate method (Casselman 1959)

FIXATION

Formal-saline or formal-calcium.

SECTIONS

10–15 μm frozen sections.

PREPARATION

Add about 1 g of oil red O to 100 cm³ of 60 per cent aqueous triethyl phosphate. *Either* heat the mixture to 95–100 °C for five minutes, stirring continuously, *or* place it in the paraffin oven for 2–3 hours, stirring occasionally. Filter the hot mixture through fluted filter paper and cool. Filter again before using.

TECHNIQUE

1. Rinse sections well in 60 per cent triethyl phosphate.
2. Immerse sections in the staining solution for 10–15 minutes.
3. Wash off excess dye in 60 per cent triethyl phosphate.
4. Rinse in distilled water.
5. Counterstain nuclei with alum haematoxylin.
6. Blue in tap water.
7. Mount the section on a slide and apply a coverslip using an aqueous mountant. Ring the coverslip.

RESULTS

Simple lipids are bright red; other lipids are less strongly stained or are unstained.

NOTES

1. Sudan black B may be used in the same way as oil red O in this method; carmalum should be the counterstain.
2. Sudan black B may be profitably applied to paraffin sections, especially if the tissue was fixed in the formal-calcium and given post-chromation. It will demonstrate those compound lipids that are resistant to paraffin embedding.

FLUORESCENCE MICROSCOPY

Primary fluorescence is exhibited by the oxidation products of lipids known as lipofuscins and by carotinoid pigments dissolved in lipids. Secondary fluorescence is exhibited by fluorochromes (e.g. phosphine 3R) dissolved in lipids.

Secondary fluorescence method (Popper 1944)

FIXATION

Formalin or formal-calcium.

SECTIONS

10–15 µm frozen sections.

TECHNIQUE

1. Wash sections in distilled water.
2. Stain for three minutes in 0.1 per cent aqueous phosphine 3R.
3. Rinse quickly in distilled water and mount in 90 per cent glycerol.

RESULTS

Simple lipids, including cholesterol esters and all compound lipids exhibit a silvery-white fluorescence; derived lipids, i.e. fatty acids and cholesterol are negative.

NOTE

This and other methods using similar fluorochromes have the advantage that the aqueous solutions used do not dissolve fine lipid droplets.

OSMIUM TETROXIDE

The mechanism of osmium reduction is as yet poorly understood and the use of this expensive and unpleasant reagent for the demonstration of lipid can in no sense be regarded as a true histochemical method. Its main value in this field is in the Marchi-type methods for degenerate myelin [p. 369] and in providing a means of demonstrating lipid in a way that will survive subsequent paraffin embedding. This last procedure is useful for the preparation of durable, non-fading sections for teaching purposes.

Osmium tetroxide method for the demonstration of lipid in paraffin sections

FIXATION

Flemming's fluid [p. 53].

SECTIONS

10–15 µm paraffin sections.

TECHNIQUE

1. Fix thin slices of tissue in Flemming's fluid for 24–48 hours.
2. Wash in running water for 12–16 hours.
3. Dehydrate in 70 per cent, 90 per cent, and absolute alcohol, clear in chloroform or toluene and embed in paraffin wax.
4. Cut sections at 5–10 µm, mount on slides and dry.
5. Remove wax with xylene and mount with a synthetic resin medium. Counterstaining with neutral red or safranin is optional.

RESULTS

Lipids are blackened as are other reducing substances.

POLARIZED LIGHT AND METHODS FOR CHOLESTEROL

It is not possible to differentiate between types of lipids by the use of polarized light. It may be useful, however, to show the presence or absence of bire-fringent material in conjunction with extraction techniques.

Fats which are present in a liquid form are usually monorefringent, but if they are cooled, they may form birefringent crystals. Cholesterol esters and some compound lipids, over a certain range of temperatures, can exist as liquid spherocrystals and exhibit Maltese-cross birefringence. If heated, they become monorefringent and if cooled below a certain point, they may assume the form of acicular crystals giving plain birefringence with four positions of extinction on rotating the stage of the microscope through 360 degrees. While glycerides and fatty acids never exist in the form of spherocrystals, absence of cholesterol esters and compound lipids cannot be presumed from the failure to demonstrate Maltese-cross birefringence.

Unstained, formalin or formal-calcium fixed frozen sections are mounted with an aqueous mountant and examined with the polarizing microscope. Sections may be warmed to 37 °C for a few moments before re-examination.

Digitonin reaction for cholesterol (after Windaus 1910)

FIXATION

Formalin or formal-calcium.

SECTIONS

10–15 μm frozen sections.

TECHNIQUE

1. Wash sections in distilled water.
2. Immerse in 0.5 per cent digitonin in 50 per cent alcohol for several hours.
3. Rinse in 50 per cent alcohol.
4. Wash in water, mount the section on a slide, apply a coverslip, using an aqueous mountant.

RESULTS

Examination under the polarizing microscope reveals crystals or rosettes of the digitonin–cholesterol complex which are birefringent.

NOTE

Differentiation between cholesterol and its esters, which are themselves bire-fringent, may be effected by counterstaining one section with Sudan III or IV and leaving another unstained. The esters are stained by Sudan and their bire-fringence disappears while the cholesterol complex remains unstained and birefringent.

Schultz (1924) reaction for cholesterol and its esters

FIXATION

Formalin or formal-calcium.

SECTIONS

20–30 μm frozen sections.

TECHNIQUE

1. Wash sections in distilled water.
2. Immerse in 2.5 per cent iron alum for three days at room temperature or for 36 hours at 37 °C. (This converts cholesterol to oxycholesterol.)
3. Rinse in water, mount on a clean slide, and drain off excess fluid.
4. Apply several drops of an equal parts mixture of concentrated sulphuric acid and glacial acetic acid, carefully apply a coverslip, blot off excess acid, and examine immediately.

RESULTS

A positive reaction is indicated by the rapid development of an intense blue or reddish-purple colour which changes to green after about 30 seconds.

NOTES

1. It is essential that all reagents, especially the acids, should be pure; if not, massive bubble formation is likely to make examination extremely difficult.
2. More rapid oxidation (stage 2) may be obtained by treatment with 20 per cent ferric chloride (Everett 1945).
3. The blue or purple colour-reaction which takes place initially is not itself characteristic of cholesterol alone; it is the terminal change to green which is diagnostic.

METHODS FOR PHOSPHOLIPIDS

Baker's (1946) acid haematein method for phospholipids

FIXATION

Formal-calcium for 6–8 hours.

SECTIONS

10 μm frozen sections.

PREPARATION

Dichromate-calcium
Potassium dichromate	5 g
Calcium chloride (anhydrous)	1 g
Distilled water	100 cm³

Acid haematein
Haematoxylin	0.05 g
Sodium iodate 1 per cent	1 cm³
Glacial acetic acid	1 cm³
Distilled water	48 cm³

Dissolve the haematoxylin and sodium iodate in the distilled water with the aid of heat, and when cool add the acetic acid.

The solution only keeps for a few hours.

Borax-ferricyanide differentiator
Potassium ferricyanide	0.25 g
Sodium tetraborate (borax)	0.25 g
Distilled water	100 cm³

Store in a dark bottle.

TECHNIQUE

1. Treat small pieces of tissue for 18 hours in dichromate–calcium at room temperature.
2. Transfer to fresh dichromate–calcium for 24 hours at 60 °C.
3. Wash thoroughly in distilled water.
4. Cut frozen sections at 10 μm (gelatine embedding optional).
5. Treat section with dichromate–calcium for one hour at 60 °C.
6. Wash in distilled water.
7. Stain in acid haematein for five hours at 37 °C.
8. Wash in distilled water.
9. Differentiate in borax–ferricyanide for 18 hours at 37 °C.
10. Wash in tap water and mount in an aqueous medium.

RESULTS

Phospholipids, sphingolipids, and nucleoproteins—dark blue.

NOTE

The method should be used in conjunction with the Baker's pyridine extraction technique (above): parallel blocks should be taken, one being extracted with pyridine before processing, thus forming a negative control.

The plasmal reaction (Feulgen and Voit 1924)

FIXATION

Nil, fresh tissue.

SECTIONS

10–15 μm frozen sections.

TECHNIQUE

1. Rinse sections in distilled water.
2. Mount on a clean slide and treat for three minutes with 1 per cent mercuric chloride.
3. Transfer to Schiff's reagent [p. 239] for not longer than 15 minutes.
4. Rinse in three changes of sulphurous acid [p. 240].
5. Wash in water and mount in an aqueous medium.

RESULTS

Acetal phospholipids and plasmalogens—magenta or red.

NOTES

1. Control sections treated only with Schiff's reagent for 15 minutes and not with mercuric chloride are essential.
2. It is imperative that the tissue should be unfixed, and that the times given be strictly adhered to. Prolonged treatment with Schiff's reagent, either of the control or test sections, can give rise to false positives.

The PAS method [p. 237]

This demonstrates carbohydrate-containing lipids (cerebrosides and gangliosides) and also those unsaturated lipids and phospholipids which contain groups that yield aldehydes on oxidation with periodic acid.

METHODS FOR ACIDIC LIPIDS

Nile blue for neutral and acidic lipids (after Cain 1947)

Although non-specific, Nile blue is of some value in distinguishing neutral and acidic lipids having a red (oxazone) component which is soluble in neutral lipid and a blue (oxazine) component which reacts with phospholipids and fatty acids.

FIXATION

Formalin or formal-calcium [p. 289].

SECTIONS

10–15 μm sections.

TECHNIQUE

1. Rinse sections in distilled water.
2. Stain in a covered dish of 1 per cent aqueous Nile blue for ten minutes at 37 °C.
3. Rinse rapidly in distilled water.
4. Differentiate in 1 per cent acetic acid until of a uniform colour.
5. Rinse in water; mount on a clean slide in an aqueous medium.

RESULTS

Neutral lipids—rose pink or red.
Acidic lipids—blue, as are also various non-lipid basiphil elements.

NOTE

Nile blue as commercially supplied consists of two components, Nile blue and Nile red. The presence of the latter, which is essential for the success of the reaction, may be confirmed by treating a few grains of the powder with xylene, the red component becoming immediately visible.

Feyrter's (1936) 'inclusion' method

FIXATION

Formalin.

SECTIONS

10–15 μm frozen sections.

TECHNIQUE

1. Wash sections thoroughly in distilled water.
2. Mount on a clean slide, allow to partially dry.
3. Apply several drops of 1 per cent thionin in 0.5 per cent tartaric acid and cover carefully with a coverslip.
4. Remove the excess stain from the edges of the coverslip with a piece of filter paper and when dry, seal the edges with asphalt varnish or paraffin wax.

RESULTS

Acidic lipids—rose pink. Epithelial and connective tissue mucins and mast cell granules also exhibit metachromasia.

NOTES

1. Metachromatic staining may appear after ten minutes, but usually reaches its maximum after 24–48 hours; sections tend to fade after several weeks.
2. The reaction may be expedited with the aid of gentle heat.

REFERENCES

BAKER, J. R. (1946). *Quart. J. micr. Sci.* **87**, 441.

BAYLISS HIGH, O. B. (1977). In *Theory and practice of histological techniques* (eds. J. D. Bancroft and A. Stevens). Churchill Livingstone, Edinburgh.

BODIAN, M. and LAKE, B. D. (1963). *Br. J. Surg.* **50**, 702.

CAIN, A. J. (1947). *Quart. J. micr. Sci.* **88**, 383.

CASSELMAN, W. G. B. (1959). *Histochemical technique.* Methuen, London.

CHIFFELLE, T. L. and PUTT, F. A. (1951). *Stain Technol.* **26**, 51.

COOK, H. C. (1974). *Manual of histological demonstration techniques.* Butterworths, London.

DADDI, L. (1896). *Arch. ital Biol.* **26**, 143.

EVERETT, J. W. (1945). *Am. J. Anat.* **77**, 3.

FELDMAN, A. T. and DAPSON, R. W. (1974). *Med. Lab. Technol.* **31**, 335.

FEULGEN, R. and VOIT, K. (1924). *Pflügers Arch. ges. Physiol.* **206**, 389.

FEYRTER, F. (1936). *Virchows Arch. path. Anat.* **296**, 645.

FRENCH, R. W. (1926). *Stain Technol.* **1**, 79.

GOMORI, G. (1952). *Microscopic histochemistry.* Chicago University Press.

HERXHEIMER, G. W. (1903). *Zbl. allg. Path. path. Anat.* **14**, 481.

HIRSCH, T. and PEIFFER, J. (1957). In *Cerebral lipidoses* (ed. J. N. Cumings). Blackwell, Oxford.

KEILIG, I. (1944). *Virchows Arch. path. Anat.* **312**, 405.

LILLIE, R. D. and ASHBURN, L. L. (1943). *Arch. Path.* **36**, 432.

LISON, L. (1960). *Histochimie et cytochimie animales.* Gauthier-Villars, Paris.

LISON, L. and DAGNELIE, J. (1935). *Bull. Histol. appl. Physiol. Path.* **12**, 85.

MARSHALL, P. N. (1977). *J. Chromat.* **136**, 353.

MICHAELIS, L. (1901). *Virchows Arch. path. Anat.* **164**, 263.

PEARSE, A. G. E. (1968). *Histochemistry: theoretical and applied*, 3rd edn., Vol. I. Churchill, London.

POPPER, H. (1944). *Physiol. Rev.* **24**, 205.

SCHULTZ, A. (1924). *Zbl. allg. Path. path. Anat.* **35**, 314.

WINDAUS, T. (1910). *Z. phys. Chem.* **65**, 110.

ZUGIBE, F. T. (1970). *Diagnostic histochemistry.* C. V. Mosby, St. Louis.

16 | Enzyme histochemistry

Enzymes are proteins that catalyse the chemical reactions which are essential for the metabolic changes that take place in living tissues. They often have a high degree of specificity and most enzymes are named after their biochemical action, together with the suffix -*ase*. There are several types of enzymes—*hydrolases* which are hydrolytic (e.g. phosphatases and esterases), *oxidoreductases* which are oxidative and remove hydrogen (oxidases and dehydrogenases), *transferases* which transfer radicles (phosphorylase) and *proteolytic* enzymes such as leucine aminopeptidase.

It has already been stressed [p. 110] that histochemistry is not a separate or distinct part of histological technique. Perls' Prussian blue reaction (for iron) and the periodic acid-Schiff reaction (for carbohydrates, mucin) are precise histochemical methods that are in everyday use. Enzyme techniques now have a place in diagnostic histology, but it must be appreciated that they differ in several respects from other histological methods. Most tissue constituents are demonstrated in sections of dead, fixed tissue by direct interaction with a dye or reagent to produce coloration of the actual tissue component. However, with enzymes the reagent is a substrate upon which the enzyme acts, and the final opaque or coloured product is derived from a change in the substrate that is produced by the active enzyme. Another important difference is the lability (instability) of enzymes, nearly all of which disappear from the tissues quickly and progressively after removal of tissues from the body and after cellular death. Special precautions must be taken to preserve enzymes, and these will be briefly described.

Historically, methods for enzymes have almost all been developed since 1939, some of the earliest and fundamental being those described by Takamatsu (1938, 1939) and Gomori (1939). Histochemical methods for enzymes have been revolutionized by the development of the refrigerated microtome (cryostat). Early enzyme techniques were often difficult, complicated or unrealiable, but the use of fresh frozen cryostat sections of fresh tissues has brought enzyme histochemistry within the reach of all histological laboratories. Many techniques for enzymes have been produced, but it is only possible to include some of the most important here. Additional information on the theoretical and practical aspects of enzyme histochemistry has been given by Pearse (1968, 1972) and in the classical works of Gomori (1952) and Lison (1953). The practical applications of histochemical methods, interpreted in their widest sense, have been briefly described by Niemi and Korhonen (1972), and in greater detail by Zugibe (1970).

THE ROLE OF ENZYME HISTOCHEMISTRY IN GENERAL HISTOLOGY

The morphologist investigating animal tissues can obtain additional information about the structure and function of cells by enzyme histochemistry.

Table 16.1 Cellular structures and their associated enzymes.

Cellular structure	Enzyme
Lysosomes	Acid phosphatase, β-glucuronidase
Membranes	Alkaline phosphatase, aminopeptidase, ATPase
Mitochondria	Dehydrogenases, diaphorases, monoamine oxidase, ATPase
Microsomes	Esterases, glucose-6-phosphatase

Enzymes are associated with certain intracellular structures and enzymes act as markers for the identification of cellular components; Table 16.1 shows some of the enzymes that are associated with intracellular organelles.

Using light microscopy, enzyme histochemistry will give indications of the types of metabolic activity that take place in a cell. These will be guides to the identity and functions of the cell, which can be valuable in abnormal tissues, and will also suggest the ultrastructural components that are present in it. Electron microscopy will confirm ultrastructure, and some enzyme histochemical methods can be carried out on ultra-thin sections for the electron microscope but these will not be described. This ability to categorize the functions of a cell in biochemical terms is used in histopathology in abnormal tissues. The enzyme histochemistry of tumour cells has been compared with that of the normal tissue from which the tumour originated in the hope that enzyme markers could be used to determine malignancy. Although only limited progress has been made with tumours, enzyme techniques can confirm their histogenesis in some instances, such as the tartrate-labile acid phosphatase in carcinoma of prostate. The loss of certain enzymes, such as succinate dehydrogenase, can be demonstrated in abnormal intestinal biopsies and enzyme techniques play an important part in the investigation of diseases of skeletal muscle since they can identify nerve endings and the types of muscle fibre as well as showing alterations in functional activity. The extent of the aganglionic segment of colon in Hirschsprung's disease can be shown by the TPNH diaphorase technique. There are many practical applications of enzyme histochemistry in histopathology and these are listed by Zugibe (1970), together with the enzyme patterns that have been found in tumours.

PREPARATION OF TISSUES FOR ENZYME TECHNIQUES

Tissues must be prepared in such a way as to preserve enzymes as completely as possible, and to retain them in their original sites. Fixation should not allow the enzymes to deteriorate or to diffuse, and the final colour reaction should be sharply precise so that exact localization of the enzyme can be obtained. Because of the difficulty of fixing enzymes in tissues without considerable loss, freeze-drying was widely used for early techniques. Fresh frozen (cryostat) sections have largely superseded sections of freeze-dried material, tissue that has been fixed in conventional fixatives and sectioned on the carbon dioxide freezing microtome or fixed tissues embedded in paraffin. Within two miniutes of obtaining fresh tissue, cryostat sections can be prepared and introduced into the substrate solution; complicated processing is avoided and a better preservation of enzyme activity is obtained. The classical fixation and embedding techniques, and that of freeze-drying, will be briefly discussed, as they still have a place in some enzyme methods, but the cryostat is now established as the method of choice for most histochemical reactions for enzymes, and is recommended for its speed, ease of handling, and versatility.

The difficulties encountered in the preservation of enzymes, and of demonstrating them in their original sites without serious loss or diffusion, makes it essential to interpret the results of enzyme histochemistry with caution. Controls must be used to determine specificity and validity of results, and these are described on page 301. Because of these pitfalls most histologists will be content with a qualitative result, but *quantitative histochemistry*, stating enzyme activity in absolute figures, can be performed. Progress is being made towards the quantitative chemical analysis of the cell in its living state and quantitation has been reviewed by Pearse (1972), Wied (1966), and Wied and Bahr (1970).

FIXATION AND TISSUE PROCESSING

Many enzymes can be preserved reasonably well after appropriate fixation and it is not always appreciated that tissue processing and embedding in paraffin may be far more destructive to enzymes than fixation. Chayen, Bitensky, and Butcher (1973) have listed the final activity of many enzymes after fixation in various fixatives for different durations at a range of temperatures; it is usually possible to preserve at least 50 per cent of enzyme concentrations by fixation in ice-cold acetone or alcohol. Since much of the remaining enzyme activity is lost in paraffin embedding the use of fresh tissue for cryostat sections is recommended, and these sections may be used unfixed or fixed for ten minutes in formal-calcium [p. 303] or acetone after cutting. Cryostat sections of prefixed tissue can also be used and formal-calcium at 4 °C gives good results with the hydrolytic enzymes and is a useful fixative for biopsy specimens; thin blocks (less than 3 mm) are fixed for 24 hours and should be impregnated for at least 24 hours with gum-sucrose [p. 304] in which they may be left over the week-end without harm. It is not easy to cut cryostat sections of tissues which have been pre-fixed in acetone. If a cryostat is not available thin blocks should be fixed in ice-cold acetone followed by very brief paraffin embedding in the vacuum oven at 56 °C, but this is not satisfactory for certain enzymes such as dehydrogenases and diaphorases for which fresh tissue is needed.

FREEZE-DRYING

Freeze-drying has been described on page 74, and one of its applications is the processing of tissues for enzyme histochemistry. Modern freeze-drying equipment is less cumbersome and delicate than earlier apparatus, and will preserve enzymes without excessive loss. By the use of thermo-electric modules (similar to those used as freezing microtome stages, page 101) tissues can be frozen and dried under a low vacuum. The electric current through the module is then reversed and the heat that is generated melts paraffin wax in which the specimen is embedded *in situ*. Although freeze-drying is an effective way of preserving enzymes, and is now easier to use, it must be repeated that it has been largely replaced by the refrigerated microtome (cryostat) for enzyme techniques. For most histological laboratories the cryostat is more useful than freeze-drying equipment, not only for the demonstration of enzymes, but also for other purposes.

SECTION CUTTING

Frozen sections of fresh tissue cut on a refrigerated microtome ᵢ
many enzyme methods and the technique of cryostat microton
on page 103. Cryostat sections of tissue fixed in cold formal-cᵤ
used [p. 303]. As only a few enzymes are partly preserved in paraffin ᵤᵢ
Gomori's (1952) methods for paraffin sections have been largely superseded
by the cryostat.

TESTS FOR SPECIFICITY AND VALIDITY OF ENZYME TECHNIQUES

The rapid disappearance of most enzymes from tissues after death makes it essential to carry out positive and negative controls in conjunction with the sections under investigation. Material known to contain the enzyme should be available for positive controls and should always be used, especially when new reagents are prepared or if the technique is only used occasionally. Negative controls (blanks) must be processed in parallel with the test sections in order to ensure specificity. The usual controls are as follows: (1) The omission of an essential step in the technique such as the replacement of the substrate by distilled water, or, in the case of alkaline phosphatase, the omission of calcium. (2) The use of specific inhibitors of enzyme activity in adequate concentration (0.1 per cent potassium cyanide, M/100 sodium fluoride, eserine, etc.). (3) The treatment of sections with a non-specific agent known to destroy the enzyme (boiling water, strong acids, oxidizing agents, etc.); these may be variable, some enzymes being more resistant to non-specific inhibitors than others. Any positive reaction that is obtained after effective enzyme inhibition or after the omission of an essential part of the technique indicates that the test is non-specific.

Use eight sections for enzyme histochemistry techniques. Stain the first and the last with haematoxylin and eosin before starting the enzyme method to ensure that the sections are of suitable tissue. Use a substrate control section with all the reagents except the substrate, and an inactivated control section with all the reagents including the substrate. Perform the method on two sections, one of which can be counterstained. The last two sections are spares in case the method requires repeating.

Accurate localization of the enzyme reaction at the original site of the enzyme in the cell is an important aspect of enzyme histochemistry, and this can be used as an additional control. Positive reactions in unusual situations may be the result of faulty technique or of non-specific staining. The product of the enzyme activity upon the substrate is usually a colourless diffusible substance, and this must be precipitated at its site of formation by another reagent. Maximum sensitivity and correct localization are dependent upon the precipitation being rapid and the precipitate being practically insoluble. False positive reactions may result from the spontaneous hydrolysis or oxidation of the substrate, if the reaction products are absorbed into the tissue of the section. Some methods depend upon the combination of calcium or other metallic ions with the breakdown products due to enzyme activity, and false positive reactions will be given by calcium or other metals in the section. Other errors may be due to incorrect interpretation of naturally occurring pigments or other compounds that resemble the final colour reaction, especially if reagents used in the technique (such as ammonium sulphide) _ause changes from the recognizable natural colour to one that is closer to that of the final reaction product.

It must be appreciated that whilst we are attempting to obtain true chemical specificity and exact tissue localization, these are not always possible with histological methods. One enzyme may attack several similarly related chemical compounds, and a single substrate may be acted upon by more than one enzyme. The optimal conditions for the activity of an individual enzyme upon a particular substrate must be determined, and when these have been found they must be carefully followed in the histochemical technique. There is less lattitude in enzyme reactions than in other histological staining methods.

THE NATURE OF ENZYME HISTOCHEMICAL REACTIONS

Most enzyme techniques depend upon the formation of a *primary reaction product* (PRP) due to the action of the enzyme upon the substrate. This is followed by the production of a coloured or opaque *final reaction product* (FRP) by combining the PRP with a second reagent, and is usually accomplished by blackening the PRP by chemical means or combination with a diazonium salt to form a diazo-dye. These two steps may take place concurrently or consecutively. In some techniques the production of the PRP and its capture as a coloured FRP take place simultaneously in one incubating medium (*simultaneous capture*), but in others the two reactions are carried out separately one after another (*post-incubation coupling or post-coupling*). An example of simultaneous capture is the diazo-technique for alkaline phosphatase; the enzyme releases a coupler from the substrate, and this combines with the diazonium salt that is present with the substrate in the incubating medium to form a coloured azo-dye. A post-coupling reaction, such as the Rutenberg and Seligman (1955) method for acid phosphatase, first produces a colourless PRP that is subsequently coupled into a coloured FRP in a separate solution. The simultaneous capture technique appears to be the one of choice, as the PRP is combined into the FRP as it is being liberated by enzyme activity, and diffusion of the PRP throughout the tissue or into the incubating medium should be prevented. Post-coupling reactions can give as accurate results if the PRP is insoluble and if the conditions of the histochemical reaction are carefully controlled.

A few histochemical methods for enzymes make use of other types of reaction. A *coloured soluble substrate* can be precipitated at the sites of enzyme activity if the enzyme renders it insoluble. Further developments in enzyme techniques may be possible by the use of colourless substrates that can undergo *molecular rearrangement* into insoluble coloured compounds due to the action of enzymes.

In summary, the successful demonstration of enzymes depends upon many factors. The enzyme must be present in the tissue in a quantity that is greater than the threshold of the technique. The enzyme must not be lost during fixation, processing or cutting of the sections, and the easiest way to ensure that enzyme activity is preserved in the tissue is by the use of fresh frozen cryostat sections. The PRP must be formed in the histochemical technique without serious diffusion or loss and the FRP should be formed at the site of the original enzyme activity. The histologist should be aware of the possibility of false positive reactions due to naturally occurring substances in tissues that are not enzymes, and will control his methods with known positive material, specific inhibitors and 'blanks'. Though these may be seen to be formidable difficulties many techniques have become quick and easy to perform, giving reliable and reproducible results.

METHODS FOR ENZYMES

PHOSPHATASES

ALKALINE PHOSPHATASE

This enzyme, or group of enzymes, hydrolyses a wide variety of mono-orthophosphate eseters in an alkaline medium (pH 9.0). Roche (1950) recommended the term 'phosphomonoesterase I' for alkaline phosphatase. The rate of hydrolysis varies with different substrates, and is increased by the presence of magnesium. There are two important histochemical methods for alkaline phosphatase. The first is a two-stage reaction using glycerophosphate as a substrate in the presence of calcium; calcium phosphate is formed and is subsequently demonstrated by a cobalt substitution technique. This method was originally described by Takamatsu (1938, 1939) and by Gomori (1939). The second method is a simultaneous coupling and capture technique using an incubating medium containing the substrate naphthyl phosphate and a diazonium salt; naphthol is liberated and combines with the diazonium salt to form an insoluble coloured azo-dye (Menten, Junge, and Green 1944; Mannheimer and Seligman 1948). Theoretically the second method should be the better, as the coloured final reaction product is formed as the naphthol is liberated, and is less soluble than the final product (cobalt sulphide) of the first method. However, in practice it is usually found that the results of the two methods are similar. The enzyme is present in many tissues, and kidney or intestine are suitable for positive controls.

The calcium phosphate method for alkaline phosphatase (from Gomori 1952)

Phosphate ions are liberated from the substrate glycerophosphate at pH 9.0 by the enzyme; these are immediately precipitated as calcium phosphate. The calcium is then substituted for cobalt and shown as opaque cobalt sulphide. False positive reactions will be given by calcium that is already present in the tissue, and by any other black pigment (carbon, etc.). Control sections, using distilled water in place of the substrate or destruction of the enzyme activity by heat (do not use fluoride), should be taken through the technique with the test section. Blackening at sites that are not blackened in the control sections can be taken to represent alkaline phosphatase activity.

FIXATION

Use fresh tissue for cryostat sections which may be post-fixed in cold (4 °C) formal-calcium or cold acetone for ten minutes after cutting.

Formal-calcium solution:
Formalin (40 per cent formaldehyde)	10 cm³
Calcium chloride	2 g
Distilled water	90 cm³

Neutralize with marble chips.

Alternatively, thin blocks of tissue (less than 3 mm) should be fixed in formal-calcium at 4 °C for 24 hours and impregnated with gum-sucrose (see below).

SECTIONS

1. Cryostat sections of fresh tissue which may be fixed after cutting (see above).
2. Cryostat sections of formal-calcium fixed tissue blocks which have been impregnated with gum-sucrose. Fix for 24 hours in formal-calcium at 4 °C and transfer to 0.88 M sucrose containing 1 per cent gum acacia at 4 °C for at least 24 hours. Tissues can be left in this for a few days without harm.
3. Paraffin sections (if cryostat is not available). Fix and dehydrate small pieces of tissue 2–3 mm thick in acetone at 4 °C. Clear in two changes of chloroform for ½–1 hour each. Infiltrate with paraffin wax for 15–30 minutes in the vacuum oven. Cut sections at 5 μm and flatten on lukewarm water and mount on albuminized slides.

PREPARATION

Solution A

Sodium barbitone	6.1 g
Calcium chloride (CaCl$_2$)	1.2 g
Magnesium sulphate (MgSO$_4$.7H$_2$O)	0.5 g
Distilled water	1000 cm^3

Keep at 4 °C.

Solution B

One per cent sodium b-glycerophosphate (BDH Ltd., page 503) in distilled water. Keep in the refrigerator.

The working substrate solution is made up of 50 cm^3 of solution A and 30 cm^3 of solution B. The pH should be 9.4; adjust with 0.1 N hydrochloric acid or 0.1 M sodium barbitone if necessary.

TECHNIQUE

1. Incubate for ½–3 hours in freshly prepared working substrate solution at 37 °C. The time required is dependent upon the amount of enzyme activity in the sections.
2. Wash for 3–5 minutes in distilled water.
3. Place slides in 2 per cent aqueous cobalt nitrate for five minutes.
4. Wash in at least three changes of distilled water for a total of 6–8 minutes.
5. Transfer to fresh 1 per cent ammonium sulphide for about one minute.
6. Wash for five minutes in running tap water.
7. Counterstain, if desired, with 0.1 per cent safranin in 0.1 per cent acetic acid.
8. Wash in running water.
9. Mount in glycerol jelly *OR* dehydrate rapidly in alcohol, clear in xylene, and mount in a synthetic resin medium.

RESULTS

Sites of alkaline phosphatase activity—brown to black.
Calcium in the tissue will be blackened.

The azo-dye coupling method for alkaline phosphatase (Pearse's (1968) modification)

The substrate is a solution of alpha-naphthyl phosphate, and contains a diazonium salt. Alpha-naphthol is liberated by the enzyme, and this couples with the diazonium salt to form an insoluble coloured final reaction product.

FIXATION

As for the previous method [p. 303].

SECTIONS

Fresh frozen cryostat sections are mounted on coverslips and allowed to dry; then cover immediately with substrate. Frozen sections of fixed material are cut at 10 μm and mounted on clean slides without adhesive; allow to dry for 1–3 hours. Paraffin sections are brought to water via absolute acetone after the removal of paraffin with light petroleum.

PREPARATION

Dissolve 10–20 mg of sodium alpha-naphthyl phosphate in 20 cm^3 stock 'Tris' buffer [p. 498] at pH 10. (The final pH of the incubating medium is reduced by the addition of the substrate and the diazo-salts.) Add 20 mg of Fast Red TR or Fast Black B and stir well. Prepare this fresh *immediately* before use.

TECHNIQUE

1. Filter the fresh substrate-diazonium salt mixture on to the slides. The solution should not be warmer than 22 °C. Leave for 15–60 minutes. Paraffin sections may require up to 12 hours with Fast Red TR and should be placed in a covered Petri dish to prevent evaporation.
2. Wash in running water for 1–3 minutes.
3. Counterstain in Mayer's haemalum [p. 139] for 1–2 minutes.
4. Wash and blue nuclei in running water for 30–60 minutes.
5. Mount in glycerol jelly.

RESULTS

Sites of alkaline phosphatase activity—brown with Fast Red TR, black with Fast Black B.

ACID PHOSPHATASE

Acid phosphatase (phosphomonoesterase II) splits mono-orthophosphate esters in an acidic medium. The optimum pH is usually around 5.0. It is not activated by magnesium, but is inhibited by fluoride. As with alkaline phosphatase, there are two important techniques for its demonstration. The lead nitrate method (Gomori 1941) demonstrates liberated phosphate as lead sulphide, and is analogous to the calcium phosphate method for alkaline phosphatase. An azo-dye method for phosphatase (Seligman and Manheimer 1949) is also basically similar to the corresponding method for alkaline phosphatase. Neither of these acid phosphatase techniques has been so reliable as those for alkaline phosphatase, and the diazo-technique gave such gross errors and non-specific staining that Gomori (1952) did not recommend it as a satisfactory method; modifications have now made both these techniques less capricious and of approximately equal reliability. The use of substituted naphthol AS phosphate compounds (Burstone 1958) gives sharp localization of the enzyme. Barka's (1960) naphthol AS-B1 phosphate method is a simultaneous coupling technique with substituted naphthols and is described by Bancroft (1975).

The lead nitrate method for acid phosphatase (modified from Gomori 1950)

The enzyme acts upon a substrate of organic phosphate in an incubating medium containing a lead salt. The phosphate that is produced forms lead phosphate as it is liberated; this is subsequently converted by ammonium sulphide into opaque lead sulphide.

FIXATION

Fresh tissue for cryostat sections which may be fixed after cutting in formal-calcium or acetone at 4 °C for ten minutes.

Alternatively, fix in formal-calcium at 4 °C for 24 hours and impregnate with gum-sucrose [p. 304] for cryostat sections.

SECTIONS

Fresh, prefixed, or post-fixed cryostat sections.

PREPARATION

Substrate solution. To 400 cm³ of 0.05 M acetate buffer at pH 5.0 add 0.53 g lead nitrate and 40 cm³ of 3 per cent solution of sodium β-glycerophosphate (BDH Ltd., page 503). Leave at 37 °C for 24 hours and filter.

TECHNIQUE

1. Incubate in the substrate solution at 37 °C for 15–30 minutes (up to four hours if needed).
2. Wash briefly and transfer to dilute (1 per cent or less) fresh ammonium sulphide for 1–2 minutes.
3. Wash and counterstain with 1 per cent aqueous eosin for five minutes.
4. Wash in tap water and distilled water and mount in glycerol jelly.

RESULTS

Sites of acid phosphatase activity—black deposits of lead sulphide.

NOTES

1. The time required in the incubating medium varies with the tissue. A series of sections can be treated and removed at regular intervals to determine the optimum time.
2. Add 0.01 M sodium fluoride to the substrate for the control section.

The azo-dye coupling method for acid phosphatase (Grogg and Pearse 1952; Pearse 1968)

The substrate is α-naphthyl phosphate; acid phosphatase releases α-naphthol, which couples with a diazonium salt to form a coloured azo-dye.

FIXATION

As for previous method.

SECTIONS

Cryostat sections of fresh tissue are mounted on slides or coverslips and allowed to dry. Use unfixed or post-fix.

PREPARATION

Dissolve 10–20 mg of sodium α-naphthyl phosphate in 20 cm³ of 0.1 M hydrochloric acid–veronal buffer mixture (Michaelis) [p. 499] at pH 5.0. Alternatively 0.1 M acetate buffer (Walpole) [p. 496] may be used. Add 1.5 g polyvinyl pyrrolidone and allow to dissolve. Add approximately 20 mg of Fast Garnet GBC salt, or Fast red ITR.

TECHNIQUE

1. Filter the incubating medium on to the sections at 37 °C. Incubating times vary: $\frac{1}{2}$–1 minute for dog prostate, 30–60 minutes for rat liver.
2. Wash in running water for two minutes.
3. Counterstain in Mayer's haemalum, 1–2 minutes.
4. Wash in running water for 30 minutes and mount in glycerol jelly.

RESULTS

Sites of acid phosphatase activity—reddish-brown.
Nuclei—blue.

SPECIFIC PHOSPHATASES

Some phosphatases act upon a single substrate whilst the alkaline and acid phosphatases have a wide range of substrates. Adenosine triphosphatase is a specific phosphatase that hydrolyses adenosine triphosphate and this enzyme can be used for the identification of the different types of voluntary muscle fibres (Dubowitz and Brooke 1973). Glucose-6-phosphatase and 5-nucleotidase are also specific enzymes and methods for these will be described.

Lead method for adenosine triphosphatase
(Wachstein, Meisel, and Niedzwiedz 1960)

ATPase acts upon the substrate adenosine triphosphate to produce phosphate. This combines with lead to form lead phosphate which is converted into lead sulphide by ammonium sulphide. Adenosine triphosphatase is present in cardiac and skeletal muscle, kidney, and prostate.

FIXATION

Use fresh tissue for cryostat sections.

SECTIONS

Cryostat sections.

PREPARATION

Mix together in the following order:

0.125 per cent disodium adenosine triphosphate	20 cm³
0.2 M 'Tris' buffer [p. 498] pH 7.2	20 cm³
2 per cent lead nitrate	3 cm³
2.5 per cent magnesium nitrate	5 cm³
Distilled water	2 cm³

TECHNIQUE

1. Incubate sections in the lead nitrate–substrate medium for 5–60 minutes at 37 °C.
2. Wash in two changes of distilled water for two minutes each.
3. Place in 1 per cent yellow ammonium sulphide for one minute.
4. Wash in distilled water for two minutes.
5. Mount in glycerol jelly.

RESULTS

Sites of ATPase activity—brownish-black.

Lead method for glucose-6-phosphatase (Wachstein and Meisel 1956)

This enzyme is bound to microsomes in tissues such as liver, kidney, and intestinal epithelium. The technique depends on the production of lead phosphate by the enzyme acting upon glucose-6-phosphate in the presence of lead. Dark lead sulphide is then precipitated by ammonium sulphide. The enzyme is found in liver, which can be used as positive control material, but is absent in von Gierke's disease.

FIXATION

Use fresh tissue.

SECTIONS

Cryostat sections 10–15 μm thick.

PREPARATION

Mix together the following:

0.125 per cent potassium glucose-6-phosphate	20 cm³
0.2 M 'Tris' buffer [p. 498] pH 6.7	20 cm³
2 per cent lead nitrate	3 cm³
Distilled water	7 cm³

TECHNIQUE

1. Place fresh cryostat sections in the incubating medium at 37 °C for 5–20 minutes.
2. Wash in two changes of distilled water for two minutes each.
3. Immerse in 1 per cent ammonium sulphide for 1–2 minutes.
4. Wash in distilled water.
5. Mount in glycerol jelly.

RESULTS

Sites of glucose-6-phosphatase activity—brownish-black.

NOTE

To ensure that false-positive results are not produced by non-specific acid or alkaline phosphatases duplicate sections should be treated in the incubating medium containing 20 cm³ of 0.125 per cent sodium β-glycerophosphate in place of the glucose-6-phosphate.

Lead method for 5-nucleotidase (Wachstein and Meisel 1957)

Like the two previous techniques, this is based upon the successive production of phosphate, lead phosphate, and lead sulphide at pH 7.5. The enzyme is present in liver, muscle, and brain.

FIXATION

Use unfixed tissue.

SECTIONS

Cryostat sections.

PREPARATION

Prepare incubating medium freshly before use.

0.125 per cent adenosine-5-monophosphate	20 cm³
0.2 M 'Tris' buffer [p. 498] pH 7.2	20 cm³
3 per cent lead nitrate	3 cm³
0.1 M magnesium sulphate	5 cm³
Distilled water	2.5 cm³

TECHNIQUE

1. Incubate sections for 30–60 minutes at 37 °C.
2. Rinse in two changes of distilled water for two minutes each.
3. Treat with 1 per cent ammonium sulphide for two minutes.
4. Wash well in two changes of distilled water.
5. Mount in glycerol jelly.

RESULTS

Sites of 5-nucleotidase activity—brownish-black.

NOTES

1. Use a duplicate section treated with 0.1 M sodium fluoride, which inhibits 5-nucleotidase, as a negative control.
2. Use a duplicate section in an incubating medium containing a similar concentration of sodium β-glycerophosphate in place of the adenosine-5-monophosphate, as alkaline phosphatases may give false-positive results.

ESTERASES

These are enzymes that hydrolyse esters of carboxylic acids. Each may be able to act upon a number of substrates and many esterases are able to hydrolyse the same substrate such as α-naphthyl acetate. These are known as *non-specific esterases*, and they may be divided into three subgroups according to the type of ester which they optimally hydrolyse—the carboxyl esterases, the aryl esterases, and the acetyl esterases. The most important specific esterases are the *cholinesterases*, of which acetyl cholinesterase ('true') hydrolyses acetylthiocholine and cholinesterase ('pseudo') acts more quickly upon esters of choline. Both are inhibited by eserine, which does not affect the non-specific esterases. It is important to appreciate that the cholinesterases are not highly specific and there is overlap with the non-specific esterases and all these enzymes will hydrolyse α-naphthyl acetate but only the cholinesterases will act upon acetylthiocholine or esters of choline. Another group of esterases is the *lipases* which hydrolyse long-chain fatty acid esters; these are also capable of hydrolysing simple esters. Histochemical methods for non-specific esterases, and the more specific cholinesterases and lipases will be described; the cholinesterases and lipases will also give positive results with the techniques for non-specific esterases. A review of the problems of identifying esterases and the diagnostic significance of esterase histochemistry has been given by Deimling and Bockling (1976).

NON-SPECIFIC ESTERASES

The α-naphthyl acetate method for non-specific esterases (after Gomori 1952)

Esterases liberate α-naphthol from the substrate and this is coupled with an azo-dye to form an insoluble coloured compound. Small intestine, liver, and kidney are suitable as positive control tissue.

FIXATION

Use fresh tissue, or formal-calcium at 4 °C [p. 303], for cryostat sections.

SECTIONS

Cryostat sections are preferred. Carefully processed paraffin sections of acetone-fixed tissue.

PREPARATION

Dissolve 10 mg of α-naphthyl acetate in 0.25 cm³ of acetone. Thoroughly mix with 20 cm³ of phosphate buffer [p. 495] pH 7.4. Add 20 mg of Fast Blue B salt. Filter onto the section and use immediately.

TECHNIQUE

1. Place sections in the incubating medium at room temperature for up to ten minutes. Cryostat sections may only require a few minutes.
2. Wash in several changes of distilled water.
3. Mount in glycerol jelly.

RESULT

Sites of esterase activity—purple.

NOTE

The use of pararosanilin hydrochloride [p. 313] in place of Fast Blue B (Davis and Ornstein 1959) may give more precise localization of the enzyme and has the added advantage that sections can be rapidly dehydrated, cleared, and mounted in a synthetic mounting medium.

The indoxyl acetate method for non-specific esterases
(Holt and Withers 1952)

In this technique the enzyme hydrolyses bromoindoxylacetate to form bromo-indoxyl. This is oxidized by potassium ferricyanide to insoluble indigo.

FIXATION

Use fresh tissues, or formal-calcium at 4 °C [p. 303], for cryostat sections.

SECTIONS

Cryostat sections.

PREPARATION

1. Dissolve 1.3 mg of 5-bromoindoxylacetate in 1 cm³ absolute ethyl alcohol.
2. Dissolve and mix

0.2 M 'Tris' buffer [p. 498] pH 7.2	2 cm³
Potassium ferricyanide	17 mg
Potassium ferrocyanide	21 mg
Calcium chloride	11 mg
Distilled water	7.9 cm³

Mix solutions 1 and 2 together and use immediately.

TECHNIQUE

1. Incubate sections in the incubating solution at 37 °C for 15–60 minutes.
2. Rinse in tap water.

3. Counterstain in carmalum [p. 428] for five minutes.
4. Rinse in tap water.
5. Mount in glycerol jelly *OR* dehydrate in alcohol, clear in xylene, and mount in a synthetic resin medium.

RESULTS

Sites of esterase activity—blue.
Nuclei—red.

CHOLINESTERASES

There are two types of cholinesterase: true or acetyl cholinesterase and pseudo-cholinesterase. Their actions have considerable histochemical similarity but their distribution differs. Acetyl cholinesterase is the most important enzyme in the nervous system, muscle, and red cells; pseudo-cholinesterase is found in many glands. The motor end-plates of muscles can be well demonstrated by the following method, due to the high concentration of acetyl cholinesterase. It is also possible to combine an acetylthiocholine iodide technique for motor end-plates with silver staining of nerves and nerve endings; the method of Beerman and Cassens (1976) demonstrates the intramuscular nerve, its subterminal axons, and the motor end-plate.

The thiocholine method for cholinesterases
(Koelle 1951; modified by Gomori 1952)

Both cholinesterases will hydrolyse acetylthiocholine and the free thiocholine is precipitated as its cupric salt.

FIXATION

Fresh unfixed tissue for cryostat sections or squashed or teased preparations. Cold formal-calcium fixation (up to 24 hours at 4 °C) for cryostat sections.

SECTIONS

Cryostat sections of fresh material or cold formal-calcium fixed tissue.

PREPARATION

Stock solution

Copper sulphate ($CuSO_4.5H_2O$)	0.3 g
Glycine	0.375g
Magnesium chloride ($MgCl_2.6H_2O$)	1.0 g
Maleic acid	1.75 g
N (4 per cent) sodium hydroxide	30 cm^3
Hot saturated (about 40 per cent) Na_2SO_4	170 cm^3

This solution keeps indefinitely though some sodium sulphate may crystallize out; this does not affect results.

For use, dissolve 20 mg acetylthiocholine iodide in a few drops of distilled water. Add 10 cm^3 of the stock solution.

TECHNIQUE

1. Incubate sections for 10–60 minutes in the incubating medium at 37 °C (30 minutes is usually satisfactory).
2. Rinse in two or three changes of saturated aqueous sodium sulphate.

3. Place in 2 per cent ammonium sulphide for two minutes.
4. Rinse in distilled water.
5. Mount in glycerol jelly *or* counterstain if required and dehydrate, clear, and mount in a synthetic resin medium.

RESULTS

Sites of enzyme activity—dark brown (cupric sulphide).

LIPASES

Commercial detergents known as the Tweens can be used as substrates, and a large number of these fatty acid esters (saturated stearic acid ester, Tween 60; saturated palmitic acid ester, Tween 40; unsaturated oleic acid ester, Tween 80; etc.) are available. The saturated compounds are satisfactory substrates for lipases of many organs, the unsaturated compounds being attacked only by pancreatic lipase. The longer-chained esters (stearates) are commonly used as they yield a finer precipitate that gives more accurate localization than the short-chain esters such as the laurates.

The Tween technique for lipases (Gomori 1945)

Fatty acids produced by enzyme action upon the substrate are precipitated as calcium salts; these are converted into lead salts and demonstrated as lead sulphide. There is a similarity to Gomori's alkaline phosphatase technique.

FIXATION

Ice-cold acetone for paraffin sections. Ice-cold formal-calcium for cryostat sections.
Lipases are not destroyed by fixation.

SECTIONS

Paraffin or cryostat sections.

PREPARATION

Stock solutions
1. 5 per cent Tween 60 (stearic acid ester) or Tween 40 (palmitic acid ester).
2. 0.5 M 'Tris' buffer at pH 7.3 [p. 498].
3. 10 per cent calcium chloride.

To prepare the incubating medium, mix 5 cm³ of buffer solution with 2 cm³ calcium chloride solution and 2 cm³ Tween solution; add 40 cm³ of distilled water.

TECHNIQUE

1. Incubate sections, mounted on slides, in the above medium for 3–12 hours at 37 °C.
2. Wash in distilled water.
3. Place in 1 per cent lead nitrate for 15 minutes at 55 °C.
4. Wash in running water for five minutes.
5. Treat with 1 per cent ammonium sulphide for one minute.
6. Counterstain (with eosin, red nuclear stain, or haematoxylin), wash, and mount in glycerol jelly.

RESULTS

Lipase activity—brownish-black.

NOTE

Use a duplicate section as a control in an incubating solution without Tween. Also use a positive control section of pancreas.

β-GLUCURONIDASE

This is a hydrolytic enzyme which acts at acid pH on glucosiduronic acids. It is associated with lysosomes of the epithelial cells of the kidney, endometrium, and other organs.

The naphthol AS–BI method for β-glucuronidase (Hayashi, Nakajima, and Fishman 1964)

This is a simultaneous coupling technique in which the enzyme releases the primary reaction product naphthol AS–BI from the substrate naphthol AS–BI glucuronide; the PRP is then coupled with hexazotized pararosanalin.

FIXATION

Thin blocks should be fixed in formal-calcium for 24 hours at 4 °C and impregnated with gum-sucrose [p. 304]. Alternatively, fresh frozen cryostat sections can be fixed for ten minutes in formal-calcium or acetone after cutting.

SECTIONS

Cryostat sections.

PREPARATION

1. Substrate solution.
   Dissolve 28 mg naphthol AS–BI glucuronide in 1.2 cm^3 of 0.42 per cent sodium bicarbonate. Make up to 100 cm^3 with 0.1 M acetate buffer (p. 496) pH 5.0.
2. Pararosanalin-HCl stock solution.
   Dissolve 1 g pararosanalin hydrochloride in 20 cm^3 distilled water and 5 cm^3 of conc. hydrochloric acid. Heat gently, cool, and filter.
3. Incubating medium.
   Add 0.3 cm^3 of freshly prepared 4 per cent sodium nitrite in distilled water to 0.3 cm^3 of the stock pararosanalin solution. After one minute, add this just before use to 10 cm^3 of substrate solution. Adjust the pH to 5.12 with N NaOH, make up to 20 cm^3 with distilled water, and filter.

TECHNIQUE

1. Incubate sections in the incubating medium at 37 °C for 20–60 minutes.
2. Wash well in distilled water.
3. Counterstain, if required, in 2 per cent methyl green (chloroform washed) for four minutes.
4. Wash quickly in tap water.
5. Dehydrate in alcohol, clear in xylene, and mount in a synthetic resin medium.

RESULTS

Sites of glucuronidase activity—red.
Nuclei—green.

OXIDASES AND PEROXIDASES

The oxidoreductase enzymes oxidize substrates and they can do this in two main ways. The oxidases catalyse a reaction between the substrate and oxygen; the dehydrogenases [p. 318] remove hydrogen from the substrate and transfer it to a hydrogen receptor.

OXIDASES

Oxidases are widely distributed in animal tissues and methods for cytochrome oxidase, DOPA-oxidase, monoamine oxidase, and peroxidases will be described.

The 'nadi' reaction for cytochrome oxidase (after Moog 1943)

Cytochrome oxidase catalyses the oxidative reaction between α-naphthol and dimethyl-*p*-phenylenediamine, forming indophenol blue. This is known as the 'nadi' reaction.

FIXATION

Use unfixed fresh tissue.

SECTIONS

Cut fresh frozen sections on the cryostat. Deliver the sections from the knife into freshly prepared 'nadi' reagent.

PREPARATION

Make up a 0.1 per cent solution of α-naphthol in 1 per cent sodium chloride and M/15 phosphate buffer at pH 5.8 [p. 495].

Prepare a fresh 0.1 per cent solution of dimethyl-*p*-phenylenediamine hydrochloride in 1 per cent sodium chloride and M/15 phosphate buffer at pH 5.8.

Immediately before use prepare the 'nadi' reagent by mixing equal parts of these two solutions.

TECHNIQUE

1. Incubate the fresh sections in the newly-prepared 'nadi' reagent at 37 °C. Five minutes may be sufficient, but up to one hour may be required.
2. Wash in 0.9 per cent sodium chloride in distilled water.
3. If required, counterstain nuclei in carmalum or other red nuclear stain.
4. Mount in 5 per cent potassium acetate in water and ring the coverslip with paraffin wax. The preparations are not permanent.

RESULTS

Sites of cytochrome activity—bluish-violet.
Nuclei—red.

NOTE

Use pre-treatment with 0.1 per cent potassium cyanide solution for a few minutes as a control, which abolishes the 'nadi' reaction.

The metal chelation method for cytochrome oxidase (Burstone 1959)

In this method the primary reaction product is a naphthol compound which combines with a phenylenediamine; this secondary reaction product is chelated to cobalt to form a well localized colour reaction which demonstrates mitochondria and may be more specific than the 'nadi' reaction.

FIXATION

Unfixed tissue for cryostat sections.

SECTIONS

Cryostat sections.

PREPARATION

1. Dissolve 10 mg of *N*-phenyl-*p*-phenylenediamine and 10 mg of 1-hydroxy-2-acetonaphthone in 0.5 cm³ of absolute ethyl alcohol. Add 35 cm³ of distilled water and 15 cm³ of 0.2 M 'Tris' buffer [p. 498] pH 7.4. Shake and filter.
2. Dissolve 5 g of cobalt acetate in 45 cm³ of distilled water and add 5 cm³ of conc. formaldehyde.

TECHNIQUE

1. Place sections in incubating solution (number 1, above) for 15 minutes to two hours.
2. Transfer to the 10 per cent cobalt acetate solution (number 2, above) for one hour.
3. Wash in distilled water.
4. Mount in glycerol jelly.

RESULT

Cytochrome oxidase activity—blue-black.

The dopa-oxidase (tyrosinase) reaction (Becker, Praver and Thatcher 1935)

Dihydroxyphenylalanine (DOPA) was thought to be a precursor of melanin, and it was assumed that DOPA-oxidase converted it into melanin; sites of DOPA-oxidase activity were considered to be sites of melanin formation. It seems more probable that the enzyme demonstrated by the DOPA reaction is a tyrosinase that converts tyrosine into DOPA and then to melanin.

FIXATION

Fresh tissue for cryostat sections which may be post-fixed in formalin. Alternatively, formalin fixation for frozen or cryostat sections.

SECTIONS

Cryostat or frozen sections.

PREPARATION

100 mg of DL.3:4-dihydroxyphenylalanine (DOPA) in 100 cm³ of 0.1 M phosphate buffer [p. 495] pH 7.4.

TECHNIQUE

1. Wash frozen sections briefly in distilled water.
2. Place sections in incubating solution at 37 °C for 45 minutes.
3. Change to a fresh incubating solution at 37 °C for at least two hours.
4. Wash in running tap water.

5. Sections may be counterstained in carmalum [p. 428] and washed in water.
6. Dehydrate in alcohol, clear in xylene, and mount in a synthetic resin medium.

RESULTS

Sites of DOPA-oxidase (tyrosinase) activity—dark brown granules.
Nuclei—red.

Tetrazolium method for monoamine oxidase (Glenner, Burtner, and Brown 1957)

Monoamine oxidase acts on short chain monoamines and reacts quickly with adrenalin and 5-hydroxytryptamine. In this technique the enzyme oxidizes the tryptamine of the incubating solution and the primary reaction product reduces the tetrazolium salt to a black formazan compound. Liver and kidney are suitable positive control tissues.

FIXATION

Fresh tissue for cryostat sections.

SECTIONS

Cryostat sections 8–16 μm thick.

PREPARATION

The incubating solution is made of 25 mg tryptamine hydrochloride, 4 mg sodium sulphate, 5 mg tetranitro-blue tetrazolium (TNBT), 5 cm^3 0.1 M phosphate buffer [p. 495] pH 7.6, and 15 cm^3 distilled water.

TECHNIQUE

1. Place sections in incubating solution at 37 °C for 45 minutes.
2. Wash in running tap water for two minutes.
3. Place sections in 10 per cent formal-saline for 30 minutes.
4. Wash well in tap water.
5. Mount in glycerol jelly.

RESULT

Sites of monoamine oxidase activity—bluish-black.

PEROXIDASES

The leuco-dye method for haemoglobin peroxidase (Lison 1938; Dunn and Thompson 1946)

Haemoglobin peroxidase is a relatively stable enzyme and will withstand fixation in formalin for not more than 48 hours. Patent Blue is reduced to a colourless leuco-dye by nascent hydrogen, and this is oxidized to the coloured dye by peroxide in the presence of peroxidase.

FIXATION

Thin blocks are fixed in neutral 10 per cent formalin for 24–48 hours.

SECTIONS

Paraffin sections.

PREPARATION

To 100 cm³ of 1 per cent aqueous Patent Blue V (acid blue 3, CI 42051) add 10 g of powdered zinc and 2 cm³ glacial acetic acid. Boil until colourless. Cool and filter. This is stable in a tightly stoppered bottle.

Immediately before use take 10 cm³ of stock solution, add 2 cm³ of glacial acetic acid and 1 cm³ of 3 per cent hydrogen peroxide.

TECHNIQUE

1. Bring sections to water.
2. Stain in the leuco-blue–peroxide reagent for 3–5 minutes.
3. Rinse in water.
4. Counterstain in 0.1 per cent safranin or other red nuclear stain for ½–1 minute.
5. Rinse in water.
6. Dehydrate, clear, and mount in a synthetic resin medium.

RESULTS

Haemoglobin—dark blue.
Oxidase granules—dark blue.
Nuclei—red.

The diaminobenzidine method for peroxidase (Graham and Karnovsky 1966)

The benzidine reaction for peroxidase (Villamil and Mancini 1947) has been a standard method, but the recognition of the carcinogenic properties of benzidine has led to the use of benzidine substitutes. Diaminobenzidine has been thought to act in a similar way; when peroxidases catalyse the transfer of oxygen from hydrogen peroxide, diaminobenzidine acts as a hydrogen donor forming an insoluble coloured polymer.

FIXATION

Formal-glutaraldehyde was recommended, but although this is important for electron microscopy formal-calcium can be used for light microscopy.

SECTIONS

Cryostat sections.

PREPARATION

Make a saturated solution of 3:3 diaminobenzidine tetrahydrochloride in 10 cm³ of 0.2 M 'Tris' buffer [p. 498] pH 7.6 and add 0.1 cm³ of 1 per cent hydrogen peroxide.

TECHNIQUE

1. Rinse sections in distilled water.
2. Place in the incubating medium at room temperature for five minutes.
3. Wash in three changes of distilled water.
4. Counterstain, if required, in 2 per cent methyl green (chloroform washed) for five minutes; wash in distilled water.
5. Dehydrate in alcohol, clear in xylene, and mount in a synthetic resin medium.

RESULTS

Sites of peroxidase activity—fine brownish granules.
Nuclei—green.

DEHYDROGENASES AND DIAPHORASES

The dehydrogenases remove hydrogen from the substrate, transferring it to a hydrogen acceptor. The hydrogen acceptor can be NAD (nicotinamide adenine dinucleotide or co-enzyme 1, formerly known as DPN), or NADP (nicotinamide adenine nucleotide phosphate or co-enzyme 2, formerly known as TPN), or a flavoprotein, or the dehydrogenase itself. Dehydrogenases can act under anaerobic conditions whereas the oxidases need oxygen and are aerobic. The diaphorases are dehydrogenases which remove hydrogen from reduced NAD or NADP (NADH → NAD + H).

It is now possible to demonstrate a large number of specific dehydrogenases and two diaphorases and an important feature of these enzyme techniques is that they use the specific natural substrate, whilst in most other enzyme histochemical reactions an unnatural substrate is employed. The reaction is therefore similar to that taking place *in vivo*. The basis of these enzyme reactions is the transfer of hydrogen from the substrate to a tetrazolium salt which is used as the hydrogen acceptor and is converted into a coloured formazan compound in the process. The following equation gives the chemical changes that take place when a colourless tetrazolium salt is reduced to a coloured compound.

$$C_6H_5.C\underset{Cl'}{\overset{\nearrow N-N-}{\underset{\searrow N=N^+}{}}} + 2H = C_6H_5.C\overset{\nearrow N-NH-}{\underset{\searrow N=N-}{}} + HCl$$

$$\text{(Colourless)} \qquad\qquad \text{(Coloured formazan)}$$

The dehydrogenases and diaphorases are now usually demonstrated by histochemical methods using the easily reduced tetrazolium salts MTT* and Nitro-BT†.

A basic method for dehydrogenases and diaphorases, using these tetrazolium salts, is applicable to enzymes which are 'bound' and do not diffuse. These include succinate and α-glycerophosphate dehydrogenases and NADH and NADPH diaphorases; β-hydroxybutyrate and glutamate dehydrogenases diffuse only slowly and can be regarded as insoluble if the incubation period is short.

Standard method for dehydrogenases and diaphorases (Pearse 1972)

This method is suitable for the following 'bound' enzymes which do not diffuse to a significant extent:

Succinate ⎫
β-Hydroxybutyrate ⎪
Glutamate ⎬ dehydrogenase
α-Glycerophosphate ⎭

NADH ⎫
NADPH ⎬ diaphorase

The rationale of the technique has been described above.

---

* 3-(4,5-Dimethylthiazolyl-2)-2,5-diphenyltetrazolium bromide.

† 2.2′-Di-*p*-nitrophenyl-5,5′ diphenyl-3,3′-(3,3′-dimethoxy)-4,4′ diphenylene ditetrazolium chloride.

FIXATION

Unfixed tissue for cryostat sections.

SECTIONS

Cryostat sections at 5 μm.

PREPARATION

The substrates and the tetrazolium solutions can be prepared and kept as stock solutions according to the following tables.

1. Stock substrate solutions.

These are made up in 8 cm³ of distilled water, neutralized to pH 7.0 with N HCl and made up to 10 cm³ with distilled water. Store at −20 °C, they will keep for several months.

Table 16.2 Stock substrate solutions

Dehydrogenase	Substrate	Amount for 10 cm³ (g)
Succinate	Disodium succinate	6.75
β-Hydroxybutyrate	Sodium-D-3-hydroxybutyrate	1.27
Glutamate	Sodium-L-glutamate (monohydrate)	1.87
α-Glycerophosphate	Disodium-α-glycerol-3-phosphate	3.15

2. Stock tetrazolium solutions.

The following stock solutions should be pH 7.0 to 7.2; adjust if necessary with the 'Tris' buffer solution or with 0.2 M HCl. Store at −20 °C; they will keep for several months.

Table 16.3 Stock tetrazolium solutions

	With MTT	With Nitro-BT
Tetrazolium salt	5 mg MTT	10 mg NBT
'Tris' buffer (pH 7.4) [p. 498]	2.5 cm³	2.5 cm³
Cobalt chloride (50 mM)	0.5 cm³	—
Magnesium chloride (5 mM)	1.0 cm³	1.0 cm³
Distilled water	5.0 cm³	5.0 cm³

3. Preparation of incubating solutions.

Make up the incubating solutions from the stock solutions according to Table 16.4. Note that in the diaphorase techniques the reduced co-enzyme is the substrate. Add the co-enzymes just before use.

TECHNIQUE

1. Mount cryostat sections on coverslips.

Table 16.4 Final incubating solutions

	Enzyme	Vol. of stock substrate (cm³)	Vol. of stock tetrazolium (cm³)	Vol. of distilled water (cm³)	Co-enzyme
Dehydrogenases	Succinate	0.1	0.9	—	—
	β-Hydroxybutyrate	0.1	0.9	—	2 mg NAD
	Glutamate	0.1	0.9	—	2 mg NAD or NADP
	α-Glycerophosphate	0.1	0.9*	—	—
Diaphorases	NADH	—	0.9	0.1	2 mg NADH
	NADPH	—	0.9	0.1	2 mg NADPH

* Stock solution should be saturated with vitamin K_3 (menadione) (see Pearse 1972).

2. Cover sections with incubating medium at 37 °C (about 0.2 cm³ is enough) for 10–60 minutes.
3. Pour off the incubating medium and place in 15 per cent formal-saline for 15 minutes.
4. Wash in distilled water.
5. Counterstain, if required. With MTT, use 2 per cent methyl green (chloroform washed) for 2–5 minutes. With Nitro-BT use carmalum [p. 428].
6. Wash in distilled water.
7. Mount in glycerol jelly (MTT) or dehydrate in alcohol, clear in xylene, and mount in a synthetic resin medium.

RESULTS

Sites of the enzyme activity—black (MTT) or purple (Nitro-BT).
Nuclei—green (MTT), red (Nitro-BT).

PEPTIDASES

The peptidases hydrolyse $-CO-NH-$ linkages, and leucine aminopeptidase hydrolyses a number of peptides that have a free amino group on leucine or a related amino-acid. It can be found in the kidney and small intestine. Leucine aminopeptidase has a broad specificity for leucyl compounds and will split leucinamide; because of this action leucyl-β-naphthylamide is used as the substrate.

Method for leucine aminopeptidase (Nachlas, Crawford, and Seligman 1957)

This is a simultaneous coupling reaction. The incubating medium contains the substrate L-leucyl-β-naphthylamide and a diazonium salt (Fast Blue B). The enzyme frees β-naphthylamine which couples with diazo-compound to produce a coloured insoluble final reaction product. If copper ions are added, after incubation, to the β-naphthylamine–Fast blue B compound, it forms a stable purple-blue copper chelate.

FIXATION

Use *fresh* tissue only.

SECTIONS

Cut cryostat sections 5–10 μm thick and mount on coverslips. Allow to dry in air and cover immediately with the incubating medium.

PREPARATION

Stock substrate solution
Dissolve 8 mg per cm³ of L-leucyl-β-naphthylamide in distilled water. (This can be stored at 0–4 °C for several months.)

Incubating medium

Stock substrate solution	1 cm³
0.1 M acetate buffer pH 6.5 [p. 497]	10 cm³
Sodium chloride (0.85 per cent)	8 cm³
Potassium cyanide (0.02 M)	1 cm³
Fast blue B salt	10 mg

Check pH and adjust to 6.5–6.8.

TECHNIQUE

1. Cover sections with incubating medium.
2. Incubate at 37 °C for 15 minutes to two hours.
3. Drain off incubating medium, rinse with saline, and leave in this for two minutes.
4. Flood section with 0.1 M cupric sulphate (1.6 per cent); leave for two minutes.
5. Rinse in saline.
6. Dehydrate in ethyl alcohol, clear in xylene, and mount in a synthetic resin medium.

RESULTS

Sites of leucine aminopeptidase activity—purplish-blue.

REFERENCES

BANCROFT, J. D. (1975). *Histochemical techniques*, 2nd edn. Butterworths, London.
BARKA, T. (1960). *Nature (Lond.)* **187**, 248.
BECKER, S. W., PRAVER, L. L., and THATCHER, H. (1935). *Arch. Derm. Syph. (Chic.)* **31**, 190.
BEERMAN, D. H. and CASSENS, R. G. (1976). *Stain Technol.* **51**, 173.
BURSTONE, M. S. (1958). *J. nat. Cancer Inst.* **21**, 523.
—— (1959). *J. Histochem. Cytochem.* **7**, 112.
CHAYEN, J., BITENSKY, L., and BUTCHER, R. G. (1973) *Practical histochemistry*. John Wiley, London.
DAVIS, B. J. and ORNSTEIN, L. (1959). *J. Histochem. Cytochem.* **7**, 297.
DEIMLING, O. V. and BOCKLING, A. (1976). *Histochem. J.* **8**, 215.
DUBOWITZ, V. and BROOKE, M. H. (1973). *Muscle biopsy, a modern approach*. W. B. Saunders, London.
DUNN, R. C. and THOMPSON, E. C. (1946). *Stain Technol.* **21**, 65.
GLENNER, G. G., BURTNER, H. J., and BROWN, G. W. (1957). *J. Histochem. Cytochem.* **5**, 591.
GOMORI, G. (1939). *Proc. Soc. exp. Biol. (N.Y.)* **42**, 23.
—— (1941). *Arch. Path.* **32**, 189.

GOMORI, G. (1945). *Proc. Soc. exp. Biol. (N.Y.)* **58**, 362.

—— (1950). *Stain Technol.* **25**, 81.

—— (1952). *Microscopic histochemistry.* Chicago University Press.

GRAHAM, R. C. and KARNOVSKY, M. J. (1966). *J. Histochem. Cytochem.* **14**, 291.

GROGG, E. and PEARSE, A. G. E. (1952). *J. Path. Bact.* **64**, 627.

HAYASHI, M., NAKAJIMA, Y., and FISHMAN, W. H. (1964). *J. Histochem. Cytochem.* **12**, 293.

HOLT, S. J. and WITHERS, R. F. J. (1952). *Nature (Lond.)* **170**, 1012.

KOELLE, G. B. (1951). *J. Pharmacol. exp. Ther.* **103**, 153.

LISON, L. (1938). *Beitr. path. Anat.* **101**, 94.

—— (1953). *Histochimie et cytochimie animales*, 2nd edn. Gauthier-Villars, Paris.

MANHEIMER, L. H. and SELIGMAN, A. M. (1948). *J. nat. Cancer Inst.* **9**, 181.

MENTEN, M. L., JUNGE, J. and GREEN, M. H. (1944). *J. biol. Chem.* **153**, 471.

MOOG, F. (1943). *J. Cell comp. Physiol.* **22**, 223.

NACHLAS, M. M., CRAWFORD, D. T., and SELIGMAN, A. M. (1957). *J. Histochem. Cytochem.* **5**, 264.

NIEMI, M. and KORHONEN, L. K. (1972). *Int. Path.* **13**, 11.

PEARSE, A. G. E. (1968). *Histochemistry, theoretical and applied*, 3rd edn., Vol. 1. Churchill, London.

—— (1972). *Histochemistry, theoretical and applied*, 3rd edn., Vol. 2. Churchill Livingstone, London.

ROCHE, J. (1950). In *The enzymes* (eds. J. B. Sumner and K. Myrbäck). Academic Press, New York.

RUTENBERG, A. M. and SELIGMAN, A. M. (1955). *J. Histochem. Cytochem.* **3**, 455.

SELIGMAN, A. M. and MANHEIMER, L. H. (1949). *J. nat. Cancer Inst.* **9**, 427.

TAKAMATSU, H. (1938). *Manshu Igaku Zasshi* **31**, 34.

—— (1939). *Trans. Soc. path. (Japan)* **29**, 492.

VILLAMIL, M. F. and MANCINI, R. E. (1947). *Rev. Soc. argent. Biol.* **23**, 215.

WACHSTEIN, M. and MEISEL, E. (1956). *J. Histochem. Cytochem.* **4**, 592.

—— —— (1957). *Am. J. clin. Path.* **27**, 13.

—— —— and NIEDZWIEDZ, A. (1960). *J. Histochem. Cytochem.* **8**, 387.

WIED, G. L. (1966). *Introduction to quantitative cytochemistry.* Academic Press, New York.

—— and BAHR, G. F. (1970). *Introduction to quantitative cytochemistry*, Vol. II. Academic Press, New York.

ZUGIBE, F. T. (1970). *Diagnostic histochemistry.* C. V. Mosby, St. Louis.

17 | Immunohistology

The demonstration of specific antigens and antibodies in tissue sections, and the localization of the exact sites of antigen–antibody reactions, have now become possible. As these are so small they cannot be demonstrated by conventional staining methods but their presence can be shown and categorized accurately in the tissue by the use of *markers*. These markers are of two main types: firstly *fluorescent dyes* and secondly *enzymes*.

FLUORESCENT IMMUNOHISTOLOGICAL TECHNIQUES

The fluorescent antibody techniques were developed by Coons and his colleagues (Coons, Creech, and Jones 1941; Coons, Creech, Jones, and Berliner 1942) and the basis of these methods depends upon the fact that it is possible to conjugate antibodies (antisera) with a fluorescent dye, whilst leaving their capacity of combining with an antigen unchanged. Coons combined antibodies with fluorescein isocyanate, thus producing a fluorescent antibody compound [Fig. 17.1].

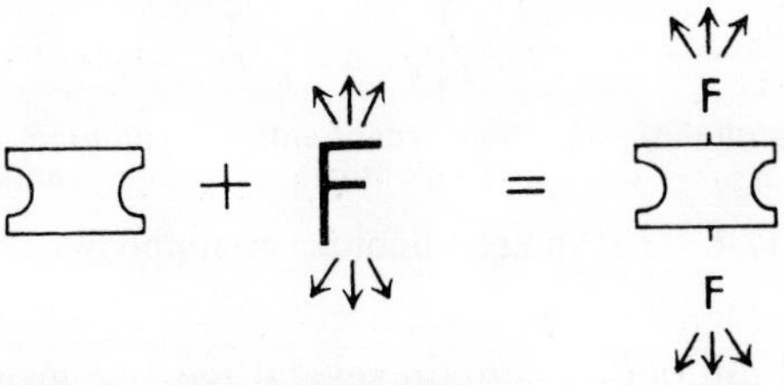

Fig. 17.1.   Conjugation of fluorescent antibody.

A section of the tissue under investigation was treated with this fluorescent antibody compound and after fluorescent antibodies had combined with all the corresponding antigens in the tissue the excess fluorescent antibody was washed off. When examined with a fluorescence microscope the sites of antigen–antibody reaction were seen as bright green fluorescence given off by the antibody [Fig. 17.2]. The principles of the fluorescence microscope and fluorescence microscopy are described in Chapter 2 [p. 22].

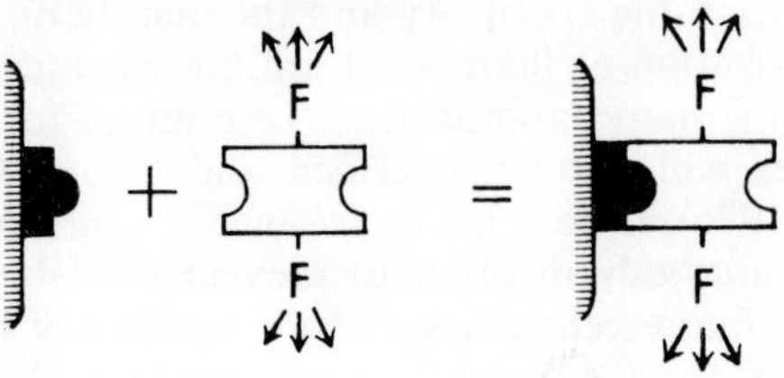

        (cell, antigen)   (fluorescent antibody)   (fluorescent antibody—
                                                          antigen reaction)
Fig. 17.2.   Demonstration of antigens with fluorescent antibody.

Fluorescein isocyanate has now been largely replaced by fluorescein and rhodamine B isothiocyanates (Riggs, Seiwald, Burckhalter, Downs, and Metcalf 1958) which are more intense, giving up to three times more fluorescence, and are easier to prepare. Another fluorescent compound used in the preparation of fluorescent antibodies is DANSYL (1-dimethylamino-naphthalene-5-sulphonyl chloride) which also gives a green fluorescence.

The direct application of fluorescent antibodies to tissue demonstrates antigens, and it might be expected that fluorescent antigens would be used for the demonstration of antibodies. This is impractical, as antigens contain larger numbers of immunologically active groups and are much less sensitive. Antibody sites can be visualized by the use of a multiple layer or sandwich technique (Weller and Coons 1954). In this, the antibodies in the tissue are first supplied with non-fluorescent antigens, and these antigens are then demonstrated with fluorescent antibody in the same way as has been described. Indirect fluorescent antibody techniques are widely used in immunohistology, fluorescent anti-gamma globulin being attached to gamma globulin that has become bound to antigenic sites [FIG. 17.3].

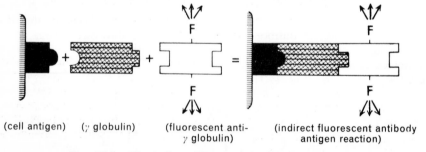

(cell antigen)   (γ globulin)   (fluorescent anti-γ globulin)   (indirect fluorescent antibody antigen reaction)

FIG. 17.3. The indirect fluorescent antibody technique.

As antigens and antibodies contain several reactive groups it is possible to build up successive layers of antigen–antibody–antigen–antibody, etc., each layer becoming larger than the last. This 'sandwich' technique increases the amount of the fluorescence in the final preparation and makes the investigation more sensitive.

With these methods it has become possible to determine the sites of many immunological processes in tissues [FIG. 17.4]. The techniques are now well developed and can be used in routine laboratories, and reliable fluorescent antisera are widely available commercially. The success of the technique is largely dependent upon the specificity and the quality of the fluorescent antibody, and the preparation of fluorescent antibody conjugates is complex and beyond the scope of many laboratories. Techniques for the preparation of antibody conjugates will not be described and details are given by Pearse (1968) and Nairn (1976). Care must be taken in the preparation and purification of fluorescent antibody in order to prevent the labelling of non-specific antibodies with the fluorescent marker. New batches of fluorescent antibody should be tested for specificity and sensitivity before being taken into use. Fluorescent antibody should be tested by specific absorption with the specific antigen; fluorescent staining does not take place if a satisfactory conjugate has been absorbed in this way. Absorption with different antigens (non-specific

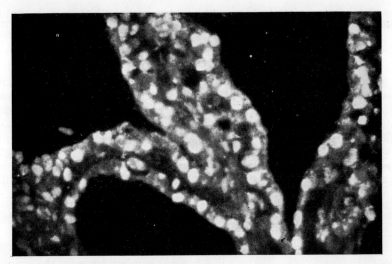

FIG. 17.4. Demonstration of anti-nuclear factor by the indirect fluorescent antibody technique. Human thyroid. × 525.

absorption) should have no effect on the staining properties of the fluorescent antibody. In a similar manner, sections for the direct technique may be controlled by absorption of reactive antigen in the tissues with unconjugated (not fluorescent) antisera, after which the fluorescent antibody should produce no staining reaction. This is the blocking technique, and a non-specific blocking test with non-specific serum should have no effect on the subsequent staining reaction of the fluorescent antibody.

When fluorescent antibody techniques are being carried out in the laboratory, control sections must be prepared in parallel with the test sections; blanks using buffer or saline instead of fluorescent antibody and known positive and negative control specimens should be put through at the same time. These controls, together with the scrupulous removal by careful washing of all ununited fluorescent antibody, should make the results of fluorescent antibody reactions reliable, but it must be appreciated that fluorescent labelling of non-specific antibodies and false reactions in tissues are difficult to prevent and there may always be auto-fluorescence in tissues. A critical approach to the method and to its results is always necessary.

The success of the fluorescent antibody techniques is dependent upon the high degree of contrast that can be obtained. Although the amount of fluorescence is small, it shows brightly against a dark background when observed with the fluorescence microscope in a dark room; the site of the fluorescence can be localized precisely under high magnification. Specimens can be photographed but need long exposures as the total amount of light coming from the specimen is very small in comparison with that of a stained section examined by normal transmitted illumination. Fluorescent antibodies techniques are not applicable to electron microscopy. In histopathology, these methods are widely used for the detection of antigen–antibody complexes in tissues such as renal glomeruli and also for the demonstration of auto-antibodies in sera [p. 331].

The direct and indirect fluorescent antibody techniques

The general features of the two methods will be described, and the indirect technique is given on page 332.

FIXATION

Use unfixed fresh tissues for cryostat sections. Dorsett and Ioachim (1978) have obtained satisfactory results using paraffin sections of tissues fixed in Bouin's solution at room temperature for 6–8 hours. Formalin-fixed tissue is not suitable, but can be used for the immunoperoxidase technique [p. 328].

SECTIONS

Use cryostat sections of fresh tissues. Paraffin sections after Bouin's fixation (see above) and freeze-dried tissue embedded in polyester or other waxes have been employed. Sections must be as thin as possible to determine the localization of the induced fluorescence.

TECHNIQUE

The direct technique
Cut cryostat sections and dry in a stream of warm air. Cover with appropriate fluorescent antiserum in a humid chamber; leave for the optimum time at room temperature or 37 °C; the antiserum may require dilution before use. Wash off all excess unattached fluorescent antibody with three changes of saline, stirring by mechanical agitation. Rinse in water and mount in buffered glycerol. Examine with a fluorescence microscope.

The indirect technique [p. 332]
This differs from the direct method in that the specific antiserum is not labelled with a fluorescent marker. After washing with three changes of saline, the specific antiserum is demonstrated by treating with an appropriate fluorescent antiglobulin conjugate. Sections are washed, mounted, and examined in the same way as for the direct method.

RESULTS

With fluorescein isothiocyanate the fluorescence is green. With rhodamine B isothiocyanate the fluorescence is orange.

NOTES

1. Control sections and blanks [p. 329] must be used with both methods.
2. The general features of fluorescence microscopy have been described [p. 22]. For immunofluorescent techniques a high intensity ultraviolet light source is required, and an incident-light fluorescence microscope is recommended. Fluorescein gives its maximum fluorescence with light of 400–520 nm, and the exciter filter should allow light of this wavelength to reach the section.

IMMUNO-ENZYME TECHNIQUES

The direct and indirect fluorochrome labelled antibody techniques of Coons [p. 324] are now fully established as a means of identifying specific antigens and antibodies in tissue sections, but these suffer from the disadvantage of requiring fresh, unfixed tissue for cryostat sections, and produce end results which are unstable and are not satisfactory for electron microscopy. The main disadvantages are listed below:

1. Fresh tissue required, fixed or paraffin embedded material unsuitable.
2. Impermanent, specimens fade.
3. Direct comparative studies difficult.
4. Special equipment and dark-room required.
5. Not easy to make photographic record of results.
6. Not applicable to electron microscopy.

These difficulties have been largely overcome by the labelling of antibodies with *enzymes*, especially horseradish peroxidase (Avrameas and Uriel 1966; Nakane and Pierce 1966). In the horseradish immuno-enzyme method the fluorochrome label of the standard immunofluorescent method is replaced by peroxidase and the peroxidase labelled antigen–antibody complex is demonstrated by the histochemical preparation of a coloured reaction-product deposited at the site of peroxidase activity. A satisfactory dark brown reaction-product can be produced by the DAB method with diamino-benzidine tetrahydrochloride and hydrogen peroxidase (Graham and Karnovsky 1966), and this is examined by ordinary light microscopy and can be rendered electron opaque with osmium tetroxide for electron microscopy. The immunoperoxidase methods have many of the advantages of high specificity and selectivity that are present in the classical immunofluorescent techniques but are free from their important disadvantages and formalin-fixed, paraffin-embedded tissue can be used, even if this is several years old. Antigens in pathological tissue, such as immunoglobulins and hepatitis B antigen [FIG. 17.5], have been demonstrated in formalin-fixed paraffin sections by immunoperoxidase methods and compared with the classical immunofluorescent technique (Burns, Hambridge, and Taylor 1974). The development of the immunoperoxidase methods has been described by Burns (1975a, c).

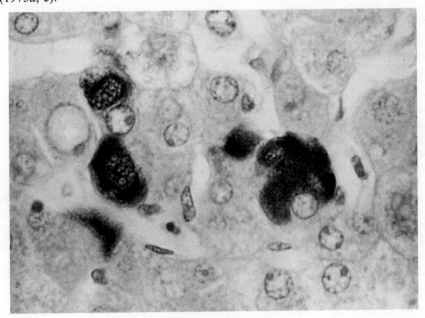

FIG. 17.5   Hepatitis B surface antigen stained by the indirect peroxidase-labelled antibody method.

PEROXIDASE-LABELLED ANTIBODY METHODS

As in the classical fluorochrome-labelled antibody techniques the peroxidase-labelled antibody methods are of two types, the *direct method* and the *indirect method*. In the *direct method* the antigen X binds with a rabbit anti-X immunoglobulin that has been labelled with horse-radish peroxidase; the horseradish peroxidase then reacts with the DAB substrate to give a brown reaction product at the site of antigen X [FIG. 17.6]. In the *indirect method* antigen X in the tissue reacts firstly with unlabelled rabbit anti-X immunoglobulin and secondly with swine anti-rabbit immunoglobulin that has been labelled with horseradish peroxidase; this is then exposed to the DAB reaction giving the same brown end-product at the site of antigen X [FIG. 17.6]. The results of these techniques may be affected by *endogenous*

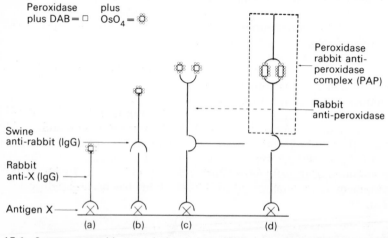

FIG. 17.6 Immunoperoxidase techniques. (a) Direct peroxidase-labelled method. (b) Indirect peroxidase-labelled method. (c) Unlabelled antibody–peroxidase bridge method. (d) Peroxidase-antiperoxidase (PAP) method.

peroxidase activity which is present in the tissue before the peroxidase-labelled antibody is applied, or by *background staining* due to uptake of the specific labelled antibody by tissue components other than the antigen which is being demonstrated. Endogenous peroxidase activity can be inhibited or removed before immunoperoxidase staining by a number of reagents, such as 0.5 per cent hydrogen peroxide in methyl alcohol for 30 minutes (Burns 1975b), or can be previously stained a different colour to that given by the DAB method; in some tissues the distribution of endogenous peroxidase is so different from that of the true positive immunoperoxidase-stained areas that they can be readily distinguished on microscopical observation. Background staining can be reduced by diluting the antiserum to its optimal strength or by absorbing the tissue with normal swine serum (Burns 1978a).

Indirect peroxidase-labelled antibody method

FIXATION

Ten per cent buffered formal-saline or acetate buffered glutaraldehyde-formalin (Garvin, Spicer, and McKeever 1976).

SECTIONS

Paraffin sections cut at 5 μm or less, mounted on glass slides, and dried at 37 °C for not more than 24 hours.

TECHNIQUE

1. Paraffin sections are dewaxed in xylene and brought to alcohol.
2. Endogenous peroxidase activity is blocked with a fresh 0.5 per cent solution of hydrogen peroxide (10 per cent solution for blocking acid haematin) in methyl alcohol for 30 minutes, or with acid alcohol for 15 minutes (cryostat sections).
3. Wash (see below).
4. Non-specific background staining is reduced with normal swine serum diluted 1:5 for 5–10 minutes. Excess serum is removed, but not washed prior to next stage.
5. Sections are treated with optimally diluted rabbit antiserum for 15–30 minutes.
6. Wash (see below).
7. Sections are treated with peroxidase-conjugated swine anti-rabbit serum immunoglobulin diluted 1:20 for 15–30 minutes.
8. Wash (see below).
9. Treat with a freshly prepared solution of 0.05 per cent 3, 3′-diaminobenzidine tetrahydrochloride (Sigma) and 0.01 per cent hydrogen peroxide in 0.05 M Tris buffer (pH 7.6) for 5–10 minutes.
10. Wash well in tap water.
11. Sections are counterstained with a weak haematoxylin, dehydrated, cleared in xylene, and mounted in a synthetic resin medium.

RESULTS

The sites of the specific antibody—dark brown.
Nuclei—lightly stained blue [FIG. 17.5].

NOTES

1. Reactions are performed in 0.5 M Tris buffer (pH 7.6) diluted 1:10 with saline. This buffer is used for all the washings, repeated three times, 5–15 minutes in all.
2. The antisera are diluted with normal swine serum 1:5 in Tris-saline.
3. Controls should always be prepared at the same time by substituting (a) normal rabbit serum, (b) absorbed immune rabbit serum for stage 7. Sections should also be stained by the DAB reaction before and after treating with hydrogen peroxide in methyl alcohol.
4. A Leitz KP 490 FITC interference filter enhances the result (Burns *et al.* 1974).

Phenylenediamine–pyrocatechol substitute for DAB in the immunoperoxidase technique (Burns 1978b)

A new alternative to 3-3′-diaminobenzidine for the demonstration of the peroxidase-labelled antigen–antibody complex has been described by Hanker, Yates, Metz, and Rustioni (1977). This is sensitive, specific, non-carcinogenic, and overcomes the difficulty of obtaining good quality DAB. The peroxidation of *p*-phenylenediamine is accelerated by pyrocatechol and produces a copolymer that is osmiophilic and darker than the DAB end-product. A pre-mixed reagent made up of one part of *p*-phenylenedia-mine dihydrochloride and two parts of pyrocatechol (PDP) is commercially available.

PREPARATION

Dissolve 7.5–15 mg of phenylenediamine–pyrocatechol reagent (PDP; Hanker–Yates reagent, Polysciences Inc., page 503) in 10 cm³ of Tris buffer pH 7.6 and add 0.1 cm³ of 1 per cent hydrogen peroxide.

TECHNIQUE

1. Proceed to the completion of step 8 of the peroxidase-labelled antibody method [p. 329].
2. Treat with the PDP reagent solution for 5–20 minutes at room temperature.
3. Rinse with 'Tris' buffer pH 7.6 and wash in water.
4. Counterstain in weak haematoxylin, dehydrate in alcohol, clear in xylene, and mount in a synthetic resin medium.

RESULTS

Similar to those obtained by using DAB, but a darker coloration of the antigen–antibody complex may be obtained.

UNLABELLED ANTIBODY PEROXIDASE METHODS

The immunoglobulin–enzyme bridge method (Mason, Phifer, Spicer, Swallow, and Dreskin 1969; Sternberger 1969) uses a bridging antibody to join the peroxidase to the antigen [FIG. 17.6]. The antigen X is first treated with unlabelled rabbit anti-X immunoglobulin and this is bound to rabbit anti-horseradish peroxidase by using unlabelled swine anti-rabbit immunoglobulin in excess as a bridge. A modification of this method (Sternberger, Hardy, Cuculis, and Meyer 1970) extends the two stages of the previous method by reacting the rabbit anti-horseradish peroxidase antibody and free horseradish peroxidase [FIG. 17.6] to form a soluble complex known as PAP (peroxidase antiperoxidase complex).

The PAP unlabelled antibody method

SECTIONS

Paraffin sections cut at 5 μm or less.

TECHNIQUE

1. Paraffin sections are dewaxed in xylene and brought to alcohol.
2. Endogenous peroxidase activity is blocked with a fresh 0.5 per cent solution of hydrogen peroxide (10 per cent solution for blocking acid haematin) in methyl alcohol for 30 minutes.
3. Wash (see below).
4. Non-specific background staining is reduced with normal swine serum diluted 1:5 for 5–10 minutes. Excess normal swine serum is removed but not washed off prior to next stage.
5. Sections are treated with optimally diluted rabbit anti-X immunoglobulin for 15–30 minutes.
6. Wash (see below).

7. Unlabelled swine anti-rabbit serum immunoglobulin diluted 1:20 for 15–30 minutes.
8. Wash (see below).
9. Rabbit peroxidase antiperoxidase complex (PAP) diluted 1:50 for 15–30 minutes.
10. Wash (see below).
11. Stain with a freshly prepared solution of 0.05 per cent 3,3′-diaminobenzidine tetrahydrochloride (Sigma) and 0.01 per cent hydrogen peroxide in 0.05 M Tris buffer (pH 7.6) for 5–10 minutes. Wash well in tap water.
12. Sections are counterstained with a weak haematoxylin, dehydrated, cleared in xylene, and mounted in a synthetic resin medium.

RESULTS

The sites of the specific antigen—dark brown.
Nuclei—lightly stained blue.

NOTES

1. For the washings use 0.5 M Tris buffer (pH 7.6) diluted 1:10 with saline.
2. The antisera are diluted with normal swine serum 1:5 in Tris saline.
3. Controls should be prepared at the same time as the technique is performed by substituting (a) normal rabbit serum, (b) homologous antigen-absorbed immune rabbit serum for the diluted immune rabbit serum of stage 5. Sections should also be stained by the DAB reaction before and after treating with hydrogen peroxide in methyl alcohol.
4. The phenylenediamine–pyrocatechol reagent [p. 329] can be used in place of DAB in step 11.

Immunoperoxidase preparations can be counterstained with haematoxylin and eosin and with many other histological staining method, though counterstaining should be light. Other non-carcinogenic substitutes for DAB have been proposed by Seligman, Shannon, Hoshino, and Plapinger (1973). For electron microscopy the DAB end-product can be rendered electron opaque with osmium tetroxide. A wide number of applications of the immunoperoxidase techniques are being developed for intracellular immunoglobulins, enzymes, and hormones as well as many antigens including tumour-associated antigens; immune complexes can be demonstrated on the basement membranes of glomeruli in kidney biopsies and their exact sites have been determined by critical light microscopy and electron microscopy (Davies, Tighe, Wing, and Jones 1977). Immunoperoxidase methods can be effectively used for the demonstration of auto-antibodies and the technique for the antinuclear test will be briefly described.

HISTOLOGICAL IDENTIFICATION OF AUTO-ANTIBODIES IN SERA

Histological laboratories are becoming more widely involved in the detection of auto-antibodies in sera by fluorescent or peroxidase techniques using fresh animal or human tissues. An auto-immune screen usually involves the detection of anti-nuclear factor and antibodies to thyroid, smooth muscle, gastric parietal cells, and mitochondria. The technique that is most widely used is the indirect immunofluorescent sandwich technique, but the indirect immunoperoxidase technique has now been developed and gives good results with less specialized equipment. The principle of these two techniques is similar in that appropriately diluted serum under investigation is applied to unfixed cryostat sections of rat liver, kidney, or stomach and cryostat sections from a block of fresh human thyroid. After appropriate washing the sections are treated with fluorescein or peroxidase-labelled anti-human globulin serum which combines with any antibodies from the serum under investigation that have reacted with the appropriate antigen in the tissue section. After further washing the fluorescein sections are examined by a fluorescence microscope. The immunoperoxidase coloured end-product is produced by the DAB technique as described earlier and examined by the light microscope.

The indirect immunofluorescent technique for auto-antibodies

FIXATION

None, fresh tissue is required.

SECTIONS

Cryostat sections are cut from a composite block of fresh rat liver, kidney, and stomach and a separate block of fresh human thyroid. Tissues may be stored in re-sealable plastic bags in the deep freeze at -40 to -70 °C. When using stored tissue the first few dried sections are discarded and sections are cut approximately 5 µm thick and collected on to clean microscope slides. With a new block the first section should be stained with haematoxylin and eosin to check the presence of the necessary tissues. The sections are air dried for 20 minutes and are ringed with a diamond marker to make orientation easier during fluorescence microscopy and by a felt-tip pen to conserve re-agents. Phosphate buffered saline, pH 7.2, is used for diluting serum and for washing sections.

TECHNIQUE

1. Test and control sera are diluted (usually 1:5 with buffer) and applied to the dried sections in a covered and moistened container for 20 minutes.
2. Wash for 15 minutes in phosphate buffer saline with mechanical agitation with at least one change of buffer.
3. Wipe off excess saline and add appropriately diluted fluorescein-labelled anti-human globulin to the sections and leave in the container for 20 minutes.
4. Wash in phosphate buffer saline for 30 minutes with at least one change of buffer.
5. Mount in buffered glycerol.
6. Examine with a fluorescence microscope.

RESULTS

Sera that contain antibodies against tissue components will produce green fluorescence at the appropriate site in the tissue [FIG. 17.4] with a black background.

NOTES

1. Do not allow sections to dry after stage 1.
2. The preparations are not permanent but may be stored in the dark at 4 °C for limited periods of time.

3. Control sections must always be prepared at the same time as the test sections. Parallel sections should be treated with known positive and negative sera and with phosphate buffered saline alone in place of stage 3 in every series of sera tested.
4. Positive anti-nuclear factor sera are usually re-examined quantitatively using doubling dilutions of the serum. The titre is reported as the last dilution that shows positive fluorescence.

Immunoperoxidase method for auto-antibodies

FIXATION

None, use fresh tissue.

SECTIONS

Cryostat sections of fresh rat liver and other tissues are used, as for the immunofluorescent technique.

TECHNIQUE

1. Pipette aliquots of suitably diluted patient serum, usually 1:5 with buffer, on to the cryostat sections and incubate for 30 minutes at 37 °C. 0.5 M Tris buffer (pH 7.6) diluted 1:10 with saline is used for diluting the sera and for washing the sections.
2. Carefully rinse off serum from each of the tissue sections with buffer and wash in four changes of buffer with gentle agitation for a total of 20 minutes.
3. Remove buffer and treat the tissues on each slide with undiluted anti-human immunoglobulin–peroxidase conjugate.
4. Carefully rinse off serum from each tissue section with buffer and wash in four changes of buffer with gentle agitation for 20 minutes.
5. The end-product is produced with 0.05 per cent 3,3′-diaminobenzidine tetrahydrochloride (Sigma) and 0.1 per cent H_2O_2 in buffer for five minutes. Wash well in tap water.
6. Do not counterstain; either mount in glycerol or dehydrate in alcohol, clear in xylene, mount in a synthetic resin medium, and examine with the light microscope.

RESULTS

Sera with autoantibodies will produce a dark brown reaction product at the appropriate site in the tissue section.

NOTES

1. For controls, substitute patient serum in stage 1 of the technique with (a) buffer, (b) known negative serum, (c) known positive serum.
2. The presence of endogenous peroxidase activity can be demonstrated by staining by DAB by itself.
3. Positive anti-nuclear factor sera should be examined quantitatively by using doubling dilutions and reporting the titre as the last dilution that shows the presence of recognizable end-product.

REFERENCES

Avrameas, S. and Uriel, J. (1966). *C. R. Acad. Sci. (Paris)* **262**, 2543.
Burns, J. (1975a). *Proc. roy. micr. Soc.* **10**, 97.
—— (1975b). *Histochemistry* **43**, 291.

Burns, J. (1975c). *Histochemistry* **44**, 133.

—— (1978a). In *Recent advances in histopathology* (eds. P. P. Anthony and N. Woolf). Churchill Livingstone, Edinburgh.

—— (1978b). *J. clin. Path.* **31**, 701.

—— Hambridge, M., and Taylor, C. R. (1974). *J. clin. Path.* **27**, 548.

Coons, A. H., Creech, H. J., and Jones, R. N. (1941). *Proc. Soc. exp. Biol. (N.Y.)* **47**, 200.

—— —— —— and Berliner, E. (1942). *J. Immunol.* **45**, 159.

Davies, D. R., Tighe, J. R., Wing, A. J., and Jones, N. F. (1977). *Histopathology* **1**, 39.

Dorsett, B. H. and Ioachim, M. D. (1978). *Am. J. clin. Path.* **69**, 66.

Garvin, A. J., Spicer, S. S., and McKeever, P. E. (1976). *Am. J. Path.* **82**, 457.

Graham, R. C. and Karnovsky, M. J. (1966). *J. Histochem. Cytochem.* **14**, 291.

Hanker, J. S., Yates, P. E., Metz, C. B., and Rustioni, A. (1977). *Histochem. J.* **9**, 789.

Mason, T. E., Phifer, R. F., Spicer, S. S., Swallow, R. A., and Dreskin, R. B. (1969), *J. Histochem. Cytochem.* **17**, 563.

Nairn, R. C. (1976). *Fluorescent protein tracing*, 4th edn. Churchill Livingstone, Edinburgh.

Nakane, P. K. and Pierce, G. B. (1966). *J. Histochem. Cytochem.* **14**, 929.

Pearse, A. G. E. (1968). *Histochemistry, theoretical and applied*, 3rd edn., Vol. 1. J. and A. Churchill, London.

Riggs, J. L., Seiwald, R. J., Burckhalter, J. H., Downs, C. M., and Metcalf, T. G. (1958). *Am. J. Path.* **34**, 1081.

Seligman, A. M., Shannon, W. A., Hoshino, Y., and Plapinger, R. E. (1973). *J. Histochem. Cytochem.* **21**, 756.

Sternberger, L. A. (1969). *Mikroskospie* **25**, 346.

—— Hardy, P. H., Cuculis, J. J., and Meyer, H. G. (1970). *J. Histochem. Cytochem.* **18**, 315.

Weller, T. H. and Coons, A. H. (1954). *Proc. Soc. exp. Biol. (N.Y.)* **86**, 789.

18 | Diagnostic cytology

Cytological techniques are now widely applied to the diagnosis of disease. Cells obtained from all parts of the body by abrasive methods, by fine needle aspiration techniques, or exfoliated into body fluids and secretions may reveal morphological characteristics associated with certain pathological states. The most common application of cytology is in the diagnosis of malignancy but information may also be obtained about endocrine effects or the types of tissue reaction. In addition, cytology specimens may reveal evidence of infestation and some specimens may be subsequently submitted for microbiological examination.

Most specimens for cytological examination are processed for examination as *smears* on a slide, but when solid matter is present in a fluid or in an aspirate then particles can be separated and sectioned. Clots which form in effusions rich in protein, when anticoagulant has not been added, may also be processed as solid tissue and the cellular content of the clot can then be examined in addition to the sediment in the fluid. Diagnostic cytology and histopathology are complementary examinations. It should be a routine for cytology reports which recommend biopsy to be followed-up and correlated with the sections. In this way discrepancies in both methods can be detected and each act as a control for the other.

The technical and interpretative aspects of general cytology have been described by Koss (1968) and Hughes and Dodds (1968).

COLLECTION OF SPECIMENS

The accuracy of the cytology report is highly dependent on the quality of the preparation of the specimen. Time spent on ensuring that the morphology of the cells is well preserved is worth while. For many cytological preparations cells are obtained by scraping or brushing directly from the site as it is being examined. For instance, with cervical smears the clinician will collect the specimen with a spatula when he visualizes the cervix and make the smear directly on to a clean glass slide which is then treated immediately with fixative. Clinicians using endoscopic techniques or taking needle aspirations may also prepare the cytology specimen. If the material is submitted to the laboratory in this way the clinician must be advised on the preparation of the smear, in particular of the need to include all the available material, to spread it thinly on one or more slides so that it can be adequately screened, and of the absolute necessity for the rapid fixation of the specimens. Each laboratory will have its own preferred methods and these should be discussed with the clinician so that the best results are obtained. Particularly important is the need for rapid fixation of the smears, unless air dried preparations are required. Clean glass slides with a frosted end for easy labelling, a soft pencil to label the slides, spatulae where appropriate, and bottles of fixative and boxes or pots for transporting the slides should be provided for the clinician.

When the material collected at the clinical examination is of such a kind or of such quantity that the preparation of the cytological specimens will be particularly complicated or time consuming, it may be preferable for one of the laboratory staff to be present. For instance, needle aspirates vary in content and consistency and this factor may alter the method of preparing the specimen which is best determined at the time of collection.

All fluid specimens will require processing in the laboratory in order to isolate the cell content, usually by centrifugation. Sputum specimens must also be prepared in the laboratory. It must always be borne in mind that these specimens, because they are unfixed before preparation for screening, are potentially infectious and thus require to be dealt with accordingly.

The following sections describe techniques of preparation of smears from material given to laboratory staff during clinical investigation or delivered directly to the laboratory.

SPUTUM

Sputum is examined in the cytology laboratory for the presence of malignant cells and exceptionally for certain organisms such as *Pneumocystis carinii*. Ideally three consecutive early morning specimens should be sent from the patient. To avoid contamination by food particles or other matter the sputum should be coughed up by the patient before the teeth are brushed or before breakfast is eaten. If more than one specimen is received on the same day they should be combined to make the smears.

The specimen is poured into a Petri dish unless the container is of wide enough a diameter to allow adequate inspection. Its appearance is recorded and if food material is present or the specimen seems to consist only of saliva further specimens should be requested. These specimens should not be rejected without examination as it may be possible to identify malignant cells in them. Smears should be made from any white areas in the specimen which are likely to come from the tumour and from any streaks of blood. If no white or blood-stained areas are apparent then the smears should be made from different parts of the specimen. The material can be picked up from the Petri dish using orange sticks or forceps and spread carefully on at least two slides. The slides are immersed immediately in 95 per cent alcohol and left to fix for at least 20 minutes before staining. Smears from each specimen should be fixed in separate containers so that there is no possibility of cells floating from one specimen to another.

It may be preferred to examine sputum specimens treated with a mucolytic agent such as methyl cysteine (Cytoclair, page 503), in this way the cell content of the whole specimen can be concentrated. Concentration of the sputum can be particularly valuable when asbestos bodies are to be looked for or when the rather watery specimen, characteristically produced by patients with oat-cell carcinoma, is received. Methyl cysteine is available as a powder and is used as a 2 per cent solution in normal saline. An equal volume of the solution is added to the sputum specimen and incubated at 37 °C for at least two hours when most specimens will have liquified. Thicker specimens may take longer and can be left for up to 18 hours without adverse effect on the cell morphology. The specimen is then centrifuged at 3000 rev/min for five minutes and the supernatant poured off. The deposit is resuspended in the fluid which runs back from the sides of the container. Using a Pasteur pipette two drops are placed on the slide and spread evenly across it using the side of the pipette. The smears are fixed with an aerosol fixative and then stained. The cells in these concentrated sputum specimens prepared in this manner have a good morphology and without the presence of mucus lie discreetly in the smear. A study has shown an improvement of 60 per cent in the pick-up rate of positive specimens using this method compared with ordinary sputum smears (Evans and Shelley 1975). Concentration does involve more handling of potentially infectious material and it may be wise to use the method in a limited way.

All sputum specimens should be regarded as potentially tuberculous and therefore should be handled in an exhaust protective cabinet. Protective clothing such as gowns and gloves should be worn whilst preparing the specimens and hands washed when the preparation is completed. Forceps or orange sticks used to make the smears should be placed in a discard jar containing a phenolic disinfectant. Used containers should be put in receptacles so they can be autoclaved or incinerated. Sputum smears should not be made by drawing the specimen through two slides as a large aerosol effect is created when this is done. Residual sputum should be retained in a labelled container in the laboratory refrigerator until the smears have been screened and reported.

Papanicolaou stain is the stain of choice for screening sputum, although methylene blue can be used to make temporary preparations. Carbol chromotrope 2R [p. 171] is useful if the eosinophil content of the sputum needs to be assessed. *Pneumocystis carinii* may be demonstrated by Grocott's method [p. 406] or by Romanowsky stains.

URINE

Cytological examination of urine specimens is carried out to detect malignancy arising in the urothelium or in the kidney. Examination of saline washings obtained during cystoscopy or retrograde pyelography may also be useful.

Preparations for cytological examination should be made from freshly voided urine, within two hours of its production. Mid-stream specimens of urine passed after the bladder has been emptied in the morning should be requested as they will contain freshly shed cells.

In screening programmes designed to detect early changes in the bladder epithelium in those populations at high risk for bladder cancer (workers in rubber and cable industries) specimens may have to reach the laboratory through the post. The urine must then be prefixed [see p. 343]. Urine which cannot be processed within two hours may be mixed with an equal quantity of a mixture of ethyl alcohol and glacial acetic acid [see p. 343].

The cell content of most urine specimens is very scanty. Preparations are easier to screen if they are made using a cytocentrifuge which concentrates the cells into a defined area on the slide (Watson 1966). The urine is first centrifuged in the conventional centrifuge for five minutes at 1500 rev/min. The resultant supernatant and the deposit are then described on the report. Unless there is a thick deposit, when smears can be made directly, enough of the supernatant is discarded to resuspend the deposit at a suitable dilution for a cytocentrifuge preparation, that is, not too thick. The concentrated specimen is then pipetted into at least two cuvettes of the cytocentrifuge and spun at 1500 rev/min for ten minutes. The slides are removed from the cytocentrifuge and the preparations are fixed immediately using an aerosol spray fixative.

Adherence of the cells to the slide in urine specimens may be assisted by adding a few drops of fixative containing Carbowax to the cuvette prior to adding the urine. A smear of albumin on to the slide before it is put in the cytocentrifuge will also prevent the loss of cells. Vacuum filter techniques (Millipore) may be used for urine specimens. Filters made of cellulose acetate with a regular pore size of 5.0 + 1.2 μm are suitable for cytological preparations. To preserve cell morphology care must be taken during filtration to avoid too high a vacuum and to break the vacuum before all the fluid is drawn through the filter, as the filter must not be allowed to dry.

BODY FLUIDS

These specimens are usually from the pleural or peritoneal cavity, but fluids may be aspirated from the pericardial sac and from cysts. Body fluids often contain protein which will form clots unless an anticoagulant is added. If clots are present they should be processed histologically and examined at the same time as the smears which are made from the remaining fluid.

To prevent clots the following anticoagulants will not affect cell morphology and may be added to the fluid;

1. Sodium citrate 3.8 per cent solution.
   5 cm³ sodium citrate to 100 cm³ fluid.
2. Heparin 2 mg or 200 units/20 cm³ fluid.
3. EDTA 20 mg/20 cm³ fluid.

On receipt in the laboratory the appearance of the fluid should be recorded. To prepare smears for examination the fluid is centrifuged at 2000 rev/min for ten minutes. The supernatant and deposit are examined and their description recorded. The supernatant is poured off and the cell button is picked up with a Pasteur pipette before the tube is set upright again. Two smears are made from the material in the pipette by putting a drop on to a slide and spreading it with the side of the pipette, these smears are quickly air dried and placed in methyl alcohol prior to staining with May–Grunwald Giemsa. Four thicker smears are prepared from the cell button in the centrifuge tube which has been slightly moistened by fluid running down the sides of the tube. These smears are immediately fixed in 95 per cent alcohol. Two smears are stained with Papanicolaou, the remaining two are kept in reserve should special stains be required, e.g. PAS with diastase digestion and Alcian blue for identification of mucus in tumour cells. Slides from each specimen should be in separate fixative jars.

If the deposit contains blood the smears may be spread using a slide as for blood films. If there is much blood in the fluid, after centrifuging, transfer the supernatant, buffy coat, and top layer of blood cells using a Pasteur pipette into a second tube and centrifuge for a second time. Then pipette off the supernatant and make smears from the buffy coat. Alternatively a density gradient method may be used to separate the red blood cells from the other cellular contents of the fluid (Spriggs 1975). The haemorrhagic fluid is collected into a tube containing anticoagulant (EDTA 2 mg per cent) and centrifuged at 2000 rev/min for ten minutes. Two cm³ of 25 per cent Hypaque [p. 503] is added to a round-bottomed tube 5 mm diameter and 100 mm long. To this is added the same volume of supernatant from the specimen. Mix the two fluids using a pipette with a bent sealed-off end until a smooth colour transition is obtained. The haemorrhagic deposit from the fluid is then pipetted on to the top of the column. Using a suitable centrifuge head the tube is centrifuged at 3000 rev/min for 15 minutes. The red blood cells will have settled below the other cellular components of the fluid which can be pipetted off, resuspended in their own supernatant, and centrifuged again and smears made from the deposit. If the cell population above the red cell layer seems scanty cytocentrifuge preparations may be made.

Body fluids may have come from patients with tuberculosis and hepatitis and must be regarded as infectious. When centrifuging these fluids the containers must be capped. It may be convenient to use a sealing tissue such as Parafilm [p. 503] for this purpose. The lid of the centrifuge should be kept shut for about five minutes after it has come to a stop so that any aerosol containing organisms can subside. Always make smears in the exhaust protective cabinet and keep them there until they are fixed.

SPECIMENS OBTAINED AT ENDOSCOPY

Specimens for cytological examination may be obtained during endoscopic examination of the stomach, oesophagus, or bronchus. These are most commonly collected under direct vision by brushing the lesion with a nylon brush. The brush is smeared firmly across at least four labelled slides which are then immediately placed in fixative. The morphology of cells in smears made in this way is excellent. In order to ensure that the whole cell sample is examined the brush may be rinsed in a container holding normal saline which may then be filtered or centrifuged to obtain the residual cells. Brushings taken during bronchoscopy require careful labelling to ensure their source is known. Bronchial epithelium exfoliates readily and it may be found that brushings provide very cellular smears which are difficult to screen; in this case it may be preferred to rinse the brush in saline and use the cell deposit to make blocks which are then prepared for histological section (Blum, Cole, and Towler 1977).

Biopsies obtained during endoscopy have been found to yield useful information if an imprint for cytological evaluation is obtained before the tissue is orientated for histological processing. The biopsy specimen is dabbed lightly on to the slide which is then sprayed with fixative (Yoshii, Takahashi, Yamaoka, and Kasugai 1970; Young and Hughes 1977).

During bronchoscopy saline washings may be collected. Each saline fraction should be put into a separate container which is clearly labelled. Smears are made from the centrifuged deposit. Bronchial aspirates may also be sent for examination. These usually have a similar consistency to sputum and can be prepared in the same way.

CEREBROSPINAL FLUID

All fluid specimens for cytological examination should be processed without delay once the specimen has been collected. It is especially important for cerebrospinal fluid to be prepared immediately as the cells quickly become fragile and their morphology deteriorates. Only small volumes of cerebrospinal fluid are available for examination and as the cell content is usually scanty the cytocentrifuge is particularly appropriate for preparation of the specimens. The appearance of the fluid should always be noted.

Approximately 0.5 cm^3 of the fluid is pipetted into two or more cuvettes of the cytocentrifuge which is then operated at 700 rev/min for five minutes. One slide is sprayed with fixative, and the second slide is air dried. Papanicolaou stain is used for the fixed slide and May–Grunwald Giemsa on the air-dried slide.

The used cuvettes of the cytocentrifuge should be soaked in Decon 75 [p. 503] overnight, rinsed in tap water followed by distilled water, and drip-dried.

FINE NEEDLE ASPIRATES

Fine needle aspiration of organs and growths is a convenient method of obtaining tissue for diagnostic purposes with only minimal trauma. Fine needle aspirations are commonly obtained from breast lumps prior to surgical intervention; other organs from which aspirates are commonly obtained are the prostate gland, salivary gland tumours, and lymph nodes.

A 22 gauge needle is attached to a 10 or 20 cm³ plastic syringe and the needle is introduced into the mass. Whilst the barrel of the syringe is gently and steadily pulled back the needle is rotated and moved back and forth within the mass. Tissue is drawn into the needle but if the mass contains fluid this will also enter the syringe. The suction on the syringe is released before the needle is withdrawn so that the tissue is not spread along the needle track and the contents do not get pulled into the barrel of the syringe. The syringe is detached from the needle, the barrel withdrawn, and the needle reattached. The material in the needle can then be gently expressed from the needle on to slides. Any solid tissue is picked up and put into formal-saline for histological processing—the remaining material may be spread on the slides. Smears may be air-dried for Romanowsky staining or wet fixed for Papanicolaou or haematoxylin and eosin stains. Rapid reports may be necessary if the needle aspirations have been done during laparotomy.

If the mass contains fluid this should be put into a container and processed as for body fluids. It may increase the cell yield if the needle is rinsed in fixative consisting of a mixture of alcohol, glacial acetic acid, and Carbowax [p. 343]. Smears may then be prepared either from the centrifuged deposit or using filtration techniques (Millipore).

JOINT FLUIDS

Examination of synovial fluid aspirated from joints may reveal crystals. These can be precisely characterized using a polarizing microscope with a quartz wedge. Anticoagulant should not be added to the fluid and if a clot has formed part of it should be included with a drop of well-mixed fluid spread on the slide. A coverslip is then placed on the fluid. Ordinary light microscopy will reveal cells and sometimes crystals. However, crystals are more easily identified when a polarizing microscopic with a quartz wedge is used, as a colour shift induced by the crystals can then be seen.

Crystals of sodium urate and calcium pyrophosphate dihydrate may be found in joint fluids and both crystals are birefringent. Urate crystals exhibit a strong negative birefringence and are yellow when their long axis is parallel with the 'slow component' (indicated on the mounting) of the quartz wedge and blue when at right angles to the slow component. Calcium pyrophosphate crystals are positively birefringent and are blue when parallel to the slow component and yellow when at right angles (Currey 1968).

The crystals may be found in the cells and lying free in the fluid.

Contaminate particles in the fluid may also appear birefringent and can lead to confusion but careful inspection of the cells to find crystals will confirm any doubtful diagnosis. If the cell content is scanty and no crystals are seen, a centrifuged deposit of the fluid should be examined. To evaluate the cell content of a joint fluid, the fluid is centrifuged and the deposit spread to make smears for examination.

AMNIOTIC FLUIDS FOR ESTIMATION OF FOETAL MATURITY

Foetal maturity can be estimated from the proportion of fat-filled foetal squames found in the amniotic fluid. Two drops of well-mixed amniotic fluid are placed on the slide. One drop of filtered 1 per cent aqueous Nile blue sulphate [see p. 296] is added and mixed using a wooden applicator stick. A coverslip is placed on the fluid and left for ten minutes. Foetal squames nucleate or anucleate blue cells or anucleate orange cells. The number of anucleate orange cells represent the degree of maturation of the foetus and the percentage of these must be estimated by counting 400 cells. The whole slide should be screened in order to ensure that the distribution of the cells on the slide has been assessed. Large clumps of orange cells are impossible to count and a rough estimate must be made. Fat droplets may also be found free in the fluid.

The count of orange cells is interpreted as follows (Brosens and Gordon 1966):

Less than 1 per cent — up to 34 weeks maturity
1–10 per cent — 34–8 weeks
10–50 per cent — 38–40 weeks
More than 50 per cent — Term

Vaginal secretions suspected of draining from ruptured membranes may be examined for foetal squames. If orange-staining cells are found the fluid will be of amniotic origin.

SEMINAL FLUID

At Stepping Hill Hospital in Stockport, these examinations (Fertility + Post Vasectomy) also carried out in the Bacteriology Dept!

Analysis of semen specimens is required as part of the investigation of infertility and in the follow-up of vasectomy cases. Semen specimens must be examined within two hours of production as one of the essential investigations is that of the sperm motility.

Motility
1. Note time of arrival of the specimen.
2. Warm a clean slide to body temperature and pipette a drop of well-mixed seminal fluid on to it. Cover with a large (40 × 20 mm) coverslip.
3. Count 100 spermatozoa using a high power objective. Note the percentage of motile forms. Repeat the count and average the results.
4. If the motility is low a separate count is made of the motile forms.
   (a) Sperm showing progression (progressive forms)
   (b) Sperm showing tail movements but no progression (non-progressive forms).

Volume
Pour all the specimen into a graduated measuring cylinder and note the volume.

Viscosity

Three grades are used to denote the viscosity of the specimen.

1. Normal.
2. Hypoviscid.
3. Hyperviscid.

Sperm count

1. Mix the specimen well and dilute it 1 in 100 with 5 per cent sodium bicarbonate in 1 per cent formalin (i.e. 0.5 cm^3 semen to 49.5 cm^3 of diluting fluid).
2. Mix well and flood a Fuchs–Rosenthal counting chamber with the diluted fluid.
3. Leave to stand'for a minute and count the number of spermatozoa in ten of the smallest squares.
4. Calculation of result:

$$\frac{\text{Number of sperms counted} \times \text{depth} \times \text{dilution}}{\text{Number of small squares}}$$

$$= \frac{\text{No. of sperms} \times 80 \times 100}{10}$$

$$= \text{No.}/\text{mm}^3$$

$$\text{No.}/\text{mm}^3 \times 1000 = \text{No. of sperms}/\text{cm}^3$$

Morphology

1. Mix four drops of semen with two drops of sodium bicarbonate diluting fluid and allow to stand for a few minutes.
2. Make two thin films from the solution and air-dry them. Fix in absolute alcohol.
3. Stain with Papanicolaou stain.

Formalin–bicarbonate diluting fluid

To: Distilled water   1000 cm^3
  add Sodium bicarbonate   50 g
        Formaldehyde   10 cm^3

FIXATION

The need for rapid fixation of smears has been stressed in the preceding section. Air drying of thin smears is only used for those specimens which require Romanowsky stains. If transport of slides in containers filled with liquid is not a problem, the most suitable fixative is 95 per cent ethyl alcohol. A plastic Coplin jar with a well-fitting screw-on lid is a suitable container. Most smears adhere well to the glass slides because they contain a certain amount of mucus and there is little danger of the cells floating off the slides into the fixative.

When the specimens are less likely to adhere to the slide a fixative may be dropped on to the slide from a dropper bottle or an aerosol spray fixative may be used. If an aerosol spray is used, which is convenient but expensive, it should be held far enough away from the slide for the fixative to fall on the slide without sufficient force to drive the smears to the slide edge. Fixatives added to urine samples or used to wash out needles used for aspiration techniques improve adherence of the cells in the centrifuged deposit of these specimens.

Fixatives containing Carbowax provide a covering film for the smear as it dries and are used in dropper bottles or sprays. The slides may be packed into suitable boxes after drying for 15 minutes and these slides may then be posted if necessary. The carbowax is removed by alcohol at the beginning of the staining procedure. Carnoy's fixative may be used for heavily blood-stained specimens, e.g. endometrial aspirates. The red blood cells are lysed by this fixative and this enables the remaining cell population to be seen more clearly.

All smears should be left to fix for at least 15 minutes before staining. Fixative solutions may be used more than once but must be filtered so that any free cells are not transferred from one specimen to another. Slides may be left in fixative for up to seven days without deterioration.

FIXATIVES

1. 95 per cent ethyl alcohol.
2. Stock dilute solution of polyethylene glycol (Carbowax 1500).

Absolute alcohol (industrial spirit)	100 cm³
Carbowax 1500	3 g
Glacial acetic acid (to pH 5.8–6.0)	0.2 cm³

   Soften the Carbowax in an incubator. Add the alcohol to dissolve the Carbowax. After cooling add the acetic acid and mix well.
3. Concentrated polyethylene glycol (Carbowax 1500) fixative. This can be put in dropper bottles for posting. Before use it is diluted with 95 per cent ethyl alcohol.

Carbowax 1500	60 g
Distilled water	100 cm³
Glacial acetic acid	4 cm³

   The Carbowax is dissolved in warm water. After cooling the acetic acid is added and the solution mixed. 1.5 cm³ of this concentrate is placed in a polythene dropper bottle (capacity 25 cm³). 23.5 cm³ 95 per cent ethyl alcohol is added before use.
4. Carnoy's fixative.

Absolute ethyl alcohol (industrial spirit)	60 cm³
Chloroform	30 cm³
Glacial acetic acid	10 cm³

5. In the previous section reference was made to a fixative for urine specimens which could not be delivered fresh to the laboratory. This is ethyl alcohol 75 cm³ and glacial acetic acid 25 cm³ and an equal volume is added to the urine.
6. Fixative for urine specimens to travel by post.

Monoethylene glycol	3500 cm³
Diethylene glycol	180 cm³
Borax pentahydrate	35 g
Glacial acetic acid	500 cm³
Distilled water	5700 cm³

   2.5 cm³ of this fixative is sufficient for up to 30 cm³ of urine.

7. Fixative for fine needle washings.

Carbowax	10 g
Distilled water	600 cm³
Absolute ethyl alcohol (industrial spirit)	400 cm³

The Carbowax is dissolved in warm water and when cool mixed with the alcohol.

STAINING METHODS

GENERAL STAINING TECHNIQUES

Papanicolaou stain, which has become the most popular stain for gynaecological cytology, was originally developed to demonstrate the cyclical changes that take place in the squamous epithelium of the female genital tract in response to alteration in hormone levels. The cytoplasm of the parabasal squamous cells stains a deep greenish-blue, intermediate cells are a pale greenish-blue, and as the cells reach full maturity as superficial cells the cytoplasm stains pink. The Orange G in the stain is selective for any keratin that may be present. The stained cytoplasm retains a degree of transparency which reduces eye fatigue and the nuclei are precisely stained with Harris' haemotoxylin. The cytoplasmic staining may be influenced by several factors including change in pH as a result of infection and also by the thickness and fixation of the smear. However, Papanicolaou stain provides a good differential stain and as a result is used widely for other routine cytology smears. It must be said that a cytologist usually gets the best results from the staining method with which he is most familiar.

Romanowsky stains are commonly used to stain the cells in pleural and peritoneal fluids and in cerebrospinal fluid (Spriggs and Boddington 1968). These smears are air dried which has the effect of flattening and enlarging the cells and the stain demonstrates the cellular elements, in particular the nucleoli. Many workers prefer Romanowsky stains for epithelial cells and they are commonly used to stain needle aspirates when it may be an advantage to use a rapid method of staining for an immediate report.

Although fixation of a specimen generally increases the adherence of the material to the slide it is known that some cells will float off during the staining procedure and adhere to other slides. Gynaecological smears should be stained separately from smears obtained from other tissues. Slides of sputum and fluids should be placed in every other slot in the slide holder during the staining procedure. Stains require filtering daily if they are to be reused and reagents may need changing or can be filtered according to their appearance. Stains will need to be changed weekly or more frequently if large numbers of slides are being stained. It is necessary to be alert to the possibility that cells may be 'carried over' from one slide to another and this contamination can occur in both manual and automatic staining procedures (Husain, Grainger, and Sims 1978).

The Papanicolaou technique (Papanicolaou 1942, 1954)

PREPARATION

1. *Orange G (OG 6)*

| Orange G stock solution (0.5 per cent in 95 per cent ethyl alcohol) | 100 cm³ |
| Phosphotungstic acid | 0.015 g |

2. *Eosin–Azure 50 (EA 50)*

Light green SF (yellowish) 0.1 per cent solution in 45 per cent ethyl alcohol	45 cm³
Bismarck brown 0.5 per cent solution in 95 per cent ethyl alcohol	10 cm³
Eosin yellowish 0.5 per cent solution in 95 per cent ethyl alcohol	45 cm³
Phosphotungstic acid	0.2 g
Lithium carbonate (saturated aqueous solution)	1 drop

OG 6 and EA 50 may be purchased commercially.

TECHNIQUE

1. Fix in appropriate fixative solution (see above) and take smears through descending grades of alcohol (80, 70, and 50 per cent in the case of strongly alcoholic fixatives) to water.
2. Stain in Harris' haematoxylin [p. 139] for about three minutes.
3. Rinse in tap water for 1–2 minutes.
4. Differentiate in acid alcohol until only the nuclei retain the stain (a few seconds).
5. Rinse in tap water and blue the nuclei in slightly ammoniated water or in 1.5 per cent sodium bicarbonate.
6. Rinse in water and transfer to 70 per cent alcohol for a few seconds, then to 95 per cent alcohol.
7. Stain in OG 6 for approximately three minutes.
8. Rinse in two changes of 95 per cent alcohol.
9. Stain in EA 50 for about 2–4 minutes until the desired intensity of colour has been obtained.
10. Rinse in two changes of 95 per cent alcohol for a few seconds in each.
11. Dehydrate in alcohol, clear in xylene, and mount in a neutral synthetic resin medium.

STAINING SCHEDULE FOR AUTOMATIC MACHINES USING PAPANICOLAOU STAIN

If an automatic staining machine is used the following schedule is appropriate:

1. 95 per cent alcohol — two minutes
2. 75 per cent alcohol — two minutes
3. Distilled water — three minutes
4. Harris' haematoxylin — three minutes
5. Running tap water — five minutes
6. 1 per cent acid alcohol — 30 seconds
7. Running tap water — five minutes
8. 70 per cent alcohol — 1½ minutes
9. 95 per cent alcohol — 1½ minutes
10. Absolute alcohol (1) — two minutes
11. Absolute alcohol (2) — two minutes
12. Orange G — two minutes
13. Absolute alcohol (1) — two minutes

14. Absolute alcohol (2)	two minutes
15. EA 36	six minutes
16. Absolute alcohol (1)	two minutes
17. Absolute alcohol (2)	two minutes
18. Absolute alcohol (3)	two minutes
19. Alcohol/xylene	two minutes
20. Xylene	two minutes
21. Xylene	two minutes
22. Xylene	two minutes

It may be found that a more crisp nuclear stain results if the haematoxylin is diluted by adding water up to a third of the total volume and a few drops of glacial acetic acid. This may be particularly useful for smears from tissues with active nuclei which stain intensely with haematoxylin.

RESULTS

Cytoplasm of superficial cells—pink.
Cytoplasm of intermediate cells—pale greenish-blue.
Cytoplasm of parabasal cells—deep greenish-blue.
Nuclei—dark blue.
Red blood cells—bright red.
White cells—pale blue cytoplasm.

The Shorr staining technique (Shorr 1941)

This gives less cytoplasmic transparency and poorer nuclear definition than the Papanicolaou stain. It may be used for endocrine cytology as it gives good cytoplasmic differentiation, but is not very satisfactory for the detection of malignant cells.

PREPARATION

Ethyl alcohol (50 per cent)	100 cm³
Biebrich scarlet (water soluble)	0.5 g
Orange G	0.25 g
Fast green FCF	0.075 g
Phosphotungstic acid	0.5 g
Phosphomolybdic acid	0.5 g
Glacial acetic acid	1 cm³

TECHNIQUE

1. Stain for 1–2 minutes in Shorr's stain.
2. Rinse in 70 per cent alcohol to remove surplus stain.
3. Rinse in industrial spirit.
4. Clear in xylene and mount in a synthetic resin mountant.

RESULTS

Similar to Papanicolaou stain.

NOTE

Better nuclear staining can be obtained by pre-staining with Harris' haematoxylin, but this lengthens the method, making it only a little less elaborate than the Papanicolaou staining technique.

Romanowsky stains (Romanowsky 1891)

May–Grunwald–Giemsa stain is commonly used for cytology specimens which have been rapidly air dried after they have been spread.

PREPARATION

1. *May–Grunwald* (May and Grunwald 1902)

   Equal parts May–Grunwald and Sörensens phosphate buffer [p. 495] pH 6.8.
   Filter into a Coplin jar.
2. *Giemsa* (Giemsa 1902)
   Giemsa   5 cm^3
   Sörensen's phosphate buffer [p. 495] pH 6.8   45 cm^3

   Mix and filter into a Coplin jar.

TECHNIQUE

1. Fix the air-dried slides in absolute methyl alcohol for 10–20 minutes.
2. Rinse in buffer pH 6.8.
3. Stain in freshly prepared May–Grunwald for eight minutes.
4. Drain off the excess stain and stain in freshly prepared Giemsa for ten minutes.
5. Differentiate in buffer pH 6.8.
6. Allow smears to dry—if necessary they can be gently blotted before mounting.

RESULTS

Cytoplasm—mauve.
Nuclei—purple.

The methylene blue wet-film technique (Philps 1954)

A rapid and simple staining method that is useful for the screening of large numbers of specimens, especially sputum. The preparations are not permanent and should be examined immediately.

TECHNIQUE

1. Place a small amount of fresh sputum, or 2–3 drops of centrifuged deposit from the body fluid, on a clean microscope slide.
2. Place an equal volume of 0.5 per cent aqueous methylene blue beside the specimen.
3. Hold the slide at least 20 cm above a bunsen flame and very gently warm the slide, at the same time mixing the stain and specimen with forceps, until the excess fluid contributed by the stain has evaporated. Do not overheat the slide or allow the smear to dry.
4. Cover with a large coverslip and examine immediately. The stain will fade after about an hour, and this technique is specially suitable for the staining and screening of specimens by one person.

RESULTS

Nuclei—shades of blue.

NOTE

Wet films may be preserved for longer periods by the addition of glycerin to the stain, or by sealing the edges of the coverslip with paraffin wax.

The acridine orange fluorescence technique
(von Bertalanffy, Masin, and Masin 1956, 1958)

This method depends upon the affinity of the fluorochrome dye acridine orange for nucleic acids. At pH 6.0 it will demonstrate DNA green and RNA red with fluorescence microscopy. Carcinoma cells have a large amount of RNA in their cytoplasm and can be easily seen by their orange or red fluorescence under low-power magnification. As with other non-permanent staining methods, positive or doubtful smears will usually require confirmation by high-power examination or Papanicolaou stained smears.

PREPARATION

1. Stock stain solution. 0.1 per cent acridine orange in distilled water. Dilute this with M/15 phosphate buffer solution at pH 6.0 immediately before use to produce a 0.01 per cent solution of acridine orange.
2. Phosphate buffer (pH 6.0).
   A. M/15 potassium acid phosphate: 9.072 g KH_2PO_4 made up to one litre with distilled water.
   B. M/15 sodium phosphate dibasic: 9.465 g Na_2HPO_4 made up to one litre with distilled water.

   For use, mix 230 cm³ of solution A with 40 cm³ of solution B.
3. Differentiator. M/10 calcium chloride (11.099 g calcium chloride in 100 cm³ distilled water).

TECHNIQUE

1. Fix smears in ether–alcohol for at least 15 minutes.
2. Pass through descending grades of alcohol (80, 70, and 50 per cent) into distilled water.
3. Rinse for a few seconds in 1 per cent acetic acid and wash in two changes of distilled water for about one minute.
4. Stain in 0.01 per cent acridine orange in phosphate buffer (pH 6.0) for three minutes.
5. Destain in the phosphate buffer solution for one minute.
6. Differentiate in M/10 calcium chloride solution for $\frac{1}{2}$–1 minute. The nuclei should be clearly outlined.
7. Remove excess calcium chloride by washing with phosphate buffer solution.
8. Mount with coverslip in a drop of phosphate buffer solution.
9. Examine with a fluorescence microscope [p. 22].

RESULTS

RNA fluoresces red (these cells are suspicious of malignancy).
DNA fluoresces green.

DEMONSTRATION OF SEX CHROMATIN

The sex chromatin body is a constant and characteristic structure of the nucleus in female cells. It was described in 1949 by Barr and Bertram as a sharply demarcated planoconvex chromatin mass 1 μm in diameter attached to the nuclear membrane.

It is now accepted that the sex chromatin mass represents the inactive X chromosome in the interphase nucleus of the female. In the male where there is only one X in the chromosome complement there is no inactive X and therefore no sex chromatin body. This is also true in phenotypic females who have Turner's syndrome and a chromosome constitution 45 XO, and in those who have testicular feminization with a chromosome constitution 46 XY. Normal females with two X chromosomes have one inactive X and a sex chromatin body as do males with Klinefelter's syndrome whose chromosome constitution is XXY. Females with a chromosome constitution of XXX or males with XXXY will have two inactive X chromosomes and the nuclei of their cells will show two sex chromatin bodies. Thus the number of sex chromatin masses demonstrable is one less than the total complement of X chromosomes in the karyotype. Size of the sex chromatin body should also be taken into account as a very small or large mass may indicate an X isochromosome or a deletion.

Assessment of the sex chromatin is the primary investigation to be carried out when patients are suspected of having a sex chromosome abnormality. A full chromosome analysis should also be carried out in these cases.

Good preparations of cells to assess sex chromatin can be made from buccal smears which are easy to obtain giving the patient no discomfort. The sex chromatin is also expressed as a drumstick protruding from the nucleus of polymorphonuclear leucocytes in the blood.

It is also possible to identify the Y chromosome using fluorescent techniques. Many chromosomes fluoresce but the long arms of the Y chromosome are especially bright.

Buccal smear preparation

The patient rinses the mouth out well with water. The inside of the cheek is scraped firmly with a spatula, the broad end of an Ayres spatula is convenient. The resultant slightly turbid fluid is spread on five glass slides, three of these are fixed immediately with spray fixative. In babies very satisfactory specimens can be obtained by rubbing the inside of the cheek with a gloved finger. The cells collected on the plastic of the glove are spread on the slides immediately.

One of the fixed slides is used for fluorescent staining the other two may be stained for permanent preparations using cresyl-fast violet or acid thionin. The unfixed slides are stained immediately with lactic acetic–orcein.

Lactic acetic orcein technique for sex chromatin (Sanderson and Stewart 1961)

PREPARATION

Stock solution:

Synthetic orcein	1 g
Glacial acetic acid	45 cm³

Boil, cool, and filter.

Working solution:

Dilute stock solution with an equal volume of 70 per cent lactic acid and filter.

TECHNIQUE

1. Immediately the buccal smear specimen has been spread on the slide pipette two drops of lactic acetic orcein on to the slide.
2. Place a coverslip on the slide thus spreading the stain over the smear.

3. Leave for 20 minutes, then blot the coverslip firmly to squash the cells and remove excess stain. Examine immediately with a high-power objective.

RESULTS

Cells stain a faint pink with nuclei slightly darker, the sex chromatic is evident as a dark red mass.

NOTE

The advantage of this method is its rapidity, and bacteria do not become stained and obscure the sex chromatin. In buccal smears from females at least 30 per cent of the nuclei should contain sex chromatin. No sex chromatin is apparent in the nuclei in normal male cells.

Cresyl fast violet method (Moore and Barr 1955; Moore 1962)

This is a rapid method which is reliable and consistent, provided a good batch of stain is used.

TECHNIQUE

1. Fix smears with a spray fixative.
2. Take to water through 70 and 50 per cent alcohol, five minutes in each.
3. Rinse in distilled water.
4. Immerse the slides in a 1 per cent aqueous solution of cresyl echt violet for five minutes.
5. Rinse in tap water.
6. Differentiate in 95 per cent alcohol. This is complete when the cytoplasm has become colourless, and may require control with the staining microscope. Thick smears need some of the cells to be left overstained to obtain areas of correct differentiation. Usual time for differentiation is 2–5 minutes.
7. Quickly dehydrate in absolute alcohol, clear in xylene, and mount in a synthetic resin medium.

RESULTS

Nuclei—pale mauve.
Sex chromatin—deeply stained.
Cytoplasm—almost colourless.

NOTES

1. Some batches of the dye are unsatisfactory.
2. This method is not easy to over-differentiate, and false-negative results are unlikely, but control smears must be used if the laboratory only examines occasional single specimens, and with all new batches of stain.
3. Contamination with bacteria from the mouth may cause difficulty. Bacteria can be reduced if a light scraping is first discarded and a second deeper scraping taken.
4. Differentiation can be avoided altogether by the use of the dye at a concentration of 0.5 per cent (Ross 1960).

The acid thionin method (Klinger and Ludwig 1957)

PREPARATION

1. *Stock thionin solution*
   1 per cent thionin in 50 per cent alcohol.

2. *Stock buffer solution*

Sodium acetate	9.714 g
Sodium barbiturate	14.714 g
Distilled water to make	500 cm³

3. *Working solution of thionin*

0.1 normal hydrochloric acid	32 cm³
Stock buffer solution	28 cm³
Stock thionin solution	40 cm³

This solution keeps for 6–8 weeks.

TECHNIQUE

1. Fix the smear with a spray fixative.
2. Transfer to a 0.2 per cent solution of celloidin in ether–alcohol for two minutes. Wipe the back of the slide, dry in the air for a few seconds, and immerse in 70 per cent alcohol for five minutes. This step attaches the cells firmly to the slide so that they do not come off during the subsequent hydrolysis.
3. Wash in two changes of distilled water for five minutes each.
4. Hydrolyse the smear for not more than five minutes in normal hydrochloric acid at 56 °C.
5. Wash in two changes of distilled water for five minutes each.
6. Stain for five minutes in the working solution of thionin.
7. Differentiate and dehydrate in 70, 95 per cent, and absolute alcohol. Usually about one minute is required for each stage, depending on the thickness of the smear. Differentiation is critical (see below).
8. Clear in xylene and mount in a synthetic resin medium.

RESULTS

As for previous method.

NOTE

It is possible to over-differentiate, with a danger of decolorizing the sex chromatin, causing a false-negative result. Known female control smears should be made and stained with the smear under investigation.

Y chromosome fluorescence (Pearson, Bobrow, Vosa, and Barlow 1971)

Use one smear of the five obtained by scraping the buccal mucosa.

TECHNIQUE

1. Fix smear with a spray fixative.
2. Rinse in tap water.
3. Stain in a 0.5 per cent aqueous solution of quinacrine dihydrochloride (Atebrin) for six minutes.
4. Wash in running tap water one minute and rinse in phosphate buffer, pH 5.5.
5. Mount in buffer at pH 5.5 and seal with a rubber adhesive.
6. Examine 100–200 cells with the fluorescence microscope for a bright fluorescent mass about 0.25 km in diameter within the nucleus.

RESULTS

The long arms of the Y chromosome fluoresce particularly brightly. In a normal male approximately 25–50 per cent of the cells will display a fluorescent Y chromosome. No Y fluorescence is evident in the normal female.

NOTE

Extraneous extracellular material may also fluoresce and cause difficulty in distinguishing the Y chromosomes.

The interpretation of buccal smears requires experience, and when it is not a routine procedure a control specimen should be prepared simultaneously for comparison. Analysis of the karyotype will always be required for patients who raise a clinical suspicion of sex chromosome abnormalities.

Elegant preparations for chromosome analysis can be prepared by using phytohaemagglutinin to transform lymphocytes in blood. Using micro-techniques enough blood for these preparations may be obtained from a baby by a heel prick. The individual parts of each chromosome may be identified by using banding techniques. Pairs of chromosomes normally display similar banding patterns common to their number. Examination of banded preparations should establish the karyotype, precisely identifying chromosome rearrangements such as translocations, deletions, and other abnormalities including extra chromosome material. Cytogenetic techniques are described by Yunis (1974), Poulding (1977), Priest (1977), and Sharp (1977).

REFERENCES

BARR, M. L., and BERTRAM, E. G. (1949). *Nature (Lond.)* **163**, 676.

BERTALANFFY, L. VON, MASIN, F., and MASIN, M. (1956). *Science* **124**, 1024.

———— ———— ———— (1958). *Cancer (Philad.)* **11**, 873.

BLUM, L. J., COLE, L., and TOWLER, G. (1977). *Histopathology* **1**, 115.

BROSENS, I. and GORDON, H. (1966). *J. Obstet. Gynaec. Br. Cwlth.* **73**, 88.

CURREY, H. L. F. (1968). *Proc. roy. Soc. Med.* **61**, 969.

EVANS, D. M. D. and SHELLEY, G. (1975). *Acta Cytol. (Philad.)* **19**, 484.

GIEMSA, G. (1902). *Zbl. Bakt., 1. Abt. Ref.* **32**, 307.

HUGHES, H. E. and DODDS, T. C. (1968). *Handbook of diagnostic cytology*. Livingstone, London.

HUSAIN, O. A. N., GRAINGER, J. M., and SIMS, J. (1978) *J. clin Path.* **31**, 63.

KLINGER, H. P. and LUDWIG, K. S. (1957) *Stain Technol.* **32**, 235.

KOSS, L. G. (1968) *Diagnostic cytology and its histopathologic basis*, 2nd edn. Pitman, London.

MAY, R. and GRUNWALD, L. (1902). *Zbl. inn. Med.*, **23**, 265.

MOORE, K. L. (1962). *Acta Cytol. (Philad.)* **6**, 1.

——— and BARR, M. L. (1955). *Lancet* **ii**, 57.

PAPANICOLAOU, G. N. (1942). *Science* **95**, 438.

——— (1954). *Atlas of exfoliative cytology*. Harvard University Press, Cambridge, Mass.

PEARSON, P. L., BOBROW, M., VOSA, C. G., and BARLOW, P. W. (1971). *Nature (Lond.)* **231**, 326.

PHILPS, F. R. (1954). *Br. J. Cancer* **8**, 67.

POULDING, R. H. (1977). *Cytological techniques for human chromosome studies. Histopathology, selected topics* (ed. H. C. Cook). Bailliere Tindall, London.

PRIEST, J. H. (1977). *Medical cytogenetics and cell culture*, 2nd edn. Lea and Febiger, Philadelphia.

ROMANOWSKY, D. (1891). *St Petersburger med. Wschr.* **16**, 297.

ROSS, A. (1960). *J. med. Lab. Technol.* **17**, 178.

SANDERSON, A. R. and Stewart, J. S. S. (1961). *Br. med. J.* **2**, 1065.

SHARP, J. A. (1977). *An introduction to annual tissue culture*. Edward Arnold, London.

SHORR, E. (1941). *Science* **94**, 545.

SPRIGGS, A. I. (1975). *Acta Cytol. (Philad.)* **19**, 470.

—— and BODDINGTON, M. M. (1968). *The cytology of effusions and cerebrospinal fluid*, 2nd edn. Heinemann, London.

WATSON, P. (1966). *J. Lab. clin. Med.* **68**, 494.

YOSHII, Y., TAKAHASHI, J., YAMAOKA, Y., and KASUGAI, T. (1970). *Acta cytol. (Philad.)* **14**, 249.

YOUNG, J. A. and HUGHES, H. E. (1977). Seventh European Congress of Cytology. Liege.

YUNIS, J. J. (1974). *Human chromosome methodology*, 2nd edn. Academic Press, London.

19 | The nervous system

The central nervous system

INTRODUCTION

No stain or combination of stains, metallic impregnation or histochemical method is capable of showing in a single preparation all the components of any tissue. This applies especially to the tissues of the central nervous system (CNS) and knowledge of the histology (both normal and pathological) of the brain and spinal cord is gained by the integration of the appearances furnished by a number of different preparations, each of which demonstrates only certain elements of the mass of cells, cell constituents, processes and fibres which make up the most complex cell organization of the body. Because of this, methods for the demonstration of the elements of the CNS are many and varied and range from electron microscopy, which is being increasingly used to reveal the fine structure of cells and fibres, to methods for light microscopy that have changed little since the late nineteenth century, are largely empirical and often capricious.

Metallic impregnation methods are extensively used in neurohistology and there is at present no way of selectively colouring axons and dendrites with dyes in routine preparations. Furthermore, a formalin fixed paraffin section stained with haematoxylin and eosin is of very limited value for the demonstration of some cell processes and fibres and special fixatives or mordants and frozen or cellulose nitrate sections are often necessary.

Reference to Table 19.1 will indicate the range of structures to be demonstrated and the methods described below have been selected for their general usefulness and reliability. Several of them entail frequent handling of sections, careful timing, and attention to detail.

Table 19.1 Structures to be demonstrated in the CNS

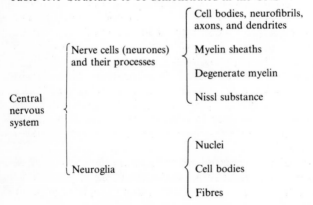

Central nervous system
- Nerve cells (neurones) and their processes
  - Cell bodies, neurofibrils, axons, and dendrites
  - Myelin sheaths
  - Degenerate myelin
  - Nissl substance
- Neuroglia
  - Nuclei
  - Cell bodies
  - Fibres

FIXATION

Although the CNS is prone to autolytic changes and prompt fixation is desirable, brains should only be cut into slices after fixation is complete. Small wedges of tumours presenting on the surface may be removed for more rapid examination and samples required for special purposes such as histochemistry or electron microscopy must be removed before fixation. Unless the organ is fixed as a whole, slices will distort and discolour during fixation rendering recognition of anatomical features difficult or impossible.

Ten per cent formal-saline is the best general purpose fixative and the entire brain should be fixed for 3–4 weeks. To prevent distortion during fixation, a string or a hook attached to a string should be passed under the basilar artery to suspend the brain in the container which should be large enough and of suitable shape to allow suspension of the specimen a few centimetres below the surface of the fixative and for it to touch neither the sides nor the base. Open the ventricular system by making a small incision in the corpus callosum. Renew the formalin after 48 hours and thereafter weekly.

The brain may be rapidly fixed by injection, as follows, and is useful if removal of the organ must be delayed.

TECHNIQUE

1. Expose the carotid artery and insert a cannula.
2. Open the external and internal jugular veins on the same side as the artery.
3. Perfuse with normal saline until the issuing fluid is almost blood-free; then run in formal-saline of two to three times the volume of the brain.
4. Either remove the brain and complete fixation by immersion, or, tie off the vessels until this can be done.

NOTE

This technique will not be successful in cases of cerebrovascular disease where vessels are occluded.

Spinal cords removed whole should be fixed suspended in vessels such as large measuring cylinders, care being taken not to bend or distort them. Traction or pressure when removing segments of nerves or spinal cord will cause artifacts which may be particularly misleading when demonstrating degenerate myelin [p. 369].

Slicing of the brain must be done with a very sharp, long, thin blade, without undue pressure. Regular slices, approximately 1 cm thick should be cut through the whole brain, usually in the frontal plane although saggital or horizontal sections may be required for some purposes. This permits the various tracts and structures to be identified and followed.

There are several devices for procuring even slices, some being similar to hand microtomes where the thickness may be varied. Hume Adams and Miller (1970) recommend the use of two right-angles made of 1-cm square brass, the longer limb being 18 cm and the shorter 15 cm. These are fitted round the brain on a non-slip surface and the knife drawn across them in long, smooth strokes, avoiding a sawing action.

Blocks of brain and spinal cord selected for sectioning may be identified by marking the surface opposite to the cutting face with Indian ink after blotting with filter paper or cloth. A 'section map' in the form of a photograph or diagram of the various slices of brain, annotated to show blocks sectioned, is useful.

PREPARATION OF SECTIONS

Paraffin sections

Tissues of the CNS are dense and rich in lipid and for these reasons not readily penetrated by processing fluids or paraffin wax. Long processing is recommended and the larger blocks required for studies of the brain may require up to 24 hours in wax although this time may be reduced by use of the vacuum embedding oven for the final changes of wax. To avoid artifacts, care should be taken to reduce pressure and to re-admit air to the chamber gradually. Rapid processing techniques are not suitable for non-neoplastic CNS tissue.

Best quality paraffin wax is essential for the production of good sections of nervous tissues and the use of waxes with 'plastic' additives [p. 61] is advantageous in reducing distortion as is the celloidin-paraffin double-embedding procedure [p. 71] although the formation of perivascular and perineuronal spaces is inevitable in formalin-fixed, wax-embedded CNS tissue.

Sections of brain and spinal cord for studies of normal structure or non-neoplastic conditions are usually cut at about 7 μm and at 15–20 μm. The use of an adhesive such as albumen or gelatine [p. 92] is desirable. When sections are as flat as possible on the water-bath they are picked up on to slides when any slight wrinkling remaining may be removed by gently blotting with moistened filter paper. Sections should be dried at 37 °C for 15–24 hours rather than at 60 °C for shorter periods.

Cellulose nitrate sections

Cellulose nitrate sections are widely used in neurohistology where larger, thicker sections are required. No special technique is necessary for embedding nervous tissue in this medium but care must be taken to ensure complete impregnation and even hardening of the block, and because of the size of the blocks and the density of the tissue a long time (up to two months) may be required for completion of the process. Rapid schedules are not applicable to this material.

Cellulose nitrate sections of CNS material are usually cut at about 15 μm and at 25–30 μm.

Frozen sections

Frozen sections are used extensively in neurohistology and certain constituents can only be demonstrated by using this type of section. Fortunately, thin sections are not usually required as many cells are only complete with their processes in thicker preparations.

Because of their high content of lipid, large pieces of brain do not freeze as readily as less fatty material and the partial enclosure of the freezing stage of CO_2 microtomes will conserve gas and hasten the attainment of a suitable temperature and consistency for cutting. Thermo-electric cooling devices [p. 101] should be tested before purchase for their suitability for use with CNS material as some may freeze too slowly. They are, however, particularly useful when a large number of serial sections are required as the tissue will remain frozen for as long as necessary. This is also true of the cryostat [p. 102] but most non-histochemical methods requiring frozen sections demand that they are stained unattached to slides and the cryostat is less useful than a thermo-electrically cooled microtome stage for the production of these sections. A cryostat is necessary for neurohistochemistry and for preparation of the rapid frozen sections of biopsy material frequently required in neuropathology.

Ralis, Beesley, and Ralis (1973) recommend soaking tissue in 30 per cent sucrose in 10 per cent formalin for two or three days before cutting frozen sections. This extends the optimum cutting temperature-range and good sections, free from cracking, are more easily obtained.

The varied, often lengthy impregnation treatments to which frozen sections of brain and spinal cord are subjected may make them brittle and difficult to handle and mounting them on to slides requires practice and patience. The use of gelatine coated slides (Ralis *et al.* 1973) is helpful. Clean slides are dipped into a warm 1 per cent gelatine solution, drained, and dried at 37 °C. Sections are mounted from distilled water, creases are floated out, and the sections are gently blotted with filter paper moistened with dilute formalin or 70 per cent alcohol. They may then be dehydrated and cleared.

Smears

Smears which may be adequate for rapid diagnosis can be made from brain tumours except for the more collagenous varieties such as some metastases.

A small fragment of unfixed tissue is squashed between two glass slides which are then slid apart leaving a smear of tissue on one or both slides. The preparations are rapidly fixed in alcohol or an alcoholic fixative and stained with 1 per cent toluidine blue or methylene blue or by a rapid haematoxylin and eosin sequence [p. 105]. Areas where the tissue has been spread into a thin sheet are the most useful for diagnosis. Material which is difficult to spread or from tumours where the diagnosis appears equivocal will need freezing and sectioning and all material for rapid diagnosis should subsequently be embedded and sectioned in paraffin wax.

STAINING AND IMPREGNATION METHODS

Although haematoxylin and eosin staining reveals little of the many specialized structures of the CNS it is nevertheless employed as the primary staining technique and much useful information can be gained from it. The nuclei of the different types of neuroglia cells differ in shape, size, and arrangement of chromatin and thus agglomerations of these cells may be recognized. Tumours, both metastatic and primary may be identified and it gives an indication of non-neoplastic lesions and conditions which may be confirmed by the use of other techniques. Van Gieson's picro-fuchsin is also used extensively in neuro-histology. Collagen fibres of small blood vessels are clearly shown, collagen and glial fibres are more easily distinguished, and when used with Weigert's iron haematoxylin, areas of demyelination may be discerned. Mallory's pho-photungstic acid haematoxylin is also commonly used, particularly for the demonstration of glial fibres.

In neurohistology and neuropathology, a general picture of the cell population of brain and spinal cord is obtained with a 'Nissl-type' stain [p. 379] which gives very precise nuclear definition as well as demonstrating Nissl substance within the neurones, thus indicating their 'state of health'.

Of the more specialized techniques, the most important are the stains for myelin and metallic impregnation methods which will demonstrate neurones, nerve fibres, neurofibrils, and the various glial cells with their processes according to the technique employed.

DEMONSTRATION OF NEURONES, NEUROFIBRILS, AXONS, AND DENDRITES

The methods given below are arranged according to the structure to be demonstrated. Most require frozen or cellulose nitrate embedded sections, some are applicable to paraffin wax or double embedded material.

The Golgi techniques (Golgi 1875, 1878)

The Golgi methods are long (some require several months), capricious, and enigmatic. Since first described, many modifications have been suggested to shorten the time and to increase reliability but the rationale of the methods is still not fully understood. At best they give a dense black impregnation of nerve cells and their processes, internal structure being obscured, while axons are usually impregnated only when devoid of myelin sheaths. Not all the neurones in the tissue are impregnated in any preparation but this, instead of detracting from their usefulness gives a clearer picture of the structure shown and is most useful for teaching and demonstrating individual cells and their processes but because of this 'selectivity', the methods are not suitable for pathological studies.

Three methods were described by Golgi, known as the 'slow', the 'rapid', and the 'mixed'. The last of these was modified by Cox (Golgi–Cox) and is recommended, having proved the most reliable of the Golgi group.

The basis of the original methods is a treatment of pieces of central nervous system with potassium dichromate (either alone or combined with osmium tetroxide), this being followed by impregnation with silver nitrate. The Golgi–Cox modification involves the use of two chromium salts and mercuric chloride, the white deposits formed being blackened by the use of ammonia or sodium carbonate.

The Golgi–Cox method (Cox 1891)

The method is applicable to whole brains of young animals and to large slices of adult human brains, preferably not more than 1 cm in thickness.

FIXATION/IMPREGNATION

Golgi–Cox solution

5 per cent potassium dichromate	10 volumes
5 per cent mercuric chloride	10 volumes
5 per cent potassium chromate	8 volumes
Distilled water	15 to 20 volumes

Mix well.

Place the tissue blocks on a layer of glass wool in a large volume of fluid. Incubate at 37 °C. Change the fluid after 24 and 48 hours. Seal the container and leave in the incubator for one to three months. Several blocks should be processed and removed at intervals during this time.

SECTIONS

1. Freehand (for assessment of impregnation).
2. Frozen sections.
3. After embedding in cellulose nitrate (50–100 μm thick).

TECHNIQUE

1. Blacken the impregnation by placing sections for about one hour *either* in 5 per cent sodium carbonate *or* in 5–10 per cent ammonia solution.
2. Wash thoroughly in distilled water.
3. Dehydrate, clear, and mount in a synthetic resin medium.

RESULTS

Nerve cells and their processes are black; neuroglia cells and processes (if demonstrated) similarly stained. The impregnation is not transparent and constituents of cells (e.g. nuclei) cannot be seen.

NOTE

It was previously thought that fading was inevitable if the preparations were mounted under a coverslip and sections were protected by the application of Canada balsam or thickened cedarwood oil only. Modern synthetic resin mountants appear to preserve the impregnation reasonably well when used with a coverslip.

Bielschowsky's (1904, 1909) method for axons and neurofibrils

This is one of the oldest and most reliable of the ammoniacal silver impregnation methods and is more suited to diagnostic material than the foregoing.

FIXATION

Ten per cent formal-saline for seven days or longer; prolonged immersion in formalin is not detrimental to impregnation. Wash in running water for some hours before sectioning.

SECTIONS

Cut frozen sections at 10 μm for neurofibrils, at 15–20 μm for micro-anatomical observations of fibre tracts. Receive sections in distilled water.

PREPARATION

Add six drops of 40 per cent sodium hydroxide to 5 cm³ of 20 per cent silver nitrate. A brown precipitate is formed. Cautiously add strong ammonia until the precipitate is almost dissolved (usually about 5 cm³ of ammonia are required). Make up to 25 cm³ with distilled water and filter through a filter paper moistened with distilled water.

TECHNIQUE

1. Wash sections in four changes of distilled water over two hours.
2. Place sections in a covered dish of 4 per cent silver nitrate, in the dark, for 24–48 hours. Sections should not be folded nor overlap one another.
3. Rinse rapidly in distilled water.
4. Place in freshly prepared ammoniacal silver solution for ten minutes or until sections are rusty brown (see Notes).
5. Wash rapidly in distilled water.

6. Reduce in 10 per cent formalin in tap water (which must not be acid) for about ten minutes. Progressive darkening of sections takes place.
7. Wash well in tap water followed by distilled water.
8. Tone in 0.2 per cent gold chloride until sections are grey (about ten minutes).
9. Rinse in distilled water.
10. Remove any unreduced silver by treatment (fixing) with 5 per cent sodium thiosulphate.
11. Wash in distilled water. (Counterstaining of nuclei with neutral red or safranin is optional at this stage.)
12. Mount sections on slides, dehydrate in ascending grades of alcohol, clear in xylene, and mount in a synthetic resin medium.

RESULTS

Neurofibrils, axons and dendrites—black.
Background—greyish.
Neuroglia and collagen may sometimes be lightly impregnated.

NOTES

1. It is common practice with this and other metallic impregnation methods to take several sections from each block. One of these is likely to show rather superior impregnation.
2. Judgement of shades of colour is subjective and practice is recommended to determine the optimum shade at stage 4.
3. Toning at stage 8 is not obligatory. Lack of treatment with gold chloride gives black nerve fibres and a golden brown background. Two or three drops of glacial acetic acid added to the toning bath result in a purplish background.

Holmes' (1947) method for axons

This method was devised as an alternative to Bodian's (1936, 1937) copper–Protargol method, Protargol being a silver proteinate of uncertain composition varying according to maker and country of manufacture.

Holmes' method is applicable to paraffin sections of both central and peripheral nervous system material.

FIXATION

Ten per cent formal-saline gives good results, primary or secondary fixation in mercuric chloride–formalin is better. Chrome or osmium-containing fixatives are not suitable.

SECTIONS

Paraffin sections of 10–20 μm thickness should be mounted on slides with an adhesive. The optimum thickness should be determined by experiment.

PREPARATION

pH 8.4 *buffer*

(a) Boric acid   12.4 g
    Distilled water   1000 cm^3
(b) Borax ($Na_2B_4O_7.10H_2O$)   19 g
    Distilled water   1000 cm^3

Impregnating solution
Mix 55 cm³ of boric acid buffer solution, (a) with 45 cm³ of borax buffer solution, (b) in a 500 cm³ measuring cylinder. Dilute to 494 cm³ with distilled water. Add 1 cm³ of 1 per cent silver nitrate and 5 cm³ of 10 per cent pyridine. Mix thoroughly.

Reducer

Hydroquinone	1 g
Sodium sulphite crystals	10 g
Distilled water	100 cm³

(The reducer can be used repeatedly, but may not keep for more than a few days.)

TECHNIQUE

1. Remove wax with xylene and take sections to water, treating with iodine to remove mercury pigment if necessary.
2. Wash for ten minutes in running water followed by distilled water.
3. Place in 20 per cent silver nitrate in the dark at room temperature for two hours. (Overnight treatment is permissible and may be preferable for thick sections.) The solution may be used repeatedly.
4. Take the slides from the 20 per cent silver nitrate and wash for ten minutes in three changes of distilled water.
5. Place the slides in the impregnating solution (not less than 20 cm³ of solution per slide) in covered glass vessels of a kind which can be kept thoroughly clean.
6. Impregnate at 37 °C until any convenient time on the following day.
7. Take out the slides, shake off the superfluous fluid, and place them in the reducer described above for not less than two minutes.
8. Wash in running tap water for three minutes: the slides should not lie back to back during this process or traces of reducer will be carried over. Rinse in distilled water. If desired the slides may be left in distilled water at this stage until it is convenient to proceed.
9. Tone in 0.2 per cent gold chloride (yellow variety) for three minutes. (This may be used repeatedly providing that it does not contain the brown clouds indicative of reduction.) Toning should be prolonged if the sections are still brown at the end of three minutes.
10. Rinse briefly in distilled water.
11. Place in the 2 per cent oxalic acid. The slides remain in this solution for 2–10 minutes and are examined at intervals under the staining microscope with daylight illumination. When the axons are blue–black the process is stopped; further treatment may result in a diminution of the contrast.
12. Rinse in distilled water and fix with 5 per cent sodium thiosulphate for five minutes.
13. Wash in tap water for ten minutes and counterstain with neutral red if desired.
14. Dehydrate, clear in xylene, and mount in synthetic resin mountant.

RESULTS

Axons—black.
Background—greyish.

NOTES

1. Unlike most silver impregnation methods, best results are obtained following mercuric chloride fixation (Rowe and Hill 1948).
2. Frozen and cellulose nitrate sections may be impregnated by the same procedure, before attachment to slides, but washing stages should be of longer duration than with paraffin sections.
3. The cross striations of skeletal muscle are well shown by this method.

Marsland, Glees, and Erikson's (1954) method for axons

This method was developed for the demonstration of axons in formalin-fixed paraffin sections of brain and spinal cord. It is less reliable for the demonstration of peripheral nerves.

FIXATION

Ten per cent formal-saline, duration not critical.

SECTIONS

Paraffin sections at 10–15 μm mounted with an adhesive.

PREPARATION

Ammoniacal silver solution
Mix 30 cm³ of 20 per cent silver nitrate with 20 cm³ of absolute alcohol. Add strong ammonia drop by drop until the resulting precipitate is just dissolved. Add an additional five drops of ammonia.

TECHNIQUE

1. Remove wax with xylene followed by absolute alcohol.
2. Cover section with a film of 1 per cent celloidin as described on page 186.
3. Wash well in distilled water.
4. Place in 20 per cent silver nitrate for 15–60 minutes at 37 °C.
5. Wash in 10 per cent neutral formalin from a drop bottle for 10–15 seconds. The white precipitate should float away and sections should be yellow.
6. Wash off formalin with ammoniacal silver solution and leave for 30 seconds.
7. Drain off silver solution and wash section with 10 per cent neutral formalin for one minute or longer. Examine with the microscope. If sections are insufficiently impregnated, stages 6 and 7 may be repeated.
8. Wash in distilled water.
9. Fix in 5 per cent sodium thiosulphate for five minutes.
10. Wash in tap water.
11. Dehydrate in alcohol and remove celloidin film.
12. Clear in xylene and mount in synthetic resin mountant.

RESULTS

Nerve cells and axons—black.
Background—golden.

For a review of the factors influencing the impregnation of nerve fibres in vertebrates, with many references, see Palmgren (1960).

MYELIN SHEATHS

Myelin is a complex mixture of lipids combined with protein and forms a sheath round nerve fibres in the central and peripheral nervous systems. These are called myelinated or medullated nerve fibres.

Demonstration of myelin is required to show the normal histology of nervous tissue and (negatively) the loss of myelin that occurs in various disease processes. Normal myelin may be demonstrated by the following groups of methods:

1. Osmium tetroxide.
2. Haematoxylin.
3. Copper phthalocyanin and other dyes.
4. Oil soluble dyes.
5. Histochemical methods.
6. Polarization and fluorescence microscopy.

Osmium tetroxide methods

The lipids of myelin reduce osmium tetroxide to a black compound and this reagent was used in some of the earliest methods for the demonstration of myelin. Because of its cost, and poor powers of penetration, however, osmium tetroxide is of little practical value for the staining of normal myelin in masses of tissue from the CNS but is used with peripheral nerves [p. 381] and for the demonstration of degenerate myelin [p. 369].

Haematoxylin methods

Weigert (1884, 1885, 1891) was the originator of the haematoxylin methods for myelin using chrome mordanted material. The principle of his methods is the reduction of chrome salts to chromium dioxide by myelin; this acts as a mordant and forms a lake with the subsequent haematoxylin stain, the chromium–myelin complex being largely insoluble in processing reagents.

Of the numerous modifications of the Weigert principle, those of Pal (Weigert–Pal method) and Kultschitsky and Wolters are of greatest utility. The former is particularly suited to the demonstration of masses of myelinated fibres in contrast to large areas of demyelination and where the loss of stain from fine fibres is of no great importance. The Kultschitsky modification is of value where it is desired to ensure retention of stain in the finest fibres, the differentiation procedure being slow and safe. With both methods, recently degenerated myelin may be heavily stained, while areas of long-standing degeneration appear unstained and white, the myelin having been removed by phagocytosis.

Weigert recommended the use of an alkaline haematoxylin solution while in the Kultschitsky modification the stain is acidified.

Other haematoxylin stains for myelin are those of Loyez [p. 365] using Weigert's solution, Woelcke (Heidenhain, page 366) where a similar but more alkaline solution is used, and Weil [p. 382]. These three methods use an iron mordant applied to the section rather than the block.

Cellulose nitrate is recommended for embedding the somewhat brittle chrome-mordanted tissue. Paraffin wax sections are suitable for unmordanted material but cellulose nitrate sections are often preferred for myelin demonstration as areas of gross degeneration are more clearly shown in thicker sections.

In the past, well ripened solutions of haematoxylin have been recommended for use with these methods but they do not always give the best results. This is particularly so in the case of Loyez's and Weil's methods and is the cause of unpleasant brown staining. The use of old, over-oxidized batches of haematoxylin powder will have the same effect.

Kultschitsky's (1890) modification of Weigert's method for myelin

Kultschitsky's method employs the Weigert principle of chrome mordanting but incorporates an acidified haematoxylin and a different method of differentiation.

FIXATION

Ten per cent formal-saline followed by 4–5 days' mordanting in Weigert's primary mordant.

SECTIONS

Cellulose nitrate sections at 15–25 μm.

PREPARATION

Kultschitsky's haematoxylin

Ten per cent haematoxylin in absolute alcohol (ripened)	10 cm³
Distilled water	90 cm³
Glacial acetic acid	2 cm³

Differentiator

Saturated aqueous lithium carbonate	100 cm³
One per cent aqueous potassium ferricyanide	10 cm³

TECHNIQUE

1. Stain in Kultschitsky's haematoxylin for 12–24 hours at room temperature.
2. Pass sections directly to the differentiating fluid where the haematoxylin lake is formed. The process is very slow and should be checked about once an hour with the staining microscope. For human cerebral cortex, about four hours' treatment is usually necessary, for human spinal cord, up to 12 hours. The white matter should be blue–black, the grey, yellowish.
3. Wash sections thoroughly in running water.
4. Mount the section on a slide, dehydrate, clear, and mount in Euparal or Canada balsam.

RESULTS

Myelin sheaths—deep blue–black to black.
Background—yellow.

NOTE

A combination of the Weigert mordanting procedure, Kultschitsky's haematoxylin, and Pal's differentiator has been described by Wolters (1890) and Kaes (1891). These have come to be known as the Kultschitsky–Pal methods and are widely used with CNS material. A slightly modified version which is especially suitable for the demonstration of myelin in peripheral nerves is given on page 382.

Loyez's (1910) haematoxylin method for myelin (after Anderson 1929)

The Weigert-type methods previously described entail special mordanting and cellulose nitrate sections. Furthermore, sections of such material are of little value for other stains, and in general pathology formalin-fixed paraffin embedded tissue is often the only material available for study.

Following the introduction of the Weigert methods, numerous alternative ways of demonstrating myelin with haematoxylin were described and a large group of methods are available. Some of these also include a chrome–salt mordanting procedure following primary fixation in formalin, but even in the absence of mordanting, not all the components of myelin are lost during paraffin embedding and formalin fixed paraffin sections stained with iron haematoxylin give an adequate representation of myelin sheaths. One of the best and most widely used of the methods in this group is that of Marie Loyez.

FIXATION

Ten per cent formal-saline. Mordanting for 24 hours at 60 °C in La Manna's (1937) solution (potassium dichromate 6 g, zinc chloride 2.5 g, distilled water 100 cm^3) is advantageous.

SECTIONS

Paraffin, frozen or cellulose nitrate sections at 15–25 µm. Although originally designed for cellulose nitrate sections, paraffin sections are commonly used and these or frozen sections mounted on slides should be covered with a film of cellulose nitrate [p. 186] to prevent their detachment by the action of the lithium carbonate during staining.

PREPARATION

Loyez haematoxylin
Dissolve 1 g haematoxylin in 10 cm^3 absolute alcohol. Add 90 cm^3 distilled water and 2 cm^3 saturated aqueous lithium carbonate. Prepare freshly and do not use an old and well ripened stock solution of haematoxylin [see p. 364].

TECHNIQUE

1. Take sections to distilled water.
2. Mordant in 4 per cent iron alum for 12–24 hours at room temperature.
3. Wash in distilled water.
4. Stain in Loyez's haematoxylin for 2–4 hours at 50–60 °C or longer at lower temperatures (see Notes).
5. Wash well in tap water.
6. Differentiate (if necessary) in 0.1 per cent HCl in 70 per cent alcohol.
7. Wash well in running tap water.
8. Dehydrate, clear, and mount in a synthetic resin medium.

RESULTS

Myelin sheaths and erythrocytes—dark greyish-blue to blue–black.
Nuclei and elastic fibres will also stain.

NOTES

1. The stain tends to be self-limiting and sections should be examined with the microscope at intervals. Room temperature is generally warm enough for adequate staining.
2. Loyez originally prescribed a preliminary differentiation in 4 per cent iron

alum until the grey matter is evident, followed by washing and final (slower) differentiation in Weigert's borax–ferricyanide differentiator (borax 2 g, potassium ferricyanide 2.5 g, distilled water 200 cm³). Very often, however, little or no differentiation is required and in these cases, treatment with iron alum would be damaging.

3. Loyez's method is less satisfactory for use with peripheral nerves.
4. A useful alternative to Loyez's method is that of Weil [p. 382] and for a full account of the Weigert and other haematoxylin methods for the demonstration of myelin see Gatenby and Painter (1937).

Woelcke (Heidenhain) method for myelin

The origin of this method is not clear; see Cox (1977). This stain is very similar to Loyez's method. It is particularly suitable for unmordanted cellulose nitrate sections and paraffin sections tend to become detached from slides by the strongly alkaline solutions even when covered with cellulose nitrate.

FIXATION

Ten per cent formal-saline.

SECTIONS

25–30 μm cellulose nitrate.

PREPARATION

Ten per cent alcoholic haematoxylin	10 cm³
Distilled water	83 cm³
Saturated aqueous lithium carbonate	7 cm³

TECHNIQUE

1. Take sections to water.
2. Mordant in 4 per cent iron alum for 12–24 hours.
3. Rinse in distilled water.
4. Place in staining solution and agitate. Leave for 20–60 minutes.
5. Rinse in distilled water and examine.
6. Repeat steps 4 and 5 until staining and differentiation are complete.
7. Wash well in distilled water followed by tap water.
8. Dehydrate, clear, and mount.

RESULTS

Myelin—blue–black.
Erythrocytes and nuclei—blue–black.
Background—pale grey.

NOTES

1. Staining and differentiation time will vary according to (a) the amount of 'carry over' of iron alum, and (b) the ratio of staining solution to sections.
2. Differentiation may be hastened by the addition of more lithium carbonate.
3. Differentiation may be completed, after washing, with 1 per cent acid alcohol (Cox 1977) or saturated aqueous lithium carbonate (Gasser 1961).

Copper phthalocyanin and other stains for myelin

The copper phthalocyanin dyes Luxol fast blue MBS and Methasol fast blue 2G in alcoholic solution, have the property of combining with and staining the phospholipid of myelin. Klüver and Barrera (1953) used the first dye and counterstained with cresyl fast violet and Pearse (1955 and 1960) used Methasol fast blue with neutral red. Both basic dyes have an enhancing effect on the staining of myelin as well as providing staining of nuclei and the Nissl substance of neurones.

Both stains are applicable to routine formalin-fixed, paraffin-embedded material although post-mordanting in chrome salt is beneficial. Paraffin sections should be fixed to slides with an adhesive.

Luxol fast blue or Methasol fast blue method for myelin

FIXATION

Ten per cent formal-saline or formal-calcium, with or without chrome mordanting.

SECTIONS

Paraffin sections at 15–20 μm. Cellulose nitrate or frozen sections may be used.

PREPARATION

Luxol fast blue MBS *or* Methasol fast blue 2G   0.1 g
10 per cent acetic acid   0.5 cm³
95 per cent alcohol   100 cm³
Filter. The stain keeps well.

TECHNIQUE

1. De-wax sections with xylene and take to absolute alcohol.
2. Stain in Luxol fast blue *or* Methasol fast blue for 8–16 hours at 60 °C.
3. Rinse in 95 per cent alcohol followed by distilled water.
4. Commence differentiation by rinsing for a few seconds only in 0.05 per cent lithium carbonate.
5. Continue differentiation in 70 per cent alcohol for 20–30 seconds.
6. Rinse in distilled water. Differentiation should be controlled microscopically and steps 4, 5, and 6 repeated as necessary. Decolorization in 70 per cent alcohol is slow and controllable and should be continued until clear distinction is seen between the blue staining of white matter and the colourless grey matter.
7. Wash well in distilled water.
8. Counterstain *either* in 0.1–0.2 per cent cresyl fast violet in 1 per cent acetic acid for ten minutes *or* 1 per cent neutral red for 5–30 minutes.
9. Rinse in distilled water.
10. Differentiate the counterstain in 95 per cent alcohol.
11. Dehydrate, clear, and mount in a synthetic resin medium.

RESULTS

Myelin and erythrocytes—deep purplish–blue.
Nuclei and Nissl substance—purplish-blue or red according to the counterstain used.

NOTES

1. Margolis and Pickett (1956) have described methods using Luxol fast blue in combination with: (1) the PAS reaction; (2) Mallory's phosphotungstic acid

haematoxylin to show neuroglia; (3) Holmes' silver method for axons [p. 360], and oil red O [p. 291] for degenerate myelin (see below).
2. A simple and quick method for the demonstration of myelin is the solo-chrome cyanine stain of Page (1970). This is applicable to both CNS and peripheral nerves, is particularly good for the latter and is described on page 383.

Oil soluble dyes

Some of the complex of lipids that go to make up normal myelin are demonstrated by the oil soluble dyes described in Chapter 15. It should be noted however, that Sudan III and IV, for example, stain normal myelin less intensely than neutral fat.

A simple and rapid method for the general demonstration of normal myelin is as follows.

Sudan black B method

Sudan black B was used for the staining of myelin by Lison and Dagnelie (1935) who used a saturated solution of the dye in 70 per cent alcohol. The tri-ethyl phosphate solvent [p. 291] is superior.

FIXATION

Ten per cent formal-saline.

SECTIONS

Frozen sections at 15–25 μm.

TECHNIQUE

1. Rinse sections in 60 per cent tri-ethyl phosphate.
2. Stain in saturated Sudan black B in 60 per cent tri-ethyl phosphate for 5–10 minutes.
3. Wash off excess stain with 60 per cent tri-ethyl phosphate.
4. Wash well in distilled water.
5. Mount in modified Apathy's gum syrup [p. 129].
6. Ring coverslip.

RESULTS

Myelin—blue–black.

Histochemical methods

In recent years, investigations have been carried out in the identification of the lipid components of myelin and related enzymes by histochemical methods (see Pearse 1960; Tuqan and Adams 1961; Adams and Tuqan 1961; Adams and Bayliss 1961; Adams 1962). A histochemical method for normal and degenerate myelin is given under methods for the latter.

Polarization and fluorescence microscopy

Normal myelin is birefringent and in fresh or formalin fixed frozen sections mounted in aqueous media it will appear alternately light and dark, four times during complete rotation of the analyser of a polarizing microscope (Maltese cross effect).

Phosphine 3 R imparts a silvery-white fluorescence to many lipids when excited by short wavelength blue, or ultraviolet light (Popper 1941; Peltier 1954), while the thioflavine T stain for amyloid of Vassar and Culling (1959) also demonstrates the myelin of peripheral nerves. There do not at present appear to be any major advantages in using these methods for the demonstration of myelin.

DEMONSTRATION OF DEGENERATE MYELIN

Injury to nerve fibres and neurological diseases cause degeneration of myelin. This results in the break-down of the lipid constituents of myelin and, eventually, their removal by phagocytosis. Before this occurs, it is possible to demonstrate degenerate myelin by positive staining and this was first described by Marchi and Algeri in 1895. The principle of their method and of the many variants ('the Marchi methods') is that normal myelin is very readily oxidized by potassium dichromate and is not then blackened by treatment with osmium tetroxide. Degenerate myelin, however, contains oleic acid which is not oxidized by potassium dichromate but reduces and is blackened by osmium tetroxide. Because the myelin of degenerate and damaged fibres is in the course of time absorbed, however, the Marchi methods do not give positive pictures of long-standing degenerations and the useful limits of these methods are from about ten days to a few months after the damage to the nerve fibre.

Useful as the original Marchi–Algeri method has proved, the occurrence of artifacts of impregnation has detracted from the validity of preparations (Smith 1956) and modifications of the original method have been designed to improve penetration of the osmium tetroxide and to reduce artifacts. Thus Busch (1898) incorporated sodium iodate in the mixture to improve penetration while Orr (1900) added acetic acid. One of the most useful of these variants is that of Swank and Davenport (1935).

Swank and Davenport's method for degenerate myelin

FIXATION

Ten per cent formal-saline for 2–7 days.

PREPARATION

Impregnating solution

1 per cent aqueous potassium chlorate	60 cm³
1 per cent aqueous osmium tetroxide	20 cm³
Glacial acetic acid	1 cm³
Formalin	12 cm³

TECHNIQUE

1. Slices of brain or spinal cord not thicker than 4 mm are transferred without washing, from formalin to the impregnating solution for 7–10 days. Tissue should be supported above the bottom of the container by a layer of glass wool and periodically agitated. Use 15 times the volume of the fluid to each volume of tissue.
2. Wash in running water for 16–24 hours.
3. Dehydrate and embed in cellulose nitrate.
4. Cut sections at 20 μm or thicker.
5. Either counterstain cells or mount directly in Euparal or Canada balsam.

RESULTS

Degenerate myelin and fat—black.

Other tissues—light yellow or greenish, or according to counterstain.

Benda (1903) and several later authors have described the combined demonstration of normal and degenerate myelin by staining frozen sections first with an iron haematoxylin to show normal myelin and then demonstrating the lipid of degenerate myelin with an oil-soluble dye such as Sudan IV or oil red.

A histochemical method for the demonstration of normal and degenerate myelin is that of Adams (1959).

Osmium tetroxide–α-naphthylamine (Otan) method

The principle of this method is that degenerate myelin reduces osmium and is blackened while the unreduced osmium tetroxide bound by normal myelin is detected by its red chelate compound with α-naphthylamine.

It should be noted that α-naphthylamine is thought to be carcinogenic.

TECHNIQUE

1. Cut frozen sections of unfixed tissue on the cryostat at 5 μm, followed by fixation of the sections for four hours in 10 per cent formal-saline. Alternatively, cut formalin fixed tissue on the freezing microtome at 10–15 μm.
2. Treat sections for 18 hours in a mixture of one part 1 per cent osmium tetroxide and three parts 1 per cent potassium chlorate. The vessel containing the sections should be filled with fluid and tightly stoppered to prevent volatilization of the osmium tetroxide.
3. Wash the sections in distilled water for 30 minutes.
4. Treat sections with a saturated aqueous solution of α-naphthylamine at 37 °C for 20 minutes (10–15 minutes for sections at 15 μm). The filtered, saturated solution of α-naphthylamine should be previously warmed to 37 °C.
5. Wash sections in distilled water for five minutes.
6. Counterstain in 2 per cent Alcian blue in 5 per cent acetic acid for 15–60 seconds.
7. Wash in distilled water.
8. Mount in glycerol jelly or modified Apathy's medium. Ring the coverslip.

RESULTS

Degenerate myelin and some lipid—black.

Normal myelin of CNS and PNS and lipid droplets in the zona glomerulosa of the adrenal—red.

Erythrocytes—light red.

Neuroglial fibres and connective tissue—shades of blue.

Axons—unstained.

NEUROGLIA CELLS AND FIBRES

Neuroglia cells and fibres form the connective or interstitial tissue of the central nervous system. They are of three main types.

1. *Astrocytes*, which are in two forms: (a) protoplasmic astrocytes; and (b) fibrous astrocytes. The protoplasmic astrocytes are found mainly in grey matter, are rather smaller than fibrous astrocytes and their processes do not normally contain fibres. Fibrous astrocytes, on the other hand, contain long, slender fibres and a proliferation of fibrous glia (gliosis) is seen in areas

of demyelinization. Astrocytes generally have terminal expansions which are applied to the walls of blood vessels (perivascular feet).

2. *Oligodendrocytes* are present in both grey and white matter but are more abundant in the latter. They are smaller than astrocytes, do not form fibres and their small round nuclei (but not the cytoplasm) are clearly seen in haematoxylin and eosin stained sections. Oligodendroglia are seen in close relationship to myelin sheaths and are the homologue of the subcapsular cells of peripheral ganglia and the sheath of Schwann cells in the peripheral nervous system.

3. *Microglia* are not true neuroglia because they are mesodermal in origin and thus belong to the connective tissue group of cells in contrast to astrocytes and oligodendrocytes, which are ectodermal in derivation. They are demonstrated by similar methods to the other types, however, and are usually included under the heading of neuroglia. Microglia were first described by del Rio Hortega in 1919 and are phagocytic (scavenger) cells. Their form varies in relation to their activity and they may be seen either as small cells with short, spinous cytoplasmic projections with a flattened or triangular nucleus, or, as larger, rounded cells with cytoplasm stuffed with lipid or debris when they are called compound granular corpuscles.

For the demonstration of neuroglia, freshness of tissue is important and the higher the temperature at which the body is kept after death, the sooner does autolysis of these delicate structures begin. Generally, however, neuroglia cells and their processes suffer before the more resistant fibres (fibrous glia).

To demonstrate all types of neuroglia cells and fibres, a variety of metallic impregnation and staining methods are required on frozen, cellulose nitrate and paraffin sections.

Cajal's (1913) gold chloride–sublimate method for astrocytes

Santiago Ramón y Cajal was a pioneer in the development of metallic impregnation methods for the demonstration of the cells and fibres of the central nervous system. His gold chloride–sublimate method for astrocytes is still widely used.

FIXATION

Fresh pieces of tissue are fixed for 2–6 days in Cajal's formalin–ammonium bromide mixture (FAB).

Formalin	15 cm³
Ammonium bromide	2 g
Distilled water	85 cm³

Or, 10 per cent formal-saline (see Globus modification below).

SECTIONS

Frozen sections at 20 μm.

PREPARATION

Impregnating solution

Mercuric chloride	0.4 g
1 per cent gold chloride	10 cm³
Distilled water	60 cm³

Prepare freshly before use.

Yellow gold chloride (sodium aurochlorate, $NaAuCl_4.2H_2O$) is generally satisfactory but brown gold chloride (chloroauric acid, $HAuCl_4.xH_2O$) is recommended.

TECHNIQUE

1. Rinse sections in two or three changes of distilled water.
2. Place sections in a covered dish of the impregnating solution in the dark, for 4–8 hours at room temperature. At temperatures below 15 °C impregnation will be very slow or may fail. Sections should be flat and unfolded and there should be about 15 cm³ of fluids available for each section.
3. When the sections are macroscopically deep-purple, rinse in distilled water.
4. Place sections in 5 per cent sodium thiosulphate for 5–10 minutes.
5. Wash in 50 per cent alcohol.
6. Float sections on to clean slides, blot with fluffless paper, dehydrate, clear, and mount in a synthetic resin medium.

RESULTS

Protoplasmic and fibrous astrocytes—opaque purplish-black.

Globus' (1927) method for formalin-fixed material

The following pre-treatment may be used for material fixed in formalin in lieu of fixation in the FAB mixture of Cajal [p. 371].

1. Cut frozen sections at 20 μm.
2. Wash in several changes of distilled water.
3. Place in a covered dish of 10 per cent ammonia (SG 0.880) for 16–24 hours at room temperature.
4. Wash rapidly through two changes of distilled water.
5. Place in a 10 per cent dilution of pure (40 per cent) hydrobromic acid for 2–4 hours.
6. Wash quickly in two changes of 0.05 per cent ammonia water.
7. Proceed with impregnation and rest of technique as in Cajal's method above.

Hortega's (1917) silver carbonate method for astrocytes

FIXATION

Fresh tissue is fixed in the FAB mixture of Cajal [p. 371] for 15–40 days, the shorter period favouring the impregnation of protoplasmic astrocytes, the longer period fibrous astrocytes.

The secondary fixation method of Globus (above) may be used for material fixed primarily in formalin.

SECTIONS

Frozen sections are cut at 15–20 μm.

PREPARATION

Silver carbonate impregnating solution
To 10 cm³ of a 10 per cent solution of silver nitrate add an equal volume of a saturated solution of pure lithium carbonate. A precipitate is formed. Pipette off supernatant fluid and wash precipitate with about 50 cm³ distilled water.

Decant supernatant fluid and replace with 15–20 cm³ distilled water. Cautiously add strong ammonia until the precipitate is just dissolved, then make up to 50 cm³ with distilled water.

TECHNIQUE

1. Wash sections in two changes of distilled water.
2. Place sections in a covered dish of the silver carbonate solution which is heated gently over a low flame or placed in an oven at 45–50 °C. Impregnation is complete when sections have become deep amber and this may be several minutes.
3. Rinse sections briefly in distilled water.
4. Reduce in 20 per cent neutral formalin for 30 seconds.
5. Wash thoroughly in distilled water.
6. Toning (optional). Place sections in a warm, 0.2 per cent solution of gold chloride until they turn dark purple.
7. Fix in 5 per cent sodium thiosulphate for 1–5 minutes. Wash well in water.
8. Mount on slides, dehydrate, clear, and mount in a synthetic resin medium.

RESULTS

Protoplasmic and fibrous astrocytes—brown to black.
Background—yellow to light brown.

Mallory's phosphotungstic acid haematoxylin

This stain is useful for the demonstration of hyperplasia and hypertrophy of fibrous astrocytes and may be used with paraffin or cellulose nitrate sections.

FIXATION

Ten per cent formal-saline.

PREPARATION

Anderson's mordant

Distilled water	100 cm³
Sodium sulphite	5 g
Oxalic acid	2.5 g
Potassium iodide	5 g
Iodine crystals	2.5 g

Dissolve in the above order, and then add 5 cm³ of glacial acetic acid. Keep in a well-stoppered bottle.

SECTIONS

Paraffin or cellulose nitrate at 10–15 μm.

TECHNIQUE A (ANDERSON 1929)

1. Mordant sections for 20–30 minutes in saturated aqueous mercuric chloride.
2. Wash quickly in distilled water and place in Anderson's neuroglia mordant for ten minutes.
3. Without washing, transfer to Lugol's iodine for 15 minutes.
4. Wash in two changes of 95 per cent alcohol until colourless.

5. Wash in distilled water and transfer to 0.25 per cent potassium permanganate for 15 minutes.
6. Wash in distilled water and transfer to 5 per cent oxalic acid until bleached.
7. Wash in two changes of distilled water and stain in phosphotungstic acid haematoxylin [p. 146] for 4–18 hours at room temperature, or a shorter time at higher temperature.
8. Transfer directly to 95 per cent alcohol for one or two minutes followed by dehydration, clearing, and mounting according to the type of section.

RESULTS

Nuclei, astrocytic glia and fibrin—deep blue, myelin may be more lightly stained.
Collagen—rose or brick red.

TECHNIQUE B (LIEB 1948)

1. Take sections to distilled water.
2. Mordant for 20–60 minutes in 4 per cent iron alum.
3. Wash well in distilled water and then proceed from stage 5, above.

Holzer's (1921) method for fibrous glia

Holzer's method is suitable for low power or even macroscopic demonstration of glial fibrosis.

FIXATION

Ten per cent formal-saline.

SECTIONS

Originally designed for frozen sections, it may be used with paraffin sections and cellulose nitrate sections but the embedding medium must be removed from the latter before staining.

PREPARATION

Mordant
0.5 per cent phosphomolybdic acid   10 cm³
95 per cent alcohol   20 cm³

   Mix immediately before use.

Alcohol–chloroform mixture
Absolute alcohol   20 cm³
Chloroform   80 cm³

Staining solution
Crystal violet   5 g
Absolute alcohol   20 cm³
Chloroform   80 cm³

   Filter immediately before use.

Differentiator
Aniline oil   40 cm³
Chloroform   60 cm³

   Shake well and filter. Add 0.3 cm³ hydrochloric acid.

TECHNIQUE

1. Sections are mounted on albumenized slides and blotted well with filter paper.
2. Flood quickly with phosphomolybdic acid mordant and leave for 1–3 minutes.
3. Blot well with filter paper and flood with alcohol–chloroform. Blot immediately with fresh filter paper damped with alcohol–chloroform and without allowing slide to dry, flood with alcohol–chloroform again.
4. Throw off the alcohol–chloroform and replace with the crystal violet stain and leave for about ten seconds.
5. Throw off the stain and replace with several changes of 10 per cent aqueous potassium bromide until no green scum appears on the solution and the surface of the section is 'wet'.
6. Blot dry and leave dry for about ten seconds.
7. Differentiate in aniline–chloroform until only the glia fibres appear stained. This may take up to 15 minutes and the section should be rocked frequently during this time.
8. Blot section and flood with xylene. Repeat several times to eliminate all traces of aniline oil.
9. Mount in a synthetic resin medium.

RESULTS

Fibrous glia—deep blue.
Collagen—blue.

NOTES

1. Cox (1977) gives optional pretreatment of sections with Anderson's mordant, followed by iodine–thiosulphate and potassium permanganate–oxalic acid sequences.
2. Cox also recommends hydrating sections through absolute and 95 per cent alcohol to water after staining (step 4).
3. Cox (1973) advocated drying sections after treatment with potassium bromide (step 6) by leaving them in sunlight, ultraviolet light, or under an electric light bulb for 30 minutes. Thorough drying at this stage is essential.
4. The best quality, pale aniline oil should be used for differentiation and care should be taken to avoid inhalation of the toxic fumes.

Hortega's (1921a) silver carbonate method for oligodendroglia

FIXATION

Cajal's FAB mixture [p. 371] for 12–48 hours, followed by treatment in a fresh bath of the mixture for ten minutes at 45–50 °C, just prior to sectioning.

SECTIONS

Frozen sections at 15–20 μm.

PREPARATION

Impregnating solution
To 5 cm³ of 10 per cent silver nitrate add 20 cm³ of 5 per cent sodium carbonate (anhydrous). Dissolve the resulting precipitate by carefully adding strong ammonia, drop by drop. Make up the volume to 45 cm³ with distilled water. Filter before use.

TECHNIQUE

1. Wash sections in 1 per cent ammonia water followed by distilled water.
2. Impregnate in the ammoniacal silver carbonate solution for 1–5 minutes, gently moving the sections about.
3. Rinse for 15 seconds in distilled water.
4. Reduce in 1 per cent neutral formalin for one minute.
5. Tone in 0.2 per cent gold chloride until the sections are grey (10–15 minutes).
6. Fix in 5 per cent 'hypo' for one minute.
7. Wash well in water.
8. Mount section on a slide, dehydrate, clear, and mount in a synthetic resin medium.

RESULTS

Oligodendroglia—black.
Background—grey, nuclei may be lightly stained.

Hortega's (1921b) silver carbonate method for microglia

FIXATION

As in the previous method, but prolonging the initial treatment with FAB to 2–4 days.

SECTIONS

Frozen sections at 15–20 μm.

PREPARATION

Impregnating solution
As in the previous method, but diluting with distilled water to give a final volume of 75 cm³ instead of 45 cm³.

TECHNIQUE

1. Wash several sections in 1 per cent ammonia water followed by distilled water.
2. Treat sections with the impregnating solution for 20 seconds to two minutes. Remove one section after about 20 seconds, another after 45 seconds, and so on up to two minutes, reducing each section immediately and directly in 1 per cent neutral formalin, gently agitating the while.
3. Remainder of the technique as in the previous method for oligodendroglia.

RESULTS

Microglia—black.
Background—pale grey.

NOTE

The similarity of this method to the previous one for oligodendroglia will be noted, and in practice, these cells, as well as microglia may be impregnated in either method.

Penfield's (1928) combined oligodendroglia and microglia method

FIXATION

Ten per cent formal-saline (duration not critical) or in FAB mixture for seven days.

SECTIONS

Frozen sections at 20 μm.

TECHNIQUE

1. Place sections in a covered dish of 1 per cent ammonia water overnight.
2. Transfer sections directly to 5 per cent hydrobromic acid (40 per cent) in distilled water for one hour at 37 °C.
3. Wash in three changes of distilled water.
4. Neutralize in 5 per cent sodium carbonate for 1–6 hours, the exact time between these limits is not critical.
5. Place sections in the Hortega weaker ammoniacal silver carbonate solution of the previous method. Remove one section after two minutes, another after three minutes and so on, up to five minutes, reducing each section immediately and directly in 1 per cent formalin with gentle agitation, checking microscopically to achieve optimum impregnation.
6. Toning, dehydration, and mounting as in the previous methods.

RESULTS

Oligodendroglia and microglia are black, the background light grey and sometimes, light staining of astrocytes if the duration of impregnation has been prolonged.

Rapid method for oligodendroglia, microglia, and astrocytes (Scott 1971)

Scott's method is most useful when all suitable material has been embedded in paraffin wax although it is equally applicable to frozen sections.

FIXATION

Ten per cent formal-saline.

SECTIONS

15–30 μm paraffin or frozen sections.

PREPARATION

To 2 cm³ of strong ammonia add 5 per cent silver nitrate until a slight permanent turbidity is obtained and the solution is orange–brown in colour.

TECHNIQUE

1. Frozen sections: place in 10 per cent ammonia for two hours. Paraffin sections: do not mount on slides but de-wax in two baths of xylene and hydrate the free sections through absolute and progressive dilutions of alcohol to distilled water.
2. Wash well in distilled water.
3. Impregnate in the ammonia–silver solution for 3–4 seconds.
4. Reduce immediately in 3 per cent formalin and agitate for approximately 30 seconds.
5. Wash well in two changes of distilled water.
6. Fix in 5 per cent sodium thiosulphate.
7. Wash in water and mount on slides.
8. Dehydrate, clear, and mount in a synthetic resin medium.

RESULTS

Oligodendroglia, microglia, and astrocytes—black.

NOTE

Re-impregnation may be carried out, repeating stages 2–5.

Weil–Davenport method for pathological glia (from Conn and Darrow 1943)

While lacking some of the selectivity and precision of impregnation methods for individual cell types, the following procedure is helpful in the demonstration of glial tumours and gliosis, especially as it is applicable to routine, formalin fixed paraffin sections.

FIXATION

Ten per cent formal-saline, duration not critical.

SECTIONS

Paraffin sections at 10 μm.

PREPARATION

Impregnating solution
Silver nitrate   8 g
Distilled water   10 cm³
95 per cent alcohol   90 cm³

Reducing solution
Pyrogallic acid   5 g
95 per cent alcohol   95 cm³
Formalin   5 cm³

TECHNIQUE

1. Remove wax with xylene.
2. Wash section in absolute alcohol and cover with a film of cellulose nitrate as described on page 186.
3. Impregnate for 6–48 hours, duration not critical.
4. Rinse very quickly in 95 per cent alcohol.
5. Reduce for about one minute, but check microscopically to control intensity.
6. Wash thoroughly in running tap water.
7. Tone in 0.2 per cent gold chloride for 5–10 minutes, wash in distilled water followed by fixing in 5 per cent 'hypo'.
8. Wash in water, dehydrate, remove cellulose nitrate film with alcohol–ether. Cellosolve or acetone, clear in xylene, and mount in a synthetic resin medium.

RESULTS

Pathological glia—grey to black.
Axis cylinders—grey or black.
Background—grey-violet.

NISSL SUBSTANCE

Nissl substance (or Nissl granules, or 'tigroid', or chromidial substance) was described by Franz Nissl in 1885 and is seen in fixed and stained neurones as intracytoplasmic clumps or granules, rich in RNA and staining readily with basic dyes. The granules, which have been shown by electron microscopy to represent the granular endoplasmic reticulum of neurones, decrease and finally disappear (chromatolysis) from nerve cells whose axons have been damaged or severed. This provides a valuable means of microscopical assessment of the condition of the cells.

Since the appearance of Nissl substance is affected by the mode of fixation, this, as well as type of section and section thickness, should be constant throughout any comparative studies.

Nissl originally prescribed alcohol fixation and freehand sections, staining them with magenta and dahlia, but numerous modifications of this method have been described employing formalin fixation, frozen, cellulose nitrate or paraffin sections, and methylene blue, toluidine blue, thionin or cresyl fast violet. The methyl green–pyronin stain [p. 163] may be used with advantage to demonstrate the high RNA content of Nissl substance.

It is likely that the originally recommended alcohol and alcohol-containing fixatives such as Carnoy give superior results and allow sharper staining of Nissl substance by removing, or partially removing, some of the obscurative lipid substance of nervous tissues, thus giving better access of the stain. Formalin-fixed frozen sections should be treated with absolute alcohol and xylene as a preliminary to staining. Failure to do so will generally result in weak, diffuse staining.

Cresyl fast violet stain for Nissl substance

FIXATION

Ten per cent formal-saline.

SECTIONS

(a) 20–30 μm cellulose nitrate sections.
(b) 15–20 μm paraffin sections.

TECHNIQUE (a) FOR CELLULOSE NITRATE SECTIONS

1. Place sections in 70 per cent alcohol for 24–48 hours at 37 °C to remove some lipid and improve subsequent staining.
2. Wash in distilled water.
3. Place in 0.1 per cent cresyl fast violet and heat gently to 50–60 °C. Allow to cool for one hour.
4. Dehydrate and partially differentiate through graded alcohols to xylene and leave in fresh xylene overnight.
5. Bring sections to 95 per cent alcohol to which has been added (a) a little cajeput oil or (b) 5–6 drops of 10 per cent acetic acid and the same quantity of chloroform per 100 cm³ of alcohol.
6. Wash in clean 95 per cent alcohol and return to xylene.
7. Repeat steps 5 and 6 if necessary.
8. Mount in Euparal or Canada balsam.

TECHNIQUE (b) FOR PARAFFIN SECTIONS

1. Remove wax with xylene and take sections to water.
2. Stain in 1 per cent cresyl fast violet for 15–30 minutes.
3. Rinse in distilled water, dehydrate, and clear in xylene. Leave for up to one hour in xylene.
4. Pass through absolute to 95 per cent alcohol to differentiate. A few drops of cajeput oil added to the alcohol will assist differentiation.

5. Wash in 95 per cent alcohol, complete dehydration, and pass to xylene.
6. Repeat steps 4 and 5 if necessary.
7. Mount in a synthetic resin medium.

RESULTS

Nissl substance—deep purple–blue.
Nuclei and some cytoplasmic processes of neurones—blue.
Background—colourless.

NOTES

1. In neuropathology, the above method is used to show the general cell pattern of brain and spinal cord rather than the display of Nissl substance exclusively.
2. Paraffin sections may be stained in 0.1 per cent cresyl fast violet in 0.25 per cent acetic acid at 56 °C for 5–6 minutes and allowed to cool before washing and differentiating in 95 per cent alcohol. This may result in more even staining.
3. Samples of cresyl fast violet (and toluidine blue and thionin) may vary in their suitability for Nissl staining and new batches of dye should be tested against control material. The variations given above may be applicable to a particular dye sample.

Einarson's (1932) gallocyanine method for Nissl substance

This is a progressive stain, requiring no differentiation. It is well suited to the bulk staining of multiple paraffin sections (Kellett 1963).

FIXATION

Carnoy's fluid was originally recommended; 10 per cent formal-saline gives adequate results.

SECTIONS

Paraffin sections at 8–10 μm mounted with an adhesive.

PREPARATION

Stain
Gallocyanine	0.3 g
Chromium potassium sulphate (chrome alum)	10 g
Distilled water	200 cm³

Dissolve the alum in the water, with heat if necessary, before adding the dye. Bring to the boil and continue boiling for 15–20 minutes. Allow to stand for 16–24 hours before filtering. The stain will keep for one month or longer if only used intermittently.

TECHNIQUE

1. Remove wax with xylene and take sections to distilled water.
2. Stain for 16–48 hours at room temperature or for 2–4 hours at 60 °C.
3. Rinse in distilled water, dehydrate, clear, and mount in a synthetic resin medium.

RESULTS

Nuclei and Nissl substance—deep blue.
Background—colourless.

The peripheral nervous system

INTRODUCTION

The principal structures to be studied under this heading are nerve fibres (myelinated and non-myelinated) and nerve endings (motor and sensory).

The methods employed for the study of nerve fibres and myelin sheaths of the CNS are not always suitable for demonstrating similar structures in the peripheral nervous system (PNS). In the latter, many small nerve bundles and individual nerve fibres meander through masses of muscle and connective tissue and differentiation from these structures is sometimes difficult, particularly when using silver impregnation methods. There are also structural differences between the myelin sheaths of the two system (Finean, Hawthorne, and Patterson 1957; Tuqan and Adams 1961) and there is evidence that more myelin is lost from peripheral nerves than from CNS material during paraffin wax processing, unless special fixation is employed [p. 363].

Degenerating myelin, however, may be demonstrated by Marchi's method, or, preferably, the Swank–Davenport modification [p. 369], as in the CNS.

STAINING AND IMPREGNATION METHODS

MYELIN SHEATHS

Osmium tetroxide

This is one of the best and simplest method for observations of both normal and degenerating myelin. The disadvantages are the cost and hazards of osmium tetroxide [p. 47].

Fresh, or formalin-fixed tissue may be used. Small pieces are placed in 0.5–1 per cent osmium tetroxide in distilled water for 3–7 days followed by thorough washing in water. Frozen sections may be cut, the specimen may be teased in a mixture of equal parts glycerol and water or taken to paraffin wax. Here, it is advantageous to prolong treatment with low-grade alcohols (12–24 hours in 70 per cent alcohol) to promote 'secondary blackening' of some fatty substances (Hoerr 1936) and to render the 'osmicated' myelin more resistant to the solvent action of high grade alcohols and clearing agent. Thereafter, treatment with alcohol, chloroform (the recommended clearing agent for this purpose), and wax, should be as brief as is consistent with adequate processing.

Paraffin sections should be dried with minimum heating and after the removal of wax, sections may be mounted directly with a synthetic resin medium or taken to water and counterstained. Normal myelin is black or dark grey, degenerate myelin is seen as black granular deposits, and most other lipid will be black. Occasionally, over-reduction occurs and a dark background is produced. This may be bleached by treating sections with dilute hydrogen peroxide or with potassium permanganate followed by oxalic acid.

Haematoxylin methods

Most haematoxylin stains for myelin may be used on peripheral nerves but for a rapid demonstration, using paraffin sections, the method of Weil (1928) is preferable to that of Loyez as sections are less likely to be removed from the slide during staining and the procedure may be completed in about one hour.

Modified Weil haematoxylin method for myelin

Berube, Powers, and Clark (1965) have made a study of this method and recommend a more dilute staining solution and a lower temperature for staining. Both Weil and Berube advise the use of ripened haematoxylin but this is not necessary and is often less reliable than a fresh preparation [see p. 364]. The staining solution itself is extremely unstable and should be used immediately the two ingredients are mixed together. Clark and Clark (1971) recommend placing the sections in a rack in an empty dish, adding the ingredients individually, and mixing by agitating the rack of slides.

FIXATION

Not critical; mordanting of formalin fixed material with a chrome salt [p. 365] is advantageous.

SECTIONS

Paraffin sections at 8–10 μm.

PREPARATION

Haematoxylin stain
Mix equal parts of 4 per cent iron alum and 1 per cent haematoxylin *immediately* before use.

TECHNIQUE

1. Remove wax with xylene and take sections to distilled water.
2. Stain for 20 minutes at room temperature in the iron haematoxylin.
3. Wash in running water.
4. Differentiate in 4 per cent iron alum until the background is grey.
5. Wash in distilled water.
6. Complete differentiation in Weigert's borax–ferricyanide mixture [p. 366].
7. Wash well in alkaline tap water.
8. Dehydrate, clear, and mount in a synthetic resin medium.

RESULTS

Myelin sheaths—dark grey to black.
Nuclei—light grey to dark grey.
Erythrocytes—black.
Connective tissue—unstained.

Gutmann and Sanders (1943) method for myelin

Gutmann and Sanders used the following modification of the Wolters (1890) method when working on measurements of myelin sheaths in peripheral nerves. It gives a superb demonstration with minimal loss or distortion of the myelin.

FIXATION

Flemming's fluid with acetic acid [p. 53] for three days.

SECTIONS

Paraffin sections at 4–10 μm. The thinnest possible sections are preferable for transverse sections of nerve trunks.

TECHNIQUE

1. Remove wax with xylene and take sections to distilled water.
2. Stain in Kultschitsky's haematoxylin [p. 364] for 24 hours at 45 °C.
3. Wash in water.
4. Place in 0.25 per cent potassium permanganate for 20–30 seconds.
5. Rinse in distilled water.
6. Decolorize in the oxalic acid–sulphite mixture of Pal for $\frac{1}{2}$–3 minutes.
7. Rinse in distilled water.
8. Repeat 4, 5, 6, and 7 until differentiation is complete.
9. Wash thoroughly in running tap water.
10. Counterstain if desired.
11. Dehydrate, clear, and mount in a synthetic resin medium.

RESULTS

Myelin—blue–black to black rings on a light background.
Degenerate myelin—black, irregular granular masses.
Most other lipid—black.
Nuclei—unstained.

Other methods

Solochrome cyanine (Page 1970)

This is a simple and fairly rapid method for myelin in peripheral nerves and gives a clear background.

FIXATION

Not critical; 10 per cent formal-saline and formal-sublimate give good results. Not suitable for use after Flemming fixation.

SECTIONS

Paraffin sections at 6–10 μm.

PREPARATIONS

Staining solution
Solochrome cyanine RS	0.2 g
Distilled water	96 cm^3
10 per cent iron alum	4 cm^3
Conc. sulphuric acid	0.5 cm^3

Mix and filter. Keeps well.

TECHNIQUE

1. Remove wax with xylene and take sections to water, removing mercury pigment if necessary.
2. Stain in solochrome cyanine solution for 10–20 minutes at room temperature.
3. Wash well in running water.
4. Differentiate in 10 per cent iron alum until nuclei are scarcely visible, controlling microscopically.
5. Wash well in running water.
6. Counterstain if desired.
7. Dehydrate, clear, and mount in a synthetic resin medium.

RESULTS

Myelin sheaths—bright blue.
Erythrocytes—blue.
Nuclei—pale blue, almost unstained.

Polarized light [p. 27] is useful for the examination of unstained frozen sections of peripheral nerves and staining with Sudan black [p. 368] is of value for the rapid demonstration of myelin in frozen or teased preparations.

NERVE FIBRES

Methods for the impregnation of nerve fibres with silver nitrate are legion, many are capricious and unreliable and it is generally necessary to find a method applicable to the particular tissue to be studied. The methods given below have been found particularly useful and reliable when used on skin, muscle, and larger nerve trunks.

Frozen sections

Frozen sections are preferable to paraffin wax for the impregnation of nerve fibres in PNS material because it is easier to cut thicker sections, thus enabling greater lengths of fibres to be seen in each preparation. Furthermore, silver methods are generally more reliable when carried out on frozen sections and deposition of precipitate is less.

Of the many modifications of Bielschowsky's method, that of Schofield has proved very successful and is particularly suitable for muscle, where the finest fibres as far as the terminal arborizations may be seen, and in skin, where various end-organs are also shown.

Thick frozen sections of formalin fixed tissue are used; very good results have been obtained with tissue which has remained in formalin for a year or more. Indeed, such material often gives a clearer picture than fresher tissue, as capillary vessels have less tendency to become impregnated.

Modified Schofield's (1959) silver impregnation method

FIXATION

Ten per cent formal saline.

SECTIONS

Frozen sections, unembedded or gelatine embedded at 50–75 μm.

PREPARATION

Ammoniacal silver solution
To about 10 cm³ of 20 per cent silver nitrate, add strong ammonia drop by drop until the precipitate is just dissolved.

Formalin
All formalin solutions are made up with tap water.

TECHNIQUE

1. Place sections in a dish of distilled water containing a few lumps of native calcium carbonate (marble chips) or, in 50 per cent alcohol containing 15 drops of pyridine per 50 cm³ for a minimum of one hour at 37 °C.
2. Rinse in distilled water.

3. Place in 20 per cent silver nitrate for 20–30 minutes at room temperature in the dark.
4. Blot the sections and pass through three baths of 10 per cent formalin and one bath of 2 per cent formalin for 30 seconds in each bath. (When the first bath becomes cloudy, discard the fluid, let the second and third baths become the first and second respectively, and replace the third with fresh formalin.)
5. Rinse rapidly in distilled water—blot.
6. Place in ammoniacal silver solution for 30–40 seconds, agitating the sections—blot.
7. Place in 1 per cent formalin and agitate until the sections are deep golden brown. Change this solution when cloudy.
8. Wash sections in tap water.
9. Fix in 5 per cent sodium thiosulphate for five minutes.
10. Wash well in water, dehydrate, and clear by passing sections through alcohol and xylene or carbol–xylene for gelatine embedded sections. Mount sections on slides and mount in a synthetic resin medium.

RESULTS

Nerve fibres—very dark brown to black.
Other tissue—light brown to dark brown.

Paraffin sections

One of the most reliable methods for use with paraffin sections is that of Palmgren (1948). Unfortunately, this method is liable to leave a heavy precipitate on the sections but the effect of this may be minimized by covering sections with a film of cellulose nitrate [p. 186] thus catching the larger granules which are washed off when the film is removed.

Palmgren's silver impregnation method

FIXATION

Ten per cent formal-saline is suitable and long storage in this is not harmful. Osmium tetroxide, chromic acid, potassium dichromate, and mercuric chloride-containing fixatives should not be used.

SECTIONS

Paraffin sections at 6–20 μm.

PREPARATION

Acid formalin
Formalin	25 cm³
Distilled water	75 cm³
1 per cent nitric acid	0.2 cm³

Silver solution
Silver nitrate	15 g
Potassium nitrate	10 g
Distilled water	100 cm³
5 per cent glycine	1 cm³

Reducer

Pyrogallol	10 g
Distilled water	450 cm³
Absolute ethyl alcohol	550 cm³
1 per cent nitric acid	2 cm³

Toning bath

Gold chloride	0.5 g
Distilled water	100 cm³
Glacial acetic acid	0.1 cm³

Intensifier

50 per cent ethyl alcohol	100 cm³
Aniline oil	two drops

Fixer
5 per cent sodium thiosulphate.

TECHNIQUE

1. Remove wax with xylene, cover sections with a film of cellulose nitrate [p. 186], and take to distilled water.
2. Treat with acid formalin for five minutes.
3. Wash in three changes of distilled water for five minutes altogether.
4. Place in silver solution for 15 minutes at room temperature (20–25 °C) or for 4–5 minutes at 35 °C.
5. Without rinsing, drain the slide a little and place in the reducer, preheated to 40–50 °C for one minute, agitating vigorously at first, then more gently. Use one jar of reducer for each section and then discard. The sections should be yellow–brown.
6. Rinse in 50 per cent alcohol.
7. Wash in three changes of distilled water during five minutes. Examine microscopically.
8. If necessary, repeat from stage 2, reducing the time in the silver solution and decreasing the temperature of fresh reducer to about 30 °C.
9. Tone in gold chloride solution until the yellow–brown tint has uniformly faded. This will take a few minutes. Examine microscopically.
10. Intensify without rinsing for 15 seconds with agitation.
11. Rinse in tap water.
12. If necessary, repeat from stage 9.
13. Fix for about five seconds.
14. Rinse in tap water.
15. Dehydrate, remove cellulose nitrate film, clear, and mount in a synthetic resin medium.

RESULTS

Black nerve fibres on a grey background.

NOTES

1. Acceptable results have been obtained by omitting the toning process altogether, thus simplifying the procedure considerably. After stage 5 (reduction), rinse well in distilled water, fix in 5 per cent sodium thio-sulphate for a few minutes, wash, dehydrate, remove cellulose nitrate

film, clear, and mount. This gives very dark brown to black nerve fibres on a yellowish-brown background.

2. Repetition of stages 2–8 or 9–12 is not always satisfactory as the background is liable to darken and contrast is not increased.

Other methods in common use for the demonstration of peripheral nerves in paraffin sections are those of Marsland, Glees, and Erikson [p. 362] a rapid but less reliable method, Rogers (1931), Bodian (1937), and Romanes (1950).

NERVE ENDINGS

Two main groups of methods are available for the demonstration of nerve endings. These are metallic impregnation methods and vital staining. The histochemical demonstration of cholinesterase will also show the sites of many of the endings, particularly the motor endings in voluntary muscle.

Metallic impregnation

Three types of nerve endings are of particular interest; these are:

1. Motor nerve endings in voluntary muscle.
2. Intramuscular spindles.
3. Sensory nerve endings in skin.

The motor endings, as far as the terminal arborizations and complete cutaneous endings can be shown by Schofield's method [p. 384]. Parts of muscle spindles may also be seen but the spindles are relatively large and teased preparations are required to demonstrate them in their entirety.

The large quantity of fat and connective tissue in skin makes the demonstration of cutaneous endings more difficult. Prolonged treatment in the pyridine solution of the Schofield technique and the de-fatting procedures recommended by Winkelmann and Schmit (1959) and Winkelmann (1960) are of value.

Modifications of the Ranvier–Loewitt technique use teased preparations and whole muscle spindles may then be demonstrated. Motor endings are also shown. Pieces of tissue were 'fixed' in fresh lemon juice in the original method. Fixation is here a somewhat misleading term for although in some respects the tissue is partially preserved, it is also partially macerated and becomes considerably swollen. Other workers have replaced the fresh lemon juice with proprietary brands of preserved juice (Zinn and Morin 1962), or citric acid (Zinn and Morin 1962) and formic acid (Carey 1942). In all these methods the tissue is then treated with gold chloride followed by formic acid which produces a black impregnation of neural elements against a pinkish-grey background and further maceration of the tissue. Microscopical preparations are made by preserving, teasing, and mounting in glycerol or glycerol–alcohol mixtures.

Barker and Ip (1963) and Gladden (1970) have described silver impregnation methods for nerve endings which are suitable for use with teased preparations.

Vital staining

Paul Ehrlich (1885, 1886) was the first to describe the staining of peripheral nerves by the injection of dilute solutions of methylene blue into living animals, and since that time, many investigators have modified the original procedure according to the material to be studied.

Coers and Woolf (1959) recommend intravital staining as a diagnostic tool, but good results have been obtained using unfixed material several hours after removal from the body and perfusion of small animals or whole limbs, immediately after death or amputation, is generally satisfactory.

Studies of the innervation of muscle have been largely superseded by histochemical methods in the diagnosis of neuromuscular disorders but vital staining still provides a means of demonstrating the innervation of muscle and skin of superb delicacy and precision. In teased or squash preparations, the full ramification of the neuromuscular innervation is shown, from bundles of axons down to their terminal arborizations and expansions. Various deformities and changes within the axons, such as beading and swellings are well demonstrated as are encapsulated endings in skin and the complex arrangement of fibres round hair follicles.

A detailed account of a reliable methylene blue method is given by Page (1970). This involves supravital injection of a dilute (0.015 per cent) methylene blue solution, exposure to oxygen followed by fixation of the dye in a solution of ammonium molybdate. After washing, tissues may be teased, squashed, or frozen and sectioned followed by dehydration, clearing, and mounting in a resinous medium. This provides an almost permanent preparation although some workers report fading of the stained elements.

CHOLINESTERASE

Cholinesterase is present at the neuromuscular junction where it destroys the activator substance (acetyl choline ester) after the transmission of the nervous impulse. A simple and reliable method for its demonstration is that of Koelle (1951) [p. 311]. This may be used on squash preparations or on frozen sections of fresh or briefly fixed tissue. It has also been satisfactorily performed on material which had been stained supravitally with methylene blue but this may cause excessive extraction of the dye (Page 1970).

Gwyn and Heardman (1965) combined a modification of Koelle and Friedenwald's (1949) method for cholinesterase with a modified Bielschowsky technique while Namba, Nakamura, and Grob (1967) used Karnovsky's (1964) modification of Koelle and Friedenwald's technique with a development of one of Cajal's silver impregnations.

In the latter method, fresh or fixed tissue is incubated in a buffered solution containing the substrate acetyl thiocholine iodide and copper sulphate; the product is visualized with potassium ferricyanide to give a red deposit at the sites of cholinesterase activity. Impregnation of the nerve fibres is carried out by treatment with silver nitrate and copper sulphate which is reduced with a hydroquinone–sodium sulphite mixture. Results at the neuromuscular junctions show black terminal arborizations surrounded by black–brown deposits of the cholinesterase reaction product.

REFERENCES

ADAMS, C. W. M. (1959). *J. Path. Bact.* **77**, 648.
—— (1962). *Devl. Med. Child Neurol.* **4**, 393.
—— and BAYLISS, O. B. (1961). *J. Histochem. Cytochem.* **9**, 473.
—— and TUQAN, N. A. (1961). *J. Neurochem.* **6**, 334.

ANDERSON, J. (1929). *How to stain the nervous system.* Livingstone, Edinburgh.
BARKER, D. and IP, M. C. (1963). *J. Physiol., Lond.* **169**, 73.
BENDA, C. (1903). *Neurol. Zbl.* **22**, 139.
BERUBE, G. R., POWERS, M. M., and CLARK, G. (1965). *Stain Technol.* **40**, 53.
BIELSCHOWSKY, M. (1904). *J. Psychol. Neurol. (Lpz.)* **3**, 169.
—— (1909). *J. Psychol. Neurol. (Lpz.)* **12**, 135.
BODIAN, D. (1936). *Anat. Rec.* **65**, 89.
—— (1937). *Anat. Rec.* **69**, 153.
BUSCH, K. (1898). *Neurol. Zbl.* **17**, 476.
CAJAL, SANTIAGO RAMÓN Y (1913). *Trab. Lab. Invest. biol. Univ. Madrid* **2**, 219, and **14**, 155.
CAREY, E. J. (1942). *Am. J. Path.* **18**, 237.
CLARK, G. and CLARK, M. (1971). *A primer of neurological staining procedures.* Thomas, Springfield, Ill.
COERS, C. D. and WOOLF, A. L. (1959). *The innervation of muscle: a biopsy study.* Blackwell, Oxford.
CONN, H. J. and DARROW, M. A. (1943). *Staining procedures.* Biotech Publications, Geneva, N.Y.
COX, G. (1973). Neuroglia and Microglia. In *Histopathology—selected topics* (ed. H. C. Cook). Baillière Tindall, London.
—— (1977). Neuropathological techniques. In *Theory and practice of histological techniques* (eds. J. D. Bancroft and A. Stevens). Churchill Livingstone, Edinburgh.
COX, W. H. (1891). *Arch. mikr. Anat.* **37**, 16.
EHRLICH, P. (1885). *Zbl. med. Wiss.* **23**, 113.
—— (1886). *Biol. Zbl.* **6**, 214.
EINARSON, L. (1932). *Am. J. Path.* **8**, 295.
FINEAN, J. B., HAWTHORNE, J. N., and PATTERSON, J. D. E. (1957). *J. Neurochem.* **1**, 256.
GASSER, G. (1961). *Basic neuropathological techniques.* Blackwell, Oxford.
GATENBY, J. B. and PAINTER, T. S. (1937). *The microtomist's vade mecum,* 10th edn. Churchill, London.
GLADDEN, M. (1970). *Stain Technol.* **45**, 161.
GLOBUS, C. (1927). *Arch. Neurol. Psychiat. (Chic.)* **18**, 263.
GOLGI, C. (1875). *Riv. sper. Freniat.* **3**, 405.
—— (1878) *Rc. Ist. Lomb. Sci. Lett.* 2nd series, **12**, 5.
GUTMANN, E. and SANDERS, F. K. (1943). *J. Physiol., Lond.* **101**, 489.
GWYN, D. C. and HEARDMAN, V. (1965). *Stain Technol.* **40**, 15.
HOERR, N. L. (1936). *Anat. Rec.* **66**, 149.
HOLMES, W. (1947). In *Recent advances in clinical pathology* (ed. S. C. Dyke). Churchill, London.
HOLZER, W. (1921). *Z. ges. Neurol. Psychiat.* **69**, 354.
HORTEGA, DEL RIO P. (1917). *Trab. Lab. Invest. biol. Univ. Madrid* **15**, 367.
—— (1919). *Bol. Soc. esp. Biol.* **9**, 68.
—— (1921a). *Bol. Real. Soc. esp. Hist. Nat.* **22**, 1.
—— (1921b). *Arch. cardiol. haematol.* **2**, 161.
HUME ADAMS, J. and MILLER, L. (1970). *Nervous system techniques for the general pathologist,* Broadsheet No. 73. Association of Clinical Pathologists.
KAES, T. (1891). *Neurol. Zbl.* **10**, 456.
KARNOVSKY, M. J. (1964). *J. Histochem. Cytochem.* **12**, 219.
KELLETT, B. S. (1963). *J. med. Lab. Technol.* **20**, 196.
KLÜVER, H. and BARRERA, E. (1953). *J. Neuropath. exp. Neurol.* **12**, 400.
KOELLE, G. B. (1951). *J. Pharmacol. exp. Ther.* **103**, 153.
—— and FRIEDENWALD, J. S. (1949). *Proc. Soc. exp. Biol. Med.* **70**, 617.
KULTSCHITSKY, N. (1890). *Anat. Anz.* **5**, 519.
LA MANNA, S. (1937). *Z. wiss. Mikr.* **54**, 257.
LIEB, E. (1948). *Arch. Path.* **45**, 559.

LISON, L. and DAGNELIE, J. (1935). *Bull. Histol. appl. Physiol. Path.* **12**, 85.

LOYEZ, M. (1910). *C. R.Soc. Biol. (Paris)* **69**, 511.

MARCHI, V. and ALGERI, G. (1895). *Riv. sper. Freniat.* **11**, 492.

MARGOLIS, G. and PICKETT, J. P. (1956). *Lab. Invest.* **5**, 459.

MARSLAND, T. A., GLEES, P., and ERIKSON, L. B. (1954). *J. Neuropath. exp. Neurol.* **13**, 587.

NAMBA, T., NAKAMURA, T., and GROB, D. (1967). *Am. J. clin. Path.* **47**, 74.

NISSL, F. (1885). *Neurol. Zbl.* **4**, 500.

ORR, D. (1900). *J. Path. Bact.* **6**, 387.

PAGE, K. M. (1970). *J. Med. Lab. Technol.* **27**, 1.

PALMGREN, A. (1948). *Acta Zool.* **29**, 377.

—— (1960). *Acta Zool.* **61**, 1.

PEARSE, A. G. E. (1955). *J. Path. Bact.* **70**, 554.

—— (1960). *Histochemistry, theoretical and applied*, 2nd edn. Churchill, London.

PELTIER, L. F. (1954). *J. Lab. clin. Med.* **43**, 321.

PENFIELD, W. (1928). *Am. J. Path.* **4**, 153.

POPPER, H. (1941). *Arch. Path.* **31**, 766.

RALIS, H. M., BEESLEY, R. A., and RALIS, Z. A. (1973). *Techniques in neurohistology.* Butterworths, London.

ROGERS, W. M. (1931). *Anat. Rec.* **49**, 81.

ROMANES, G. J. (1950). *J. Anat., Lond.* **84**, 104.

ROWE, M. and HILL, R. G. (1948). *Bull. Inst. med. Lab. Technol.* **14**, 49.

SCHOFIELD, G. (1959). In *Leprosy in theory and practice* (ed. R. G. Cochrane). Wright, Bristol.

SCOTT, T. (1971). *J. clin. Path.* **24**, 578.

SMITH, MARION C. (1956). *J. Neurol. Psychiat.* **19**, 74.

SWANK, R. L. and DAVENPORT, H. A. (1935). *Stain Technol.* **10**, 87.

TUQAN, N. A. and ADAMS, C. W. M. (1961). *J. Neurochem.* **6**, 327.

VASSAR, P. S. and CULLING, C. F. A. (1959). *Arch. Path.* **68**, 487.

WEIGERT, C. (1884). *Fortschr. Med.* **2**, 120, 190.

—— (1885). *Fortschr. Med.* **3**, 236.

—— (1891). Dtsch. med. Wschr. **17**, 1184.

WEIL, A. (1928). *Arch. Neurol. Psychiat., Lond.* **20**, 392.

WINKELMANN, R. K. (1960). *Nerve endings in normal and pathological skin.* Thomas, Springfield, Ill.

—— and SCHMIT, R. W. (1959). *Stain Technol.* **34**, 193.

WOLTERS, M. (1890). *Z. wiss. Mikr.,* **7**, 466.

ZINN, D. J. and MORIN, L. P. (1962). *Stain Technol.* **25**, 165.

20 | Bacteria and viral inclusions

Methods for bacteria

THE PREPARATION AND FIXATION OF TISSUES

The histological method is not the one of choice for the identification of bacteria; morphology is inferior to culture. In all cases requiring bacteriological investigation a swab from the tissue or an unfixed piece of the tissue should be submitted in a sterile container to the microbiologist. Part should be retained for histology, but in many instances the whole specimen will be sent for histology if the possibility of a bacterial infection has not been seriously considered, and sections from these may have to be stained for bacteria. With tuberculous tissues the time required for culture is lengthy and it is usually possible to make a definite histological diagnosis of tuberculosis more quickly by the type of tissue reaction, though this should be confirmed by the identification of acid-fast bacilli and by culture.

Tissues can be fixed in 10 per cent formal-saline. Prolonged fixation in formalin may diminish the staining of acid-fast bacilli with carbol-fuchsin, but this is seldom a serious disadvantage and normally-fixed material is satisfactory. Formal-sublimate is a suitable fixative, and 2 per cent acetic acid with formal-saline can be used. Tissues should be dehydrated, cleared and impregnated with paraffin wax in the usual way. Sections must be thin (3–5 μm) since prolonged microscopical examination of thick sections with the ×40 or ×100 objective (that have a very small depth of focus) is difficult and tiring.

Care must be taken to avoid the contamination of tissues with bacteria or fungi after they have been taken for histology, and bacteria must be prevented from growing in mounting media, etc. Perfectly clean slides are essential. Bacteria in infected tissues will continue to grow after removal from the body or after death until they are fixed; if fixation cannot be immediate the tissue should be kept cool or refrigerated, though not deep-frozen because of the risk of ice-crystal artifacts. Specimens that have been left in warm laboratories or operating theatres often contain large numbers of bacteria and even small bubbles of gas due to gas-producing bacteria; these are of limited value for bacteriology or histology, though they may suggest that some of the bacteria were originally present in the tissue. *Pathogenic* bacteria produce a tissue reaction but *saprophytic* bacteria or *contaminants* do not.

STAINING METHODS FOR BACTERIA

GRAM'S METHOD

This is the classical method of the bacteriologist (Gram 1884). It divides bacteria into two groups: *Gram-positive* bacteria retain the stain after treatment with alcohol or acetone, while *Gram-negative* bacteria are decolorized. Bacteria with similar morphology can be distinguished from each other if their reaction to Gram's stain is different (Table 20.1). The method is a regressive one; both Gram-positive and Gram-negative bacteria are first stained with a powerful basic aniline dye, then treated with iodine solution and differentiated until only Gram-positive bacteria retain the stain. In order to see the Gram-negative bacteria a counterstain (neutral red, dilute carbol fuchsin, safranin) is applied after differentiation.

Table 20.1 Gram-positive and Gram-negative bacteria

Morphology	Gram-positive	Gram-negative
Cocci	*Staphylococcus* *Streptococcus* *Pneumococcus*	*Neisseria*
Cocco-bacilli		*Brucella* *Haemophilus*
Bacilli	*Bacillus anthracis* *Clostridia* *Corynebacterium* *Mycobacterium* *Lactobacillus* and other non-pathogens	*Escherichia* *Klebsiella* *Pasteurella* *Proteus* *Pseudomonas* *Salmonella* *Shigella* *Vibrio*

This method is based upon the differential solubility of the Gram stain in alcohol or acetone when the stain is absorbed by different bacteria. The addition of iodine after initial staining either acts as a mordant between the bacteria and the dye, or precipitates the stain in the protoplasm of Gram-positive bacteria; in either case the differentiating fluid extracts the stain from the Gram-negative bacteria more readily than from the Gram-positive bacteria. However, it must be appreciated that it is possible to decolorize Gram-positive bacteria by over-differentiation and this is apt to take place in sections; bacteria are small in comparison with the thickness of the section and by the time the differentiating fluid has fully penetrated the whole section some bacteria may be over-differentiated; bacteria in a section may appear to be either Gram-positive or Gram-negative for this reason. In addition to the problem of differentiation, it is not always easy to stain all the Gram-negative bacteria in a section, though Gram-positive bacteria stain more easily. The classical Gram and Gram–Weigert techniques will be described, and the Gram–Twort modification, which gives elegant colour contrast in tissues, is also given. Because of the difficulties that may be encountered with Gram staining of bacteria in tissue sections, many modification have been developed (Brown and Brenn 1931; Humberstone 1963; Taylor 1966; the MacCallum–Goodpasture method—Luna 1968; Brown and Hopps 1973). All methods should be interpreted critically, and control sections should be used.

Gram's technique for bacteria in sections (after Gram 1884)

This depends upon the fact that different types of bacteria retain an aniline dye–iodine complex in varying degrees when differentiated with alcohol or acetone (see above).

FIXATION

Formalin or other fixatives.

SECTIONS

Thin (3–5 µm) paraffin sections.

PREPARATION

1. Crystal violet solution for Gram's stain:

Crystal violet	2 g
95 per cent alcohol	20 cm³
Ammonium oxalate	0.8 g
Distilled water	80 cm³

This solution (Lillie 1928) is made by dissolving the dye in the alcohol and the oxalate in the water and mixing the two solutions. It has the advantage of being stable for two or three years.

2. Gram's iodine:

Iodine crystals	1 g
Potassium iodide	2 g
Distilled water	300 cm³

This solution may weaken and lose its colour after many months.

3. Aniline–xylene:

Aniline	2 parts.
Xylene	1 part.

TECHNIQUE

1. Take paraffin sections to water.
2. Stain with crystal violet for 2–3 minutes.
3. Wash off the stain with Gram's iodine; then flood the slide with Gram's iodine and leave for 2–3 minutes.
4. Decolorize the section in absolute alcohol or acetone (see Note 1).
5. Stain for 2–3 minutes, direct from the absolute alcohol, in a 1 per cent aqueous solution of neutral red (see Note 4).
6. Rinse rapidly in water.
7. Blot dry and rapidly dehydrate in aniline–xylene.
8. Clear in xylene and mount in a synthetic resin medium.

RESULTS

Gram-positive bacteria—blue–black.
Gram-negative bacteria—red.
Tissues are generally Gram-negative (red), but keratin, fibrin, and calcium may be blue–black.

NOTES

1. Gram's stain is easily under- or over-differentiated. Under-differentiation stains Gram-negative bacteria blue. Over-differentiation stains

Gram-positive bacteria red. Practice and experience are needed to obtain the correct degree of differentiation. Alcohol or acetone should be dropped on the slide until stain ceases to come out and the specimen is almost completely decolorized on naked-eye examination. With alcohol this may take up to half a minute, but with acetone a few seconds is enough (usually 1–2 seconds). It is essential that differentiation is uniform throughout the whole section.

2. Control sections are usually necessary to be sure that differentiation is correctly carried out. Sections of pathological material known to contain both Gram-positive and Gram-negative bacteria (appendix, intestine) should be stained concurrently with the section under investigation. In difficult cases a control section may be cut and mounted upon the same slide as the test section, thereby ensuring that both receive identical differentiation. The use of the Gram–Twort method (see below) is recommended because of the greater control of differentiation. Uneven or excessive differentiation are common faults of sections stained with Gram's method.

3. Adams (1975) has shown that the addition of iodine to alcohol increases the rate of extraction of crystal violet by alcohol from Gram-negative organisms, but delays the extraction of the dye from Gram-positive organisms. Stain with crystal violet and differentiate with a solution of 0.1 per cent safranin, 0.1 per cent basic fuchsin, and 0.06 per cent iodine in 95 per cent alcohol for about 20 seconds. Gram-positive organisms—violet; Gram-negative organisms—pink.

4. Improved staining of Gram-negative bacteria can be obtained by counter-staining with methyl green–pyronin and light green (Sowter and McGee 1976).

The Gram–Weigert technique for bacteria and fibrin
(Weigert 1887; modified by Conn, Darrow, and Emmel 1960)

This differs from the classical Gram method in that counterstaining is carried out before the Gram reaction and differentiation is more slowly performed with aniline–xylene.

FIXATION

Formalin or other fixatives.

SECTIONS

Thin (3–4 μm) paraffin sections.

PREPARATIONS

1. Lithium–carmine. Dissolve 4 g carmine in 100 cm³ saturated lithium carbonate solution and boil for 10–15 minutes. When cool add 1 g thymol. Filter before use.
2. Crystal violet solution. As for Gram method (see above).
3. Gram–Weigert iodine. Iodine 1 g; potassium iodide 2 g; dissolve in 100 cm³ distilled water.

TECHNIQUE

1. Take paraffin sections to water. It is not strictly necessary to treat mercury-fixed tissue with iodine and 'hypo' as mercury is removed by the Gram–Weigert iodine.

2. Stain for five minutes in lithium–carmine solution.
3. Transfer directly to acid alcohol for a few seconds (this holds the red colour in the section during subsequent staining).
4. Wash thoroughly in tap water.
5. Using a slide staining rack, pour crystal violet solution on the slides and leave for 2–3 minutes.
6. Drain and blot with filter paper.
7. Pour Gram–Weigert iodine solution over the slides and leave for 30 seconds.
8. Drain and blot with filter paper.
9. Differentiate in a mixture of equal parts of aniline oil and xylene from a dropping bottle. Blot and pour on fresh aniline-xylene several times until the section is well differentiated and no more purple colour washes out.
10. Blot; rinse in several changes of xylene to remove the aniline.
11. Mount in a synthetic resin medium.

RESULTS

Gram-positive bacteria and fibrin—blue–black.
Gram-negative bacteria—red.
Nuclei—red.

The Gram–Twort modification for bacteria in sections

The following modification of the Twort (1924) method for bacteria has the advantages of easier differentiation and a better colour contrast compared with the other Gram techniques (Ollett 1947, 1951). The sections are easy to examine for long periods without eye-strain.

FIXATION

Formalin; other fixatives can be used.

SECTIONS

Thin (3–5 μm) paraffin sections.

PREPARATION

Modified Twort's stain
Make a stock solution of:

0.2 per cent absolute alcoholic neutral red   90 cm³
0.2 per cent absolute alcoholic fast green FCF   10 cm³

    For use, dilute one volume of stock solution with three volumes of distilled water.

TECHNIQUE

1. Stain in 1 per cent aniline–crystal violet or crystal violet [p. 393] for 3–4 minutes.
2. Wash quickly in distilled water.
3. Treat with Gram's iodine, three minutes.
4. Wash quickly in distilled water and blot absolutely dry.
5. Decolorize with 2 per cent acetic acid in absolute alcohol until no more colour comes away (about ten minutes.) The section should be a dirty straw colour at this stage.
6. Wash quickly in distilled water.

7. Counterstain in the modified Twort's stain for five minutes.
8. Wash quickly in distilled water.
9. Decolorize in 2 per cent acetic acid in absolute alcohol until no more red colour comes away (about ten seconds).
10. Clear in xylene and mount in a synthetic resin medium.

RESULTS

Gram-positive bacteria—dark blue.
Gram-negative bacteria—pink.
Nuclei—red.
Cytoplasm—light green.
Red blood corpuscles—green.

THE STAINING OF ACID-FAST BACILLI

The identification of tubercle bacilli is one of the most important techniques for bacteria that is used by the histopathologist. In some patients the diagnosis of tuberculosis is not seriously considered when material is taken at operation, and unfixed material is not available for culture; the demonstration of tubercle bacilli in sections is then the only means of diagnosis of tissues that show histological changes suspicious of tuberculosis. In addition, the similarity between tuberculous lesions and those of sarcoid or other granulomata makes the identification of tubercle bacilli essential for final diagnosis.

The classical method for acid-fast bacilli is the *Ziehl–Neelsen* technique. This may necessitate the staining and examination of many sections, a time-consuming and laborious process that may not always be absolutely reliable; in chronic tuberculous lesions the number of bacilli may be small and difficult to identify. A laboratory that handles a large amount of routine diagnostic material requires a rapid screening method for the preliminary examination of doubtful material. The *fluorescence method* for the microscopic identification of tubercle bacilli (Clegg and Foster-Carter 1946) is very valuable; suitably stained sections or smears are examined by ultraviolet light, and acid-fast bacilli fluoresce brilliantly. They can be easily identified with the × 10 (16 mm) objective, enabling large areas of tissue or large numbers of slides to be examined in a short time.

The fluorescence method for acid-fast bacilli

The detection of acid-fast bacilli in tissue sections by fluorescence microscopy is discussed in detail by Matthaei (1950) and Kuper and May (1960). The principles and the use of the fluorescence microscope are described on page 22. Preparations are not permanent and must be examined immediately as the specific fluorescence of acid-fast bacilli fades within a few days and non-specific fluorescence develops. A completely black background is not advisable as it will be necessary to use the fine adjustment of the microscope and the section can be inadvertently focused-out unless the tissue can be seen. This is a useful technique for confirming the presence of acid-fast bacilli in tuberculoid granulomata in sections. The bacilli appear to be larger than usual, due to the fluorescent glow, but retain their morphology and can be more easily seen in sections or smears (Silver, Sonnenwirth, and Alex 1966) than by the Ziehl–Neelsen method. The finding of fluorescent bacilli in tissues that do not have suspicious cellular changes, or bacilli with atypical morphology or weak fluorescence, should not be accepted without confirmation by the Ziehl–Neelsen technique.

FIXATION

Formalin or other fixatives.

SECTIONS

Thin paraffin sections are suitable.

PREPARATION

Auramine–rhodamine staining solution

Auramine	1.5 g
Rhodamine B	0.75 g
Glycerol	75 cm³
Phenol crystals (liquefied at 50 °C)	10 cm³
Distilled water	50 cm³

This will keep about two months.

Acid-alcohol differentiator
0.5 per cent hydrochloric aicd in 70 per cent alcohol.

TECHNIQUE

1. Take sections to water.
2. Flood sections with staining solution and stain on a rack for 10–30 minutes at 60 °C.
3. Wash in tap water.
4. Differentiate in acid alcohol for two minutes.
5. Wash in tap water.
6. Counterstain for 1–3 minutes in 0.5 per cent potassium permanganate; the section should be very slightly brown.
7. Sections may be examined with the fluorescence microscope [p. 22] unmounted, but it is better to blot and very rapidly dehydrate in alcohol, clear in xylene and mount. The preparations do not keep well, and with synthetic resin media such as DPX considerable background fluorescence may develop. This can be diminished by the use of a fluorescence-free mountant such as Fluormount.

RESULTS

Acid-fast bacilli fluoresce brilliantly as a golden colour against a dark background.

NOTES

1. Sections are examined with the × 10 and × 40 (16 and 4 mm) objectives; the oil immersion objective is not needed for this method, but a high-dry (× 63) objective may be useful for final identification.
2. The morphology of the bacilli is well retained, but atypical bacilli can be marked, decolorized, and overstained with the Ziehl–Neelsen technique; this is seldom necessary.
3. This technique may be combined with acridine orange [p. 405] in order to stain fungi as well as acid-fast bacilli (Mote, Muhm, and Gigstad 1975).
4. Lepra bacilli can be demonstrated [p. 399].

The Ziehl–Neelsen technique for acid-fast bacilli
(Ziehl 1882; Neelsen 1883)

The histological method is similar to the classical bacteriological technique that depends upon the resistance of certain bacilli, after staining by hot carbol-fuchsin, to decolorization with alcohol or acids. The waxy lipid capsules of the Mycobacteria make them difficult to stain, but when they have been stained the lipid makes removal of the stain a slower process than in other bacteria. *M. tuberculosis* is the commonest acid-fast pathogen and is highly resistant to decolorization by mineral acids and alcohol; *M. leprae* is less acid-fast and a slightly different technique may be required to demonstrate the causative organisms of leprosy; non-pathogenic mycobacteria are acid-fast but are not usually alcohol-fast. Acid-fast bacilli can be stained by this method in tissues that have been decalcified by the usual agents, but not after treatment with 2.5 M hydrochloric acid; the commercial decalcifying agent Rapid Decalcifer (RDC) contains hydrochloric acid and is unsuitable (Anderson and Coup 1975).

FIXATION

Most fixatives can be used. Avoid Carnoy, which removes lipid from the bacilli and makes them less acid-fast. Formalin, especially when prolonged, is said to reduce acid-fastness, but specimens usually stain perfectly satisfactorily. The treatment of formalin fixed sections with 0.5 per cent ammonium hydroxide before staining may improve the brightness of the colour of acid-fast bacilli, but this is seldom necessary and may detach the sections from the slide.

SECTIONS

Thin (3–5 µm) paraffin sections.

PREPARATIONS

1. Carbol-fuchsin:

Basic fuchsin	1 g
Absolute alcohol	10 cm³
5 per cent phenol in distilled water	100 cm³

Dissolve the basic fuchsin in the alcohol, then mix with the phenol solution. Filter.

2. Acid-alcohol:

1 per cent hydrochloric acid in 70 per cent alcohol.

3. Counterstain:

Methylene blue	1 g
Glacial acetic acid	1 cm³
Absolute ethyl alcohol	20 cm³
Distilled water	80 cm³

TECHNIQUE

1. Take sections to water.
2. *Either*, flood the slide with carbol-fuchsin, after placing a rectangle of filter paper over the section to prevent precipitation of the stain. Warm the slide until the stain begins to steam; this can be conveniently done by the flame from a throat swab soaked in spirit. Leave for 10 minutes. *Or*, place the

slide in a warmed vessel of carbol-fuchsin for at least one hour in the 37 °C incubator or 30 minutes at 60 °C.

3. Rinse in tap water.
4. Decolorize with acid-alcohol until the section is pale pink and no more colour comes away (about 1–3 minutes). A further decolorization is recommended in neutral 70 per cent alcohol for the exclusion of non-pathogenic acid-fast bacilli (see Note 1).
5. Rinse in water.
6. Counterstain in acidified methylene blue for one minute.
7. Rinse in water.
8. Dehydrate and differentiate the counterstain until blue with absolute alcohol.
9. Clear in xylene and mount in a synthetic resin medium.

RESULTS

Acid-fast bacilli—red.
Other bacteria—blue.
Cells and their nuclei—blue.
Red blood corpuscles should retain a slight red colour.

NOTES

1. Since this method involves the use of both acid and alcohol decolorization, the risk of mistaking the non-pathogenic acid-fast bacilli for the tubercle bacillus is decreased. In sections the tubercle bacilli will be found in the abnormal areas (tubercles) and this risk is slight. The non-pathogenic acid-fast bacilli that are found in butter, milk or cerumen are seldom alcohol-fast, but the smegma bacillus may require prolonged alcohol decolorization.
2. Counterstaining should be light, especially in sections containing much nuclear material, such as lymphoid tissue. Heavy counterstaining makes the identification of acid-fast bacilli difficult and may colour them purple. Pathological tissues often contain mycobacteria in small numbers and these are most easily seen if the sections are thin and absolutely flat, a little residual pink stain is present and counterstaining is light. Several sections from the paraffin block should be stained and the tuberculous foci are examined with the × 40 dry objective. Prolonged search with the × 100 oil immersion objective is seldom needed.
3. Basic fuchsin specified for Schiff's reagent may not give satisfactory results.
4. Control sections of known positive tuberculous material with abundant acid-fast bacilli are valuable in that they indicate that the staining technique is satisfactory when several negative sections are being examined. They also give an idea of the colour of the acid-fast bacilli; this may vary from a light to a dark red.
5. If sections are stained with Victoria blue R in place of basic fuchsin, and counterstained with tartrazine in Cellosolve [p. 401], acid-fast bacilli are blue against a yellow background. This is satisfactory for colour-blind microscopists.

Methods for leprosy bacilli in paraffin sections

The *leprosy bacillus* is more easily decolorized than the tubercle bacillus as it is less acid- and alcohol-fast; differentiation must be very carefully controlled. A faint residual red colour in the tissues is especially important, and sections that do not show this may be unreliable for the exclusion of leprosy. The use of strong solutions of acids must be avoided and alcohol should not be used for differentiation of the stain, nor for taking paraffin sections to water or for final dehydration.

Lepra bacilli can be demonstrated by the fluorescent method [p. 396] but may be differentiated with 0.5 per cent hydrochloric acid without alcohol. Blot dry, and dry off the section in the 56 °C oven before mounting. With Ziehl–Neelsen staining, acid-fastness is improved if the bacilli are protected from oil solvents. The Fite–Faraco modification (Faraco 1938; Fite, Cambre, and Turner 1947) for leprosy bacilli is similar to the standard Ziehl–Neelsen technique, but the paraffin wax is removed from the sections with two changes of a mixture of one part of groundnut oil, cotton seed oil, or olive oil and two parts of xylene for ten minutes each. Wade (1952) used two parts of rectified turpentine and one part of liquid petrolatum for the same purpose. After either of these variants the sections are drained, blotted until opaque, and placed directly in water; the residual oil in the sections helps to prevent shrinkage.

In many leprosy specimens the bacilli stain easily, but if difficulty is experienced the Wade technique, together with avoidance of alcoholic differentiation and dehydration, will improve Ziehl–Neelsen staining. In old paraffin blocks lepra bacilli may be impossible to stain, but Sutter (1965) has shown that they retain their characteristic morphology and are well demonstrated by Gomori's hexamine–silver method [p. 270].

Methods for viral inclusions

Individual viruses are too small for demonstration by light microscopical techniques. Viral inclusion bodies within the cells of infected tissues may be large and numerous, as in molluscum contagiosum, and these can be stained by various methods. Many staining techniques were developed for the Negri bodies of human and canine rabies when this disease was commoner than it is now, but they are not always reliable and better results may be obtained in a well differentiated haematoxylin–eosin section. Viral inclusions (Negri, Guarnieri, and Kurloff bodies; herpes, varicella, and molluscum inclusions, etc.), stain differently, variably, and non-specifically. They cannot be accurately classified or identified by their staining reactions, and viruses are far less satisfactory than bacteria in this respect. The methods described below are designed to show viral inclusion bodies selectively, but they also stain other tissue components. A viral disease can only be suspected in histological sections for light microscopy by the presence of intracellular inclusions in association with characteristic cellular changes in certain recognized situations. Electron microscopy is often the best method of identification.

STAINING METHODS

Phloxine–tartrazine stain for inclusion bodies (Lendrum 1939, 1947)

This is dependent upon the phloxinophilia of certain structures (inclusion bodies, nucleoli of some tumour cells, Paneth cell granules, etc.). These retain the red stain when differentiated with a yellow tartrazine solution.

FIXATION

Formal-sublimate is recommended, but other fixatives (except bichromate) are satisfactory.

SECTIONS

Paraffin sections.

TECHNIQUE

1. Bring sections to water. Treat with iodine and sodium thiosulphate to remove mercury deposits if necessary.
2. Stain nuclei with alum haematoxylin; Mayer's is recommended, but any haematoxylin may be used.
3. Wash and blue the nuclear stain with running water.
4. Stain with a solution of 0.5 per cent phloxine in 0.5 per cent aqueous calcium chloride for 30 minutes.
5. Rinse in water, drain almost dry and replace by a saturated solution of tartrazine in Cellosolve (2-ethoxyethanol) from a drop bottle, controlling microscopically.
6. Rinse in 95 per cent alcohol, dehydrate in alcohol, clear in xylene, and mount in a synthetic resin medium.

RESULTS

Inclusion bodies—bright red.
Nuclei—blue.
Cytoplasm and collagen—yellow.

NOTES

1. Paneth cell granules, Russell bodies in plasma cells, and fibrin stain red, though less intensely. The degree of staining can be controlled by the time of differentiation, and it is possible to retain an orange–red colour in muscle, keratin, and red blood corpuscles if desired.
2. Negri bodies are not brightly stained by this method. Lists of viral inclusions which give good results, and those that give poor results, are in the description of the method (Lendrum 1947).

Schleifstein's stain for Negri bodies (Schleifstein 1937)

As originally described this is a rapid technique whereby sections are ready for examination about eight hours after the removal of the brain. Tissues processed in the usual way may be used.

FIXATION

Zenker's fluid; tissues fixed in other fixatives should be post-chromed in 3 per cent potassium dichromate for 24–48 hours and well washed.

SECTIONS

Thin (3–5 μm) paraffin sections.

PREPARATION

Staining solution A

Basic fuchsin	1.8 g
Methylene blue	1 g
Glycerol	100 cm³
Methyl alcohol	100 cm³

Shake for several minutes. This solution keeps indefinitely.

Staining solution B
Potassium hydroxide 1 : 40 000 aqueous solution.

The working staining solution is a mixture of ten drops of solution A and 20 cm³ of solution B.

TECHNIQUE

1. Take sections to water and remove mercury precipitates with iodine and thiosulphate.
2. Wash in running water and rinse in distilled water.
3. Place slides on a staining rack and flood with freshly prepared staining solution; warm the slides until they steam and leave for five minutes.
4. Decolorize and differentiate each slide separately with 90 per cent alcohol until the section is a faint violet colour.
5. Pass rapidly through absolute alcohol, clear in xylene, and mount in a synthetic resin medium.

RESULTS

Negri bodies—deep magenta.
Cytoplasm—bluish-violet.
Red blood corpuscles—copper.

REFERENCES

ADAMS, E. (1975). *Stain Technol.* **50**, 227.
ANDERSON, G. and COUP, A. J. (1975). *J. clin. Path.* **28**, 744.
BROWN, J. H. and BRENN, L. A. (1931). *Bull. Johns Hopkins Hosp.* **48**, 69.
BROWN, R. C. and HOPPS, H. C. (1973). *Am. J. clin. Path.* **60**, 234.
CLEGG, J. W. and FOSTER-CARTER, A. F. (1946). *Br. J. Tuberc.* **40**, 98.
CONN, H. J., DARROW, M. A., and EMMEL, V. M. (1960). *Staining procedures: used by the Biological Stain Commission*, 2nd edn. Williams and Wilkins, Baltimore.
FARACO, J. (1938). *Rev. bras. Leprol.* **6**, 177.
FITE, G. L., CAMBRE, P. J., and TURNER, M. H. (1947). *Arch. Path.* **43**, 624.
GRAM, C. (1884). *Fortschr. Med.* **2**, 185.
HUMBERSTONE, F. D. (1963). *J. med. Lab. Technol.* **20**, 153.
KUPER, S. W. A. and MAY, J. R. (1960). *J. Path. Bact.* **79**, 59.
LENDRUM, A. C. (1939). *J. Path. Bact.* **49**, 590.
—— (1947). *J. Path. Bact.* **59**, 399.
LILLIE, R. D. (1928). *Arch. Path.* **5**, 828.
LUNA, L. (1968). In *Manual of histologic staining methods of the Armed Forces Institute of Pathology*, 3rd edn. McGraw-Hill, New York.
MATTHAEI, E. (1950). *J. gen. Microbiol.* **4**. 393.
MOTE, R. F., MUHM, R. L., and GIGSTAD, D. C. (1975). *Stain Technol.* **50**, 5.
NEELSEN, F. (1883). *Zbl. med. Wiss.* **21**, 497.
OLLETT, W. S. (1947). *J. Path. Bact.* **59**, 357.
—— (1951). *J. Path. Bact.* **63**, 166.
SCHLEIFSTEIN, J. (1937). *Am. J. publ. Hlth* **27**, 1283.
SILVER, H., SONNENWIRTH, A. C., and ALEX, N. (1966). *J. clin. Path.* **19**, 583.
SOWTER, C. and McGEE, Z. A. (1976). *J. clin. Path.* **29**, 433.
SUTTER, E. (1965). *Stain Technol.* **40**, 49.
TAYLOR, R. D. (1966). *Am. J. clin. Path.* **46**, 472.
TWORT, F. W. (1924). *J. State Med.* **32**, 351.
WADE, H. W. (1952). *Am. J. Path.* **28**, 157.
WEIGERT, C. (1887). *Fortschr. Med.* **5**, 228.
ZIEHL, F. (1882). *Dtsch. med. Wschr.* **8**, 451.

21 | Fungi and spirochaetes

Methods for fungi

CLASSIFICATION AND TISSUE REACTIONS

The recognition of many types of fungi in hospital patients and animals has led to an increased interest in the identification of fungi in tissues. Fungi may be *saprophytic* or *pathogenic*, and some fungi which are normally not pathogenic may become so in tissues that have been damaged by other diseases. *Opportunistic* fungal infections can occur in normal tissues if immune defence systems are impaired by immunosuppressive, cytotoxic, or steroid treatment. Most pathogenic fungi have a predeliction for certain organs, of which skin, lymph nodes, and lung are often affected, but most organs and tissues can be the site of fungal diseases.

Fungi can be classified according to their morphology in living animal tissues into three groups, (Table 21.1). (1) those with filaments (hyphae) only; (2) those with rounded bodies only; and (3) those with both filaments and rounded bodies. Most fungi can be cultured, and as with the bacterial diseases, suspect tissues should always be submitted for culture as well as for histology. Some fungi cannot be cultured (*Rhinosporidium, Pneumocystis*), and a few like *Pneumocystis* are thought by some workers to be protozoan parasites rather than fungi.

Table 21.1 Classification of pathogenic fungi

1. Filaments (hyphae) only	Actinomyces Nocardia asteroides
2. Rounded bodies only	*Cryptococcus neoformans* *Blastomyces dermatitidis* and *B. brasiliensis* *Histoplasma capsulatum* *Sporotrichum schenkii* *Coccidioides immitis* *Rhinosporidium seeberi* *Pneumocystis carinii*
3. Both filaments and rounded bodies	*Candida albicans* *Aspergillus* spp *Rhizopus. Mucor* *Madurella* spp *Trichophyton*

In some instances the demonstration and identification of fungi in sections may be easy, but in other cases (especially those with rounded bodies only) it can be difficult to show fungi clearly, and even more difficult to exclude their presence in a tissue with certainty. A combination of knowledge of the most likely sites of fungi in tissues, their morphology, and their staining reactions, will help the histologist to choose the most suitable staining methods and to examine sections for fungi with accuracy. Table 21.2 gives some of the tissue reactions that may be seen around pathogenic fungi (Symmers 1960); these reactions are variable, but as the successful search for tubercle bacilli must be concentrated upon parts of the section, so must the search for fungi be directed at the most likely places in the tissue.

Table 21.2 Tissue reactions of pathogenic fungi

Cryptococcus, *Rhizopus*	No reaction
Histoplasma	Within histiocytes
Histoplasma, Cryptococcus	Within giant cells
Rhinosporidium, Cryptococcus	Chronic inflammation without suppuration
Actinomyces, Nocardia Madurella, Aspergillus	Acute and chronic suppuration
Sporotrichum, Blastomyces Coccidioides	Suppurating tuberculoid granuloma
Blastomyces, Coccidioides Histoplasma, Cryptococcus	Tuberculoid granuloma
Dead fungal material	Foreign body giant cells
Monilia, Aspergillus	Occasional pyaemic abscesses
Pneumocystis	Plasma cell pneumonia

SOURCES OF ERROR IN THE EXAMINATION OF TISSUES FOR FUNGI

The histologist who is not continually handling tissues containing fungi is liable to make errors of identification unless he is constantly aware of the variable morphology of pathogenic fungi and of the normal structures that may resemble fungi. The intracellular organisms of histoplasmosis can closely resemble those of leishmaniasis or blastomycosis. Even more important is the recognition of nuclear debris, Russell bodies, foreign material, intracellular vacuoles, or droplets of mucin, and the 'stainable bodies' found in Flemming's germinal centres of lymphatic tissue; all these may resemble the yeast-like rounded fungi. Some of these may be Gram-positive and stain brightly with the PAS reaction or Gridley's stain, and an infected lung or a hyperplastic lymph node may contain many suspicious intracellular bodies. Asteroid bodies and calcified spheroids (Schaumann bodies) which are found in old tuberculous processes and in sarcoidosis, and larger corpora amylacea [p. 227], either hyaline (eosinophilic) or calcifying (basiphilic) in the lung, prostate, or brain may be confused with fungi. Contamination with non-pathogenic fungi can occur during histological processing or staining; since a tissue reaction is not always seen in fungal diseases the absence of changes in the tissue is not a reliable indication that fungi are contaminants. The accurate recognition of fungal disease is usually based upon typical morphology of the fungus and a characteristic tissue reaction in an organ which is known to be commonly affected. If these criteria are not satisfied, the observations should be interpreted with caution.

GENERAL STAINING METHODS FOR FUNGI IN SECTIONS

It is essential to avoid contaminating tissues or slides with non-pathogenic fungi. Extraneous fungi may reach tissues from dirty specimen jars, or from the atmosphere if jars are left uncovered; fungi may contaminate water taps, rubber tubing, paraffin wax or mounting media. If there are fungi on the fingers these can be transferred to clean slides when glycerol–albumen is spread upon them. There are no special problems in fixation, and paraffin sections are suitable for almost all staining methods. Thin sections are needed for the small rounded fungi, such as cryptococci; thicker sections may be more suitable for filamentous hyphae.

Most fungi stain sufficiently with haematoxylin and eosin to be recognizable. Gram's method and its modifications [p. 393] can be used to demonstrate fungi, most of which are Gram-positive. Giemsa [p. 426] is especially valuable for the small causal organism of histoplasmosis. The mucoid capsules of cryptococci can be shown by metachromatic staining; toluidine blue or thionin (1 : 1000) for 30 seconds will stain cryptococci violet, other tissue components being blue. Cryptococci often have a particular affinity for mucicarmine, and Southgate's mucicarmine [p. 244] has been found to be superior to any other mucin stain. The periodic acid–Schiff reaction [p. 237] is recommended for mycelial and rounded fungi in tissues, especially if they are scanty or difficult to identify; Gridley's modification is described below. Most fungi can be demonstrated by one of the silver impregnation methods for reticulin [p. 186], though the Hortega method [p. 372] has been used with greater success for *Pneumocystis*; the Grocott modification of the Gomori hexamine–silver method (see below) gives a very clear picture of most fungi. Chick (1961) has described the fluorescence of fungi with acridine orange, using a technique similar to that of Hicks and Matthaei (1958) for mucin [p. 253]; this method can be combined with the Ziehl–Neelsen technique for acid-fast bacilli [p. 398], which is useful for demonstrating the cause of tuberculoid granulomata in tissue sections.

Gridley's stain for fungi (Gridley 1953).

This is similar to the periodic acid–Schiff reaction [p. 237], but uses chromic acid as the oxidizing agent. The aldehydes that are produced recolour Schiff's reagent and this is then reinforced by staining with aldehyde–fuchsin.

FIXATION

Any well fixed tissue.

SECTIONS

Thin paraffin sections.

Aldehyde–fuchsin solution

Basic fuchsin	1 g
70 per cent alcohol	200 cm^3
Paraldehyde	2 cm^3
Concentrated hydrochloric acid	2 cm^3

Stand at room temperature until the solution turns a deep purple colour (three days). Keep in refrigerator, filter and warm to room temperature before using. This solution lasts about three months and should be discarded when staining time becomes unduly long.

Sulphurous acid rinse

Ten per cent aqueous potassium metabisulphite	5 cm^3
0.1 N hydrochloric acid	5 cm^3
Distilled water	100 cm^3

Prepare fresh before use.

TECHNIQUE

1. Take sections to distilled water.
2. Place in 4 per cent chromic acid for one hour.
3. Wash in running water for five minutes.
4. Place in Schiff's reagent [p. 239] for 15 minutes.
5. Rinse three times in sulphurous acid solution for two minutes in each.
6. Wash in running water for 15 minutes.
7. Place slides in the aldehyde–fuchsin solution for 15–45 minutes.
8. Rinse off excess stain with 95 per cent alcohol.
9. Rinse in running water for five minutes.
10. Counterstain lightly with 0.25 per cent metanil yellow made up in 0.25 per cent acetic acid in distilled water.
11. Rinse in running water.
12. Dehydrate in 95 per cent and absolute alcohol.
13. Clear in xylene and mount in a synthetic resin medium.

RESULTS

Fungi—deep red or purple with blue mycelia.
Background—yellow.
Elastic tissue and mucin also stain deep blue.

Grocott's modification of Gomori's hexamine silver method (Gomori 1946; Grocott 1955)

Chromic acid oxidation causes the formation of aldehydes from carbohydrate compounds in fungi. The aldehydes reduce a hexamine–silver nitrate solution to a black metallic silver compound.

FIXATION

Ten per cent formal-saline.

SECTIONS

Paraffin, celloidin, or frozen sections.

PREPARATION

Hexamine–silver nitrate solution

Stock solutions
1. 5 per cent sodium tetraborate (borax) in distilled water
2. 5 per cent silver nitrate in distilled water   5 cm³
    3 per cent hexamine (methenamine) in distilled water   100 cm³

    A white precipitate will form, but this dissolves on shaking. Clear solutions will keep for several months at 4 °C.

Working solution
Mix 2 cm³ of the borax stock solution (No. 1, above) with 25 cm³ of distilled water. Add 25 cm³ of the hexamine–silver nitrate stock solutions (No. 2, above). Use freshly prepared.

TECHNIQUE

1. Take sections to water.
2. Oxidize in 5 per cent chromic acid for one hour.
3. Wash in running water.
4. Rinse briefly in 1 per cent sodium bisulphite to remove residual chromic acid.
5. Wash in tap water for five minutes.
6. Wash in at least three changes of distilled water.
7. Place in preheated working hexamine–silver nitrate solution in the oven at 56 °C for 30–60 minutes. The section should be yellowish-brown (see Note 1, below). The time required will vary with the fixative of the tissue.
8. Rinse in six changes of distilled water.
9. Tone in 0.1 per cent gold chloride solution for 2–5 minutes.
10. Rinse in distilled water.
11. Place in 2 per cent sodium thiosulphate ('hypo') solution for 2–5 minutes to remove the unreduced silver.
12. Wash thoroughly in water.
13. Counterstain with light green solution (light green SF 0.2 g, glacial acetic acid 0.2 cm³, distilled water 500 cm³) for 30 seconds.
14. Dehydrate, clear, and mount in a synthetic resin medium.

RESULTS

Fungi—sharply outlined in black.
Mucin—grey.
Background—pale green.

NOTES

1. It is advisable to check the colour of the sections after step 7 with the microscope and a control section known to contain fungi should always be run at the same time.
2. Reticulin fibrils and threads of fibrin will be blackened by this method, and must not be confused with fungi.
3. Modifications of this technique for the rapid identification of *Pneumocystis carinii* and fungi in smears and sections have been described by Cherukian and Schenk (1977) and Pintozzi (1978). The latter has reduced the time required to ten minutes by heating the chromic acid and the methenamine–silver solutions in a water-bath at 80 °C.

Methods for spirochaetes

GENERAL METHODS OF EXAMINATION

FRESH PREPARATIONS

Blood spirochaetes, particularly *Spirochaeta recurrentis* of relapsing fever, may be seen by high-power examination with direct illumination. The active movements and the consequent agitation of the adjacent red blood corpuscles catch the eye. For diagnostic purposes by far the best method is that of *dark-ground illumination*, which gives good details of the shape and movements of spirochaetes. Use the dark-ground condenser as described on page 21, and examine thin preparations on slides of the correct thickness. Suitable optical combinations for searching for spirochaetes are:

1. A × 40 (4 mm) objective and a high-power eyepiece (e.g. a 4 mm apochromatic objective and a × 12 compensating eyepiece). In many respects these are the most convenient.
2. × 100 (2 mm) oil-immersion objective, provided with the proper stop, and a low- or medium-powered eyepiece.
3. A × 60 (3.4 mm) oil-immersion objective gives excellent definition with the dark-ground condenser. Owing to its low numerical aperture a stop is not necessary. High-power eyepieces can be used with it successfully.

FILMS AND SMEARS

Leishman's and Giemsa's stains, used according to the standard technique, stain many spirochaetes. Make films and fix, without allowing them to dry, in the vapour of 2 per cent osmium tetroxide for one minute. Then place the slide in absolute alcohol for 15 minutes. Stain in Giemsa or Leishman. Wash in water, if necessary differentiate in dilute alcohol and rinse in water again, and allow to dry. Examine with the oil-immersion objective without mounting.

NOTE

Dobell found that his material (*Cristispira veneris*) underwent distortion if the films were allowed to dry before fixation with osmium tetroxide, or if they were fixed direct in absolute alcohol.

METHODS FOR THE DETECTION OF *TREPONEMA PALLIDUM*

This important spirochaete, the pathogenic organism of syphilis, is very slender, has a refractive index close to that of plasma and is resistant to stains. It was not demonstrated until 1905, when Schaudinn and Hoffmann succeeded in staining it with Giemsa's stain. Ordinary stains are not successful with films or sections.

DARK-GROUND ILLUMINATION OF LIVING SPIROCHAETES IN FILMS AND SECTIONS

This is the best method for diagnostic purposes. Staining methods are only recommended when dark-ground illumination is not possible. The apparatus must be set up as described on page 21. Clean slides and coverslips of the correct thickness must be available.

The examination of a syphilitic chancre is conducted as follows:

1. Moisten a swab in alcohol and roughly rub the lesion until it is quite clean. A clear fluid exudate will appear after a few minutes from the abraded surfaces.
2. Take up a drop of exudate from the periphery of the lesion with a platinum loop or capillary pipette and deposit this on the slide.
3. Add a coverslip and gently press it down with the handle of the platinum loop.
4. Examine for spirochaetes with dark-ground illumination, bearing in mind the following:
    (i) The examination must be systematic—i.e. field by field—and is done with a mechanical stage.
    (ii) The *depth* of the exudate must be examined by continuous focusing up and down with the fine adjustment. The uppermost layers tend to be the richest in spirochaetes.
    (iii) Attention should be paid to the fluid immediately adjacent to air-bubbles in the preparation. Sometimes spirochaetes are more abundant here than elsewhere.
    (iv) Experience alone enables one to distinguish between *Treponema pallidum* and other spirochaetes.
    (v) At least two slides should be carefully examined before pronouncing a given specimen negative.

NOTES

1. The technique described above is only applicable when patient and dark-ground are adjacent. If the specimen of tissue fluid has to be transported, the most satisfactory plan is to take up the exudate with a fine Pasteur pipette, seal the end, and transport it in a plugged test-tube or piece of wide glass tubing.
2. The same combination of objective and eyepiece should always be used, since the distinction between the syphilitic and other spirochaetes is partly one of size.
3. Mucous patches in the mouth and cutaneous eruptions require scraping and the exudate is examined in the same way. Fluid for dark-ground examination can be obtained from lymph nodes by aspiration with a syringe.

STAINING TREPONEMA PALLIDUM IN FILMS

Giemsa's stain

A good sample of stain is essential. It is best bought ready made up. The spirochaetes are collected as described above.

TECHNIQUE

1. Fix dry smears of the fluid or other material suspected to contain spirochaetes in absolute alcohol for 10–20 minutes.
2. Dry with filter paper.
3. Add ten drops of the undiluted (stock) Giemsa solution to 10 cm³ of pure distilled water in a measuring cylinder. The previous addition of 5–10 drops of a 1 per cent solution of sodium carbonate to the distilled water

intensifies staining and is recommended. Mix with the minimum of shaking. Pour the staining mixture over the slide and leave for 10–30 minutes. The older the preparation, the longer the time required to stain syphilitic spirochaetes.

4. Rinse by holding the slide, smear downwards, under the tap for a few seconds.
5. Dry with filter paper. Examine with oil-immersion objective without mounting.
6. In the case of old, air-dried films, staining may often be advantageously prolonged (time permitting) to several hours or even overnight.

RESULTS

Spirochaetes—reddish-violet.
Red blood corpuscles, leucocytes, pus cells, etc., stained as in a blood film, but more deeply.

NOTES

1. The distilled water must be pure and glass-distilled.
2. All glassware must be scrupulously clean.
3. If the film is overstained (a rare occurrence), differentiate for 1–5 minutes in a dish of distilled water. Then blot and examine as above.
4. The diluted staining solution loses its strength after use; therefore never attempt to use it again.

Hage–Fontana silver method (Fontana 1925–6)

A silver impregnation method that is useful on account of its rapidity. Make thin smears of suspected material and allow to dry in air without warming.

FIXATION

Fix for one minute in Ruge's fluid:

Concentrated formaldehyde (40 per cent)	20 cm³
Glacial acetic acid	1 cm³
Distilled water	100 cm³

PREPARATION

Mordant

Phenol	1 g
Tannic acid	5 g
Distilled water	100 cm³

TECHNIQUE

1. Remove from the fixative and wash very rapidly (about ten seconds) in running water.
2. Flood the slide with mordant and warm over a flame until steam just rises; leave for 20–30 seconds.
3. Wash in running water for 30 seconds; rinse in distilled water.
4. Flood slide with 0.25 per cent aqueous silver nitrate and add one drop of concentrated ammonia. Warm over a flame for 20–30 seconds. A brownish scum should be formed.
5. Rinse in distilled water.
6. Blot and examine dry.

Spirochaetes—black.
Background—yellow.

STAINING SPIROCHAETES IN SECTIONS

There are a number of problems in staining sections for spirochaetes. The methods are silver impregnation techniques and if they are overstained it is possible to confuse threads of fibrin, or fine fibrils such as reticulin or elastica, with spirochaetes. A successful preparation should have black spirochaetes against a light brown background and this is not easy to achieve in the Levaditi method as the tissue blocks are stained before they are sectioned. The recognition of spirochaetes in sections is less easy than in smears as they are not flat on the slide and may be in any plane of the section; vertical or oblique spirochaetes may be incomplete and impossible to resolve. Positive control sections are highly desirable but tissue is difficult or impossible to obtain. Elias and Schnitzenbaumer (1976) have recommended commercial preparations of lyophilized spirochaetes, used for the immunological detection of syphilis, as control material for sections; smears of the reconstituted material were fixed in formaldehyde vapour and gave good results with silver impregnation methods. Finally the fluorescent antibody technique [p. 326] can be used for demonstrating leptospirae in smears made by scraping the surface of tissue blocks (Cook, Coles, Garner, and Luna 1971).

Levaditi's method (Levaditi and Mamouelian 1906)

This variant has the great advantages over the original method of: (1) not staining connective tissue; and (2) greater reliability. Spirochaetes are stained in the tissue blocks; these should be thin (about 1 mm).

FIXATION

Fix in 10 per cent formal-saline for 24 hours. Longer fixation may be satisfactory.

TECHNIQUE

1. Wash for several hours in running water.
2. Transfer to 95 per cent alcohol for 24 hours.
3. Place in distilled water until the tissue sinks.
4. Impregnate with 2 per cent aqueous silver nitrate for 3–5 days in the dark at 37 °C.
5. Wash well in several changes of distilled water.
6. Reduce in 1 per cent hydroquinone in 50 per cent alcohol for 12–24 hours.
7. Complete dehydration in several changes of ascending grades of alcohol.
8. Clear in cedar wood oil and embed in paraffin.
9. Cut sections at 5 μm. Remove the wax with xylene and mount in balsam or a synthetic resin medium.

RESULTS

Spirochaetes—black.
Tissues—yellow or light brown.

NOTES

1. All traces of formalin and alcohol must be removed before stage 4.

Thorough washing is also required before stage 6 to avoid precipitation of silver in the tissues as well as on the spirochaetes.

2. The spirochaetes appear larger than they really are.
3. Baceteria and fungi can be seen by this method.

The Warthin–Starry method (Warthin and Starry 1920)

A good method for paraffin sections after fixation in formal-saline. The intensity of the staining is more controllable than in the Levaditi technique by variations of the development time and pH (see Notes, below).

FIXATION

Ten per cent formal-saline.

SECTIONS

Thin (5 μm) paraffin sections.

PREPARATIONS

1. *Buffer solution*
   Stock solutions:
   (i) M/5 sodium acetate solution; 16.4 g sodium acetate made up to a litre with distilled water.
   (ii) M/5 acetic acid; 11.8 cm³ of glacial acetic acid made up to a litre with distilled water.

   For pH 3.6, take 1.5 cm³ of solution (i) and 18.5 cm³ of solution (ii); mix and add 480 cm³ of distilled water. *Use this for all solutions.*

2. *Developer solution*
   Make a fresh solution of 0.3 g hydroquinone in 10 cm³ of buffered water. Take 1 cm³ of this solution and mix with 15 cm³ of warmed 5 per cent Scotch glue (carpenter's glue); keep in the 40 °C incubator. Take 3 cm³ of a 2 per cent silver nitrate solution, warm to about 55 °C, and keep in the incubator. Mix the two solutions immediately before use.

TECHNIQUE

1. Take paraffin sections through xylene and alcohol to buffered water.
2. Impregnate with 1 per cent silver nitrate in buffered water at 55–60 °C for one hour.
3. Whilst the sections are incubating, prepare the developer. Place the slides in the fresh solution at 55 °C for 3½ minutes. The sections should become a golden-brown colour.
4. Pour off the developer and rinse for 2–3 minutes in warm (55–60 °C) tap water and then in cool buffer solution.
5. Dehydrate, clear, and mount in a synthetic resin medium.

RESULTS

Spirochaetes—black.
Tissues—pale yellowish-brown.

NOTES

1. Under-development gives pale thin spirochaetes and a pale background. Over-development gives dark thick spirochaetes, but the background may be very dark and may contain precipitates.

2. Spirochaetes are denser if a buffer solution of pH 3.8 is used (2.4 cm³ of solution (i) and 17.6 cm³ of solution (ii) with 480 cm³ of distilled water). Tissue staining is also more dense at this pH, and a pH of 3.6 is usually more satisfactory.
3. Young (1969) has stressed that the temperatures of the developer is critical and must not fall below 55 °C. Heat the developer solution to 60 °C and place in a staining jar in a water-bath.

REFERENCES

CHERUKIAN, C. J. and SCHENK, E. A. (1977). *Am. J. clin. Path.* **68**, 427.
CHICK, E. W. (1961). *Arch. Derm. Syph. (Chic.)* **83**, 305.
COOK, J. E., COLES, E. H., GARNER, F. M., and LUNA, L. G. (1971). *Stain Technol.* **46**, 271.
ELIAS, J. M. and SCHNITZENBAUMER, S. (1976). *Stain Technol.* **51**, 55.
FONTANA, A. (1925–6). *Derm. Z.* **46**, 291.
GOMORI, G. (1946). *Am. J. clin. Path.* **16** (technical section), 177.
GRIDLEY, M. F. (1953). *Am. J. clin. Path.* **23**, 303.
GROCOTT, R. G. (1955). *Am. J. clin. Path.* **25**, 975.
HICKS, J. D. and MATTHAEI, E. (1958). *J. Path. Bact.* **75**, 473.
LEVADITI, C. and MANOUELIAN, Y. (1906). *C. R. Soc. Biol. (Paris)* **60**, 134.
PINTOZZI, R. L. (1978). *J. clin. Path.* **31**, 803.
SYMMERS, W. ST. C. (1960). In *Recent advances in clinical pathology* (ed. S. C. Dyke), Series III. J. and A. Churchill, London.
WARTHIN, A. S. and STARRY, A. C. (1920). *Am. J. Syph.* **4**, 97.
YOUNG, B. J. (1969). *J. med. Lab. Technol.* **26**, 248.

22 | Protozoa and parasitic worms

Protozoa

In protozoological technique the sectional method is largely subordinated to the study of films or smears, though it will be seen that some of the staining techniques for films or smears are similar to those used for tissue sections. The direct microscopic identification of living protozoa is also of great importance, and fresh preparations of unfixed material form the basis of clinical protozoology. Body fluids, such as blood and lymph or faeces are the commonest specimens that are examined for evidence of systemic or intestinal protozoal infections. It will not be possible to include a comprehensive account of all methods for all protozoa found in animal tissues in this chapter, but a guide to the methods for the recognition of the commoner protozoa found in the blood (malarial parasites, trypanosomes, etc.) and in the faeces (amoebae, etc.) will be given.

As protozoa are small, and recognized by minute structural details, a high-power binocular microscope which will give good resolution without eye-strain is required, and a mechanical stage is an absolute necessity. Artificial light, suitably screened, is preferable to daylight for protozoology. It must be stressed that the light should be reduced for the examination of fresh preparations of protozoa as diagnostic features are lost in a blinding glare. This is best achieved by partially closing the substage iris diaphragm.

GENERAL METHODS FOR PROTOZOA

The techniques adopted for the demonstration of protozoa are more dependent upon the specimen than upon the type of parasite. Some protozoa are regularly present in the blood (malaria parasites, trypanosomes) and almost all can be demonstrated by staining thin or thick films. Other protozoa are usually or only present in the intestine (amoebae, *Balantidium coli*, *Giardia lamblia*, etc.) and can be found in smears made from intestinal swabs or from faeces. Some are always present in tissues (*Leishmania tropica*, coccidia, etc.), and smears may be made from aspirates from these lesions or sections can be prepared from excised tissues. It must be realized that many protozoa are found in the tissues as well as in the blood or intestine, and the type of specimen that can be examined will depend upon the accessibility of the disease process; for instance, it may be difficult to obtain diagnostic material from an amoebic abscess of the liver, but it is easier to perform a rectal biopsy and even simpler to examine faeces for amoebae. Table 22.1 lists the more important protozoa that can be found in humans and in other animals, together with the sites in which the parasites can be found, and the methods that are most suitable; this table may help the laboratory worker to use the techniques that are likely to give the best results. Always bear in mind the facts that protozoa

Table 22.1 The commoner pathogenic protozoa, their usual sites, and laboratory techniques

Type of protozoa DISEASE	Present in	Technical methods	
		Preparations	See pages
Entamoeba histolytica AMOEBIASIS	Faeces Intestine	Fresh preparations Smears Sections	420 421 425
	Liver	Smears Sections	421 425
Trypanosomes TRYPANOSOMIASIS	Blood	Fresh preparations Smears	415 416
	Tissues	Sections	425
Leishmama donovani KALA-AZAR	Blood	Smears	415
	Tissues	Sections	425
Leishmania tropica TROPICAL SORE	Tissues	Smears of aspirate Sections	417 425
Trichomonas vaginalis VAGINITIS	Vagina	Fresh preparations Smears	419 421
Giardia lamblia	Faeces	Fresh preparations Smears	419 421
Coccidia COCCIDIOSIS	Tissues	Smears Sections	421 425
Plasmodia MALARIA	Blood	Fresh preparations Smears	415 416
	Tissues	Sections	425
Balantidium coli BALANTIDIASIS	Faeces	Fresh preparations Smears	419 421

are usually small, delicate, and may be difficult to identify; they may stain lightly (leishmaniae), lose their motility, and degenerate quickly (amoebae), be susceptible to artifacts (trypanosomes, etc.), be present only at certain times (plasmodia), or have a patchy distribution (amoebae, etc.). The techniques and staining methods will be described under three main headings—protozoa in the blood, faeces, and tissue sections.

METHODS FOR PROTOZOA IN THE BLOOD

The following methods, though specially described for malaria parasites, are largely applicable to other types of haemosporidia, to trypanosomes and to Leishman-Donovan bodies.

FRESH PREPARATIONS

When examining fresh preparations for the presence of motile protozoa, the use of a warm stage is advantageous and in the case of amoebae is essential.

BLOOD FILMS

The examination of Romanowsky-stained blood films is a standard laboratory method for all haemosporida. The stains of Leishman, Giemsa, and Wright all stain the parasites admirably. Stain in the standard way or by Field's buffered Giemsa technique [p. 417]. The unmounted film is examined with the × 100 (2 mm) oil-immersion objective and a low-power eyepiece. Searching for 'crescents' (the sexual forms of *Plasmodium falciparum*) can be carried out more quickly with × 40 (4 mm) dry objective and a film mounted in cedarwood oil or balsam. A × 60 (3.5 mm) oil-immersion objective is a useful compromise between these two magnifications, and the final magnification and size of field is controlled by the eyepiece.

THICK FILM METHOD

An invaluable adjunct to the standard thin film method when searching for malaria parasites. It is also useful for the spirochaetes of relapsing fever and for blood parasites.

1. Take up a large drop of blood on the centre of a slide, then spread it out with a needle so as to form a square or circle of 1–1½ cm diameter. Print should be just visible when seen through the spread droplet.
2. Allow the slide to dry at room temperature, or in a current of warm air or in the incubator. The slide should be horizontal during the earlier stages of the drying process.
3. Dehaemoglobinize and stain simultaneously by Field's rapid method or the buffered Giemsa method (see below).
    or
   Dehaemoglobinize the film by placing it face downwards on two glass rods, or on a curved tile, in cold distilled water.
4. Fix in absolute ethyl or methyl alcohol for 5–15 minutes.
5. Stain in Giemsa's stain diluted in the standard proportion (i.e. one drop of stain for every millilitre of distilled water) for 10–30 minutes. Rinse rapidly in distilled water. Blot *around* the film and dry at room temperature or in a current of warm (but not hot) air.
6. Examine with the × 100 (2 mm) oil-immersion objective and a low-powered eyepiece.

   Gametocytes (of benign tertian and quartan) and the 'crescents' (of subtertian malaria) are well shown by the thick film method. The younger trophozoites ('rings') are less easy to distinguish by this method. For the microscopical appearance of a dehaemoglobinized film see page 418.

NOTES

1. The time required for drying is obviously dependent on temperature and humidity.
2. The film must be protected from dust and from flies both during and after the drying process.
3. One function of drying is the obvious one of preventing subsequent detachment of the film, but drying also imparts some degree of auto-fixation to unfixed parasites and white cells, though not sufficient to impede the subsequent lysis of the red cells.
4. *Unstained* thick films cannot be kept for more than a few days: staining

deteriorates and lysis of the red cells becomes more difficult owing to progressive autofixation. Why this occurs is not known.

5. The thick film is not a 'thick drop'; it is a smear spread to a thickness of 50 μm or less. Only by practice can the correct thickness be learnt: when made, it should be possible to see vaguely the hands of a watch through it. A useful method is to graduate the thickness of the film when it is spread so that one end is too thick, the other too thin. If after staining the film is held to the light, the thick end will appear a deep purplish-blue, the thin end greenish. Select the zone where the purplish area is just becoming greenish and mark it with a drop of immersion oil. The parasites will be seen most clearly in this zone (personal communication, Dr J. C. Gregory).

6. Trypanosomes in human blood are usually scanty, and prolonged examination of blood films is necessary. In cases of sleeping sickness, puncture of the enlarged cervical lymph glands often confirms the diagnosis. The fluid of the gland is taken up with a *dry* hypodermic needle and syringe, spread on slides, dried, and then stained by Leishman's or Giemsa's method.

7. In kala-azar (caused by *Leishmania donovani*), the parasite may be obtained by *splenic, hepatic, inguinal, or sternal puncture* when ordinary methods fail to reveal it. The latter is the least dangerous. The needle must be absolutely dry; if it contains water, the endothelial cells and the parasites within them will be greatly distorted. Smears are made on slides and then stained with Leishman or Giemsa stains. A leucopenia—e.g. one of 2000–3000 per mm^3—is the rule. A differential leucocyte count shows the relative numbers of the white cells not far removed from the normal. These two points are of aid in establishing a differential diagnosis between kala-azar and malaria.

8. In *tropical sore* (= Delhi boil, etc.) the parasite (*Leishmania tropica*) can only be obtained from the actual lesion. This should be scraped or punctured, the material spread on slides, and stained with Leishman's or Giemsa's stains. Another method is to perform a biopsy, and fix, section, and stain it.

THE STAINING OF BLOOD FILMS FOR PROTOZOA

Romanowsky stains

Thin films are stained by the Romanowsky techniques used by haematologists.

Field's buffered Giemsa method (modified by Vigo 1941)

A good method for thick blood films. The film is dehaemoglobinized and stained at the same time.

PREPARATION

(A) *Buffer solution (pH 7.1)*

Disodium hydrogen phosphate, Na_2HPO_4 (anhydrous)	0.68 g
Potassium dihydrogen phosphate, KH_2PO_4	0.32 g
Distilled water	1000 cm^3

(B) *Giemsa's stain*
This is best bought in solution from a reliable source. It must be kept well stoppered.

TECHNIQUE

1. Place unfixed thick films on a staining bridge or back to back in a slide trough.
2. Mix sufficient solution A and B together in a test-tube or measuring cylinder in the proportion of two parts of buffer solution A to one part of stain B. Pour mixture over slides and leave for three minutes.
3. Wash by immersing briefly in distilled water. Do not wash under the tap and do not blot.
4. Stand the slides on end to dry.

RESULTS

Background of lysed cells—mottled grey.
Cytoplasm of malarial parasites—pale blue and their chromatin red.
Nuclei of leucocytes—purple–blue.
Granules of eosinophils—pink.
Platelets (often occurring in groups)—pale purple.

Field's rapid method for thick blood films (Field 1941)

A large drop of blood is placed near the centre of a slide and spread with a needle over an area about 2 cm in diameter. Allow to dry in the air without fixation. This staining method dehaemoglobinizes and stains in less than 15 seconds.

PREPARATION

Stain A

Methylene blue (medicinal)	0.8 g
Azur I	0.5 g
Disodium hydrogen phosphate (anhydrous)	5 g
Potassium dihydrogen phosphate	6.25 g
Distilled water	500 cm^3

Stain B

Eosin (the yellow water soluble variety is suitable)	1g
Disodium hydrogen phosphate (anhydrous)	5 g
Potassium dihydrogen phosphate	6.25 g
Distilled water	500 cm^3

Dissolve the phosphate salts in the distilled water and then add the stain. Stand the stain solutions A and B for 24 hours, then filter.

TECHNIQUE

1. Dip the film into stain A for 1–2 seconds.
2. Wash for a few seconds in distilled water.
3. Shake to remove excess water.
4. Dip for one second into stain B.
5. Wash in water for 1–3 seconds.
6. Stand slides on end to dry.
7. Examine unmounted with oil-immersion × 100 (2 mm) objective.

RESULTS

Parasite cytoplasm—blue; chromatin, puplish-red.
Leucocyte nuclei—deep blue; cytoplasm, pale blue.
Eosinophil granules—dull red and well defined.

Neutrophil granules—pale and rather indistinct.
Background of film—pale pink.

NOTE

Dye samples sometimes vary, and slight readjustment of the above timing may be required.

Practical notes on the examination of malarial blood

1. *Thin films*. The field of a × 100 (2 mm) oil-immersion lens is so small that a large number of fields must be examined. A mechanical stage is essential, and both edges and ends of the film should be scanned.
2. *Thick films*. With experience, the four different species of human plasmodia can be distinguished in spite of some distortion and the lysis of the red cells. Malarial pigment is better seen in thick than in thin films. Always examine the margins of the film.
3. *Artifacts*. In thin films the only common artifact sometimes mistaken for the intercellular parasite is a platelet lying on top of a red cell.

    In thick films errors of interpretation are more easily made; they comprise:

    (a) *Platelets*. Often simulate trophozoites of *P. vivax* or *P. malariae*. The pigment of the parasites is, however, pathognomonic.
    (b) *Howell–Jolly bodies*. Sometimes mistaken for young trophozoites and appear as chromatoid debris.
    (c) *Reticulum of immature red cells*. May be taken for trophozoites of *P. vivax*.
4. *Pigmented leucocytes*. The presence of these is practically pathognomonic of malarial infection and when present the parasites also are usually abundant. They are especially well seen in fresh preparations. The type of cell is generally the large mononuclear, occasionally the polymorph. The pigment in leucocytes and parasites is doubly refractile.

METHODS FOR INTESTINAL PROTOZOA

The most important protozoa that may be present in faeces or the intestinal tissue are the various species of amoebae and their cysts. Others that may be found, and for which the following methods are suitable, include *Balantidium coli* and *Giardia lamblia* (see Table 22.1). Vaginal specimens for *Trichomonas vaginalis* may also be stained by these methods, but Trichomonas is difficult to stain and is best recognized in wet films by its motility.

The general scheme for the examination of faecal specimens for protozoa is shown in Table 22.2. The specimen must always be examined immediately after leaving the body. It should be checked macroscopically, and if mucus is seen this material should be examined first. Fresh preparations of mucus or faeces diluted with physiological saline are prepared; if no protozoa are found in these unstained preparations by microscopic examination using a warm stage 1 per cent eosin in physiological saline may be used to stain background material, and iodine will stain the cysts of pathogenic amoebae.

UNSTAINED FRESH PREPARATIONS

Both active amoeboid and encysted forms can be observed by dissociating fragments of infected tissue in 0.9 per cent NaCl or in Ringer–Locke solution.

Table 22.2 Scheme for the examination of faecal specimens for protozoa

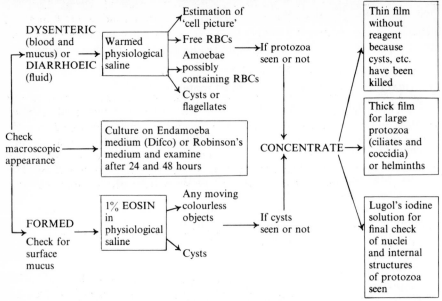

In the case of faeces, these must be diluted so as to reduce the amount of vegetable debris, etc., and to increase the transparency.

To make a fresh preparation from faeces, place a drop of physiological saline on a slide with a pipette (do not use water); take up some faeces with a wooden bacteriological swab stick or similar rigid object and make a dilute emulsion in the saline. Lower a square coverslip on to the mixture without making air-bubbles. Examine with reduced illumination. Such preparations must be thin and the use of a warm stage is essential.

STAINED FRESH PREPARATIONS

Fresh eosin preparations

Unless the observer has had considerable experience in this work it is often difficult to differentiate between protozoa and particles of debris which closely simulate these organisms. If no obvious protozoa are seen, it is useful to make a second fresh preparation in 1 per cent eosin in physiological saline. This solution has the property of staining all other materials pink except live protozoa; these stand out clearly as white objects in the pink background and can easily be seen with the low power objective.

Fresh iodine preparations

When cysts have been seen by one of the methods described above iodine preparations may be of value.

Prepare a fresh unstained specimen using a large drop of Lugol's solution [formula, p. 243] in place of the saline. The nuclei of cysts are more easily seen after fixation and partial staining by this method. It is particularly useful in clinical pathology where it is important to distinguish between the cysts of pathogenic amoebae and those of harmless commensals of the intestine, but unfortunately the iodine stain may obliterate the chromatoid bodies that are of paramount importance in the diagnosis of the cysts of *Entamoeba histolytica*.

CONCENTRATED PREPARATIONS

After fresh preparations have been made it may be advisable to concentrate the faeces in order to discover as many positive cases of protozoal or helminthic infections as possible. Many techniques have been developed, but the following adaptation of the formal-ether technique, based on Ritchie's (1948) and Ridley and Hawgood's (1956) methods, has four advantages over earlier concentration methods: it concentrates all cysts and ova without exception; it does not distort them; it destroys blastocysts; it takes little more than five minutes to perform.

The formal-ether method of concentrating faecal cysts and ova (modified from Ridley and Hawgood 1956)

TECHNIQUE

Emulsify with a pestle and mortar approximately 2 g faeces in about 10 cm³ of distilled water. This will dispose of any blastocysts. Strain through a wire sieve (40 mesh to an inch) into a centrifuge tube. Centrifuge for three minutes at approximately 2500 rev/min to obtain a deposit. Pour off the supernatant fluid, add 10 per cent formal-saline to within 2.5 cm of the top of the tube, and mix with a swab stick or glass rod. Add about 3 cm³ of ether, cork, and shake vigorously. Centrifuge again, regulating the acceleration so that 2000 rev/min is attained in two minutes; then switch off and allow to come to rest slowly.

Loosen the fatty debris at the interface of the liquids with a swab stick, and pour away the whole of the supernatant fluid together with the debris. Wipe clean the inside of the tube. Shake the deposit at the bottom of the tube with the last drop of fluid. Extract a drop with a pipette, mount on a slide under a coverslip, and examine. Cysts and ova should be concentrated 20–30 times.

NOTES

1. As a fixative has been used, the cysts will not respond to the eosin reaction, but will stain with Lugol's iodine solution.
2. The usual precautions should be taken when the ether is exposed to the air.

STAINED SMEARS

A standard method is to make coverslip smears. Never put coverslip preparations face upwards in any stain or reagent as deposits may fall upon the surface of the film and be difficult or impossible to remove. Coverslip preparations can be floated face downwards on fluids which contain less than 50 per cent of alcohol. In higher grades of alcohol, in xylene, and in any reagents in which coverslips sink, watch-glasses or 10-cm porcelain staining dishes with ribbed serrations should be used. The ridges prevent the coverslips from lying flat on the bottom of the dish, allow a sufficient quantity of the reagent to be in contact with the film at all times, and make it easy to manipulate the coverslips freely.

Preparation of the Film
Make thin smears with a match or bacteriological swab stick. Do not dilute the material or it will not remain attached to the coverslip.

Fixation
Drop the coverslip (or place the slide) face downwards on to the fixative. Do not allow the film to dry at any time. Films which are allowed to dry produce distortion—especially in unencysted amoebae. With practice, several films can be dealt with simultaneously in one dish.

Fix for 10–30 minutes in:

Mercuric chloride, concentrated aqueous solution	2 parts
Absolute industrial spirit	1 part
Glacial acetic acid	5 per cent by volume

Modified Heidenhain's iron haematoxylin

A standard method for the protozoologist. Fine details of amoebae and their cysts are well shown. The following short method (Wheatley 1951) gives good results in one hour.

TECHNIQUE

1. Fix preparations as described above.
2. Wash briefly in 70 per cent alcohol.
3. Remove mercury pigment with iodine and thiosulphate [p. 45].
4. Wash in distilled water.
5. Mordant for 2–3 minutes in a 5 per cent aqueous solution of iron alum at 56 °C.
6. Wash briefly in distilled water.
7. Stain for 1–2 minutes in:

10 per cent alcoholic solution of haematoxylin	1 cm^3
Glacial acetic acid	2 cm^3
Distilled water	100 cm^3

8. Wash for 10–15 minutes in running tap water until the film is blue.
9. Dehydrate with ascending grades of alcohol and absolute alcohol.
10. Clear in clove oil, wash in xylene, and mount in a synthetic resin medium.

RESULTS

Nuclei—black.
Cytoplasm—shades of grey.

Phosphotungstic acid haematoxylin

This gives good results with all protozoa, is simple, and requires no experience. Differentiation is not usually needed, and coverslips can be passed through the various reagents with ample latitude. Cooper's modification for staining intestinal protozoa is described.

PREPARATION

Distilled water   80 cm³
Haematoxylin   0.1 g

Dissolve the haematoxylin by heat in a little of the water, cool, then add the remainder. Add 20 cm³ of 10 per cent phosphotungstic acid and allow to ripen for several months. Ripening can be accelerated by the addition of 10 cm³ of 0.25 per cent aqueous potassium permanganate.

TECHNIQUE

1. Make preparations and fix as described above.
2. Wash briefly in 70 per cent alcohol.
3. Remove mercury pigment with iodine and thiosulphate [p. 45].
4. Wash briefly in 70 and 90 per cent alcohol.
5. Place in absolute alcohol for five minutes to harden the protozoa.
6. Pass through 70, 50, and 30 per cent alcohol to distilled water. Leave in each for approximately one minute.
7. Immerse face downwards in covered dish of stain for 12 hours or overnight. If freshly made stain is used, staining is helped by leaving the dish in a 37 °C incubator for a similar period.
8. Wash briefly in tap water and dehydrate rapidly by passing through 25, 50, and 70 per cent alcohol to absolute alcohol.
9. Clear in clove oil, wash in xylene, and mount in a synthetic resin medium.

RESULTS

Nuclei and cytoplasmic structures—shades of blue.

Ehrlich's haematoxylin

This can be used and may be satisfactory for rapid work. It is not recommended for cysts, which may collapse during the staining process. Proceed as for sections [p. 140] after removing mercury deposits from the film. Control with the staining microscope, remembering to invert the coverslip (face upwards) on a slide.

Mann's methyl blue–eosin

Dobell's modification gives excellent results with amoebae and their cysts.

PREPARATION

1 per cent aqueous methyl blue   35 cm³
1 per cent aqueous eosin   45 cm³
Distilled water   100 cm³

This solution keeps indefinitely.

TECHNIQUE

1. Make preparations and fix as described above.
2. Stain for 4–12 hours in the methyl blue–eosin solution.

3. Rinse in distilled water for a few seconds.
4. Differentiate, controlling with the microscope, in the following solution:

70 per cent alcohol   100 cm³
Saturated aqueous solution of orange G   10 drops

5. Dehydrate in ascending grades of alcohol, clear in xylene and mount in a synthetic resin medium.

RESULTS

Nuclei—blue.
Cytoplasm—pink to blue.

MIF (merthiolate–iodine–formalin) method for the examination of faeces by direct smear

On certain occasions it may be necessary to preserve specimens of faeces containing protozoa for teaching purposes, for a second opinion or because of pressure of work. The merthiolate–iodine–formalin method is a stain preservation technique (Sapero and Lawless 1953) that can be used for the direct examination of faeces or for the preservation of faeces.

1. Mix one part of commercial formalin with six parts of 1 : 1000 Merthiolate tincture (Lilly) No. 99. Immediately before use add one part of 5 per cent iodine in 2 per cent aqueous potassium iodide. If a black deposit forms the mixture must be discarded and a fresh one made.
2. Place one drop on a slide and dilute with one drop of distilled water.
3. Emulsify faeces in this solution, cover with a coverslip, and examine. The iodine stain gradually fades leaving a pink colour for the final checking of morphological structures.

MIF method for the preservation of infected faeces

Mix together:

Merthiolate, 1 : 1000   200 cm³
Formalin   25 cm³
Glycerol   5 cm³
Distilled water   250 cm³

and immediately before use add 25 cm³ of 5 per cent iodine in 2 per cent aqueous potassium iodide.

Emulsify faeces in this preservative, using narrow tubes. Cork and allow to settle. Material for examination is pipetted from the interface layer between the faecal deposit and the supernatant fluid. Amoebae, cysts, and flagellates are fixed in a life-like manner, and appear to be concentrated at the top layer of the faecal deposit.

NOTES ON THE EXAMINATION OF FAECAL PREPARATIONS FOR PROTOZOA

1. In cases of suspected amoebic dysentery, systematic examination must be made of several fresh unstained and eosin preparations. If the stool is not homogeneous preparations from the different portions should be examined. A negative examination should be repeated—if possible, daily—until a definite diagnosis is made.

2. The fresher the stools the better. Amoebae degenerate rapidly after the specimen is passed.

3. In the tropics the fluid used for diluting faeces should be filtered (or sterilized), to ensure against protozoal contamination of the faeces from this source. Furthermore, if a specimen of stool be kept for more than 24 hours in very warm weather, free-living protozoa may appear in it. This is by development from previously encysted forms.

4. An eyepiece micrometer is especially useful in dealing with protozoal cysts, since the identification of these is often partly based on their dimensions. The micrometer should be calibrated for a given objective (preferably the × 100 (2 mm) oil-immersion objective), and the same tube-length always used.

METHODS FOR PROTOZOA IN TISSUE SECTIONS

It has already been seen that pathogenic protozoa are usually recovered from the blood or from faeces, and in the majority of diseases the examination of blood smears or faecal specimens should be the method of choice. Protozoa may be present in tissue sections, and some infections, such as *Leishmania tropica* (tropical sore), are confined to tissues. In most cases a more rapid and precise diagnosis can be made from fresh preparations or from stained smears than from tissue sections; cells are larger and flatter in smears than in sections, and plasmodia (malaria) or Leishman-Donovan bodies (kala-azar) are more easily seen and can be identified with greater accuracy. Fresh preparations, and some smears, give better morphological details than sections, which always have some artifacts due to fixation and paraffin embedding.

With these provisos in mind, there is no fundamental difficulty in preparing tissue sections for the demonstration of protozoa. Good results can be obtained with small biopsy specimens or excised organs if fixation is immediate and thorough. Post-mortem material is less likely to be successful, and material removed many hours after death may be completely unsatisfactory; the diagnosis of some haematological diseases requires fine cellular detail, as do the smaller protozoa, and specimens that have autolysed will not show minute cytological structure.

FIXATION

The most important aspect of fixation is that it must be carried out at once, be thoroughly completed, and that thin tissue slices, not thick blocks, be used. If all these are done, most fixatives can be used and will give adequate results.

For malaria parasites and other haemosporidia, and for Leishman-Donovan bodies, the most suitable fixatives are those that preserve red blood corpuscles. Zenker-formal [p. 52] is a good fixative and is compatible with most stains, and neutral formal-saline is usually satisfactory; this may produce formalin artifact pigment, which is an acid haematin similar to that of malaria pigment. This may cause some confusion and diagnostic dificulty, as formalin pigment is likely to be present in post-mortem tissues and in some biopsies in exactly the same parts of the tissue (blood vessels, spleen, liver, etc.), that will be examined for malaria parasites or malaria pigment. Moreover, the methods for the removal of formalin pigment will also remove malaria pigment.

Although both give similar staining reactions, malaria pigment is intracellular and formalin pigment is extracellular; therefore they can usually be distinguished by their situation. Primary mercuric chloride or Carnoy fixation should be avoided, but secondary fixation with mercuric chloride [p. 54] is not contra-indicated, as red blood cells are still preserved and cellular detail may be considerably improved.

For trypanosomes, coccidia, amoebae, and the larger protozoa the preservation of red blood corpuscles is not so important and thin pieces of tissue may be fixed in mercuric chloride–acetic acid:

Mercuric chloride, saturated aqueous solution	95 cm^3
Glacial acetic acid	5 cm^3

Most other fixatives may be used, including Zenker, Bouin, mercuric chloride-formal, and formal-saline.

SECTIONS

Paraffin sections are satisfactory, provided they are thin (5 μm or less).

STAINING OF TISSUE SECTIONS

Routine haematoxylin and eosin staining should be carried out for the preliminary screening of sections for protozoa, and a well stained carefully differentiated H and E will often give perfectly satisfactory results, even of the smaller protozoa such as Leishman-Donovan bodies. Some artifact is unavoidable in sections of amoebae. Phosphotungstic acid haematoxylin [p. 146] is also suitable. Heidenhain's iron haematoxylin is a classical protozoological stain, and the standard method [p. 143] may be combined with light green–picric acid counterstain; dip the section into the following for a few seconds:

Light green	1 g
Picric acid	0.5 g
Absolute alcohol	100 cm^3

Differentiate the counterstain during dehydration in absolute alcohol, which must be rapid. The periodic acid–Schiff reaction [p. 237] will demonstrate the cytoplasm of some protozoa. Giemsa's stain may be capricious with sections but the method of Bayley (1949) is quick and easy and may give good results; it can be varied by alteration of the composition of the acetic acid–Giemsa stain [see p. 216]. The following modification of Giemsa staining will demonstrate protozoa in tissue sections.

1. Stain in Giemsa's solution, diluted in the proportion of one drop of stain for every millilitre of carbon dioxide-free distilled water, for 24 hours.
2. Rinse rapidly in water.
3. Differentiate rapidly in 0.5 per cent acetic acid until the section is pink.
4. Rinse in distilled water. Blot.
5. Dehydrate very rapidly in absolute alcohol.
6. Xylene.
7. Mount in a synthetic resin medium.

Nuclei—purple.

Red blood corpuscles—pink.
Malarial parasites—bluish; their chromatin, red.

NOTE

A modification which gives excellent results is the following: suppress stages 3 and 4; transfer from 5 to a slide jar of 0.2–0.5 per cent colophonium in absolute alcohol. Move the slide about in this and control differentiation with the staining microscope. Eliminate any traces of colophonium by rapid treatment with absolute alcohol. Then clear and mount. The reason why colophonium facilititates differentiation in this and most other methylene blue–eosin methods is unknown.

Parasitic worms

Parasitic worms are divided into three classes—Trematodes (flukes), Cestodes (tapeworms), and Nematodes (roundworms). Their presence in the body is usually diagnosed by finding their ova in faeces, blood, or tissues.

As with the protozoa, only the methods applicable to the more important parasitic worms that are found in man or in other animals will be considered. The techniques are largely dominated by the following factors: (1) special pre-cautions may be necessary to avoid extreme contraction during fixation; (2) identification may be based upon the study of the whole parasite, stained or unstained, rather than on sections; and (3) the examination of the ova of parasitic worms, in faeces or in urine, is important as the various species may be recognizable by their ova.

To observe the movements of living parasites, place them in physiological saline at 37 °C. Cestodes, especially, become very sluggish at temperatures much below that of the body.

METHODS FOR TREMATODES

The parasites should be freed from tissue or alimentary debris by washing in physiological saline.

FRESH PREPARATIONS

Examine the adult parasite between a coverslip and slide (if small) or between two slides (if large). Or examine in a little saline with the dissecting micro-scope.

FIXED WHOLE PREPARATIONS

Place the parasites in a test-tube of normal saline. Shake vigorously for a few seconds in order to straighten the worms. Quickly decant half of the saline and fill up with the fixative. The most suitable fixatives for general use are formal-saline or 70 per cent alcohol to which has been added 3 per cent acetic acid.

An alternative method which may give better results is as follows. With large specimens place the parasite between two glass slides or plates and gently press to flatten the worm. Slip a rubber band over each end to maintain pressure and drop into a beaker of the acetic acid–70 per cent alcohol fixative.

Small specimens may be flattened if necessary by placing the parasite on a slide and carefully lowering on to it a coverslip with a small dot of petroleum jelly at each corner. By gentle pressure the specimen can be flattened to the desired degree and will be held by the petroleum jelly in this position during fixation. Fix as for the larger specimens.

Kirkpatrick's carmalum staining method

PREPARATION

Cochineal or carmine	25 g
Glacial acetic acid	25 cm³
Potassium alum	25 g
Distilled water	1000 cm³

Powder the cochineal or carmine in a mortar; add the acetic acid and 100 cm³ of water; allow to soak for 20 minutes. Then boil gently or place in a Koch sterilizer for one hour. Meantime dissolve the alum in 500 cm³ of water and add it to the cooled cochineal or carmine solution. Repeat the heat treatment for one hour. Cool and filter. Add 1 g salicylic acid (or some thymol crystals) to inhibit the growth of moulds. The stain keeps for at least a year.

TECHNIQUE

1. Stain the worms for 12 hours or longer.
2. Differentiate in acid-alcohol; this may take several hours.
3. Dehydrate in ascending grades of alcohol (50, 70, and 90 per cent) leaving for at least half an hour in each grade.
4. Complete dehydration in absolute alcohol or industrial spirit (two hours to overnight).
5. Clear in beechwood creosote.
6. Mount in balsam, which must not be too fluid if the object is thick. Harden the mount on a hot-plate.

RESULTS

The worm should be a transparent red; the various organs in shades of red.

NOTE

With very thick objects that tend to curl under the coverslip a weight or clip should be used to keep the preparation flat while the balsam is drying.

Mayer's haemalum staining method

PREPARATION

See page 139.

TECHNIQUE

1. Take the worms to water and stain for 1–24 hours depending on the thickness of the specimen.
2. Differentiate in 0.5 per cent hydrochloric acid and blue in running tap water.
3. Dehydrate, clear, and mount as for carmalum.

RESULTS

The internal organs are stained in shades of blue.

SECTIONS

Fix in formal-saline or in any standard fixative of good penetrative power—
Susa, Bouin's fluid, or Carnoy. Stain by standard histological methods such as
haematoxylin and eosin [p. 143], or Heidenhain's iron haematoxylin [p. 143].

LARVAL FORMS (MIRACIDIA, SPOROCYSTS, REDIAE, CERCARIAE)

Fix in 10 per cent formal-saline, 70 per cent alcohol, or Bouin's fluid. Stain as
described for whole preparations (above) or make transparent preparations
by clearing in glycerol–alcohol (method as for nematodes, page 430). The
observation of the living larvae often reveals detail that is lost in fixed
specimens.

Owing to their small size, the times for fixation, dehydration, etc., may be
greatly reduced. Mount beneath a coverslip supported by some device to
avoid crushing.

OVA

In faeces
In cases of heavy infestation direct smears may be made by emulsifying a wire-
loopful of faeces with a little physiological saline on a slide. Add a coverslip
and examine with a × 10 (16 mm) objective. In light infections the stool should
be concentrated by the formal-ether technique [p. 421].

In urine
Allow the urine to stand in a conical urine-glass. Then take up a little of the
deposit with a fine pipette. Examine between slide and coverslip as above. In
cases of suspected infection with *Schistosoma haematobium* (bilharzia), if examination by the above method is negative, use the following procedure: In-
struct the patient to pass urine. Then to pass a few drops by straining. Collect
the latter separately and examine with the microscope. The ova are usually
present, if the urine is so examined, in cases of urinary schistosomiasis.

METHODS FOR CESTODES

FRESH PREPARATIONS

These may be examined in physiological saline between slide and coverslip if
they are small. Larger cestodes should be examined alive in a dish of saline
with the dissecting microscope.

WHOLE PREPARATIONS

Wash the worms in saline, transfer to a dish of tap water, and allow the
worms to become thoroughly relaxed. This may take between one and 12
hours. Fixation can be carried out with the worm between two glass plates as
for trematodes, wound around glass plates or cut into suitable lengths, and
fixed in a suitable container. Acetified 70 per cent alcohol or formal-saline
are both satisfactory fixatives. Store in glycerol–alcohol or stain as for

trematodes. Times of fixation will depend on the size of the worm, but at least 24 hours are needed when fixed between glass plates. Stain as for trematodes.

SECTIONS

As for trematodes [p. 429].

LARVAL FORMS

Cysticerci may be fixed between glass plates as for the adult forms. The scolex of living cysticerci can be evaginated by placing in a 30 per cent solution of ox bile in saline for half an hour at 37 °C. Press between glass plates and fix. Clear the cysticerci in glycerol–alcohol or after dehydration in beechwood creosote. No staining is necessary.

OVA

In some species of cestodes the ova are very scanty in the faeces. It is then necessary to take samples from several different parts of the stool and concentrate by the formal-ether technique [p. 421].

METHODS FOR INTESTINAL NEMATODES

The techniques for dealing with these parasites are specialized. This is the result of: (1) the impermeable cuticle of these worms; (2) the difficulty of fixing them in extension; and (3) the fact that the tough chitinous cuticle makes section cutting difficult.

FRESH PREPARATIONS

Examine between slide and coverslip after washing the worms in normal saline. Do not apply pressure or the worms will rupture.

WHOLE PREPARATIONS

1. Wash the worms thoroughly by shaking in normal saline. Pour off the supernatant and replace with clean saline, just sufficient to cover the worms.
2. Carefully heat some 70 per cent alcohol to 60 °C.
3. Quickly pour the worms into the hot alcohol and immediately remove the source of heat. The worms will die in extension. It is important to use the smallest amount of saline to avoid the rapid cooling of the alcohol.
4. If it is wished to store the parasites, keep them in 5 per cent glycerol in 70 per cent alcohol.
5. Clear the specimens by placing them in a wide-mouthed tube, watch-glass, or dish containing 5 per cent glycerol in 70 per cent alcohol. Allow the water and the alcohol to evaporate slowly; when these have all disappeared the specimen will be cleared and transparent.
6. Mount in pure glycerol or glycerol jelly [p. 129]. It is advisable to ring the coverslip.

NOTES

1. Large nematodes may be fixed in 10 per cent formal-saline.
2. Occasionally, shrinkage will occur soon after the worms are placed in 5 per

cent glycerol in 70 per cent alcohol; in such cases the glycerol must be decreased.

3. In the case of thick nematodes the following more powerful clearing method should be used. Dehydrate in ascending grades of alcohol up to absolute alcohol. Clear in beechwood creosote and mount in balsam. Prolonged immersion in creosote stains the worms dark brown and makes them unsatisfactory for microscopical examination.
4. Lacto-phenol of Amann may be used in place of glycerol for clearing.

Phenol crystals	10 g
Lactic acid	10 g
Glycerol	20 g
Distilled water	10 cm³

Dilute with equal parts of 70 per cent alcohol and allow to evaporate slowly. Mount in glycerol jelly.

Rubin's method for clearing and mounting

This clears and mounts simultaneously. Specimens may be placed in the following solution direct from formalin or alcohol fixatives.

Dissolve 15 g of polyvinyl alcohol in 100 cm³ distilled water. Use a water bath at 80 °C to facilitate solution.

Polyvinyl alcohol (stock solution)	56 cm³
Lactic acid	22 cm³
Phenol crystals	22 cm³

This is the mountant and is kept in a dark glass bottle.

Mount nematodes or their ova in this on the slide. As the medium retracts, add a little more every 48 hours. Clearing is progressive. Ring the coverslip if permanent preparations are desired. The initial stages may be done in a tube. This technique can be applied to cestodes; several weeks' immersion will be required before mounting.

SECTIONS

Fix in 10 per cent formal-saline, hot 70 per cent alcohol, or warm Carnoy's fluid. The chitinous cuticle of nematodes tends to splinter and disintegrate the underlying tissues during section cutting. Consequently the following precautions should be observed.

1. After fixation, either cut the worm into segments or incise the cuticle in several places to assist penetration. Dehydrate in 90 per cent and absolute alcohol. Clear in cedar wood oil (not xylene, which increases the brittleness of nematodes). Remove the cedar wood oil with toluene for $\frac{1}{4}$–$\frac{1}{2}$ hour. Embed in hard paraffin wax (56–60 °C), or one of the 'plastic waxes' [p. 61] or ester wax [p. 68].
2. If the material fragments during sectioning paint the surface of the block with celloidin [p. 95] or use the Sellotape method [p. 95].
3. Double embedding (Peterfi's method, p. 71) is often very successful when other methods fail to give good results.
4. Standard methods for staining the sections are employed. Haematoxylin and eosin [p. 140] is satisfactory.

LARVAL FORMS

The larvae are collected and fixed as for adult worms. Clearing and mounting can be carried out in a similar way. Owing to the thinness of the cuticle they may also be stained. Mayer's acid haemalum has the advantage of penetrating well. Stain as follows.

1. Fix larvae in 70 per cent alcohol and stain in Mayer's acid haemalum [p. 139] in a test-tube for 3–24 hours.
2. Pipette off the stain and differentiate with 0.5 per cent aqueous hydrochloric acid. Control by examining a few larvae with the staining microscope. When sufficiently differentiated:
3. Wash larvae in 70 per cent alcohol to which has been added a few drops of ammonia. When the larvae are blue

Either
4. Transfer to the glycerol–alcohol mixture and clear according to the technique for whole preparations [p. 430].
5. Mount in glycerol or in glycerol jelly.

or
4. Dehydrate in 90 per cent and absolute alcohol.
5. Clear in beechwood creosote.
6. Mount in balsam.

NOTE

The best detail is obtained by the glycerol method, since the balsam clears the transparent and delicate larval tissues too powerfully.

Fixation in Carnoy's fluid should facilitate staining.

Ehrlich's haematoxylin, preferably after fixation in 70 per cent alcohol acidulated with acetic acid, stains the larvae fairly well. But it should be used dilute and the staining-time prolonged (12–24 hours). Differentiate in an 0.5 per cent aqueous solution of hydrochloric acid, blue by immersion in tap water, and mount in balsam. Glycerol jelly is not suitable for mounting, since the haematoxylin fades in this medium.

OVA

Nematodes may be identified by their ova in the faeces.

Fresh preparations

These afford the readiest means of clinical diagnosis. Emulsify with the platinum loop a little of the faeces in saline or water on a slide. The amount of water required to dilute the material depends on its consistency: the more solid the stool the more it must be diluted. Then add a coverslip and examine systematically (a mechanical stage is necessary) first with the × 10 (16 mm) and then with the × 40 (4 mm) objectives. The light should be reduced, preferably by lowering the condenser, since the outlines of the ova are rendered sharper.

Several such preparations must be carefully examined before regarding a given specimen of faeces as free from nematode infection.

Preservation of ova

Fix in 10 per cent formal-saline, preferably hot, as this prevents further development of the ova. Permanent preparations of ova are often not very satisfactory. If 1–2 per cent glycerol is added to the fixative and this is left to evaporate slowly the ova can be mounted in glycerol jelly. This method is particularly satisfactory with the thick-shelled ova. Staining methods are not very successful, and more detail is seen in unstained ova.

Concentration of ova

When direct examination of the stool fails to reveal any ova, sedimentation and concentration should be carried out. Most methods of concentration depend on the fact that helminth ova are comparatively heavy and tend to sink more rapidly than other material when the stool is diluted with water or normal saline.

Diarrhoeic stools. Mix with equal quantity of water or saline, pass through a sieve having a mesh of 60 to the inch into a measuring cylinder or urine glass. Allow to stand for at least half an hour. Decant the supernatant fluid. Refill with water or saline and allow to stand for another half hour. Decant the supernatant and examine the deposit.

Solid stools. Emulsify the stool in water or saline using a pestle and mortar and proceed as above.

Formal-ether concentration method [p. 421] is recommended for helminth ova of all parasitic worms.

Flotation methods. These are very successful for the non-operculate ova (with the exception of schistosomes). (1) Emulsify the stool in water. (2) Pass through a 60 mesh sieve. (3) Centrifuge some of the fluid for 2–3 minutes at 2000 rev/min. (4) Decant the supernatant fluid. (5) Partly fill the centrifuge tube with one of the following solutions: (a) saturated aqueous sodium chloride; *or* (b) 33 per cent aqueous zinc sulphate; *or* (c) 450 g of sugar in 335 cm³ of water. (6) Gently stir the deposit into the solution and fill the tube completely with additional solution. (7) Centrifuge the tube for three minutes at 2000 rev/min. (8) Carefully touch the meniscus with a 7–8 mm diameter wire loop and transfer the contents of the loop on to a slide. It will be found that ova will have risen to the surface and faecal material sunk to the bottom of the tube.

METHODS FOR NEMATODES OF THE BLOOD AND BODY FLUIDS

ADULT FORMS

Use the same techniques as for the intestinal nematodes. To study the worms *in situ* (lymph nodes, etc.) excise the tissue and fix as for histological specimens. Embed in paraffin and section in the usual way; standard histological stains are satisfactory.

LARVAL FORMS (MICROFILARIAE)

The technique for studying the larval forms in the blood is largely haematological.

Fresh preparations

Make a fresh preparation of the patient's blood. If it is intended to keep the specimen for any time it should be ringed with petroleum jelly. Examine with the × 10 (16 mm) and × 40 (4 mm) objectives. Systematic search of such a preparation easily reveals the presence of microfilariae, which in a properly ringed specimen will remain alive for many hours.

Thick films

Make thick films by placing a large drop of blood in the centre of a slide. Spread the blood until it is about 15 mm in diameter. Stain by one of the following methods. (1) Dehaemoglobinize the film by placing it face downwards in a dish of distilled water for a few minutes. (2) Harden by immersion in absolute methyl or ethyl alcohol for 5–10 minutes. (3) Stain in Giemsa by the standard techniques [p. 416]. *Or* (1) Dehaemoglobinize and harden as above. (2) Place on a staining rack and cover with Ehrlich's haematoxylin. (3) Gently warm over a flame until steam just begins to rise; stain for 8–10 minutes. (4) Wash in tap water until blue. (5) Stand the film upright in a rack until dry; do not blot. (6) Examine dry with × 60 (3.5 mm) oil-immersion objective and a low-power eyepiece; *or* make a temporary mount with cedar wood oil and examine with dry objectives; *or* mount in green Euparal. In balsam the preparation will eventually fade.

Thin films

Make these as for the standard technique for blood films. Do not make too large a film, and ensure that the edges and ends of the blood film are clear of the sides and ends of the slide; this is because microfilariae are usually found at the borders of the film. Stain without dehaemoglobinization with Giemsa or haematoxylin. Mount and examine as for thick films. This method is only of use when the parasites are abundant.

NOTES

1. For rapid diagnosis, either examine the patient's blood in a fresh preparation, or make a thick film and stain it after dehaemoglobinization. By these methods you diminish the area of blood to be examined.
2. *Wuchereria bancrofti.* The larvae are most numerous in the peripheral blood during the evening, whereas they are scanty or absent from blood films made during the day; 22.00 is a good time to make the blood examination.
3. *Loa loa.* The periodicity is reversed. Therefore make blood films from 10.00 onwards.
4. The sheath of *Loa loa* embryos will not stain with Giemsa, but that of *Wuchereria bancrofti* will.
5. The sheath of both *Loa loa* and *Wuchereria bancrofti* embryos will stain with haematoxylin.

Concentration of microfilariae

1. Add 2 cm³ of blood to 8 cm³ of distilled water.
2. Centrifuge for three minutes at 2000 rev/min.
3. Carefully pipette off the supernatant fluid.
4. Add a drop of 1 per cent methyl violet, diluted if necessary so that the final colour is not too deep, to the deposit.

5. Gently mix and place upon a slide. Examine under a coverslip as a wet preparation.

Unsheathed microfilariae will soon become stained; sheathed microfilariae will be seen as white threads in a mauve background.

REFERENCES

BAYLEY, J. H. (1949). *J. Path. Bact.* **61**, 448.
FIELD, J. W. (1941). *Trans. roy. Soc. trop. Med. Hyg.* **35**, 35.
RIDLEY, D. S. and HAWGOOD, B. C. (1956). *J. clin. Path.* **9**, 74.
RITCHIE, L. S. (1948). *Bull. U.S. Army med. Dep.* **8**, 326.
SAPERO, J. J. and LAWLESS, D. K. (1953). *Am. J. trop. Med. Hyg.* **2**, 613.
VIGO, A. W. (1941). *Gradwohl Laboratory Digest* **5**, 2.
WHEATLEY, W. B. (1951). *Am. J. clin. Path.* **21**, 990.

23 | Quantitative methods

It has become increasingly apparent that a mere qualitative expression of histological structure is inadequate. The examination of tissue sections may give an impression of the relationship between the structure of the component parts of an organ and its function, but it is clearly of benefit to be able to define this in absolute terms. Lord Kelvin expressed the desirability of quantitation when he stated in 1883, 'I often say that when you can measure what you are speaking about and express it in numbers, you know something about it; but when you cannot express it in numbers your knowledge is of a meagre and unsatisfactory kind.'

Some of the early quantitative methods that were applied to histology were designed to measure such entities as the area of the absorbing surface of the lung (Aeby 1880; Zuntz 1882; Schulze 1906) or to count components within an organ, such as the glomeruli of the kidney (Kittleson 1917). The techniques which were developed were often inaccurate or extremely laborious and interest in quantitation diminished. More recently, similarities have been demonstrated between the problems facing geologists and histologists and the estimation of the relative volumes of different mineral components in a sample of rock presents the same difficulties as the determination of the volumes of the cell types within a tissue. The application of principles of geometrical and statistical probability have brought renewed interest to quantitative techniques in histology. Early attempts at detailed morphometry were thwarted by methods of examining organs in enormous detail using techniques which were inflexible and slow; the exactitude gained was often outweighed by the labour and expense of obtaining it. Current methods are quicker and more flexible and are based upon a series of justifiable sampling techniques and assumptions. The results are approximate, but the limits within which the true answer lies may be specified statistically, and the degree of accuracy may be verified by a repetition of differential sampling.

It is the purpose of this chapter to describe the preparation of biological material so that the required measurements may be made with meaning and accuracy, to discuss the general principles and application of the techniques available for quantifying histological observations, and finally to examine the theoretical basis of the methods used and the assumptions made. Examples of some of the methods are given, but it is not within the scope of this chapter to provide a detailed account of all the specific techniques for each individual tissue.

METHODS OF PREPARATION OF MATERIAL

The best methods of tissue preparation for morphometric studies are those which preserve the geometric relationship between tissue components, even if some loss in preservation of fine tissue structure occurs. For the purpose of a quantitative histological approach it is first necessary to fix the organ intact so that the fixed morphology resembles as closely as possible that of the normal state of function. In certain cases this necessitates special fixation procedures, for example the lung and the kidney. For other tissues the immersion of the entire organ into fresh fixative may be adequate.

FIXATION

LUNGS

The lungs present a particular problem of a vast loculated air–fluid interface. The often used technique for the fixation of lungs is the installation of a liquid fixative (either formaldehyde or gluteraldehyde solution) into the airways. This procedure, however, drastically alters one of the important natural conditions of the lung by substituting fluid for air as the content of the airways, and it has become increasingly evident that it is necessary to employ a more natural fixation technique by the introduction of the fixative in the form of a vapour into the airways if the lungs are to be used for morphometric analysis. The reasons for this are two-fold: firstly, among the many changes that may occur are the abolition of the important forces generated by surface tension at the air–liquid interface of the alveolar surface. Secondly, the heavy fluid mass tends to cause distortions of the architecture and of the peripheral lung structures. Several methods have been developed, using compressed air or cold formaldehyde fumes, to fix lungs in an expanded state. These techniques are generally time-consuming and several days are necessary for fixation; they also have the undesirable consequence of providing a dry lung. Weibel and Vidone (1961), therefore, developed a technique of lung fixation by means of warm concentrated formalin-steam which they applied to the lung through the airways at a controlled degree of gaseous inflation. This technique was an improvement on simple 'total immersion', but the steam still condensed in the lungs so that the water in which the formaldehyde was dissolved accumulated in the air spaces causing the distortion already mentioned. Despite some fixation by formalin gas, the method was one of wet fixation. Two important complications arose from this technique. The first was that fluid collected in the dependent parts of the lung, causing distortion of architecture, and the apices did not satisfactorily fix. The second was that the lung became fixed from the inside only, and thus allowed time for the outer parts to begin to decompose before fixation occurred. Wright, Slavin, Kreel, Callan, and Sandin (1974) have developed a fixation apparatus for lungs which ventilates them with formalin vapour while they hang in a closed atmosphere saturated with formalin. Fixation occurs in the inflated state and gives good overall preservation of lung architecture together with a satisfactory preservation of fine detail. The time required is usually five to six hours.

PLACENTA

Aherne and Dunnill (1966) have found the following simple method satisfactory for morphometric examination of the placenta. The intact placenta is collected fresh and the membranes carefully trimmed from the edge. The cord is cut to within 2 cm of its insertion. The placenta is weighed, and the volume determined by water displacement [p. 439]. Fixation is then carried out by immersing the entire organ in 10 per cent buffered formal-saline in a large container for at least seven days. It has been shown that the degree of shrinkage which occurs during fixation is less than 1 per cent and may be considered negligible. Further preparation is by placing the foetal surface downwards and cutting into slices, each 1 cm in thickness. These sections may remain in the fixative to be used for quantitative studies as required.

KIDNEY

Although the fundamental function of the kidney has been well defined since the original work of Bowman (1842), the manner in which that function is performed has been satisfactorily investigated only since the use of detailed morphometry. Elias and Hennig (1967) used kidneys removed at necropsy, performed on patients dying 1½–8 hours previously. Volume determination was satisfactorily performed by immersion in water in a graduated cylinder, after all connective tissue had been stripped from the organs. Fixation was by immersion in buffered formal-saline for 48 hours, a few cuts first having been made into the kidney to allow penetration to the fixative. These investigations showed that, in distinction to most other tissues, kidney (being hypertonic) neither shrinks nor remains isovolumetric during fixation. Instead it normally expands by 5–10 per cent.

Although renal tissue fixes in a generally satisfactory manner by this technique, the presence of random cuts into the organ has the effect of disturbing the fundamental morphology and also causing local variations in fixation. A different technique, which leaves an intact kidney, so that a truly random selection of tissue blocks may be obtained, is that of perfusion followed by immersion. The kidney is removed from the body and stripped of fat and adherent connective tissue, with the vein and artery carefully preserved so that they may be cannulated. After initial volume determination has been performed, fresh buffered 10 per cent formal-saline is gently perfused via the artery and at the same time the kidney is suspended in a similar medium. Twelve hours processing in this manner will yield satisfactory results, although a full 24 hours is recommended. By this method, uniform fixation occurs and results in an intact kidney which may be thinly sliced, and tissue blocks chosen randomly for further processing.

VOLUME DETERMINATION

As most preparative procedures induce some change in the dimensions of the organ, and of the individual tissue components, it is essential to determine the absolute dimensions of the fresh organ prior to fixation and processing. In order to infer accurate quantitative results from those determined on the final preparations it is necessary to estimate the degree of dimensional changes introduced by the preparatory procedures and to derive appropriate conversion factors. It is therefore of utmost importance to determine the overall dimensions of the organ—its weight and its volume, for example. Aherne (1970) has estimated the shrinkage of rat kidney slices due to processing and has shown that this is generally negligible during fixation with formal-saline over a period of 20 hours. During dehydration, and particularly during wax embedding, a volume change to approximately half natural size usually occurs. There is a variation between different tissues and for precise morphometric analyses a 'standard' shrinkage factor for a particular type of tissue should be measured for each individual specimen.

WATER DISPLACEMENT

This simple method is suitable for estimating the volume of most organs, but in those instances where the organ is too small (for example the pituitary), or where deformation of the organ is likely to occur due to compression (for example the lung) the volume can be determined by using *Simpson's rule*.

SIMPSON'S RULE

This gives a good approximation of the volume of an organ, and is as reliable as water displacement. To carry out this procedure, the organ is first cut into slices of equal thickness and the area of one face of each slice is measured. For large organs, the simplest procedure is to lay each slice on a sheet of clean graph paper, trace its outline, and measure the area with a planimeter or by a square-counting technique. If smaller organs are to be measured, then sections of the organ are taken at given equal intervals and are projected at a suitable known magnification onto a screen. The outline may then be traced, and the area measured as above. It may be demonstrated mathematically that if n slices are taken and the area of each slice is A_0, A_1, A_2, etc., and the thickness of each slice is h, then the volume of the organ (V) is calculated from eqn 23.1.

$$V = \tfrac{1}{3}h[(A_0 + A_n) + 4(A_1 + A_3 + \dots A_{n-1}) + 2(A_2 + A_4 + \dots A_{n-2})]$$

(23.1)

It may appear strange to define the first area as A_0 and not A_1, but this is done to preserve the convention which is established in the mathematical derivation of the expression. The use of the equation will become clear in the following example.

Example: Simpson's rule

An organ has been fixed as described previously and cut into six (n) slices, each 1 cm thick (h). The following data were obtained.

Slice	A_0	A_1	A_2	A_3	A_4	A_5
Area (cm²)	110	200	240	300	315	290

Then, from eqn 23.1,

$$V = \tfrac{1}{3} \times 1 \times [(110 + 290) + 4(200 + 300 + 290) + 2(240 + 315)]$$
$$V = \tfrac{1}{3}[400 + 3160 + 1110]$$
$$V = \tfrac{1}{3} \times 4670$$

So $V = 1557$ cm³

SAMPLING FOR HISTOLOGICAL ANALYSIS

Two methods of sampling are available for histological analysis. The first is *systematic sampling* and involves the taking of blocks of tissue at given intervals throughout an organ. Its disadvantage is that if an organ has a natural periodicity of structure (for example the glomerular arrangement in a kidney), or if the sampling pattern is affected by areas of disease, then the sample will be unrepresentative of the organ as a whole. The second and preferred method is one of *random sampling*. This is the selection of samples using random number tables which are unrelated to any structural component within the organ. This technique has the advantage of obtaining a small group of blocks of tissue which possess the same characteristics of the organ as a whole.

That morphometry makes extensive use of statistical procedures has already been indicated. By its nature statistics asks, in most instances, for random conditions in the substrate analysed in order to provide reliable and representative data about the whole population. However, biological structures possess an extremely high degree of organization and it may therefore appear impossible to apply statistical procedures in such situations. Three assumptions, therefore, need to be drawn in the application of random sampling to biological material (Weibel 1963).

(1) Random distribution of structures in space can be assumed if the units under investigation do not exhibit any stratified array in the unit tissue volume even though they may be well organized into units of higher order. In other words, sections in all directions of space must yield identical pictures.

(2) Randomness of distribution of structures refers only to a well specified part of the tissue: alveoli for example, are randomly distributed only with respect to lung parenchyma.

(3) If randomness of distribution cannot be assumed then ordinary statistical procedures cannot be employed. It will be necessary to define the underlying lattice and then to devise appropriate statistics based on systematic sampling.

Technique of random sampling

A simple technique of stratified random sampling is to use a transparent grid made up of squares of known dimension. The size of the squares should be matched to the size of the organ under investigation—for example, 1 cm squares are adequate for an organ of the size of the lung. The squares are then numbered and the grid is placed over each slice of the organ and blocks of tissue are selected by means of a random number [FIG. 23.1]. It is important in sampling to avoid ragged or oblique-angled blocks. The blocks are taken in the standard manner using a sharp scalpel and ones of approximately $2.0 \times 1.0 \times 0.5$ cm are convenient. The area of the face of each block is accurately measured.

The blocks of tissue are then processed in the usual manner, which should be standard for all tissues which are to be compared, embedded in paraffin wax, and sections cut. The area of each section is measured and the ratio of the area of the block of fixed tissue to the area of the corresponding section gives a measure of the shrinkage that has occurred during processing. It has already been mentioned that Aherne (1970) has obtained a factor of 0.5 as the shrinkage factor for rat kidney dehydration and wax embedding. Similarly Dunnill (1964) has shown that the shrinkage factor from fixed to fully processed human lung is 0.75. If it is assumed that condition (1) above is valid then the values for linear shrinkage L, and volume shrinkage L^3, may easily be calculated and will be valid for that particular tissue.

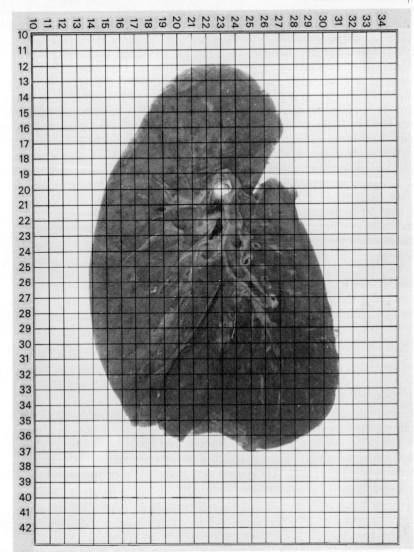

Fig. 23.1. Appearance of 1 cm square grid used to select blocks of lung by random number method. The co-ordinates represent the upper left-hand corners of the blocks defined by the random numbers.

QUANTITATIVE ANALYSIS OF HISTOLOGICAL SECTIONS

The primary objective of quantitative methods in histology is the accurate numerical description of an organ or tissue in terms of the precise components being investigated. This may be *number*, *volume*, or *proportion*, but in all cases necessitates the three-dimensional integration of information obtained from a flat surface of a sample of that tissue with a volume, the determination of which has already been discussed.

Viewed microscopically, a histological section may be regarded as a mosaic in which the mosaic blocks are the individual particles of interest. It is not necessarily the size and number of the individual particles which are of interest but instead their contribution to the total volume. Since the direct measurement of volume is not possible, the principle advanced by Delesse (1848) is adopted. In solving geological problems of differential volume determination he stated: 'If a section is placed through a tissue volume containing a given component, the fraction of the section area covered by transections of the component will be equal to the fraction of the volume occupied by that component.' The validity of this theorem (in which the geological terms have been replaced by histological terms) presupposes a large enough quantity of test material, or at least a representative sample of the population as a whole: and the task of differential volume determination thereafter resolves itself into the determination of areas, or ratios of areas, of various components on a cut surface.

It may be demonstrated mathematically that the volume frequency (vc) of a given tissue component (c) is reflected on sections of the tissue in occupying a corresponding average fraction of the section area (ac) by the relationship:

$$ac = vc \qquad (23.2)$$

In other words, a tissue section is a quantitatively representative two-dimensional sample of a three-dimensional system of randomly distributed structures within that tissue. In mathematical terms the identical relationship between the area (a) of a component in a section and its volume (v) in the tissue is independent of the shape and distribution of the individual structural components.

POINT-COUNTING

The above relationship has given rise to the point-counting method of determining the proportional area occupied by a given component in a section. It is a simple procedure which depends upon the fact that a number of random points falling on a particular tissue component is proportional to the area of the component [FIG. 23.2]. If (P) points are randomly superimposed on the field (S), and (p) points fall on the component (s), it follows that:

$$\frac{s}{S} = \frac{p}{P} \qquad (23.3)$$

The application of this principle to the volumetric study of biological tissues by analysis of histological sections was first proposed in 1943 by Chalkley who used a system of five points in an eyepiece. Originally the procedure using this eyepiece was rather cumbersome, but two later modifications have since opened the way to very efficient and accurate point counting. Haug (1955) designed a graticule with a square lattice of 121 points [FIG. 23.3a]. Although potentially very accurate, because of the large number of reference points, the density of these points concentrated together over a fraction of the field of view tends to make heavy claims on the concentration and performance of the operator. Hennig (1959) designed an eyepiece arranged as an hexagonal lattice of 25 measuring points [FIG. 23.3b] which may be easily managed and yet yield 100 expressions for only four settings. The network points represent the centres of overlapping circles of equal size packed closely together on the plane, and can cover an entire field in a uniform manner. For a given volume of tissue, the collective proportion occupied by a particular component may

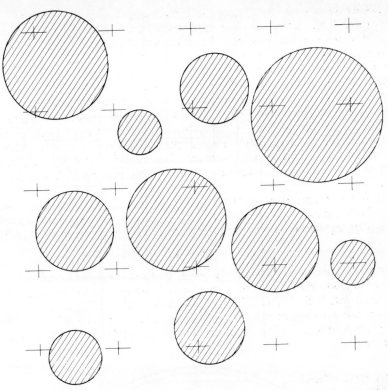

FIG. 23.2. A section taken through a cube containing randomly distributed spheres of uniform size. Points are superimposed on the cut surface, the number of points falling on the spheres being proportional to their surface area.

be calculated by superimposing a grid of points randomly and repeatedly, and counting the proportion of points which fall on to that component. After consideration of the Delesse principle, it will be apparent that the relationship:

$$\rho = \frac{h}{h + m} \qquad (23.4)$$

(where ρ = volume proportion of the component, h = number of points falling on the component, and m = number of points falling elsewhere) will represent not only the area proportion, but also the volume proportion of that component.

It is important to note that the resolution or accuracy of the point-counting method is not determined by the number of points counted in a single field, but rather by their total number and their distribution. Theoretically a single point per field would be adequate and would have the advantage of allowing a more random distribution of the points over a wider area of the section. In practice this procedure would be extremely tedious, and one of the major advantages of the random sampling techniques, discussed earlier, would be lost. The total number of points that must be counted in order to estimate the volumetric proportion of the component under investigation will depend upon

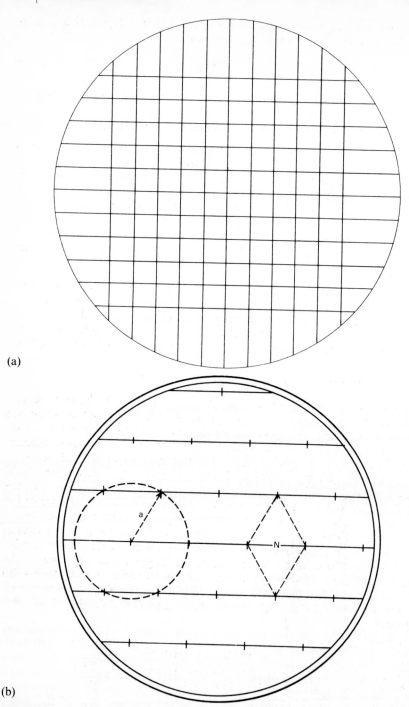

(a)

(b)

FIG. 23.3 (a) Square-lattice graticule of 121 points designed by Haug (1955). (b) Hexagonal lattice of Hennig (1959) which became the integrating eyepiece I of Zeiss. Interval between points $= a$. The area apportioned to each point (or network value) $N = a^2 \times \frac{3}{2}$. The total area of the entire field is $25N$.

the volumetric proportion (ρ) itself. The standard error (Ep) which is to be expected if (n) points are counted can be shown to be

$$Ep = \frac{\rho(100-\rho)^{\frac{1}{2}}}{n\rho} \tag{23.5}$$

As has already been shown, (ρ) is also the percentage of the points lying on the particular component counted.

Two important conclusions may be drawn from this relationship:

1. The smaller the proportion to be analysed, the larger the number of points to be counted for a given standard error.
2. If it is desired to halve the standard error it is necessary to increase the numbers of points counted four times, since the error depends upon the inverse square root of the number of points counted (Anderson and Dunnill 1965). The number of counts increases with the degree of inhomogeneity of distribution of the component being analysed, which thus influences the number of sample fields required for significant sampling.

The statistical analysis of the data obtained by point-counting is generally restricted to a calculation of the arithmetic mean and standard deviation. The usefulness of the point-counting technique may be demonstrated by considering two examples which are separated by two orders of magnitude. Nevertheless, it will become apparent that the same tenets hold for both situations.

Example 1. Enumeration of glomeruli within a kidney

The kidney was removed immediately after death and displaced a volume of 136 cm³ of water. The organ was fixed by immersion and simultaneous perfusion in buffered 10 per cent formal-saline. After 48 hours the kidney was removed from the fixative, blotted carefully, and the new volume displacement estimated. The volume change was considered negligible and hence no correction was required for fixation. The organ was sliced longitudinally and rectangular blocks cut and carefully measured. These were processed in the normal manner and embedded in paraffin. The ratio of the dimensions of the fixed tissue to the sections yielded a factor (f) which is an expression of the shrinkage due to processing. The sections were stained using haematoxylin and eosin and examined with a graticule, designed according to Weibel [FIG. 23.4], in which each line represented a length (l) of 1400 μm at the magnification used. Counts were made of the number of hits falling on glomeruli [FIG. 23.5] by line end points (h) hits elsewhere on the kidney (m), and intersections of glomeruli by the lines (c). The following data were obtained:

Original volume of kidney	136 cm³
Length of measuring lines at magnification used (l)	1400 μm
Shrinkage of kidney sections due to processing (f)	0.65
Hits by line end points falling on glomeruli (h)	80
Hits elsewhere on the kidney (m)	1460
Intersections of glomeruli by lines (c)	1388

The volume of the processed organ (Vp) is calculated by multiplying the original volume by the shrinkage factor (f):

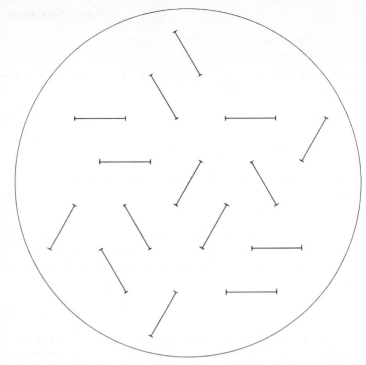

FIG. 23.4.   Graticule designed according to the specifications of Weibel (1963). The 15 lines connecting the vertices of a regular hexagonal point network ensure an even distribution of the end points.

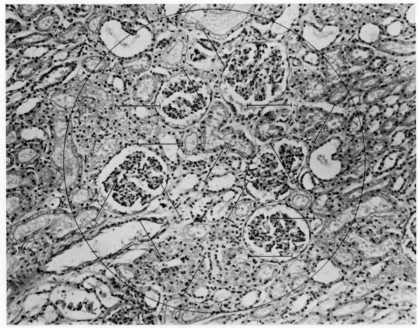

FIG. 23.5.   Section of kidney with Weibel point-counting graticule superimposed, as used in Example 1.

$$Vp = 136 \text{ cm}^3 \times 0.65$$
$$= 88 \text{ cm}^3.$$

The volume proportion of the glomeruli is obtained from the theorem of Delesse (eqn 23.4):

$$\rho = \frac{h}{h + m} \tag{23.4}$$

$$\rho = \frac{80}{80 + 1460} = \frac{80}{1540} = 0.052.$$

The collective volume of the glomeruli (Vc) is given by

$$Vc = Vp \times \rho \tag{23.6}$$
$$Vc = 88 \times 0.05$$
$$= 4.58 \text{ cm}^3 \text{ or } 4.58 \times 10^{12} \text{ μm}^3.$$

Assuming that the shape of the glomeruli approximates to a series of spheres, then the ratio of the volume to the surface of each structure is a constant (k) and is defined as:

$$k = \frac{v^{\frac{2}{3}}}{s} \tag{23.7}$$

where v = individual volume, s = surface area, and r = radius.

Hence, $k = \dfrac{(\frac{4}{3}\pi r^3)^{\frac{2}{3}}}{4\pi r^2}$

so, $k = 0.2064$ for all spheres.

Now, the total number of glomeruli (Nc) can be determined from the aggregate volume (Vc) by the following equation:

$$Nc = Vc\left(\frac{k}{Z}\right)^3 \tag{23.8}$$

where Z is defined as the volume/surface area ratio.

The mean volume/surface ratio (Z) has been shown by Chalkley, Cornfield, and Park (1949) to be expressed in the following relationship:

$$Z = \frac{h \times l}{4 \times c} \tag{23.9}$$

$$Z = \frac{80 \times 1400}{4 \times 1388}$$

$$Z = 20.$$

So, from eqn 23.8,

$$Nc = 4.58 \times 10^{12} \times \left(\frac{0.2064}{20}\right)^3$$

$$= 4.58 \times 10^{12} \times (1.032 \times 10^{-2})^3$$
$$= 4.58 \times 10^{12} \times 1.1 \times 10^{-6}$$
$$= 50 \times 10^5 \text{ glomeruli.}$$

Total number of glomeruli = 50×10^5 per kidney.

Example 2. Enumeration of mitochondria in tumour cells

This example of the point-counting technique has been included to demonstrate the usefulness of the method when considering structures at the subcellular level. An oncocytoma, or mitochondrioma, is characterized by vast numbers of morphologically normal mitochondria within the cytoplasm of each cell. The precise number of these subcellular organelles may be defined quantitatively in the following manner.

The mitochondria of the tumour examined were three times as long as broad, giving a coefficient of shape $(k) = 0.1740$. The volume of each cell was computed from the paraffin sections of the tumour viewed by light microscopy and approximated to 300 μm^3. Electron micrographs of the tumour were made at initial magnification and enlarged to give a final working magnification of 16 000.

Counts were recorded in the same way as in Example 1, except that the graticule was constructed on a transparent plastic film, and superimposed randomly on the electron micrographs [FIG. 23.6]. Each line represented a

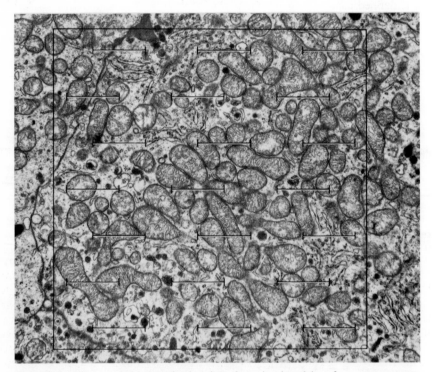

FIG. 23.6 Electron micrograph showing the mitochondria of an oncocytoma (magnification × 16 000) with Weibel-plate superimposed. See point-counting Example 2.

length (l) of 4 μm at micrograph magnification. The following data were obtained:

Hits by line end-points on mitochondria (h)	610
Hits elsewhere on cytoplasm (m)	231
Intersections of lines with mitochondria (c)	3270

Mean cell volume (Vp) of a tumour cell   3000 μm^3
Processing factor (f)   1.0
Coefficient of shape of mitochondria (k)   0.174
Length of each graticule line at micrograph magnification (l)   4 μm

Now the volume proportion of mitochondria (pm) is determined by the equation

$$\rho = \frac{h}{h + m} \tag{23.4}$$

$$\text{so } \rho = \frac{610}{610 + 231}$$

$$\rho = 0.725.$$

The aggregate volume of the mitochondria (Vm) is given by the product of the volume proportion of mitochondria (ρ) and the mean volume of a tumour cell (Vp)

$$Vm = \rho \times Vp \tag{23.6}$$

$$Vm = 0.725 \times 3000$$

$$\text{therefore } Vm = 2175 \ \mu m^3.$$

The volume/surface ratio $Zm = \dfrac{lh}{4c}$ (23.9)

$$Zm = \frac{4 \times 610}{4 \times 3270}$$

$$= 0.1865.$$

The number of mitochondria $Nm = Vm\left(\dfrac{k}{Z}\right)^3$ (23.8)

$$= 2175 \left(\frac{0.174}{0.1865}\right)^3$$

$$= 1766 \text{ mitochondria per cell.}$$

LINEAR INTEGRATION

A major advance in solving the problem of differential volumetry was made by Rosiwal in 1898 when he demonstrated that the fraction of a line passing through a randomly distributed tissue component is approximately equal to the fraction of the volume occupied by this component. The statement of this theorem marked the discovery of the classical integration process by which linear measurements made directly under the microscope are possible, and from which more sophisticated techniques have evolved. Rosiwal also demonstrated that the line along which the transections of the tissue components are recorded need not be straight, but could have any shape, provided that its course is not biased by the underlying array of transections. Two types of integrating eyepiece have been developed for this work. The first is based upon the linear integration principle of Rosiwal and is manufactured by E. Leitz, Wetzlar. This eyepiece allows the measurement of the sum of the portions of random lines lying on given components of tissue within histological sections to be made with relative ease. In practice a point (hairline cross) is moved vertically along a reference line of fixed length (Lr), recording being made as the point passes into and out of a certain tissue component. The process is repeated as often as necessary (N) to obtain a total length ($N \times Lr$) which is adequate for statistical interpretation. The linear fraction (ψc) for that component is then obtained by the relation:

$$\psi c = \frac{Lf}{N \times Lr} \qquad (23.10)$$

where Lf is the sum of the length of the fractions of the components measured.

Mechanical integrating stages, however, lack accuracy, particularly at high magnifications. The main reason for this inaccuracy lies in the mechanism which drives the stage and displaces the specimen itself along a hairline cross in the eyepiece. This is sensitive to slight movements, and in practice it becomes easy to introduce errors through use. The second system is that designed by Schuchardt (1954), to overcome this problem. He used a series of six wedges [FIG. 23.7], each with a micrometer control which is independently

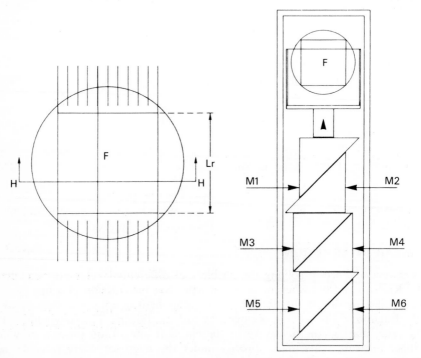

FIG. 23.7. Arrangement of mechanical integration stage designed by Schuchardt. Movements of the micrometers (M1–M6) push the wedges laterally and cause a forward movement of the reference hairline (H–H) over the field (F) for a finite length (*Lr*).

and accurately calibrated in terms of the vertical movement of a horizontal hairline. By manipulating the micrometer screws, each assigned to a particular tissue component, the wedges are pushed medially and the reference hairline is caused to traverse the field. When a sufficient total length of the section has been traversed by the hairline (*Lr*) then the linear fraction for each component (ψc) will be:

$$\psi c = \frac{Mc}{Lr} \qquad (23.11)$$

where Mc is the final distance moved by micrometer M recording component c.

An extension of the Rosiwal theory was made by Campbell and Tomkeieff (1952) who showed that if a number of lines of known length traverse a series of convex bodies then the internal surface area of the convex bodies per unit volume (Sv) may be calculated from the following relationship:

$$Sv = \frac{4 \times \text{number of intercepts}}{\text{total length of traversing lines}} \qquad (23.12)$$

If the length of the traversing line is (t) and if this line is randomly distributed across the lung and intersects the alveolar septa (m) times, and this process is repeated (c) times then the 'mean linear intercept' (L) of the lines with the alveolar septa becomes

$$L = \frac{c \times t}{m} \qquad (23.13)$$

From eqn 23.12 above

$$Sv = \frac{4 \times \text{sum of intercepts on all traverses}}{\text{number of fields} \times \text{length of single traverse}}$$

$$= \frac{4 \times m}{c \times t}$$

From eqn 23.13, $c \times t = L \times m$, therefore

$$Sv = \frac{4 \times m}{L \times m} = \frac{4}{L} \qquad (23.14)$$

For fixed and processed lung tissue the total internal alveolar surface area (Sa) would become:

$$Sa = \frac{4}{L} \times \lambda \times Vp \times f \qquad (23.15)$$

where λ = fraction of lung occupied by alveoli, Vp = volume of processed lung, and f = constant to correct for fixation and processing.

The application of the fundamental principles underlying the techniques of linear integration, together with the methodology involved, will become apparent if the following example is considered.

Example: Determination of the total alveolar surface area in human lungs

The lungs from a patient with known emphysema were removed at necropsy and fixed, using the inflation fixation technique. After 48 hours the volume of each of the fixed lungs was estimated by Simpson's rule or water displacement, and tissue blocks were randomly selected from the sliced organs. Following preparation, the processing correction factor was obtained.

VOLUME PROPORTIONS

The volume proportions (ρ) of the alveolar air, respiratory duct air, blood vessels, and lung tissue were estimated using a point-counting method (examples of the technique have already been demonstrated—see Point Counting Technique, Example 1). Eqn 23.4 is again used.

$$\rho = \frac{h}{h + m} \tag{23.4}$$

NUMBER OF ALVEOLI

Using a graticule with a hairline cross, similar to that produced by Leitz [FIG. 23.7], a square of standard dimensions contained a moveable horizontal hairline (HH) was successively superimposed on the sections of lung and the number of intersections with the alveolar septa counted [FIG. 23.8].

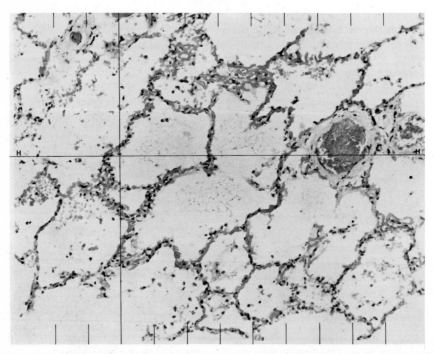

FIG. 23.8. Appearance of the field in the example used to demonstrate the determination of the number of alveoli in an emphysematous lung. The horizontal hairline of the integrating eyepiece is shown (HH).

Approximately 500 points were counted on each slide, and at least ten slides were counted for each lung. The total area of the sum of the squares within which the counting was performed is known and the number of alveoli (N) per unit volume is given by the relationship:

$$N = \frac{n^{\frac{3}{2}}}{\beta \times \rho^{\frac{1}{2}}} \tag{23.16}$$

where n = number of alveolar septal transections, β = coefficient of configuration (defined on page 455), and ρ = volume proportion of the alveoli.

Although yielding a good approximation, this formula may be further improved to account for the distribution of the component being analysed within the organ. This aspect will be dealt with in the subsequent section on Estimation of Errors.

Area of counting square	$= 9.13 \times 10^{-3}$ cm^2
Volume of fixed lung	$= 2650$ cm^3
Conversion factor for fixed-processed tissue	$= 0.75$
$n =$ alveolar transections per cm^2	$= 2.992 \times 10^4$
$\beta =$ coefficient of configuration	$= 1.55$

Substitution in eqn 23.16 gives the number of alveoli:

$$N = 94 \times 10^6 \text{ alveoli.}$$

This value is acceptable for an emphysematous lung, a healthy adult lung containing in the order of 300×10^6 alveoli.

ALVEOLAR SURFACE AREA

It has been shown in eqn 23.14 that, by the theory of tissue intercepts, the internal surface area (S) of a component may be determined from the relationship:

$$S = \frac{4Vr}{L} \qquad (23.17)$$

where $S =$ alveolar surface area, $Vr =$ volume of respiratory portion of processed lung, and $L =$ mean linear intercept.

A graticule containing a line, or lines, of known length can be used to measure the mean linear intercept (L) of the alveolar membranes since:

$$L = \frac{c \times t}{m} \qquad (23.13)$$

where $c =$ number of times line is projected across section, $t =$ length of reference line, and $m =$ number of intersections obtained.

With these data, the mean linear intercept (L) is calculated. With this, and the volume of the respiratory portion of the processed lung (Vr), the surface area of the alveoli is given by eqn 23.17.

CONSIDERATION OF ERRORS INVOLVED IN USING HISTOLOGICAL SECTIONS OF FINITE THICKNESS

There are two principal groups of error which are introduced with the preparation of histological sections. These deserve consideration and, if possible, correction.

The first group depends upon the *fundamental composition* of the material being examined and includes such parameters as the shape of the tissue components. Despite being good approximations, glomeruli are not spheres, and mitochondria are not ellipsoids. The next correction in this category is one required to compensate for the non-randomness of component distribution within a tissue. In the normal physiological state, the alveoli at the lung apices do not possess the same morphology as those in the bases and similarly glomeruli are neither scattered randomly through the entire kidney, nor even the cortex.

The second group of errors comprise those which are *introduced* during the physical process of preparing the tissues, cutting the sections, and taking the morphometric readings. As will be discussed later, however carefully the material is handled and the sections are prepared such factors as section thickness relative to component size become of fundamental importance.

Providing the following limitations are taken into account when making theoretical considerations about particular morphometric analyses, then the final approximations to the *in vivo* situation become valid.

FUNDAMENTAL ERRORS DUE TO COMPOSITION

Consider a number (N) of granules of equal shape and size, each with an individual volume (v) randomly suspended in a finite volume (V). By definition they occupy a volumetric fraction (ρ). From the principle of Delesse:

$$\rho V = Nv. \tag{23.18}$$

If this structure is now transected by a plane, such that a surface area (S) is obtained then:

$$\rho S = Ns \tag{23.19}$$

where s = mean cross sectioned area of granule.

Then the volume of an individual component may be expressed as:

$$v = \beta \times s^{\frac{3}{2}} \tag{23.20}$$

where β = coefficient of configuration.

From eqns 23.18, 23.19, and 23.20 we derive the following relationship between the total number of components (N) of equal size and shape contained in unit volume and the number of components transected (n) by the plane:

$$N = \frac{n^{\frac{3}{2}}}{\beta \times \rho^{\frac{1}{2}}} \tag{23.16}$$

However, histological components are not of equal shape or size, but may be sub-grouped into classes (i) with similar characteristics but different dimensions (D). Within each class there is a uniform relationship between the individual volume and the cube of the dimensions ($Vi \propto Di^3$). In each class of histological component there will be a definite total number (Ni) with a particular volumetric fraction (ρi) and configuration (βi). The total number of components (Nt) is equal to the sum of the components in the individual classes

$$Nt = (Ni_1 + Ni_2 + \ldots + Ni_n) \tag{23.21}$$

and it has been shown (Weibel 1963) that

$$Ni = \frac{n^{\frac{3}{2}}}{\beta i \times \rho i^{\frac{1}{2}}} \times \left[\frac{D_3}{D_1} \right]^{\frac{3}{2}} \tag{23.22}$$

where $\left[\dfrac{D_3}{D_1} \right]^{\frac{3}{2}}$ is the distribution coefficient (K) of the particular component within the volume. D_1 and D_3 are the first and third moments of the distribution of the characteristic linear dimension (D) of the component. Elias, Hennig, and Elias (1961) have shown that for glomeruli K is 1.014, thus giving an error of 1.4 per cent if it is ignored. Weibel (1963) has pointed out that for many practical cases the value for K of 1.05 may be assumed.

The coefficient of configuration (β) has already been defined as a relation between the average cross-section area of a component and its volume. For bodies with an axis of rotational symmetry, such as spheres, cylinders, or ellipsoids this value can be quantified relatively easily. In these situations the shape of the bodies may be defined as the ratio (ε) of rotated axis to axis of rotation. Thus, for cylinders $\varepsilon = D/L$ (D = diameter, L = length) and for spheres $\varepsilon = D/D = 1$. Other configurations may be calculated and are given by the relationship shown in FIG. 23.9. Thus, β (sphere) is 1.382.

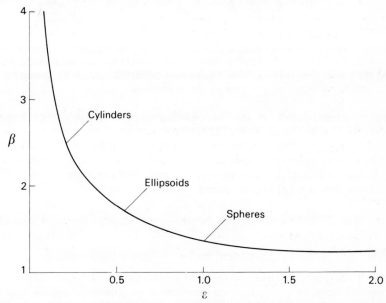

FIG. 23.9. Relationship between the dimensionless coefficient of configuration (β) for various bodies, and the ratio of rotated axis to axis of rotation (ε) for those bodies.

ERRORS DUE TO TECHNICAL PROCESSES

Unlike the polished surface of a composite rock, a histological section cannot be considered as an infinitely thin layer, and the principle of Delesse, although a good approximation, does not hold entirely true. Microscopic sections are slices of composite material of finite thickness, and when observed by transmitted light all solid structures which are contained within the section space may be projected into the plane of view [FIG. 23.10]. At low magnifications, where the magnitude of the field of view is relatively large in comparison to the thickness of the section, this source of error becomes relatively small. On the other hand, when higher magnifications are employed, for counting particular cell types or when applied to electron microscopy, then the error could be considerable. For the correct application of the principles of Delesse and Rosiwal it is necessary to consider only those structures which are sectioned by either the upper or the lower surface plane. The projection of structures deeper to the upper plane, or lying above the lower plane, will lead to an overestimation of the volume-proportion of that component, and conversely

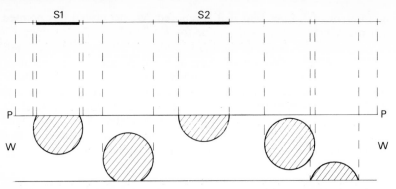

FIG. 23.10.   Section (W) contains spheres which are small in comparison to the section thickness. Although morphometric theory refers only to the components enclosed in the infinitely thin plane (P–P), all solid structures within the section become projected on to the plane. Only surface S2 is represented correctly, surface S1 appearing larger than its true dimension.

to an under-estimation of the surrounding structures. Geologists know this source of error as the Holmes (1927) effect.

The necessary correction for the errors introduced by section thickness will depend mainly upon the cross-sectional shape of the structures being investigated. For spherical bodies between parallel surfaces viewed vertically the volumetric fraction (ρ) is determined by the equation:

$$\rho = \frac{4r}{4r + 3w} \tag{23.23}$$

where r = radius of component and w = section thickness.

Consider the tissue component (a renal glomerulus or a respiratory alveolus) the overall shape of which may be assumed to be spherical, and of approximately 100 μm diameter, and let this component be enclosed within a concentric shell (capsule or septum) of mean thickness 10 μm. FIGURE 23.11 shows a scale drawing of the appearances of this component when it is included within two different histological sections (w), each of thickness 7 μm.

It may be deduced that the appearance of a component will depend upon the position of the section relative to the centre of that component. Since each position stands the same chance of occurring, there is a specific correction factor which can be expressed as

$$S^1 = S \times \theta \tag{23.24}$$

where S^1 = apparent size, S = true size, and θ = specific correction factor.

In his study of the lung, Weibel (1963) has found this alveolar component correction factor to be about 0.66. From these considerations, it will have become evident that if accurate results are to be obtained a knowledge of section thickness will be of paramount importance. A rough approximation may be obtained from the microtome reading when the sections are cut, but this can lead to the introduction of significant errors. The reasons for this are threefold. First, the microtome micrometers are not engineered sufficiently accurately for such fine measurements to be made. Second, unless specially

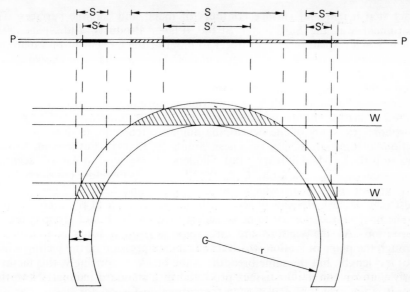

FIG. 23.11. The Holmes effect. Sections (W) cut the capsule of a spherical tissue component at two levels. Despite being a large structure compared to the section thickness, the apparent surfaces (S) are much larger than the true surfaces (S') when projected on to the visual plane (PP).

adapted, and even then unless motor-driven (Te Velde, Burkhardt, Kleiverda, Leenheers-Binnendijk, and Sommerfeld 1977), microtomes are inclined to 'chatter' their way through a cut, thus giving local variations in thickness within a single section. Finally, microtomes tend to compress the block below the knife producing alternately one thin section and one thick section, neither of which is the desired thickness nor the thickness recorded by the microtome. Marengo (1944) devised a method of measuring section thickness in which alternate sections were used for component-counting, while the intervening ones were collected together and melted, one upon another, on to a separate block of wax. This block was then trimmed edge-on and a section taken through the laminar structure so that the thickness of the individual sections could be measured with an eyepiece micrometer. Unfortunately, as already stated, the use of adjacent sections is insufficiently precise for accurate morphometry. A further advance is the optical method devised by Brattgard (1954) in which the fine adjustment of the microscope is used to focus through from the lower to the upper surface of the section. The true thickness of the section (w) is then given by the relationship:

$$w = \frac{a_2 \times b}{a_1} \tag{23.25}$$

where a_1 is the refractive index of the immersion oil, a_2 is the refractive index of the tissue (1.5 to 1.6 according to Brattgard), and b is the reading on the microscope micrometer. Other optical methods based on refractive index differences (Casperson 1956), and interference methods (Richards 1947), have been developed.

Recently, Pearse and Marks (1974) have attempted to reduce the errors due to section thickness using an instrument originally designed to measure the exact step height and surface contours of metal and ceramic surfaces. The instrument was the Surfometer SF100 (Planer Products, Ltd., page 503), which uses a displacement transducer to monitor the movement of a diamond stylus traversing the surface under analysis. Their results have shown an extremely wide divergence between the observed true section thickness and the microtome settings. All tissues examined showed similar, but not identical, differences of a factor of three or four thus confirming a potentially enormous source of error. The instrument was later used by Gadsdon (1976) for the morphometric study of the developing human cerebellum, in order to obtain sections of precisely 12 μm thickness. Similarly, Livesey, Sutherland, Brown, Swanson-Beck, MacGillivary, and Slidders (1978) have obtained accurate 7 μm sections of lymph nodes using the SF100. It is therefore considered that this type of instrument, which combines speed and accuracy, provides the most reliable measurement of section thickness available at the present time.

The final source of error to be considered within this broad group is that of truncation. As the sections are cut, so a horizontal force is transmitted through the plane of section which results in compression of the section which is of less length, but the same breadth, as the block. Surprisingly, this factor is fairly uniform for similar tissues processed in a standard manner. Nevertheless, it is the principal reason why the correction factors for linear area and volumetric changes due to processing cannot be taken from the sections, and must be taken from the finally processed blocks prior to section cutting. If *absolute* morphometry is to be performed (i.e. a morphometric study which will eventually relate components in the processed tissue to absolute units in the *in vivo* physiological situation) then the truncation factor becomes important. If, however, *relative* morphometry is sufficient, then this does not apply.

AUTOMATED TECHNIQUES

Morphometry is now losing little time in following the universal trend of becoming automated. Mechanized methods of fixing the lungs have been described, and the advantages of an accurate automated technique to measure the thickness of histological sections have been discussed.

The three major factors which initially thwarted the development of precise morphometry as a routine histological technique may be avoided by the use of modern analytical methods. Thus, a large quantity of tissue may be analysed using a system which counts an extremely high number of points per field, and without the disadvantage of observer fatigue. Although several such systems exist, it is considered to be outside the scope of this chapter to discuss in detail their individual merits. The Quantimet 720 Image Analyser (Cambridge Instruments Ltd., page 503) is the latest of a series of instruments originally manufactured for the petrological field, but which has since been adapted to fill a growing demand within the life sciences. Similarly, Leitz (Wetzlar, page 503) the company which has already played a major role in the development of the early manual techniques of morphometry, has now also produced systems for semi-automatic or fully automatic quantitative image analysis.

The basis of the automatic image analysing systems is the transfer, by projection, of the classic histological image as seen by light microscopy on to a light-sensitive layer of a selected Plumbicon tube and this is scanned line by line. Plumbicon tubes are outstanding in their linear transfer characteristic with good homogeneity of the light sensitive layer and practically negligible dark current. Different brightnesses in the image, which depend upon the differential staining of the histological sections to be analysed, are transformed, without distortion, into electrical signals for quantitative processing. The tissue components to be analysed may be selected in two fundamental ways, depending upon the objective of the analysis and the instrument employed. The component may be selected on the basis of light intensity—so that a narrow range of density which coincides with the component is selected—to the rejection of everything else. Alternatively, a 'light-pen' may be used to outline the components on the display screen [FIG. 23.12], the output of the

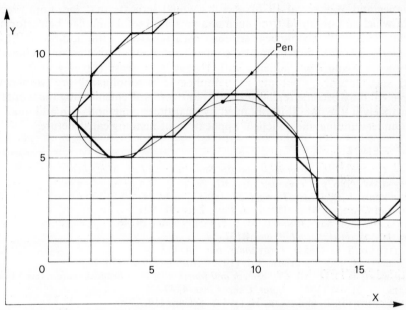

FIG. 23.12. Electronic automatic image analysis. A 'light-pen' is used to outline a contour (thin line) and this is represented as a series of approximate co-ordinates (thick line).

display electronics specifying the location of the pen as the co-ordinates of the grid closest to the current pen location. The output from the display is automatically transferred to an on-line computer facility which has been pre-programmed according to the analysis required. Information may then be stored for continuous assessment or to be retained for later comparison with data from other sections. An added sophistication to these systems is the coupling of the mechanical stage on the microscope to the computer so that each histological section may be scanned and analysed, automatically, in a predetermined manner without the necessity of operator intervention.

CONCLUSION

The evolution of morphometric methods has been described and the application of these techniques within histology has been discussed. It will have become apparent that, within the space of a few years, this branch of tissue analysis has progressed to an extent that it now ranks high in terms of sophistication and automation. The laborious hand-counting techniques, which at best were capable of giving only good approximations of tissue morphometry, have been superseded in such a manner that a very precise morphometric analysis of all tissues is now possible. As in other branches of science, the techniques which are most applicable to the requirements of the histologist lie somewhere between the two extremes, and it should emphatically *not* be assumed that meaningful morphometry can only be performed when the facilities of a fully automated image analysis system are available. Useful comparative morphometry, for example, has been performed on gastro-intestinal biopsy specimens in the assessment of malabsorption (Dunnill and Whitehead 1972; Skinner and Whitehead 1976). Results would indicate that the more precise data which are obtained from such analyses are useful, and can be performed upon the routine histological sections with relatively little additional effort. Similarly, *absolute* morphometric studies have been conducted on sections of lymphatic tissue from patients with Hodgkin's disease (Livesey *et al.* 1978) and such intuitive concepts as 'lymphocyte predominant' or 'lymphocyte depleted' may become replaced by absolute terms. Remembering the words of Lord Kelvin, the data thus obtained by quantitative methods can add much to the understanding and practical application of histological structure.

REFERENCES

AEBY, C. (1880). *Der Bronchialbaum der Saugetiere und des Menschen.*
AHERNE, W. (1967). *J. roy. micr. Soc.* **87**, 493.
—— (1970). *J. med. Lab. Technol.* **27**, 160.
—— and DUNNILL, M. S. (1966). *J. Path. Bact.* **91**, 123.
ANDERSON, J. A. and DUNNILL, M. S. (1965). *Thorax* **20**, 462.
BOWMAN, W. (1842). *Phil. Trans.* **B132**, 57.
BRATTGARD, S. O. (1954). *J. roy. micr. Soc.* **74**, 113.
CAMPBELL, H. and TOMKEIEFF, S. I. (1952). *Nature (Lond.)* **170**, 117.
CASPERSON, T. O. (1956). *Cell growth and function. A cytochemical study.* New York.
CHALKLEY, H. W. (1943). *J. nat. Cancer Inst.* **4**, 47.
—— CORNFIELD, J., and PARK, H. (1949). *Science* **110**, 295.
DELESSE, M. (1848). *Annales des Mines* **13**, 379.
DUNNILL, M. S. (1964). *Thorax* **19**, 443.
—— and WHITEHEAD, R. (1972). *J. clin. Path.* **25**, 243.
ELIAS, H. and HENNIG, A. (1967). In *Quantitative methods in morphology* (eds. E. R. Weibel and H. Elias). Springer-Verlag, Berlin.
—— —— and ELIAS, P.M. (1961). *Z. wiss Mikr.* **65**, 70.
GADSDON, D. R. (1976). *Med. Lab. Sci.* **33**, 299.
HAUG, R. (1955). *Z. Anat. Entwickl.-Gesch.* **118**, 302.
HENNIG, A. (1959). *Zeiss Werkzeitschrift*, No. 30. Carl Zeiss, Oberkochen, W. Germany.
HOLMES, A. H. (1927). *Petrographic methods and calculations.* Murby, London.
KITTLESON, J. A. (1917). *Anat. Rec.* **13**, 385.
LIVESEY, A. E., SUTHERLAND, F. I., BROWN, R. A., SWANSON-BECK, J., MACGILLIVARY, J. B., and SLIDDERS, W. (1978). *J. clin. Path.* **31**, 551.
MARENGO, N. P. (1944). *Stain Technol.* **19**, 1.
PEARSE, A. D. and MARKS, R. (1974). *J. clin. Path.* **27**, 615.
RICHARDS, O. W. (1947). *Medical physics* (ed. O. Glasses). Chicago.
ROSIWAL, A. (1898). *Verh. Königlich-Kaiserliches Geol. Reichsamt (Wien)* 143.
SCHUCHARDT, E. (1954). *Z. wiss. Mikr.* **62**, 9.
SCHULZE, F. E. (1906). *Beitrage zur Anatomie der Saugethierlungen.*
SKINNER, J. M. and WHITEHEAD, R. (1976). *J. clin. Path.* **29**, 564.
TE VELDE, J., BURKHARDT, R., KLEIVERDA, K., LEENHEERS-BINNENDIJK, L., and SOMMERFELD, W. (1977). *Histopathology* **1**, 319.

WEIBEL, E. R. (1963). *Lab. Invest.* **12**, 131.
—— and VIDONE, R. A. (1961). *Am. Rev. resp. Dis.* **84**, 856.
WRIGHT, B. M., SLAVIN, G., KREEL, L., CALLAN, K., and SANDIN, B. (1974). *Thorax* **29**, 187.
ZUNTZ, N. (1882). *Hermann's Handbuch der Physiologie*, Vol. IV, p. 90. Berlin.

24 | Photomicrography

The photography of microscopical preparations plays an essential part in teaching, research, and scientific publications. In the past, apparatus for photomicrography was constructed by photographers and used in the dark-room, but modern equipment is designed for use in the laboratory in daylight and good results can be obtained by the histologist. Details of photomicrographic technique will not be described here, but it is essential that all histologists know how to prepare sections that are ideal for photography and be aware of the general principles of photomicrography. Good descriptions of photomicrography, with full details of simple techniques, are given by Lawson (1972). Advice for users of high quality microscopes with 35-mm camera attachments are given by Fawkes and Lendrum (1977). Kodak technical publications on photomicrography (P2 1974) and photomacrography (N.12B 1969) describe the theory and practice of photography of stained sections and of specimens for lower power magnification.

THE PREPARATION OF STAINED SECTIONS FOR PHOTOGRAPHY

Theoretically, the perfectly cut and stained section should be suitable for microscopical examination, for use with the microprojector, and for photomicrography. This is not wholly true in practice, as different thicknesses of the section and different intensities of staining may be required for various purposes; in addition, in the busy routine laboratory it may not be possible to strive for perfection in every section. The human eye can make allowances for slight defects in a stained section that may be suitable for teaching or for diagnosis, but the camera makes no such compromises and tends to emphasize technical imperfections.

The tissue must be free from cracks, since these will appear in the section; it must be fresh, with no significant autolysis, and be well fixed. Fixation artifacts should be avoided. The sections must be complete, with no creases, tears, or scores. For high magnifications thin sections (5 μm or less) are essential but very thin sections are undesirable for low-power work. Some sections 10–15 μm thick should be cut if low-power photomicrographs are required. Staining must be clear and precise, but the exact intensity is not as important as might be imagined. Good contrast is needed for colour photography and for low-power monochrome, but filters are used to increase or diminish colours in black and white photographs. Mounting of the sections must be on perfectly clean slides, with clean mountant and coverslips; dust and epithelial squames can ruin an otherwise perfect section. Keep the section well away from the ends and sides of the slide, as the stage clips or the movable stage may prevent parts of the slide from being brought into view. The section must be absolutely flat on the slide; if it lifts it may fold or be out of focus. A large amount of adhesive should be avoided, since this can produce background coloration.

Do not use a large amount of mounting medium; the clearance between the coverslip and the high-power objective is very small in microprojectors and some photographic equipment. Remember that high-intensity light sources of microprojectors and photographic apparatus can burn or decolorize small areas in a section if it is left under the illumination for high-power magnification for a long time.

THE MARKING OF SELECTED FIELDS

The histologist must select the exact field for photomicrography. Coverslips can be spotted with Indian ink or with a fibre-tipped pen, but these marks are often rubbed off when the slide is cleaned. Diamond marks are best avoided as the coverslip is permanently scratched. The England Finder (Graticules Ltd., page 503) is a convenient means of relocating a field in a section. This is a 75 × 25 mm glass slide marked with a square grid at 1 mm intervals; each square is sub-divided into a central circle and four outer segments, all of which are numbered. The stained section is placed upon the movable stage of a microscope and the selected field is centred. Without moving the position of the stage the section is replaced by the England Finder and the reference number is recorded. By reversing this procedure the selected field can be relocated on the same or on a different microscope. If the histologist is not in a position to find the exact field for the photographer one of these methods must be used, and for high-power work a small sketch of the desired area is necessary.

OPTICAL CONSIDERATIONS

The objectives should be flat-field apocromats and are widely available for colour photomicrography. The Zeiss × 40 oil immersion objective is valuable as it is not affected by coverslip thickness, giving the exact focus chosen by the eye on the photographic film. Compensating eyepieces that match the objectives are necessary and a fully corrected matching condenser is essential for medium and high power magnifications. Illumination is particularly important as uneven illumination is emphasized by photomicrography and poor results will be obtained if the illumination is incorrectly aligned. For colour photography colour matching will be unsatisfactory unless the colour temperature of the lamp is correct; colour balance is described by Vetter (1974). Tungsten-halogen lamps have a colour temperature at their indicated voltages of about 3400 °K and are excellent light sources which do not vary in colour temperature with age. Daylight colour films are balanced for a colour temperature of 5500 °K and as tungsten melts at 3643 °K filters are necessary to convert tungsten illumination to daylight quality. Light balancing filters 80A and 80B can be used to convert tungsten light of 3200 and 3400 °K to daylight quality and small changes in colour temperature can be brought about by filters 82, 82A, 82B, and 82C which add 100, 200, 300, and 400 °K respectively to the colour temperature of the light. Light balancing filters which reduce the colour temperature of the light are available but are rarely needed. To achieve correct alignment proceed as follows:

1. Centre the lamp according to the manufacturer's instructions.
2. Place the stained slide on the stage and focus the section on the screen using the required objective.
3. Close the substage condenser diaphragm.

4. Close the field diaphragm of the lamp condenser.
5. Adjust the substage condenser to bring the edge of the field diaphragm into sharp focus.
6. Centre the ring of the field diaphragm, using the two centring screws on the substage condenser.
7. Open the field iris until the aperture clears the field of view.
8. Open the substage condenser diaphragm and close until sharpness and colour are well preserved and refractility is absent. Note, or mark, this position for future use.

Before the exposure is made a final adjustment of focus is carried out with the substage condenser diaphragm open and using a dim light with reduced voltage. The substage iris is then closed (see 8) and the voltage brought to the proper level for correct colour temperature and the exposure is made.

Automatic photomicroscopes and those with exposure meters may not give correct exposures with specimens of uneven tissue. Often the only way to alter the exposure is by changing the film speed rating but fine control of exposure can be achieved by the use of neutral density filters, such as Kodak Wratten NDO.1 and NDO.2 which have 80 and 60 per cent light transmission. Alteration to the exposure by changing the voltage is impractical with colour photomicrography as this will reduce the light temperature and will give unsatisfactory colour in the transparency. Colour photomicrographs for printing should be taken at the normal exposure and also at a reduced exposure so that a dense transparency is available.

Photography of specimens with the fluorescence or polarizing microscope raises problems due to the reduced amount of light which reaches the camera film. Fluorescence photomicrography is discussed by Koch (1972) and although prolonged exposures may be needed they should be kept as short as possible as the specimens progressively fade due to the destruction of the fluorescent dye by the exciting light. A fast colour film should be used. With the polarizing microscope the background should not be at maximum darkness; slight rotation of one of the polarizing screens is desirable so that there is a visible background which will demonstrate where the birefringent material is situated in the tissue.

Complete absence of all movement and vibration is essential and simple attachment cameras suffer from the lack of this. They also suffer from the disadvantage of possible vibration from the shutter of the camera. Photographic equipment needs a rigid stand and a solid bench. Vibration from equipment in the laboratory from passing traffic must be avoided or absorbed; in some cities this is so great that photomicrography can only be carried out during quiet evenings or week-ends. Most equipment needs to be carefully calibrated and standardized and it is essential to keep full records of every exposure taken with a photomicroscope. With automatic photomicroscopes there is a tendency to think that a perfect picture can be taken of every field that is seen through the eyepieces, but this is seldom if ever achieved. Careful record of the exact conditions under which each exposure was taken will allow the operator to identify the cause of failures and be able to reproduce successful colour photomicrography with regular reliability. Photomicrography, like histology, calls for time and patience in order to obtain a satisfactory standard technique, and failures can often only be identified and corrected by the systematic control of all variable factors.

LOW-POWER PHOTOMICROGRAPHY (PHOTOMACROGRAPHY)

This can be defined as the range of magnifications that are given by objectives with numerical apertures of less than 0.25. It is not always appreciated that there are difficulties on obtaining good low-power photomicrographs. High-power work (over × 400) may be easier than low-power (× 40) and photography with really low magnification (× 20 or less) may be impossible, as the objective will not cover a large enough field. Moreover, it is theoretically desirable that the magnification is sufficiently great that the smallest distance between two points resolvable as separate images covers ten times the grain of the plate. Working with a photographic plate with a grain size of 0.01 mm the following table gives the minimum magnifications that will permit satisfactory photomicrography.

Table 24.1 Minimum magnification for photomicrography

Objective		Approximate minimum magnification
Magnification	NA	
× 4	0.12	× 35
× 10	0.28	× 85
× 40	0.74	× 225
× 100	1.3	× 380

Acceptable results can be obtained with × 4 objectives if the top lens of the condenser can be swung out or unscrewed, but this still gives a field which may only cover part of a section. Special apparatus that will go as low as one to one magnification, thereby photographing the whole area of the coverslip, is available from the microscope manufacturers (Leitz Aristophot, Zeiss Tessovar, Nikon Multiphot) and described by Hill (1974). Transparency copiers such as the Illumitran (Bowens Ltd., page 503) may be satisfactory provided the lens gives a flat field. Sections must be thick, free from creases or other flaws, and well stained to give contrast. Small specimens, rather than stained sections, or parts of larger specimens can be photographed with 35-mm cameras using extension rings and tubes for close-up work between the camera body and the lens.

REFERENCES

FAWKES, R. S. and LENDRUM, A. C. (1977). *Photomicrography*. Broadsheet 86, Association of Clinical Pathologists, Journal of Clinical Pathology, BMA House, Tavistock Square, London WC1H 9JR.

HILL, B. (1974). *Med. biol. Ill.* **24**, 153.

KOCH, K. F. (1972). *Fluorescence microscopy. Instruments, methods, applications.* English edition, 512/123a/Eng. Leitz.

KODAK PUBLICATION N.12B (1969). *Photomacrography*. Eastman Kodak Company, Rochester, New York.

—— P2 (1974). *Photography through the microscope*, 6th edn. Eastman Kodak Company, Rochester, New York.

LAWSON, D. (1972). *Photomicrography*. Academic Press, London.

VETTER, J. P. (1974). *Med. biol. Ill.* **24**, 74.

25 | Autoradiography

Autoradiography demonstrates the sites and amounts of radioactivity in tissues. The radioactivity may be of two types—naturally occurring or artificially introduced as an *isotope*. The use of radioactive isotopes has led to the development of highly sensitive autoradiographic techniques that will accurately localize the situation of the radioactive material in the cells of the tissues. Similar methods can be combined with electron microscopy but the techniques for histological sections for light microscopy will be considered in this chapter. The specimen is placed in contact with a photographic plate or emulsion and left for sufficient time for the radioactivity to ionize and reduce some of the silver-halide grains of the emulsion. The exposed emulsion is developed and fixed in the usual photographic way and black grains indicate radioactivity. By comparison with the specimen the sites of radioactivity in the tissues can be determined, and the number of black grains is proportional to the amount of radioactivity.

An autoradiograph of a large specimen, an ash tree seedling, is shown in FIGURE 25.1. The plant was placed in a weak solution of radioactive phos-

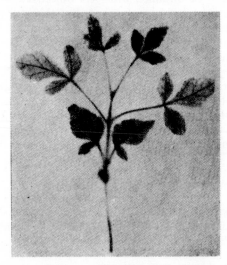

FIG. 25.1. Autoradiography of ash tree seedling using ^{32}P.

phorus (^{32}P) for several hours. Blackening in the autoradiograph indicates that the young leaves have taken up more isotope than the oldest pair of leaves. The most actively growing cells in any living tissue will take up materials in this way, and autoradiography demonstrates active tissues and will selectively pick out certain types of cell that have a particular affinity for an isotope.

With large specimens the photographic plate can be removed
specimen and compared later, but with small specimens and tissue se
is highly desirable that the section and the emulsion are permanently atta
each other. Both are exposed, developed, stained, and mounted togethe,
the section is examined through the emulsion; the emulsion is mainly tran:
ent but contains the black granules that are above the section and will be i _ a
different plane of focus. For high-power microscopy each must be focused
separately. With lower magnification it is possible to show the blackened
emulsion and the stained section in the same photomicrograph. FIGURE 25.2 is

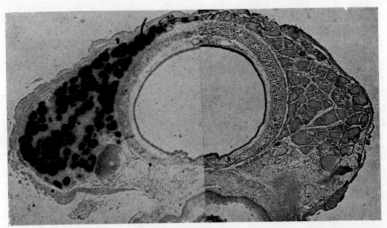

FIG. 25.2. Autoradiograph (left) and normal HE structure (right) of thyroid gland
after administration of radioactive iodine.

a compound photomicrograph showing a contact autoradiograph of the left
lobe of the thyroid gland after administration of radioactive iodine compared
with the normal H and E appearance of the right lobe of the thyroid.

THEORETICAL AND PRACTICAL ASPECTS OF AUTORADIOGRAPHY

Radioactive isotopes are unstable, and emit radiation, usually β-radiators.
They have a fixed life span which is highly variable and is measured as the
half-life, which is the time taken for half the radioactivity to decay. Precautions must be taken to prevent danger to health from over-exposure to the
radiation of isotopes and others should not be put at risk. Many isotopes are
in use in research or for diagnostic procedures and they also vary in energy.
Tritium (^3H) has a low kinetic energy, iodine (^{125}I) has rather more, whilst
^{14}C and ^{35}S are far more active.

There are two main methods for contact autoradiographs, the stripping film
technique (Pelc 1947) and the coating technique (Bélanger and Leblond 1946),
both of which use photographic emulsions which are permanently attached to
the specimen. The success of these methods is largely dependent upon their
resolving power. *Resolution* is higher with low energy isotopes, as high energy
particles will travel a greater distance, blackening a wide area of the emulsion.
In addition the emulsion should be in direct contact with the section and
FIGURE 25.3 shows how resolution decreases if the specimen and the emulsion

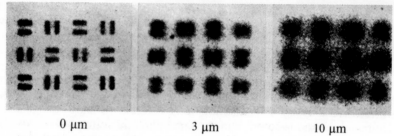

0 μm   3 μm   10 μm

FIG. 25.3. Effect of distance between the emulsion and the specimen.

are not in close contact. The same effect may be produced by thick emulsions and thick sections, but a resolution of 1 μm can be obtained with a low energy isotope (such as ^{3}H or ^{125}I) in a thin section that is in direct contact with a thin emulsion.

All procedures prior to and including the photographic development must be carried out in the dark-room. The time needed for exposure will vary according to the amount and nature of the isotope in the tissues, but may be long (several weeks). In the finished preparation the amount of blackening in the photographic emulsion is determined by the amount of isotope present in the section. *Quantitative autoradiography* can be performed by counting the blackened grains in the emulsion, and although this may be accurate it is a tedious process. Grain counting and other techniques are discussed by Pelc (1957); simpler methods such as the counting of labelled nuclei can be used, but the easiest and most accurate results are obtained with a photometric densitometer.

The applications of autoradiography are extremely wide. Not only will the method demonstrate isotopes that have been supplied to the tissue and taken up in the same way as naturally occuring non-radioactive elements, but the fate of complex compounds containing a labelled element can be followed in experimental animals. The persistence of radioactivity has already been seen to be extremely variable in different isotopes, and the penetration of some isotopes is much greater than others. This differential penetration has been used by Dawson, Field, and Stevens (1962) to demonstrate sites of radio-activity in tissues containing two radioactive isotopes, tritium (^{3}H) and radio-active carbon (^{14}C); by the use of a two-layer emulsion, only one of which was penetrated by tritium, the cells containing each isotope were identified separately.

AUTORADIOGRAPHIC TECHNIQUES

Of the two main types of contact autoradiograph the stripping film method is most widely used in Great Britain, but the coating technique will also be described. Theoretical aspects have already been briefly considered, and are discussed in more detail by Gahan (1972) and Rogers (1973). Some factors, such as fixation and staining, are common to both methods.

FIXATION AND STAINING

As in other histological techniques, fixation must prevent the loss of the target material, in this case the radioactive isotope. It must also preserve the tissue and allow it to be stained. In addition the fixative must not interfere with the photographic emulsion, but some of the common fixatives, such as mercury, can activate crystals of the emulsion whilst others, like formaldehyde and glutaraldehyde, inhibit the process. Because of these chemographic effects of fixatives Doniach and Pelc (1950) recommended absolute ethyl alcohol and Rogers (1973) preferred methyl alcohol or Carnoy's fluid. None of these are good tissue preservers, and Appleton (1972) states that small blocks can be briefly fixed in a mixture of 25 per cent acetic acid and 75 per cent ethyl alcohol for one hour, followed by formal-saline for 24 hours. It is advisable to process tissue that does not contain the isotope in a similar way and use this for control sections in order to ensure that fixation does not adversely affect the photographic emulsion.

Staining may be carried out before the autoradiographs are prepared or after they have been completed and processed. Most stains can be used for pre-staining, but unstained sections should be processed as controls to determine whether staining has affected the emulsion or caused any loss of radioactive material. Post-staining has to be achieved through the gelatin emulsion which covers the section and with the stripping technique this is 15 μm thick. Haematoxylin, with or without eosin, can be used, but staining times must be prolonged (about 20 minutes with Harris', 30 minutes with Ehrlich's haematoxylin).

The stripping film technique (after Pelc 1947)

In this technique the photographic emulsion is stripped off a plate and applied to the section on a slide. Special plates with thick gelatine layers that make the emulsion sufficiently robust for handling are made by Kodak Ltd. for this purpose (see Note 1 [p. 471]). Kodak fine grain autoradiographic stripping plate AR 10 has an emulsion 5 μm thick mounted on a gelatine layer 10 μm thick.

FIXATION

See above.

SECTIONS

Most types of sections have been used for autoradiography. Paraffin embedded material is best for the preparation of thin sections. Cryostat and freezing microtome sections are used for rapid processes and for water-soluble isotopes.

PREPARATION

1. Glass slides must be 'subbed' (coated with a thin layer of gelatine) to ensure good adhesion of the emulsion when the autoradiographs are processed. Clean the slides in chromic acid made up as follows: dissolve 100 g of potassium dichromate in 1000 cm³ of water and very slowly add 100 cm³ of concentrated sulphuric acid, stirring continuously. Wash in distilled water and dip in the following solution at about 20 °C.

Gelatine	5 g
Chrome alum	0.5 g
Water to	1000 cm³

   Drain the slides on a rack and allow to dry.

2. Strip the emulsion from a special plate in the dark-room, using a safelight. The emulsion and gelatine layer are incised with a scalpel and one corner of

the emulsion is raised with fine forceps; the emulsion with the gelatine base is carefully removed from the glass plate. Rectangles of film approximately 2 × 4 cm are floated with the emulsion surface downwards on absolutely clean cold water [FIG. 25.4]. The emulsion will swell, and should be picked up on to the slide and section within 3–5 minutes (see below).

TECHNIQUE

1. The sections are picked up on the specially prepared 'subbed' slides and allowed to dry.
2. Staining may be carried out at this stage (see above).
3. The slide and section are placed at the bottom of a dish containing filtered

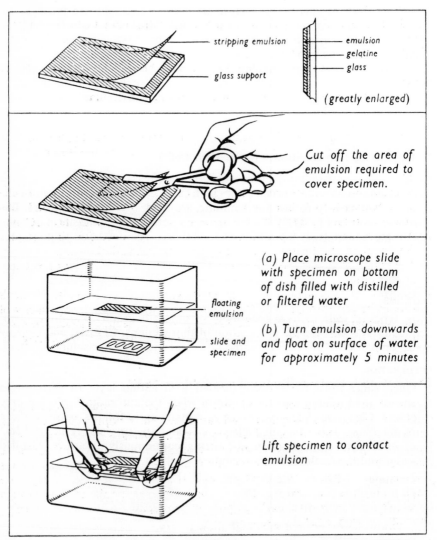

FIG. 25.4. Procedure involved in autoradiographic technique when using 'Kodak' autoradiographic plates.

distilled water and the emulsion is applied to the section as shown in FIGURE 25.4.

4. The piece of emulsion must be large enough to cover the section and to overlap the sides of the slide. This overlap will help to keep the emulsion in place when it dries.

5. The emulsion is floated on the surface of the water with the gelatine layer on top. Leave for at least three minutes so that the emulsion has stretched out flat.

6. Pick up the slide with the emulsion covering the section.

7. Dry the slide with section and contact emulsion in a stream of dry air (not above 21 °C).

8. Place the slide in a light-proof box and leave in the 4 °C refrigerator for the desired time for exposure.

9. Develop and fix the emulsion according to the manufacturer's instructions.

10. Rinse in distilled water.

11. Stain the section, if this has not already been done in stage 2 (see above).

12. Dehydrate, clear, and mount in a synthetic resin medium.

RESULTS

Radioactivity is shown as black granules in the emulsion over the section. The blackening is directly over the part of the tissue containing the isotope.

NOTES

1. Information about special stripping film for autoradiography is available from Messrs Kodak Ltd., Wealdstone, Harrow, Middlesex, England. Details of autoradiographic technique are given in Kodak data sheet SC 10.

2. All procedures with the emulsion up to and including the photographic development and fixation must be carried out in the dark-room.

3. The emulsion is very easily scratched and must be handled with great care at all times.

4. Control sections should be compared with the test sections. Controls should be put through with the radioactive tissues to ensure specificity of the photographic emulsion results, and unstained sections should be compared with the stained sections in case there is loss of silver during the staining.

The coating technique (Kopriwa and Leblond 1962)

Sections are mounted on slides and dipped into a liquid photographic emulsion. This method is quicker and easier than the stripping film technique, but it is not possible to control the thickness or evenness of the emulsion to the same degree of accuracy. Quantitative results from grain counting will be less accurate than with the stripping film technique. The coating method gives close contact between the emulsion and the section, and if a very thin emulsion layer is prepared it is easy to stain and examine the section through the emulsion. Electron autoradiographs can be prepared by this method, using an emulsion with a small crystal size.

FIXATION

Absolute ethyl alcohol or other fixatives [p. 468].

SECTIONS

Thin paraffin sections (less than 5 μm).

PREPARATION

Commercial emulsions for autoradiography are available from Kodak Ltd. or Ilford Ltd. Both Kodak (series NTB, NTE for electron microscopy) and Ilford emulsions are supplied with a choice of sensitivities appropriate for different isotopes. Ilford liquid emulsions may require dilution with glycerol before use according to the manufacturer's instructions.

TECHNIQUE

1. Take sections on 'subbed' slides [p. 469] to distilled water and allow to dry. If pre-stained, they should be overstained to avoid subsequent decolorization. At least one unstained section must be put through as a control. Sections from similar tissue that is free from the radioactive isotope should also be processed as negative controls.
2. Place the photographic emulsion in a water-bath at 40 °C in the darkroom with an appropriate safelight.
3. Transfer the melted emulsion to a 100 cm³ beaker in the water-bath and keep this at 40 °C. Make sure it is free from air bubbles.
4. Sections should be warmed to 40 °C on a hot-plate. Dip the slide and sections in the emulsion for one second. Drain excess emulsion by touching the lower end of the slide on to damp filter paper. Wipe the back of the slide and allow to dry at 25 °C in the vertical position in the dark. Drying should take about one hour; avoid very rapid drying.
5. Expose the emulsion by leaving for the appropriate time in a lightproof box in the 4 °C refrigerator. If a number of sections are prepared one can be examined at intervals until the correct time is determined.
6. Process the slides in the way recommended by the maker of the emulsion.
7. Wash in running water for 15 minutes and post-stain, if required [p. 469].
8. Dehydrate in alcohol and clear in xylene.
9. Place in a staining jar containing a synthetic resin mounting medium and leave for at least one hour. Wipe the slides and mount in fresh medium.

RESULTS

Radioactivity is shown by black grains in the emulsion, similar to the previous technique.

The wire-loop coating technique (George and Vogt 1959; Jenkins 1972)

The use of a wire-loop containing a thin layer of diluted emulsion to coat specimens has been mainly used in electron autoradiography. The method has been applied to light microscopy, especially for smears and thin films, and thin sections can be studied by this technique. In the method previously described, in which the slides are dipped in the emulsion, the coating may be wedge-shaped, thicker at the base than at the top, and the thickness and evenness of the film is not so constant as that obtained by the stripping technique. The wire-loop gives a very thin coating of emulsion that is remarkably uniform. By the following method the emulsion was shown to be 0.4 ± 0.02 μm thick.

FIXATION

See page 468.

SECTIONS

This technique is suitable for thin resin embedded sections [p. 73].

PREPARATION

Liquefy two parts of emulsion in a rectangular glass container at least 10×5 cm in size in a water-bath. Use the dark-room with a suitable safelight. Add one part of 0.1 per cent 'Dreft' and stir gently.

TECHNIQUE

1. Place the slide with mounted specimen on a cork stopper so that it is flat and about 3 cm above a glass plate.
2. Use a rectangular wire-loop that is slightly larger (8.8×3.6 cm) than the slide to be coated. Stir the warmed diluted emulsion with the loop and withdraw the loop with it parallel to the surface of the liquid. The loop will now contain a thin film of emulsion.
3. Immediately place the loop over the slide and lower it so that the film is broken by the slide.
4. Leave the loop below the slide and transfer the slide to a slide warmer at 37 °C for 1–10 minutes.
5. Expose the coated emulsion for the appropriate time in a lightproof box at 4 °C. Develop, fix, and mount as described in the previous technique.

RESULTS

Radioactivity is shown by black grains in the emulsion.

REFERENCES

APPLETON, T. (1972). In *Autoradiography for biologists* (ed. P. B. Gahan). Academic Press, London.
BÉLANGER, L. F. and LEBLOND, C. P. (1946). *Endocrinology* **39**, 8.
DAWSON, K. B., FIELD, E. O., and STEVENS, G. W. W. (1962). *Nature (Lond.)* **195**, 510.
DONIACH, I. and PELC, S. R. (1950). *Br. J. Radiol.* **23**, 184.
GAHAN, P. B. (1972). *Autoradiography for biologists*. Academic Press, London.
GEORGE, L. A. and VOGT, G. S. (1959). *Nature (Lond.)* **184**, 1474.
JENKINS, E. C. (1972). *Stain Technol.* **47**, 23.
KOPRIWA, B. M. and LEBLOND, C. P. (1962). *J. Histochem. Cytochem* **10**, 269.
PELC, S. R. (1947). *Nature (Lond.)* **160**, 749.
—— (1957). *Exp. Cell Res.* suppl. **4**, 231.
ROGERS, A. W. (1973). *Techniques of autoradiography*, 2nd edn. Elsevier, Amsterdam.

26 | Museum and injection techniques

Museum techniques

Every histologist must be able to prepare rare or important specimens for permanent preservation and display. The need for this must always be kept in mind when accepting a specimen for histology, and colour photographs should be taken whilst it is still fresh. Monochrome photographs will also be required if they are for publication. With large specimens it is often possible to use one half for histology and to preserve the other half intact. With smaller specimens it may be difficult to obtain enough tissue for histology and still leave sufficient for mounting; in these cases it is necessary to decide whether histological diagnosis or macroscopic display have the higher priority, but in most instances both can be accomplished. Medical museums have contained intact specimens which were mounted with an incorrect diagnosis that has only been corrected when histology was carried out many years later. Only a brief description of the more common techniques will be described. Fuller details are given in specialized books (Tompsett 1970; Edwards and Edwards 1959), the review by Pulvertaft (1950) and in the references quoted.

The successful museum specimen, like the good histological preparation is dependent upon many minor technical points, and calls for an artistic presentation. The specimen must never be allowed to dry, and must be kept away from water, which causes haemolysis and discoloration. Specimens may be washed in normal saline solution. Dissection should be neat, with no ragged or irregular tissue edges, and bisection requires a long (30 or 35 cm) very sharp knife, so that an absolutely flat cut surface is obtained. Treat the specimen with as much care as a histological section, and remember that there can be only one specimen for mounting, whilst additional sections are usually available from the paraffin block.

Formalin fixation is the basis of museum work, as this allows the colour of the specimen to be restored. Early museum specimens were preserved in alcohol, which distorted and permanently bleached the tissue. Only two methods are now in general use, the classical Kaiserling technique and the more modern dithionite method of colour restoration. Formalin may cause dermatitis, and formalin vapour produces sinusitis and conjunctivitis. The room used for storage and preparation of specimens for mounting should be well ventilated, and an extractor fan is required. All specimens must be in closed jars or containers with lids.

COLOUR RESTORATION TECHNIQUES FOR MUSEUM SPECIMENS

Kaiserling's method (Kaiserling 1897)

1. Fix the specimen for at least two weeks in solution No. I. Fixation must be

absolutely complete, and large specimens may take many weeks; organs should be injected with the solution whenever possible.

Kaiserling solution No. I.

Formalin (40 per cent)	400 cm^3
Potassium nitrate	30 g
Potassium acetate	60 g
Tap water	2000 cm^3

2. After fixation has been completed it is now possible to wash the specimen in gently running water. Then transfer to Kaiserling solution No. II for restoring the colours that have been lost during fixation. This solution consists of 80 per cent industrial alcohol; watch the specimen carefully during this stage, and remove it from the alcohol when maximum colour contrast has been obtained. This is usually after $\frac{1}{2}$–1 hour, though up to four hours may be required. If the correct time is exceeded colours will begin to fade and cannot be brought back.

3. Wash again in running water and place in Kaiserling solution No. III.

Formalin (40 per cent)	50 cm^3
Potassium acetate	1500 g
Glycerol	3000 cm^3
Distilled water	9000 cm^3

Adjust the pH of this solution to pH 8.0 with N sodium hydroxide. Specimens may be kept in this until they are ready for mounting in a museum jar. The jar is filled with freshly filtered, clear solution No. III.

NOTES

1. Keep specimens separate to avoid contamination or staining with diffusible substances, such as bile. Use containers that are large enough to avoid the specimen touching the sides. Specimens may be supported or hung in the solutions to avoid distortion.

2. The pH of the mounting fluid (No. III) is important. Colours will be preserved well at pH 8.0, but tend to fade if the pH changes. Colours can often be revived if the mounting fluid is drained, the specimen washed for five minutes in running water, and remounted in fresh fluid.

3. Specimens fixed in 10 per cent neutral buffered formal-saline (in place of K.I) often give satisfactory results with K.II and K.III.

The dithionite method (Pulvertaft 1936; Wentworth 1938, 1942, 1957)

This method was developed from the observation that faded specimens of chloroma could be restored by the addition of dithionite to the mounting medium; it is thought that the colour is lost during oxidation and that the reducing agent overcomes this.

1. Fix for 1–3 months in Kaiserling solution No. I, or in the following; neutralization is not necessary.

Formalin (40 per cent)	100 cm^3
Sodium acetate	40 g
Tap water	1000 cm^3

Fixation must be complete; if in doubt, give longer.

2. Trim and resurface the specimen if necessary; weigh it and transfer to

Formalin	10 cm³
Sodium acetate	100 g
Glycerol	200 cm³
Water to	1000 cm³

Adjust the pH to 7.5 with disodium hydrogen phosphate (Na_2HPO_4): approximately 1 g per litre will be needed.

Leave in this solution for several days, and if the pH is still 7.5, the specimen is mounted in a fresh filtered sample of the same composition, to which 3 g of sodium dithionite per 1000 g of tissue in the specimen is added at the time of mounting in the museum jar. It is advisable to measure the volume of mounting fluid in the jar, as the final concentration of sodium dithionite should be about 0.4 per cent. Higher concentrations may cause a white precipitate to form.

NOTES

1. As soon as the jar is firmly sealed it should be rocked to ensure even diffusion of the dithionite.
2. Colour restoration occurs within a day or so, but may take several weeks to be complete. Colours are usually revived better by this method than by the classical Kaiserling technique.
3. Specimens have been preserved in this way for 25 years, and the colours are well maintained. As in the previous method, permanent preservation of the correct pH is important.
4. This method was used and developed in the Second World War, and specimens were mounted without the use of alcohol or glycerol, both of which were in short supply. The addition of glycerol to the mounting medium increases the refractive index and improves brilliancy.

Modified Kaiserling method using liquid paraffin (Israel and Young 1978)

Pure liquid paraffin can be used in place of a solution of glycerol in the final mounting fluid. This reduces the staining of the fluid by pigments from the specimen. The optical density of liquid paraffin gives a lifelike appearance to the mounted specimen. Specimens that were mounted in the classical K. III glycerol-containing fluid can be remounted in liquid paraffin; discoloration from pigments such as bilirubin, haemoglobin, and melanin is prevented.

1. The fixative solution consists of:

Formalin	100 cm³
Potassium nitrate	11 g
Potassium acetate	21 g
Water	1000 cm³

2. Restore the colour of the specimen in 95 per cent ethyl alcohol, but do not exceed six hours.
3. Mount in pure liquid paraffin.

STAINING METHODS FOR MUSEUM SPECIMENS

Certain tissue components can be well demonstrated in museum specimens by staining techniques that are similar to those used with tissue sections.

AMYLOID

Iodine technique

1. Fix slices of tissue in formal-saline or in Kaiserling solution No. I. Wash for several hours in gently running water.
2. Leave overnight in the following solution:

Iodine	1 g
Potassium iodide	2 g
Concentrated sulphuric acid	1 cm^3
Distilled water to	100 cm^3

3. Differentiate in industrial spirit, watching the specimen carefully for maximum contrast.
4. Drain the excess spirit off the surface of the specimen and rinse in water.
5. Leave in liquid paraffin for several (usually at least eight) weeks until thoroughly impregnated. Mount in liquid paraffin.

Congo red technique

1. Fix in formal-saline or in Kaiserling solution No. I.
2. Place in 1 per cent aqueous Congo red for two hours.
3. Transfer to saturated aqueous lithium carbonate for two minutes.
4. Differentiate in 80 per cent industrial alcohol until only the amyloid is coloured red.
5. Mount in Kaiserling solution No. III, or in dithionite solution [p. 475].

HAEMOSIDERIN AND FREE IRON

This is demonstrated by Perls' Prussian blue reaction, as in tissue sections [p. 264].

1. Fix in formal-saline or in Kaiserling solution No. I. Rust or iron-containing fluids must not contaminate the specimen or the fixing fluids. Wash in running water and rinse in distilled water.
2. Place the specimen in a mixture of equal parts of 5 per cent potassium ferrocyanide and 2 per cent hydrochloric acid in distilled water until blue coloration is well developed (usually 15–20 minutes).
3. Wash in running water and mount in 10 per cent formalin. Fading may take place, but the colour can be quickly restored by washing with 20 per cent hydrogen peroxide and remounting in fresh fluid.

FAT

1. Fix slices in formal-saline or in Kaiserling solution No. I.
2. Rinse in water and stain with a saturated alcoholic solution of Sudan III or oil red O for two hours.
3. Differentiate in 70 per cent industrial spirit, wash in water, and mount in 10 per cent formalin.

Fat droplets may escape from fatty specimens and will adhere to the inside of the jar. These specimens may require remounting. Small specimens can be coated with a thin layer of gelatin [p. 479] to prevent this.

FAT NECROSIS

The sites of fat necrosis, as in breast or pancreas, can be selectively coloured blue by copper acetate (Benda's test).

1. Fix in formal-saline or in Kaiserling solution No. I. Wash in water.
2. Transfer to an aqueous solution of 5 per cent copper acetate until a blue colour has developed (usually about ½–1 hour).
3. Wash in water and mount in 10 per cent formalin.

NOTE

This technique can be used for the immediate demonstration of fresh specimens in the post-mortem room, laboratory, or class room.

TUMOURS

Cellular tumours may be stained blue–black with haematoxylin in order to increase colour contrast in pale tissues such as breast. This is not applicable to tumours that are necrotic, or rich in mucin, keratin, etc. Haematoxylin may be combined with other staining techniques, such as those for fat. Specimens can be stained with Alcian blue to demonstrate respiratory epithelium and mucous membranes (Watt, Gregory, and Stell 1975). Immerse in 1 per cent Alcian blue in 1 per cent acetic acid for five minutes if the specimen is unfixed, three minutes if fixed. Rinse in running water. Staining is permanent in Kaiserling or Wentworth treated museum specimens.

MOUNTING IN MUSEUM JARS

Plastic museum jars, made of 'Perspex', are recommended. They are light, strong, and free from optical distortion. It is seldom worth while manufacturing museum jars from 'Perspex' sheet in the laboratory, as these can be purchased in a wide range of sizes at a cost which is usually less than that of the time and materials of jars made in the laboratory. Commercial jars are supplied with an accurately cut, transparent back-plate, but supplies of black, white, and coloured 'Perspex' should be kept so that an opaque back-plate can be cut if this is required. Opaque back-plates are better for specimens with only one surface for examination, and an opaque centre-plate allows two specimens to be mounted in the same jar, one on each side. Brightly coloured back-plates can increase contrast and make a more striking visual impact.

The specimen is sewn on to the back-plate with clear transparent nylon thread which is passed through pairs of 1.5 mm holes drilled close together through the plate. When the specimen is securely fixed, the specimen and back-plate are inserted upside down into the jar; the plate can be positioned by small plastic stops cemented on the inside. The mounting fluid is run in to within 1 cm of the top, and the base-plate cemented on with chloroform or 'Perspex' cement. A hole 3 mm in diameter is drilled in the base, which is left under a weight for one hour; the jar is then completely filled with mounting fluid with a Pasteur pipette (this can be attached to a burette). A 'Perspex' spigot is used to close the hole in the base temporarily, and this is withdrawn after 48 hours to remove air-bubbles that have collected and to top up with mounting fluid; the last bubbles can be expressed by squeezing the sides of the jar, and then allowing fluid to run in through the hole as pressure is relaxed. The jar is finally closed with a short piece of 3 mm 'Perspex' rod and a drop of cement. Some air-bubbles may continued to collect, especially from lungs, and these can be removed later by drilling another hole in the base and topping up. If the mounting fluid becomes turbid or stained, it indicates faulty technique, usually from inadequate fixation [p. 474]; the fluid in plastic jars can easily be drained and replaced through a small hole in the base and sometimes this produces a permanent improvement.

A quicker, simpler method is to mount specimens in polythene bags. Sew the specimen on to a sheet of thin 'Perspex' (Haynes 1968) or 500 gauge polythene (Halton and Clark 1976) and seal in a bag of polythene tubing. This technique is less permanent than mounting in rigid jars.

SPECIALIZED MUSEUM TECHNIQUES

Cysts and cavities should be filled with gelatin in order to preserve their original shapes. Friable specimens or loose particles such as small calculi can be covered with a thin layer of gelatin. Prepare the gelatin as follows:

Boil 20 g of arsenious acid with 1 litre of distilled water for two hours, using a reflux condenser in a fume cupboard. Cool, make up to 1 litre with distilled water, and add 120 g of gelatin. Steam for 1–2 hours, and filter through sand and paper pulp whilst hot. Add 100 cm^3 of glycerol and 0.5 per cent Victoria blue until the mass is faintly blue, but still colourless in a test-tube. Store in the dark and add 0.4 cm^3 of 40 per cent formaldehyde per 100 cm^3 of the mixture immediately before use in order to convert the gelatin into an insoluble gel.

Techniques for the maceration of bones have been described by Wagoner and Nuckols (1935). Rapid results are obtained by boiling large dense bones in a pressure cooker or autoclaving in 4 per cent sodium hydroxide solution for up to ten minutes. Small bones may be damaged by this technique, but can be treated with more dilute solutions of sodium hydroxide at lower temperatures (i.e. 90 °C); alternatively they may be heated to the same temperature in water containing a biological detergent washing powder such as 'Ariel'. Putrefaction gives good results, if facilities are available for keeping specimens whilst this is proceeding.

The preparation of transparent specimens and the demonstration of calcified bone structure by staining with alizarin are not difficult but take a long time. A satisfactory method is given below.

Modified Dawson's method for staining foetal skeletons (Richmond and Bennett 1938)

1. The fresh embryo is eviscerated through a small midline abdominal incision. This permits the free access of reagents, and prevents the liver pigments from staining the final mounting solution. The brain is not removed. The specimen is fixed in 95 per cent alcohol for two weeks or more. The longer it is fixed the less likely it is to macerate in the potassium hydroxide. Formalin fixed specimens may be cleared by varying the procedure as indicated.
2. Clear the soft parts by placing the specimen in 1 per cent KOH for ten days or longer until the bones are plainly visible through the soft tissues. (Formalin fixed embryos will require 10 per cent KOH for about a month.) If the tissues become too soft in the clearing solution the appendages may break away. This is remedied by hardening the preparation in a solution of

equal parts of glycerol, 95 per cent alcohol and water for 12–24 hours, after which the specimen may be returned to the clearing solution with safety. The KOH may be reduced to 0.5 per cent for the last few days of clearing.

3. Wash in running tap water for 12 hours.
4. Stain for 30–60 minutes by immersing the specimen in a freshly prepared 0.1 per cent aqueous solution of alizarin red S to which 6–10 drops of 1 per cent KOH is added.
5. Wash in gently running tap water for 30 minutes.
6. Decolorize the soft parts, which will be stained a deep purple, by immersing the specimen in an aqueous solution of 20 per cent glycerol and 1 per cent KOH. The KOH is reduced to 0.5 per cent for small specimens. Decolorization may require 1–2 weeks before the soft tissues become entirely transparent, showing the ossified skeleton stained a deep red.
7. At this stage, the specimen is mounted on a suitable glass or plastic frame and dehydrated by passing slowly through increasing strengths of alcohol and glycerol according to the following scheme.

Solutions	1	2	3	4	5
95 per cent alcohol	10	20	30	40	50
Glycerol	20	20	30	40	50
Water	70	60	40	20	—

8. The specimen jar is sealed with the foetus in the final glycerol–alcohol.

NOTES

1. Fading of the stain will occur if the specimen is exposed to prolonged bright light.
2. This method is highly satisfactory for embryos and foetuses up to 18 weeks. Larger ones are more prone to disintegrate in the KOH.
3. Toluidine blue has been combined with alizarin for the staining of cartilage (Williams 1941; Burdi 1965) while Wassersug (1976) used Alcian blue for staining cartilage and alizarin for demonstrating bone in formalin fixed specimens.

THE RECOGNITION AND CORRECTION OF FAULTS IN MUSEUM SPECIMENS

Museum specimens on permanent display deteriorate and need inspection and attention. Faults may be fundamental, due to lack of care or inadequate knowledge of the points that need to be displayed at the time of first fixation. The decisions concerning the size, shape, and presentation of specimen must be taken at the outset, so that it can be dissected, fixed, and processed in suitably sized containers to avoid distortion.

Fixation is of the greatest importance and must be complete. Greyish areas may be due to incomplete fixation caused by the specimen resting against the container and brown 'bacon-rind' patches result from air-drying before fixation. The specimen must be kept submerged in the fixative solution and away from the sides and floor of the container; some specimens can be suspended by thread, others need supporting on wet cotton wool and covering with soft cloth, ensuring that the cotton wool does not adhere to the surface or the weave of the cloth does not leave pressure marks. Solid organs need very long fixation (several months) and it may be impossible to fix large solid organs containing much blood, such as spleen. Slices 2–3 cm thick may be necessary and if one surface is imperfect an opaque coloured back-plate in the museum jar will ensure that the better surface is on display.

Friable specimens break up and this can be diminished by covering with gelatin [p. 479]. Air in the specimen will escape, and although this does not change the mounting fluid it makes the specimen less easy to examine. Lungs can be placed in a (cool) vacuum oven under reduced pressure to extract air before mounting and if mounted specimens in plastic museum jars accumulate air it can be removed by drilling the base and topping up with additional mounting medium. Droplets of fat which come from fatty specimens such as bone marrow, breast, or subcutaneous tissues may adhere to the walls of the museum jar or rise to the surface of the mounting medium. Complete fixation reduces this, and the mounting fluid should be completely cold, or chilled, before it is added in the final stage of preparation. The growth of fungi in museum specimens can be prevented by adding a few small crystals of thymol to the mounting fluid.

Discoloration of the mounting fluid may be due to haemolysis caused by washing in water, or air-drying, before fixation. These can be avoided, but it is difficult to prevent the discoloration of mounting fluids by the haemoglobin which is present in infarcts and haematomas, by chromaffin pigment in adrenal tumours, or by melanin. The use of liquid paraffin as the final mounting fluid has been proposed [p. 476] by Israel and Young (1978). This is stated to prevent or greatly reduce the seeping of coloured pigments from the specimen, and if an old specimen has stained the fluid it can be remounted in liquid paraffin. Limited improvement can be anticipated from painting the surfaces with gelatin [p. 479]. Bile staining is reduced if the fresh specimen is fixed in Jore's (1913) solution, washed in water, and mounted in the usual mounting fluid.

Jore's fixing solution:

Sodium sulphate	55 g
Potassium sulphate	2.5 g
Sodium chloride	22 g
Sodium bicarbonate	45 g
Formaldehyde (40 per cent)	125 cm^3
Saturated aqueous chloral hydrate	125 cm^3
Distilled water	2500 cm^3

Mounted specimens which have caused green discoloration of the mounting fluid can be transferred to 10 per cent aqueous calcium chloride for 18 hours, rinsed in water, and remounted in fresh mounting fluid.

Specimens tend to fade with time, and restoration of colour is sometimes difficult. Draining and remounting in fresh fluid at the correct pH can be effective, though very old specimens fixed or over-recolorized in alcohol will not respond to this treatment. Remounting in dithionite mounting fluid [p. 475] can be tried if remounting in the original mounting fluid is not successful. Sunlight and heat accelerate the fading of colours as well as other faults; do not stand specimens over radiators or in direct sunlight.

LARGE PAPER-MOUNTED SECTIONS

Whole organs may be sectioned and mounted on paper by the methods of Gough and Wentworth (1948, 1949; Gough, James, and Wentworth 1949). These preparations provide valuable information on the structure of the whole organ and serve as intermediate links between the mounted museum specimen and the histological section of a small piece of an organ.

PREPARATION

Solution A

Formaldehyde (40 per cent)	500 cm³
Sodium acetate	200 g
Water	5000 cm³

Solution B

Gelatin	250 g
Propylene phenoxetol	10 cm³
or Phenoxetol	20 cm³
or Cellosolve	40 cm³
Capryl alcohol	5 cm³
Water	850 cm³

Solution C

Gelatin	75 g
Glycerol	70 cm³
Cellosolve	40 cm³
Water	850 cm³

TECHNIQUE

1. Fix the organ in solution A for two days or longer. Lungs should be fully distended by running the fixative into the bronchial tree. Cut a slice of the organ about 18 mm thick. Wash this in running water for at least 72 hours to remove the formalin (the addition of one part of copper sulphate per million is advisable, since this reduces enzyme action that may digest the gelatine in the following stage).
2. Place the slice in solution B heated to about 60 °C, under reduced pressure in a bell jar; with an efficient water-pump sufficient air can be extracted from the specimen in an hour, during which time the gelatin solution remains liquid. Place the specimen, in the gelatin solution, in a 35 °C incubator for 48 hours.
3. Cast the specimen in the gelatin solution B by allowing it to cool and fix the cast to the block holder of a large sledge microtome. Put in a refrigerator (preferably at −15 °C) for several hours or overnight.
4. Cut as thawing takes place (as a frozen section) at 300–400 μm; put the sections in solution A for 24–48 hours to harden the gelatin. Wash for 1–2 hours in water.
5. Pour some warm solution C over a sheet of acrylic resin such as Perspex. Place the section flat on the Perspex, and cover with a sheet of Whatman's No. 1 filter-paper. Remove air-bubbles and surplus gelatin solution by running a soft rubber roller over the paper. Allow the gelatin to set and dry in an X-ray drying cabinet or at 35 °C, and strip the paper with the section attached from the Perspex sheet.

6. Staining may not be necessary, but may be carried out before mounting the section on paper. Haematoxylin and eosin will bring out pale tissue such as neoplasms. Amyloid and haemosiderin can be well shown. Staining solutions should be more dilute than those used for ordinary histological sections.

Injection methods

Coloured insoluble substances can be injected into blood vessels, lymphatics, bronchi, bile ducts, and many other anatomical structures for the production of demonstration specimens or research purposes. Casts are produced which may be examined in the intact specimen if it is sufficiently translucent (mesentery, lung, intestine, etc.). When a radiopaque injection medium is used the specimen can be X-rayed and details of small blood vessels are seen on naked-eye examination or by low-power magnification of radiographs. Plastic resins set into a solid mass and are ideal for the preparation of corrosion casts of vascular or other structures; these are recovered intact by maceration of the tissue with strong acids.

Modern materials for injection such as neoprene latex, stabilized solutions of barium sulphate, and synthetic plastic resins are injected into the specimen at room temperature, but the classical gelatin injection materials solidify on cooling and must be injected as a warm solution in which a coloured dye or a radiopaque material has been added. Satisfactory gelatin injection masses must be colloidal; if the particles are too large the capillaries will not be filled, while a true solution is liable to diffuse through the vessel walls.

POLYESTER RESINS FOR INJECTION AND CASTING

Synthetic unsaturated polyester resins are excellent injection materials for corrosion casts obtained by macerating the specimen with strong mineral acids. Specimens which are translucent can be retained intact or dissected after the cast has set. Techniques have been developed by Tompsett (1952, 1970), but the availability of materials has recently changed in Britain. The following details are for Scott-Bader resins which are supplied by Trylon Ltd. [p. 503]. As the materials are flammable and unstable, export orders cannot be fulfilled. Overseas workers may be able to arrange supplies through the company's agents and overseas licensees; alternatively an unsaturated medium exotherm polyester casting resin which is available locally can be used as the basis of an injection or casting medium with a suitable viscosity and setting-time (pot life).

Animals and organs should not be injected immediately after death with these resins as they cause a violent muscular spasm which can interfere with the injection. Store the specimen overnight at 4 °C before perfusing the blood vessels with 2 per cent saline solution which has stood for at least 48 hours to remove excess dissolved air. Vascular injections may be obstructed by blood clots and saline perfusion within 12 hours will minimize these. It is essential to remove organs for injection without damage as any cut or break will leak resin.

PREPARATION

The specimen must be prepared, dissected if necessary, and glass or plastic cannulae inserted before the resin injection medium is made up. Large solid organs need support by floating or suspending in water to avoid lack of filling due to pressure on the lower surface. Scott-Bader Crystic resin 191E (PA), which is Trylon resin CL 201 (PA), is recommended for small injections; Scott-Bader Crystic resin 406 (PA), which is Trylon resin SP 701 (PA), should be used for larger injections, as it is less exothermic.

Polyester resin for small injections:

Crystic resin 191 E PA (Trylon CL 201 PA, page 503)	100 g
Monomer C (Trylon thinners)	20 cm³
Catalyst paste H (Trylon catalyst paste)	12 g
Accelerator E (Trylon activator)	3 cm³

If the resin is not 'PA' (pre-activated) use 6 cm³ of accelerator instead of 3 cm³.

Mix the resin with the monomer, making sure that there are no air bubbles in the mixture. Appropriate colour pastes (up to 6 per cent) can also be added. Cool to 20 °C. Dissolve the catalyst paste in the resin. This catalysed resin is usable for up to two hours. Add the accelerator immediately before use.

Polyester resin for large injections and casts: use Crystic resin 406 PA (Trylon SP 701 PA) with the same monomer, colours, catalyst paste, and accelerator in the same quantities as for small injections (see above).

These resin mixtures set in about 18 minutes. If very small blood vessels or other structures are to be filled more activator is needed and this will reduce the 'pot life' to about 12 minutes; an additional 10 per cent of monomer (Trylon thinners) will reduce viscosity and make it easier to fill fine vessels without the need for high injection pressures which can cause tissue impregnation. Failure of the resin to set before tissue impregnation, causing a solid mass of resin in which details are lost, is minimized by injecting the resin mixture about four minutes before the temperature rise that indicates that the resin is about to set. A preliminary test should be made before the first injection is performed, in order to obtain an indication of the viscosity and setting time of the mixture.

TECHNIQUE

1. For vascular injections the organ is prepared by cannulating the arterial vessels, suspending in water, and perfusing with 2 per cent saline (see above).
2. Mix the resin, monomer, colour, catalyst, and accelerator as described above, cooling to 20 °C.
3. Inject the resin when it reaches a temperature of about 26 °C, shortly before it is due to set. This can be done with disposable syringes; do not use excessive pressure. The resin will be seen to fill blood vessels; completion of injection can be judged by naked-eye examination or by increased resistance.
4. If the injection is made in the body, the organ is removed two hours after the resin has set. It is strong but flexible at this stage. Leave the injected specimen in cold water (for corrosion specimens) or Kaiserling I (for mounted specimens) for about eight days, by which time it is fully cured.

5. If a corrosion cast is required, transfer the specimen to an acid bath containing enough commercial grade concentrated hydrochloric acid to cover the specimen. Use a fume cupboard and avoid exposure of hands and eyes to acid splashes and fumes.
6. Wash the corrosion cast in running water until clean. Final immersion in industrial spirit or acetone will remove any bloom, and colour can be revived by leaving overnight in water containing a little ammonia and hydrogen peroxide.
7. Casts can be pruned by removing resin that has leaked or over-filled. Breaks are repaired with resin cement. Appearances are improved by a final spraying with a 10 per cent mixture of the original resin medium in acetone; this can be done with an atomizer immediately after the accelerator has been added.
8. Casts can be protected by mounting in a 'Perspex' museum box, or embedded in a solid block of transparent resin. Trylon resin EM 301/300 PA is suitable; for details see Tompsett (1970) and Trylon technical data sheet T.78.

NOTE

The storage life of resin injection materials at 4 °C is two years or more, but only a few months at room temperature.

NEOPRENE LATEX FOR INJECTION

Neoprene latexes are colloidal dispersions of chloroprene polymers which look like milk. For injecting anatomical specimens DuPont [p. 504] neoprene latex No. 572 is recommended and coloured latex is available from Harris Biological Supplies [p. 504]. The fluid is alkaline (pH 12) and it sets immediately it becomes acidic. When completely cured the solid latex is highly elastic and fairly strong; although polyester resins usually produce more elegant preparations the elasticity of latex casts is an advantage compared with the brittleness of resin casts. Blocks of latex-injected tissue can be processed for histology and satisfactory stained sections prepared by the usual techniques.

Latex should not be stored at less than 16 °C and is best used within a few months as older latex may set prematurely. Injection should follow the general principles described in the previous section on resin injection, but as it is less viscous it has a greater tendency to leak from damaged vessels or to impregnate tissues. Small leaks can be stopped by applying a cotton wool swab soaked in 10 per cent acetic acid which causes the latex to set. After injection the organ can be fixed in a formalin fixing fluid in which it will set, and this is hastened by the addition of 1 per cent acetic acid. Small blood vessels and lymphatics set quickly, usually in less than 20 minutes, but large amounts in vessels such as aorta or vena cava may take up to a month to set completely. This is hastened if the specimen is cooled to −20 °C for 48 hours.

RADIOPAQUE MATERIALS FOR INJECTION

Radiography of specimens that have been injected with radiopaque contrast media gives excellent results and radiopaque materials can be added to coloured latex [p. 504] and gelatin injection media [p. 486]. 'Colorpaque' (Garmanson Chemicals Ltd., page 504) has been developed for the radiographic demonstration of blood vessels of anatomical specimens; it is available in a range of colours (white, red, blue, yellow), withstands chemical corrosion, fixing and clearing agents, and may be combined with gelatin so that it sets and remains in place in dissected specimens and tissue sections. Particle size is approximately 1 μm. Viscosity is such that arterioles and venules will be filled but dilution with an equal volume of water reduces the viscosity to near that of blood and allows passage through the capillary bed; 'Colorpaque' neutral medium of high viscosity can be used if only major vessels are to be filled.

'Colorpaque', diluted with up to an equal volume of water (to reduce viscosity) or neutral medium (to increase viscosity) can be injected cold with a syringe or a constant-pressure apparatus [p. 485] using a pressure of 120–150 mm of mercury. To produce a radiopaque coloured injection medium for blood vessels or other anatomical structures that will solidify and permit dissection and section cutting proceed as follows. Dissolve 5 g of gelatin in 35 cm^3 of equal parts of 'Colorpaque' neutral medium and water on a water-bath at 40 °C. Warm 120 cm^3 of 'Colorpaque' to the same temperature and gently stir into the gelatin solution, avoiding air bubbles. Immediately before use add 2 cm^3 of 40 per cent formaldehyde to toughen the gelatin and inject with the medium and the specimen at 40 °C. Allow to cool and chill the specimen before cutting specimens; a freezing microtome may be needed for thin sections.

GELATIN INJECTION METHODS

Gelatin can be combined with insoluble dyes to form colloidal injection masses which are introduced as warm solutions. Radiopaque contrast medium can also be added if the organ is for X-ray examination. A constant-pressure apparatus in which the bottle containing the injection mass is placed in a water-bath is suitable for warm gelatin injections [FIG. 26.1].

Carmine–gelatin

1. Add a little distilled water to 150 g of powdered carmine and make a paste. Place in a bottle or flask and add 75 cm^3 of distilled water. Shake well and add concentrated ammonia until the carmine has dissolved; 10–15 cm^3 are usually needed.
2. Soak 250 g of gelatin in 750 cm^3 of distilled water. Complete solution by stirring on a water-bath, keeping the temperature at about 60 °C.
3. Warm the carmine solution to 60 °C and add to the gelatin solution.
4. Filter and pour in 30 per cent acetic acid, 1 cm^3 at a time, continuing to stir. Using a pH meter, stop when a pH of 7.2 has been reached. Add a crystal of thymol.

NOTES

1. If over-acidified, the injection mass is granular under the low-power of the microscope and is useless. If alkaline, the dye will diffuse into the tissues surrounding the vessels. When correctly prepared the carmine is in the colloidal state.
2. It seems impossible to specify the volume of acetic acid required to neutralize the ammoniacal mass. This is because samples of gelatin appear to vary in their acidity.

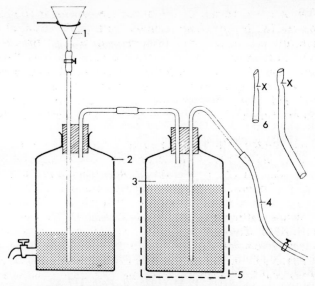

FIG. 26.1. Injection apparatus of Toldt.

1. Funnel fitted to a tall glass tube. The length of this need not be more than 15 cm since this will give a pressure of over two metres of water, which is more than enough for all injection work.

2. Mercury flask supplying the air pressure for:

3. Flask containing the injection mass.

4. Tubing connecting the contents of 3 with the cannula.

5. Water-bath. For gelatin injection masses this is filled with hot water to melt the mass. The temperature may be kept up by a small flame beneath the water-bath.

6. Cannulae for injection. Note the neck (x) on these; this constriction is essential in order that the cannula may be securely tied into the vessel or duct.

A screw clamp should be interposed beneath the mercury funnel and another near the cannula. The injection pressure is regulated by varying the height of the mercury funnel; the rate of outflow of the injection mass is controlled by the screw clamps. For most work flask 3 is duplicated so as to allow of a preliminary perfusion with saline.

Prussian (or Berlin) blue

This pigment is formed when a solution of potassium ferrocyanide is mixed with one of ferric chloride. If the potassium salt is in excess the precipitate can be dissolved in water to form a dispersed colloid. This is termed *soluble* Prussian blue and is the kind used for injection. The insoluble variety is formed when the ferric salt is in excess: it is useless for injection, only a coarse suspension (which rapidly settles) being obtainable in water. Ranvier and other histologists prepared their own Prussian blue. But it is best bought in powdered form and the mass is prepared as follows:

1. Make a 2 per cent solution of *soluble* Prussian blue in distilled water. Warm it to 40 °C.

2. Warm the gelatin prepared as above to 60 °C.

3. Add 1 to 2, stirring continuously, in the proportion of one volume of Prussian blue to three volumes gelatin.

4. Add a large crystal of thymol or 2 per cent chloral as a preservative.

5. Filter as for carmine-gelatin into a glass-stoppered bottle.

REFERENCES

BURDI, A. R. (1965). *Stain Technol.* **40**, 45.

EDWARDS, J. J. and EDWARDS, M. J. (1959). *Medical museum technology.* Oxford University Press, London.

GOUGH, J. and WENTWORTH, J. E. (1948). *Proceedings of the 9th International Congress of Industrial Medicine*, London.

—— —— (1949). *J. roy. micr. Soc.* **69**, 231.

—— JAMES, W. R. L., and WENTWORTH, J. E. (1949). *J. Fac. Radiol. (Lond.)* **1**, 28.

HALTON, A. R. and CLARK, J. V. (1976). *Med. Lab. Sci.* **33**, 325.

HAYNES, D. W. (1968). *J. med. Lab. Technol.* **25**, 101.

ISRAEL, M. S. and YOUNG, L. F. (1978). *J. clin. Path.* **31**, 499.

JORES, L. (1913). *Münch. med. Wschr.* **60**, 976.

KAISERLING, C. (1897). *Virchows Arch. path. Anat.* **147**, 389.

PULVERTAFT, R. J. V. (1936). *J. techn. Meth.* **16**, 27.

—— (1950). *J. clin. Path.* **3**, 1.

RICHMOND, G. W. and BENNETT, L. (1938). *Stain Technol.* **13**, 77.

TOMPSETT, D. H. (1952). *Thorax* **7**, 78.

—— (1970). *Anatomical techniques*, 2nd edn. Livingstone, Edinburgh.

WAGONER, G. and NUCKOLS, H. H. (1935). *J. techn. Meth.* **14**, 35.

WASSERSUG, R. J. (1976). *Stain Technol.* **51**, 131.

WATT, J., GREGORY, I., and STELL, P. M. (1975). *J. Path.* **117**, 89.

WENTWORTH, J. E. (1938). *J. techn. Meth.* **18**, 53.

—— (1942). *J. Path. Bact.* **54**, 137.

—— (1957). *J. med. Lab. Technol.* **14**, 194.

WILLIAMS, T. W. (1941). *Stain Technol.* **16**, 23.

Appendix 1

SI Units

The Système International d'Unités (SI) is becoming the approved means of expressing units of measurement in all branches of science and technology including medicine. Laboratories all over the world have adopted SI units (Young 1974) and the development of the use of SI units in laboratories is described by the *Journal of Clinical Pathology* (1970) and Baron (1973) and Baron *et al.* (1974). Guides for the use of SI units, their symbols and abbreviations are published by the Royal Society of Medicine (1972) and the World Health Organization (1977).

The basis of SI units is the use of prefixes for decimal multiples and submultiples of units according to Table A1.1.

Table A1.1 Prefixes and symbols used in SI units

Multiple	Prefix	Symbol	Submultiple	Prefix	Symbol
10^1	deca	da	10^{-1}	deci	d
10^2	hecto	h	10^{-2}	centi	c
10^3	kilo	k	10^{-3}	milli	m
10^6	mega	M	10^{-6}	micro	μ
			10^{-9}	nano	n
			10^{-12}	pico	p

Multiples and submultiples are used in steps of 10^3. Compound prefixes are not used; thus 10^{-9} metre is nanometre (nm) not millimicrometre (mμm). All the symbols used are on normal typewriters with the exception of μ; one key can be changed to μ at low cost.

THE APPLICATION OF SI UNITS TO HISTOLOGY

LENGTH

The basic unit of length is the metre (m). The micron (μ) as the name for a unit of length of 10^{-6} m is now obsolete; the correct name is the micrometre (μm). The Ångström unit (Å) which is one-tenth of a nanometre should no longer be used and the measurement should be converted to nanometres ($1 \text{ Å} = 10^{-1}$ nm).

VOLUME

The basic unit is the cubic metre (m^3). Squared and cubed are to be expressed as numerical powers and not by abbreviations; thus a square centimetre is cm^2

not sq. cm. The working unit is the litre (l) which is an alternative name for the cubic decimetre (dm^3). The lambda (λ) as the name for the unit of volume 10^{-6} l is now obsolete and the correct name for this unit is the microlitre (μl). Per cent (%) means 'per hundred parts of the same'; thus 'mg %' means 'milligrams per hundred milligrams' and does not mean 'milligrams per hundred millilitres' which differs by a factor of 1000.

MASS

The basic unit is the kilogram (kg) and the working unit is the gram (g). Multiples and submultiples are of the gram and not of the kilogram. It has been agreed that the spellings kilogram and gram are accepted for use in Britain. The gamma (γ) as a name for a unit of mass (10^{-6} g) is obsolete; the correct name for this unit is the microgram (μg). Concentration of solutions are expressed as mass concentration in multiples and submultiples of grams per litre or as molar concentrations in mol/l.

TIME

The basic unit is the second (s). Other working units are minute (min), hour (h), day (d), year (y).

REFERENCES

BARON, D. N. (1973). *J. clin. Path.* **26**, 729–30.
—— BROUGHTON, P. M. G., COHEN, M., LANSLEY, T. S., LEWIS, S. M., and SHINTON, N. K. (1974). *J. clin. Path.* **27**, 590–7.
JOURNAL OF CLINICAL PATHOLOGY (1970). *Editorial,* **23**, 818–19.
ROYAL SOCIETY OF MEDICINE (1972). *Units, Symbols and Abbreviations.* Royal Society of Medicine, London.
WORLD HEALTH ORGANIZATION (1977). *The SI for the health professions.* WHO, Geneva.
YOUNG, D. S. (1974). *New Eng. J. Med.* **290**, 368–73.

Appendix 2

Atomic weights

Aluminium	Al	27		Manganese	Mn	55
Antimony	Sb	122		Mercury	Hg	201
Arsenic	As	75		Molybdenum	Mo	96
Barium	Ba	137		Nickel	Ni	59
Bismuth	Bi	209		Nitrogen	N	14
Boron	B	11		Osmium	Os	190
Bromine	Br	80		Oxygen	O	16
Cadmium	Cd	112		Phosphorus	P	31
Calcium	Ca	40		Platinum	Pt	195
Carbon	C	12		Potassium	K	39
Chlorine	Cl	$35\frac{1}{2}$		Silicon	Si	28
Chromium	Cr	52		Silver	Ag	108
Cobalt	Co	59		Sodium	Na	23
Copper	Cu	64		Strontium	Sr	88
Gold	Au	197		Sulphur	S	32
Hydrogen	H	1		Tin	Sn	119
Iodine	I	127		Titanium	Ti	48
Iron	Fe	56		Tungsten	W	184
Lead	Pb	207		Uranium	U	238
Lithium	Li	7		Yttrium	Y	89
Magnesium	Mg	24		Zinc	Zn	65

These are sufficiently accurate for histological purposes, but not for analytical work.

Appendix 3

Molecular weights

A molar solution contains the molecular weight in grams of the dissolved substance in 1 litre of solution. The molecular weight is determined from the formula of the substance, whose constituent atomic weights are added together. This weight in grams of the substance is dissolved in distilled water and made up to 1 litre in a volumetric flask. A decimolar solution (0.1 M or M/10) contains one-tenth of the substance in a molar solution.

Acetic acid, CH_3COOH	60
Ammonia, NH_3	17
Borax (sodium tetraborate), $Na_2B_4O_7.10H_2O$	381
Boric acid, H_3BO_3	62
Formic acid, $HCOOH$	46
Hydrochloric acid, HCl	$36\frac{1}{2}$
Nitric acid, HNO_3	63
Potassium dihydrogen phosphate, KH_2PO_4	136
Potassium chloride, KCl	$74\frac{1}{2}$
Potassium hydroxide, KOH	56
Sodium acetate (anhydrous), CH_3COONa	82
Sodium acetate crystals, $CH_3COONa.3H_2O$	136
Sodium barbiturate, $C_8H_{11}O_3N_2Na$	206
Sodium chloride, $NaCl$	$58\frac{1}{2}$
Sodium dihydrogen phosphate, $NaH_2PO_4.H_2O$	138
Sodium hydroxide, $NaOH$	40
Sodium phosphate, dibasic, Na_2HPO_4	142
Sulphuric acid, H_2SO_4	98
Veronal sodium (see sodium barbiturate).	

Appendix 4

Normal solutions

A normal solution contains one gram-equivalent of the substance in one litre of the solution, a gram-equivalent being the amount of the substance capable of reacting with or being substituted for one gram-atom (1.008 g) of hydrogen. A practical way of determining the weight of the substance in a normal solution is to divide the molecular weight by the valency, which gives the amount of the substance in one litre of solution. Thus hydrochloric acid (HCl, molecular weight $36\frac{1}{2}$) contains $36\frac{1}{2}$ g of acid in one litre of normal solution. A normal solution of sulphuric acid (H_2SO_4, molecular weight 98) contains 49 g of acid in a litre of normal solution. Remember that acids are in solution and are heavy and a normal solution of sulphuric acid is *not* 4.9 per cent of the concentrated acid in distilled water. The weight of acid in solutions can be roughly determined from the concentration and the specific gravity—70 per cent nitric acid of SG 1.42 contains about 944 g of acid per litre.

For exact preparation of normal solutions of acids it is necessary to titrate approximate solutions against normal solutions of alkali, accurately weighed out. For most histological purposes the following approximations may be adequate.

ACETIC ACID

CH_3COOH. Molecular weight 60. SG 1.05. Valency one. 99.5 per cent acetic acid contains about 1046 g of acid per litre. 57.4 cm³ of concentrated acetic acid contain about 60 g of acid. Therefore a normal solution is made up of about 57.4 cm³ of concentrated acid per litre. N/10 acetic acid is approximately 5.7 cm³/litre.

HYDROCHLORIC ACID

HCl. Molecular weight $36\frac{1}{2}$. SG 1.18. Valency one. 36 per cent hydrochloric acid contains about 425 g/litre. 85 cm³ contain $36\frac{1}{2}$ g of acid. Therefore a normal solution of hydrochloric acid contains approximately 85 cm³ of concentrated solution per litre. N/10 HCl contains about 8.5 cm³/litre.

NITRIC ACID

HNO_3. Molecular weight 63. SG 1.42. Valency one. Concentrated (70 per cent) nitric acid contains about 994 g/litre. 63 cm³ of concentrated nitric acid contain about 63 g of acid. Therefore a normal solution of nitric acid contains about 63 cm³ of concentrated solution per litre. N/10 HNO_3 is approximately 6 cm³/litre.

SULPHURIC ACID

H_2SO_4. Molecular weight 98. SG 1.84. Valency two. 99 per cent concentrated sulphuric acid contains about 1800 g/litre, and 27 cm^3 contain 49 g of acid. Therefore a normal solution is approximately 27 cm^3 of concentrated sulphuric acid made up to one litre. N/10 H_2SO_4 is about 2.7 cm^3 of concentrated acid/litre.

Appendix 5

Buffer solutions

PHOSPHATE BUFFER (SÖRENSEN)

M/15 sodium phosphate, dibasic; Na_2HPO_4 (MW: 142). Dissolve 9.465 g in distilled water and make up to one litre.

M/15 potassium acid phosphate; KH_2PO_4 (MW: 136). Dissolve 9.08 g in distilled water and make up to one litre.

M/10 solutions may be used, but these give slightly lower pH values; these differences are not usually of significance in histological techniques.

Take the amounts of each solution as shown in Table A5.1. The mixtures may be diluted with distilled water up to one litre.

Table A5.1

pH	$M/15\ KH_2PO_4$ (cm^3)	$M/15\ Na_2HPO_4$ (cm^3)
8.0	4	96
7.6	12	88
7.2	27	73
6.8	50	50
6.4	71	29
6.0	88	12
5.6	95	5

SODIUM ACETATE–HYDROCHLORIC ACID BUFFER (WALPOLE)

M/1 sodium acetate; $CH_2COONa.3H_2O$ (MW: 136). Dissolve 136 g of sodium acetate crystals in distilled water and make up to one litre.

N/1 hydrochloric acid; HCl (MW: 36.5). Approximately 85 cm³ of concentrated hydrochloric acid/litre. Titrate against a N alkali solution.

Take 50 cm³ of sodium acetate solution and add the appropriate amount of hydrochloric acid solution as shown in Table A5.2. Make up to 250 cm³ with distilled water.

Table A5.2

pH	M/1 Sodium acetate (cm³)	N/1 Hydrochloric acid (cm³)
1.0	50	75
1.5	50	61
2.0	50	52
2.6	50	50
2.9	50	49
3.2	50	48
3.6	50	45
4.0	50	39
4.4	50	30
4.8	50	18
5.2	50	10

ACETIC ACID–SODIUM ACETATE BUFFER (WALPOLE)

N/10 acetic acid; CH_3COOH (MW: 60). N/10 acetic acid contains 6.0 g of acid/litre. Accurate solutions should be made by titrating against 0.1 N alkali. (N/5 acetic acid contains 12 g/litre; N/20 acetic acid contains 3 g/litre.)

M/10 sodium acetate; $CH_3COONa.3H_2O$ (MW: 136). Dissolve 13.6 g in distilled water and make up to one litre. (M/5 sodium acetate crystals contains 27.2 g/litre; M/20 contains 6.8 g/litre.)

Take the appropriate amounts of each solution as shown in Table A5.3.

Table A5.3

pH	N/10 Acetic acid (cm³)	M/10 Sodium acetate (cm³)
3.2	194	6
3.6	185	15
4.0	165	35
4.4	126	74
4.8	80	120
5.2	42	158
5.6	19	181
6.0	8	192

'TRIS' BUFFER (GOMORI)

0.2 M tris(hydroxymethyl)aminomethane; $(CH_2OH)_3CNH_2$ (MW: 121). Dissolve 24.2 g in distilled water and make up to one litre.
0.1 N hydrochloric acid; HCl (MW: 36.5). About 8.5 cm^3 of concentrated hydrochloric acid per litre. Titrate against N/10 alkali.

Take the appropriate amounts of each solution as shown in Table A5.4 and make up to 100 cm^3 with distilled water.

Table A5.4

pH	0.2 M 'Tris' (cm^3)	0.1 N Hydrochloric acid (cm^3)
7.2	25	45
7.5	25	40
7.8	25	35
8.0	25	30
8.1	25	25
8.3	25	20
8.5	25	15
8.7	25	10
9.1	25	5

BORIC ACID–BORATE BUFFER (HOLMES)

M/5 boric acid; H_3BO_3 (MW: 62). Dissolve 12.4 g in distilled water and make up to one litre.
M/20 sodium tetraborate (borax); $Na_2B_4O_7 10H_2O$ (MW: 381.4). Dissolve 19.1 g in distilled water and make up to one litre.

Mix the following quantities of the two solutions as shown in Table A5.5.

Table A5.5

pH	M/5 Boric acid (cm^3)	M/20 Borate (cm^3)
7.4	180	20
7.6	170	30
7.8	160	40
8.0	140	60
8.2	130	70
8.4	110	90
8.7	80	120
9.0	40	160

VERONAL ACETATE–HYDROCHLORIC ACID BUFFER (MICHAELIS)

N/10 hydrochloric acid; HCl (MW: 36.5). About 8.5 cm³ of concentrated hydrochloric acid per litre. Titrate against a N/10 alkali.

Veronal acetate solution:

Sodium acetate crystals; $CH_3COONa.3H_2O$	19.4 g
Sodium diethyl barbiturate (veronal)	29.4 g

Dissolve in distilled water and make up to one litre.

To prepare the buffer solutions take the following quantities of veronal acetate solution, N/10 hydrochloric acid solution and distilled water.

Table A5.6

pH	Veronal acetate solution (cm³)	N/10 Hydrochloric acid (cm³)	Distilled water (cm³)
3.2	5	15	5
3.9	5	13	7
4.4	5	11	9
4.9	5	9	11
5.3	5	8	12
6.1	5	7	13
7.0	5	6	14
7.4	5	5	15
7.9	5	3	17
8.2	5	2	18
8.6	5	1	19

Index of dyes

The Colour Index Numbers of the dyes mentioned in this book are given below. The synonyms of certain of these dyes are also given as an aid to precise identification.

CI Number	Dye	Synonym
42685	Acid fuchsin	acid magenta, acid violet 19
46005	Acridine orange	basic orange 14
45000	Acridine red	
74240	Alcian blue 8GX	Ingrain blue 1
—	Alcian green 2GX	Ingrain green 2
58005	Alizarin red S	mordant red 3
42755	Aniline blue WS	water blue, soluble blue, acid blue 22
41000	Auramine	basic yellow 2
52005	Azur A	
52010	Azur B	
—	Azur C	
—	Azur I	
—	Azur II	
42510	Basic fuchsin	magenta, basic violet 14
26905	Biebrich scarlet	acid red 66
21000	Bismarck brown Y	basic brown 1
16250	Brilliant crystal scarlet 6R	acid red 44, crystal ponceau 6R, naphthalene scarlet 6R, ponceau 6R
75470	Carmine	natural red 4
75470	Carminic acid	
51050	Celestine blue B	mordant blue 14
28160	Chlorantine fast red	Sirius red 4B
16570	Chromotrope 2R	acid red 29
22120	Congo red	direct red 28
—	Cresyl fast violet	cresyl echt violet
42555	Crystal violet	
42530	Dahlia	Hofmann's violet
—	Direct blue 109	Durazol brilliant blue B
74180	Durazol fast blue 8G	
45400	Eosin B	eosin, bluish, acid red 91
45380	Eosin Y	eosin, yellowish, acid red 87
45430	Erythrosin B	acid red 51
	Diazonium salts	
37245	Fast black B	
37235	Fast blue B	
37210	Fast garnet GBC	
37150	Fast red ITR	
37085	Fast red TR	
42053	Fast green FCF	Food green 3
45350	Fluorescein	acid yellow 73
51030	Gallocyanin	mordant blue 10

CI Number	Dye	Synonym
75290	Haematein	
75290	Haematoxylin	natural black 1
11050	Janus green B	
—	Kernechtrot	nuclear fast red
14895	Kiton red S	acid red 7, azofuchsin 33
45100	Kiton rhodamine B	lissamine rhodamine B, acid red 52
42095	Light green SF	acid green 5
17045	Lissamine fast red B	
44090	Lissamine green B	wool green, acid green 50
—	Luxol fast blue MBSN	solvent blue 38
42000	Malachite green	basic green 4
10315	Martius yellow	naphthol yellow, acid yellow 24
13065	Metanil yellow	acid yellow 36
—	Methasol fast blue	solvent blue 38
42780	Methyl blue	acid blue 93
42585	Methyl green	
42535	Methyl violet 2B	basic violet 1
42555	Methyl violet 6B	basic violet 3
52015	Methylene blue	basic blue 9
18950	Milling yellow	acid yellow 76
44530	Naphthochrome green G	mordant green 31
50040	Neutral red	basic red 5
42520	New fuchsin	basic violet 2
51180	Nile blue	Nile blue sulphate, basic blue 12
26125	Oil red O	solvent red 27
16230	Orange G	acid orange 10
—	Orcein	natural red 28
42045	Patent blue V	acid blue 1
45410	Phloxine B	acid red 92
46045	Phosphine	basic orange 15
10305	Picric acid	trinitrophenol
16150	Ponceau 2R	ponceau de xylidine
27195	Ponceau S	acid red 112
24400	Pontamine sky blue 5BX	Niagara blue 4B, direct blue 1
58205	Purpurin	alizarin purpurin
45005	Pyronin Y	pyronin G
45170	Rhodamine B	basic violet 10
45440	Rose Bengal	acid red 94
75100	Saffron	natural yellow 6
50240	Safranin O	basic red 2
43820	Solochrome cyanine RS	Eriochrome cyanine R
42755	Soluble blue	aniline blue, acid blue 22
26100	Sudan III	solvent red 23
26105	Sudan IV	scarlet R, scharlach R, solvent red 24
26150	Sudan black B	solvent black 3
19140	Tartrazine	acid yellow 23
49005	Thioflavine T	basic yellow 1
52000	Thionin	Lauth's violet
52040	Toluidine blue	basic blue 17
23850	Trypan blue	direct blue 14
42563	Victoria blue 4R	basic blue 8

Index of suppliers

Item	Supplier
Apex food pads	W. W. Chamberlain & Sons Ltd., Wood Street, Higham Ferrers, Northants, NN9 8HH, England.
Phenoxetol	Nipa Laboratories Ltd., Nipa Industrial Estate, Llantwit Fardre, Pontypridd, Mid Glamorgan, CF38 2SN, Wales.
Tissue-Tek II Process/Embedding cassette and Embedding centre	Ames Company, Division of Miles Laboratories Ltd., PO Box 37, Stoke Court, Stoke Poges, Slough, SL2 4LY, England.
Peelaway embedding moulds	Schuco International (London) Ltd., Halliwick Court Place, Woodhouse Road, London, N12 0NE, England.
Ester wax; SO_2 gas; Poly (methylmethacrylate) low molecular weight, natural beads	BDH Chemicals Ltd., Poole, Dorset, BH12 4NN, England.
Durofix cellulose adhesive (Domestic grade)	The Rawlplug Co Ltd., London Road, Kingston-upon-Thames, Surrey, England.
Hyaluronidase	Sigma London Chemical Co Ltd., Fancy Road, Poole, Dorset, BH17 7NH, England.
Sialidase	Koch–Light Laboratories Ltd., Colnbrook, Bucks., SL3 0BZ, England.
Decon 75	Decon Laboratories Ltd., Ellen Street, Portslade, Brighton, BN14 1EQ, Sussex, England.
PDP	In USA—Polysciences Inc., Paul Valley Industrial Park, Warrington, Pennsylvania, USA. In UK—International Enzymes Ltd., Vale Road, Windsor, Berks., England.
Hypaque (sodium diatrizoate)	Winthrop Laboratories, Winthrop House, Surbiton-on-Thames, Surrey, KT6 4PH, England.
Parafilm (sealing tissue)	A. Gallenkamp & Co Ltd., PO Box 290, Christopher Street, London, EC2P 2ER, England.
Cytoclair (methyl cysteine)	Sinclair Pharmaceuticals Ltd., Ockford Road, Godalming, Surrey, England.
Millipore filters	Millipore (UK) Ltd., Millipore House, Abbey Road, Park Royal, London, NW10 7SP, England.
Integrating eyepiece, ASM & TAS image analysers	E. Leitz (Instruments) Ltd., 48 Park Street, Luton, LU1 3HP, England.
Integrating disc II	Carl Zeiss (Oberkochen) Ltd., 31 Foley Street, London, W1P 8AP, England.
Surfometer SF100	Planer Products Ltd., Windmill Road, Sunbury-on-Thames, Middlesex, England.
Quantimet 720 image analyser	Cambridge Instruments, Melbourn, Royston, SG8 6EJ, England.
England finder graticule	Graticules Ltd., Sovereign Way, Botany Industrial Estate, Tonbridge, Kent, TN9 1RN, England.
Illumitran	Bowens Ltd., 72 Dean Street, London, W1V 6DQ, England.
Scott-Bader Resins	Trylon Ltd., Thrift Street, Woolaston, Northants, England.

Item	Supplier
Colorpaque	Garmanson Chemicals Ltd., Willow Road, Brackley, Northants, England.
Coloured latex	Harris Biological Supplies Ltd., Oldmixon, Weston-Super-Mare, Somerset, England.
Neoprene latex 572	DuPont Company (UK) Ltd., Elastomer Chemicals Department, Marylands Avenue, Hemel Hempstead, Herts, England.

Index of names

Index of subjects